Cardiac Problems in Pregnancy

Cardiac Problems in Pregnancy
Diagnosis and Management of Maternal and Fetal Disease

Edited by

Uri Elkayam, M.D.
Director, Inpatient Cardiology
Department of Medicine, Section of Cardiology
Los Angeles County–USC Medical Center
Assistant Professor of Medicine
University of Southern California
Los Angeles, California

Norbert Gleicher, M.D.
Chairman, Department of Obstetrics and Gynecology
Mount Sinai Hospital Medical Center of Chicago
Professor of Obstetrics and Gynecology
Assistant Professor of Immunology/Microbiology
Rush Medical College
Chicago, Illinois

Alan R. Liss, Inc., New York

Address all Inquiries to the Publisher
Alan R. Liss, Inc., 150 Fifth Avenue, New York, NY 10011

Printed in the United States of America.

Library of Congress Cataloging in Publication Data

Cardiac problems in pregnancy.

Includes bibliographical references and index.
1. Pregnancy, Complications of. 2. Heart--Diseases. 3. Fetal heart. 4. Fetal heart--Diseases. I. Elkayam, Uri. II. Gleicher, Norbert. [DNLM: 1. Heart diseases--In Pregnancy. 2. Pregnancy complications, Cardiovascular--Diagnosis. 3. Pregnancy complications, Cardiovascular--Therapy. WQ 244 C266]
RG580.H4C37 1982 618.3 82-9938
ISBN 0-8451-0216-8 AACR2

To my parents, Dvora and Mordechei, my wife, Batia,
and my children, Ifaat and Yehonatan.
U.E.

To Elizabeth.
N.G.

In memory of our friend and colleague Stephen A. Landes, M.D.,
who gave his life trying to save the lives of others.

Contents

FETAL SECTION

Contributors

Eugene Ainbender, M.D.
Associate Professor of Pediatrics, Department of Pediatrics, Division of Neonatology and Infectious Diseases
Mount Sinai School of Medicine of the City University of New York
New York, NY 10029

Louis Aledort, M.D.
Professor of Medicine
Vice Chairman, Department of Medicine
Mount Sinai School of Medicine of the City University of New York
Attending in Medicine
Mount Sinai Hospital
New York, NY 10029

Page A.W. Anderson, M.D.
Associate Professor of Pediatrics
Associate Professor of Physiology
Duke University Medical Center
Durham, NC 27710

Thomas J. Benedetti, M.D.
Assistant Professor
Obstetrics and Gynecology
University Hospital
Seattle, WA 98185

Lee B. Berman, M.D.
Clinical Instructor in Medicine
Mount Sinai School of Medicine of the City University of New York
Senior Clinical Assistant in Medicine
Mount Sinai Hospital
New York, NY 10029

Robert S. Bressler, Ph.D.
Associate Professor, Department of Anatomy
Mount Sinai School of Medicine of the City University of New York
New York, NY 10029

Edwin G. Brown, M.D.
Associate Professor of Pediatrics
Mount Sinai School of Medicine of the City University of New York
Director, Division of Neonatology
Mount Sinai Hospital
New York, NY 10029

Thomas C. Cesario, M.D.
Associate Professor of Medicine, Department of Medicine, Division of Infectious Diseases
University of California Irvine Medical Center
Orange, CA 92668

Tyson C. Cobb, M.D.
Assistant Clinical Professor of Medicine
University of California Irvine Medical Center
Chief in Cardiology
St. Joseph Hospital
Orange, CA 92668

Yoel Donchin, M.D.
Senior Lecturer, Obstetrics Anesthesia Unit
Hadassah University
Jerusalem, Israel

Jan I.M. Drayer, M.D.
Associate Professor of Medicine
University of California Irvine Medical Center
Orange, CA 92668
Associate Chief, Section of Clinical Pharmacology and Hypertension
Veterans Administration Medical Center
Long Beach, CA 90822

Uri Elkayam, M.D.
Assistant Professor of Medicine
University of Southern California
Director, Inpatient Cardiology, Department of Medicine, Section of Cardiology
Los Angeles County–USC Medical Center
Los Angeles, CA 90033

Burton W. Fink, M.D.
Clinical Professor, Pediatrics
University of California Los Angeles
Director, Pediatric Cardiology
Cedars Sinai Medical Center
Los Angeles, CA 90048

William H. Frishman, M.D.
Associate Professor of Medicine
Albert Einstein College of Medicine
Chief of Medicine
Hospital of the Albert Einstein College of Medicine
Bronx, NY 10461

Julius M. Gardin, M.D.
Assistant Professor of Medicine
University of California, Irvine
Director, Cardiology Noninvasive Laboratory
Division of Cardiology, Department of Medicine
University of California Irvine Medical Center
Orange, CA 92668
Acting Chief, Cardiology Division
Veterans Administration Medical Center
Long Beach, CA 90822

Alan Gazzaniga, M.D.
Professor of Surgery
University of California, Irvine
Director, Trauma Service
Director, Medical/Surgical Intensive Care Unit
University of California Irvine Medical Center
Orange, CA 92668

Fredda Ginsberg-Fellner, M.D.
Professor of Pediatrics
Director, Division of Pediatric Endocrinology and Metabolism
Mount Sinai School of Medicine of the City University of New York
New York, NY 10029

Norbert Gleicher, M.D.
Professor of Obstetrics and Gynecology
Assistant Professor of Immunology/Microbiology
Rush Medical College
Chairman, Department of Obstetrics and Gynecology
Mount Sinai Hospital Medical Center of Chicago
Chicago, IL 60608

Martin E. Goldman, M.D.
Clinical Assistant in Medicine
Mount Sinai School of Medicine of the City University of New York
Associate Director, Noninvasive Cardiac Laboratories
Mount Sinai Hospital
New York, NY 10029

Warren D. Johnston, M.D.
Assistant Professor of Medicine
University of California, Irvine
Director, Coronary Care Unit, Division of Cardiology, Department of Medicine
University of California Irvine Medical Center
Orange, CA 92668

Neal A. Klein, M.D.
Division of Cardiology, Department of Medicine
Albert Einstein College of Medicine
Bronx, NY 10461

Niels H. Lauersen, M.D.
Associate Professor of Obstetrics and Gynecology
Mount Sinai School of Medicine of the City University of New York
New York, NY 10029

Joseph B. Lessing, M.D.
Instructor in Obstetrics and Gynecology
Sackler School of Medicine, Tel Aviv University
Municipal-Government Medical Center Tel Aviv
Tel Aviv, Israel 69978

Andrés Manring, Ph.D.
Assistant Medical Research Professor, Department of Physiology
Duke University Medical Center
Durham, NC 27710

Jose Meller, M.D.
Associate Professor of Clinical Medicine
Mount Sinai School of Medicine of the City University of New York
Director, Noninvasive Cardiac Laboratories
Mount Sinai Hospital
New York, NY 10029

James H. Moller, M.D.
Professor of Pediatrics
Dwan Cardiovascular Learning Center and Department of Pediatrics
University of Minnesota
Minneapolis, MN 55455

Yuji Murata, M.D.
Associate Professor of Obstetrics and Gynecology
University of California, Irvine
St. Joseph Hospital and University of California Irvine Medical Center
Orange, CA 92668

Joyce Newman, M.D., Ph.D.
Instructor, Department of Obstetrics and Gynecology
Mount Sinai School of Medicine of the City University of New York
New York, NY 10029

Kenneth L. Noller, M.D.
Associate Professor of Obstetrics and Gynecology
Mayo Medical School
Consultant, Department of Obstetrics and Gynecology
Mayo Clinic
Rochester, MN 55901

Celia M. Oakley, M.D.
Honorary Senior Lecturer, Department of Medicine
Royal Postgraduate Medical School
Consultant Cardiologist
Hammersmith Hospital
London, England W12 0HS

Mary Ella Mascia Pierpont, Ph.D., M.D.
Assistant Professor of Pediatrics
Dwan Cardiovascular Learning Center and Department of Pediatrics
University of Minnesota
Minneapolis, MN 55455

William F. Rayburn, M.D.
Assistant Professor of Obstetrics and Gynecology
The University of Michigan
Director, Obstetrics Service, Department of Obstetrics and Gynecology
Women's Hospital
Ann Arbor, MI 48109

Hillel S. Ribner, M.D.
Assistant Professor of Medicine
Northwestern University School of Medicine
Director, Coronary Care Unit
Veterans Administration Lakeside Medical Center
Associate Attending
Northwestern Memorial Hospital
Chicago, IL 60611

Mortimer G. Rosen, M.D.
Professor, Department of Reproductive Biology
Case Western Reserve University
Director, Department of Obstetrics and Gynecology
Cleveland Metropolitan General Hospital
Cleveland, OH 44109

Kenneth D. Rosenman, M.D.
Clinical Assistant Professor, Department of Environmental and Community Medicine
College of Medicine and Dentistry of New Jersey, Rutgers Medical School
Director, Environmental and Occupational Health Service
State of New Jersey Department of Health
Trenton, NJ 08625

Heschi H. Rotmensch, M.D., M.S.
Assistant Professor of Medicine and Pharmacology
Jefferson Medical College
Assistant Director, Division of Clinical Pharmacology
Thomas Jefferson University Hospital
Philadelphia, PA 19107

Lawrence Santora, M.D.
Clinical Instructor of Medicine, Division of Cardiology
University of California, Irvine
Orange, CA 92668
Staff Physician
Venice Hospital
Venice, FL 33595

Ralph I. Silverman, M.D.
Assistant Professor of Medicine, Division of Cardiology
Albert Einstein College of Medicine
Bronx, NY 10461

Yoram Sorokin, M.D.
Assistant Professor, Department of Reproductive Biology
Case Western Reserve University, and
Perinatal Clinical Research Center
Cleveland Metropolitan General Hospital
Cleveland, OH 44109

Pradub Sukhum, M.D.
Assistant Professor of Medicine, Division of Cardiology
University of Minnesota School of Medicine
Minneapolis, MN 55455
Director, Noninvasive Cardiac Laboratory, Department of Medicine, Section of Cardiology
St. Paul-Ramsey Medical Center
St. Paul, MN 55101

Jonathan M. Tobis, M.D.
Assistant Professor of Medicine, Division of Cardiology
University of California, Irvine
Director, Cardiac Catheterization Laboratory
University of California Irvine Medical Center
Orange, CA 92668

Kent Ueland, M.D.
Professor of Gynecology and Obstetrics
Stanford University School of Medicine
Chief, Section of Maternal-Fetal Medicine
Stanford University Medical Center
Stanford, CA 94305

Michael A. Weber, M.D.
Associate Professor of Medicine
University of California Irvine Medical Center
Orange, CA 92668
Chief, Section of Clinical Pharmacology and Hypertension
Veterans Administration Medical Center
Long Beach, CA 90822

Archie Wilson, M.D., Ph.D.
Professor of Medicine and Physiology
University of California, Irvine
Vice Chair, Department of Medicine
Chief, Pulmonary and Critical Care Medicine
University of California Irvine Medical Center
Orange, CA 92668

Robert N. Wolfson, M.D., Ph.D.
Assistant Professor, Department of Reproductive Biology
Case Western Reserve University
Director, Obstetrical Diagnostic Ultrasound Unit, Department of Obstetrics and Gynecology
Cleveland Metropolitan General Hospital
Cleveland, OH 44109

Bruce K. Young, M.D.
Professor of Obstetrics and Gynecology
Director, Division of Maternal-Fetal Medicine
New York University School of Medicine
Chief, Obstetrical Service
Bellevue Hospital Center
New York, NY 10016

Preface

Over the past decade, the field of cardiology has made rapid progress, largely as a result of the development of new technology and its application to more sophisticated diagnosis and therapy. These developments have led to vast improvements in the medical care available to cardiac patients of all ages; in the female patient this will of course include the period of pregnancy. Although absolute maternal morbidity and mortality from such cardiac diseases as rheumatic heart disease have been declining steadily in the more developed countries, these diseases have still maintained their relative importance as major complicating factors in modern obstetrical care. This is due in part to the even greater decline in total maternal mortality, which has rendered maternal cardiac disease, despite its absolute decline, a relatively more important cause of maternal morbidity and mortality. In addition, it is now possible for cardiac patients who some years ago would have been advised against becoming pregnant, or encouraged to have an early abortion, to carry pregnancies to full term. All of these factors have contributed to maintaining cardiac disease in pregnancy as a major topic in maternal-fetal medicine. *Cardiac Problems in Pregnancy* represents an attempt to summarize in one volume all aspects of maternal cardiac disease in pregnancy as they are presently recognized, and to review diagnosis and therapy in light of the most modern methods.

In addition, the second section of this volume covers a more recently defined field, that of fetal cardiology. With its increasing diagnostic sophistication, fetal cardiology is maturing into a well recognized and established entity in its own right. Intrauterine diagnosis and, more recently, intrauterine therapy are becoming commonplace in most major medical centers. We attempt in this second section to summarize the experience to date in fetal cardiology and to outline possible future directions in this young and exciting field.

Finally, this volume contributes a new dual point of view to the study of maternal-fetal medicine—that is, organ review in both mother and fetus within one volume. This concept was inspired by the idea that basic knowledge and expertise in maternal and fetal organ systems will be mutually applicable. In view of the continuous growth of maternal-fetal medicine, a specialty that draws physicians from various fields of medicine, this unifying approach of combining fetal and maternal issues in one volume made sense to the editors and publisher; and it is their hope that such an approach will enhance the concept of maternal-fetal medicine as a unified field. It is hoped that this volume will encourage in adult and pediatric cardiologists a greater interest in fetal cardiology, while at the same time giving perinatologists, at the other, obstetric end of the spectrum, a detailed understanding of maternal cardiology and its increasing relevance to their work. Such is the goal of these two editors, who do in fact represent both ends of the spectrum and who have benefited from just this exchange between fields of expertise.

Uri Elkayam, M.D.
Norbert Gleicher, M.D.

MATERNAL SECTION

Physiologic Changes During Normal Pregnancy and the Puerperium

M.I

Cardiovascular Physiology of Pregnancy

Uri Elkayam, MD, and Norbert Gleicher, MD

I. INTRODUCTION

The fascinating process of pregnancy is involved in significant adaptation of the cardiovascular system (Table M.I.1). Maternal heart disease can significantly interfere with this process and therefore have an important effect on both mother and fetus. The increased circulatory burden of pregnancy may unmask some previously unrecognized heart disorders and make them progress rapidly to a potentially lethal condition. The recognition and management of heart disease in pregnancy is

Cardiac Problems in Pregnancy, pages 5–26

TABLE M.I.1. Cardiocirculatory Changes During Normal Pregnancy

Blood volume	Increased
Cardiac output	Increased
Stroke volume	Increased
Heart rate	Increased
Systemic blood pressure	
Systolic	Slightly decreased
Diastolic	Decreased
Pulse pressure	Increased
Systemic vascular resistance	Decreased
Oxygen consumption	Increased
Left ventricular volume	Increased
Left ventricular function	No change or somewhat improved

not always straightforward. The absence of well-defined guidelines and the scanty literature do not make it easier for the practicing physician. A comprehensive understanding of the cardiocirculatory adaptation during pregnancy, labor, and puerperium is therefore essential for a logical and rational management of the normal pregnant patient as well as the patient with cardiovascular disorders.

II. HEMODYNAMIC CHANGES DURING PREGNANCY

A. Blood Volume

One of the major cardiocirculatory changes occurring during pregnancy is that of the blood volume. The changes in blood volume have been studied by numerous investigators,[1–14] and although there has been a general agreement that blood volume increases significantly during pregnancy, there has been disagreement about the total increment and the pattern of changes throughout pregnancy. The increase in blood volume starts to be noticed as early as at the sixth week of pregnancy. A rapid increase takes place until mid-pregnancy, when the volume continues to rise but at a much slower rate.[7] A considerable individual variation in the degree of volume increase during pregnancy, ranging from 20% to nearly 100% of the nonpregnant values has been reported.[6] Rovinsky and Jaffin reported a 33% increase in blood volume at 21–24 weeks of gestation and then a progressive rise to a peak increase of 49% at 33 to 36 weeks, followed by plateau for the last 8 weeks of pregnancy.[5] Other investigators reported a slight decrease or a slow increase in volume during the last several weeks before term.[10–13] In general, most studies agree in showing a continuous blood volume increase during pregnancy up to a maximal value about 50% higher than the nonpregnant level.[3–13] Expressed in ml/kg, the mean recorded blood volume value ranged from 73 to 96 ml/kg.[1–3,5,7] The rise in blood volume during pregnancy was found by Hytten and Paintin to correlate directly with fetal weight.[4] Rovinsky and Jaffin found a positive relationship between the degree of plasma volume increment near-term and placental mass and interpreted the findings as a proof for the influence of the placenta as an arterial venous shunt on the maternal vascular compartment.[5] Ueland showed a general correlation between total blood volume and both the weight of the products of conception and the neonatal weight and suggested a correlation between the maternal weight and the total blood volume. An interesting observation was reported by Pritchard and Rowland, who stated that, in spite of a considerable variation in the intensity of hypervolemia from subject to subject, the same degree of hypervolemia usually develops with subsequent pregnancies in the same subject.[6] Other investigators have found that blood volume increments seem to be higher in multigravidas than in primigravidas, and blood volume is also greater in twin pregnancies than in single pregnancies.[14,17] It should be concluded, therefore, that these situations impose a substantially greater demand on the cardiocirculatory system, which may be overburdened in a case of heart disorder.

Although red blood cell mass increases concomitantly with blood volume during pregnancy, the latter shows a more rapid and significant rise. The predominance of plasma volume increase results in a fall in hemoglobin concentration during pregnancy, a situation that has been called the "physiologic anemia of pregnancy," with hematocrit levels as low as 33–38% and hemoglobin levels of 11–12 gm/100 ml.[16,17] A regular administration of iron is followed by rise in hemoglobin concentration, sometimes to nonpregnant levels, and results in an increase in the oxygen-carrying capacity of the maternal blood.[18,19] Treatment of pregnant women with iron in the last trimester of gestation also results in a significant rise in hemoglobin.[20]

1. Mechanism of hypervolemia in pregnancy

The exact cause and mechanism of hypervolemia in pregnancy is still not entirely understood. Some of the changes in maternal plasma volume may be attributable to changes in fluid balance, which is probably mediated by the steroid hormones of pregnancy. The plasma levels of renin and aldosterone are elevated during gestation, owing to the action of both estrogens and progesterone. This increase is associated with sodium retention and an increase in total body water.[21–24] The fact that other conditions that are associated with increased production of aldosterone, such as primary hyperaldosteronism, are also accompanied by increased blood volume may demonstrate the importance of this factor in the genesis of hypervolemia in pregnancy.[25] In addition, it has been suggested that the growth hormone-like substance in the placenta also plays a role in the genesis of hypervolemia during pregnancy.[26] An individual factor that determines the presence of high, average, or low plasma volume during pregnancy and is further modified by hormonal and vascular factors has been suggested by Lund and Donovan.[7]

It is interesting to note that a fetus is not essential for the development of hypervolemia during pregnancy. This situation has also been associated with cases of hydatiform mole (50% increase).[26] Chesley and Duffus demonstrated the effect of posture on the apparent plasma volume in late pregnancy. Volume declined in the supine position, probably because the enlarged uterus produces occlusion of the inferior vena cava and trapping of blood in the legs.[27]

Although the mechanism of hypervolemia in pregnancy is still not fully understood, it seems that the increase in volume serves to meet the metabolic demands of the enlarged uterus and protects the fetus from the impaired venous return and reduced cardiac output caused by the mechanical pressure of the enlarged uterus on the inferior vena cava. In addition, the hypervolemia acts as a safeguard against maternal blood loss at delivery. For these reasons, the normal pregnant woman can usually withstand hemorrhage equal to the volume of blood added to the circulation during normal pregnancy without gross physiologic embarrassment.

B. Cardiac Output

One of the more significant hemodynamic phenomena during pregnancy is the change in cardiac output. The assessment of changes in cardiac output dates to 1915, when Lindhard reported an increment of 50% in cardiac output during pregnancy.[28] This study was followed by numerous investigations into the effect of pregnancy on cardiac output. Several techniques have been applied for this purpose, including the direct Fick principle,[29–33] dilution techniques,[14,34–37] and most recently, echocardiography.[38,39]

It is generally agreed that cardiac output begins to rise during the first trimester, probably around the 10th week of pregnancy. The peak increment in cardiac output has been seen by most investigators by the 20th to the 24th week of gestation.[37,40,41] The rise in cardiac output is rapid in the first trimester and is followed by a slower increase during the second trimester, which continues until peak cardiac output is reached by the 20th to 24th week of pregnancy.[35,37,40] The increase in cardiac output during pregnancy is estimated to be 30–50% over the values in the nonpregnant state.[39] After reaching its peak, the cardiac output seems to be maintained at its elevated level.[35,40] Early studies performed with patients in the supine position resulted in a general agreement that the elevated cardiac output falls in the last few weeks of pregnancy. This impression, however, was challenged by some investigators who measured cardiac output with patients in the lateral recumbent position and did not observe the terminal fall in cardiac output.[42,43] In 1969, however, Ueland et al were able to show a decline in cardiac output between the 38th and 40th weeks of gestation not only when the patients were supine but also when they were sitting and in lateral recumbency. The fall in cardiac output, however, was statistically significant only in the supine position.[40] It seems, therefore, that there is a slight reduction in cardiac output toward term, especially when the mother lies supine, which is explained by the mechanical compression of the gravid uterus on the inferior vena cava and a decreased venous return to the heart.

Cardiac output is the product of stroke volume and pulse rate. The rise in cardiac output early in pregnancy is disproportionately greater than the increase in heart rate and, therefore, attributable to augmentation of the stroke volume. As pregnancy advances, heart rate increases and becomes the more predominant factor increasing the cardiac output.[44] The stroke volume is declining at the late stages of pregnancy to values within the normal, non-pregnant level.[40]

A unique and important hemodynamic phenomenon during pregnancy is the fluctuation in resting cardiac output that occurs with changes in position.[38–40,43] The compression of the inferior vena cava by the enlarged gravid uterus in the supine position results in a decrease in venous blood return to the heart and, thereby, in a significant decrease in cardiac output. The effect of maternal posture on cardiac output was demonstrated by several investigators. A significant decrease (25–30%) in cardiac output when measured by dye dilution technique was demonstrated in the supine position between 38 and 40 weeks of pregnancy.[40,43] In contrast, no changes were present when the study was performed before the 24th week of gestation. These findings were recently confirmed by echocardiographic studies.[38,39] As heart rate did not seem to be affected by the positional changes, the decline in cardiac output was a result of a decreased stroke volume. The decrease in cardiac output was also not associated with a significant change in blood pressure, probably owing to an increase in peripheral resistance.[45]

C. Effect of the Gravid Uterus on the Circulation

The effect of the gravid uterus was first alluded to in 1953 by Howard et al,[46] who showed an elevated pressure in the femoral vein in pregnant women. Radiologic studies have demonstrated an obstruction of the vena cava in approximately 90% of women studied in the supine position.[45,49] Lifting the uterus away from the vena cava during laparotomy resulted in a significant fall in caval pressure. The same effect was noted when a lateral recumbent position was assumed.[45] The maternal posture changes were found to be diminished when the fetal head was engaged in the pelvis, probably because of restriction of uteral mobility.[47] The remarkable degree of caval compression by the gravid uterus in late stages of pregnancy was demonstrated by Kerr et al,[45,47] who showed that caval pressures recorded in the supine position before delivery were comparable to pressures obtained by complete manual obstruction of the vena cava applied during surgery under direct vision. These investigators also found that a paravertebral collateral circulation develops during pregnancy, permitting the blood from the legs and the pelvic organs to pass by the occluded inferior caval vein.[47] Studies of simultaneous pressure recording obtained by direct method from different arteries have given highly persuasive evidence that vascular compression exerted by the uterus involves not only the inferior vena cava but also the aorta and its branches.[48] Bieniarz et al in 1968 used angiographic techniques and demonstrated an aorto-iliac compression in late pregnancy.[49] The aorta was found to be laterally displaced, and during uterine relaxation, less densely opacified at the region of lumbar lordosis L4 to L5. The aortic displacement was increased during uterine contraction, and the common iliac artery crossing vertebrae L4 and L5 was transiently occluded. The right renal artery was found in some cases to be stretched, elongated, blurred, and less opaque at the point where it crossed the convexity of the vertebra. Other aortic branches crossing the spine to the right side such as the ovarian and lumbar arteries, were similarly blurred and less dense.

D. Supine Hypotensive Syndrome of Pregnancy

The postural fall in cardiac output is normally followed by a compensatory increase in peripheral resistance and therefore no significant change in systemic blood pressure or heart rate.[45] Occasionally, however, a signficant decrease in heart rate and blood pressure can be seen, resulting in symptoms such as weakness, lightheadedness, nausea, dizziness, or even syncope.[45,50,51] This phenomenon described as the "supine hypotensive syndrome of pregnancy" or "the uterocaval syndrome"[52] is usually relieved promptly when the supine position is abandoned.[53–55]

The incidence of the supine hypotensive syndrome ranged in different reports from 0.5 to 11.2%.[46,47,52,55] It has been widely assumed that this syndrome derives from acute occlusion of the inferior vena cava owing to the pressure exerted by the pregnant uterus in the supine position.[46] The supine caval occlusion, however, is a common occurrence in late pregnancy and is found whether or not the patient shows a tendency to develop the supine hypotensive syndrome. A recent experimental study showed that ligation of the iliac veins in pregnant and nonpregnant animals resulted in no major change in heart rate and blood pressure, confirming the assumption that the supine hypotensive syndrome is not solely caused by mechanical compression of the inferior vena cava.[56] It is therefore unlikely that this is the only explanation for this phenomenon. It has been assumed by some investigators that women developing the supine hypotensive syndrome have a poorly developed collateral system of the paravertebral circulation, possibly associated with a strong tendency toward vasovagal attacks.[41,57] In studying two women with supine hypotensive syndrome, Kerr in 1968 showed an initial fall in cardiac output of 25–30% when they were turned to the supine position. This fall in cardiac output, however, was not associated with an immediate alteration in either heart rate or arterial pressure. Maintaining the patients supine for four to six minutes then resulted in an abrupt drop in heart rate with further fall in cardiac output and a dramatic fall in blood pressure associated with fainting.[41] In 1979 Kjeldsen described the clinical presentation of two patients with supine hypotensive syndrome and did not observe the bradycardia found by Kerr.[52] A possible explanation is that observation by Kjeldsen was discontinued before the beginning of the bradycardic phase.

The fact that, despite supine caval compression and falling cardiac output, there is usually no acceleration of heart rate is interesting and probably is unique to caval occlusion. Kerr showed that manual occlusion of the caval vein in nonpregnant patients undergoing laparotomy can also cause a reduction of cardiac output and sometimes a fall in blood pressure without an increase in heart rate.[45] Howard et al demonstrated that signs of supine hypotensive syndrome seen between contractions normalized during the following contraction.[46] It has been postulated that changes in the shape of the uterus during contraction are associated with a relief of caval compression.[48,49,58]

E. Heart Rate

Heart rate rises during pregnancy with a mean increase of about 10–20 beats per minute (bpm) at term, with mean values varying from 78 to 89 bpm.[29,36–39,52,59,60] Twin pregnancies are associated with earlier acceleration of the heart rate and peak increase up to 40% above the nonpregnant level near term.[15] The heart rate decreases slightly with a change from the supine position to the lateral position,[52] and it is higher in the sitting position (10–15 beats per minute faster than in the other positions).[40] The rise in heart rate was found by some investigators to occur early in pregnancy and to remain similarly elevated later and at term.[38] Other studies have shown a gradual increase in pulse rate with a peak at the third trimester.[39,40]

F. Systemic Arterial Blood Pressure

Rubler et al have recently shown no significant change in blood pressure between nonpregnant women and women in different stages of pregnancy.[38] However, most of the studies observing the same group of women as they advance through their pregnancies have shown a slight fall of the systolic arterial blood pressure in pregnancy associated with a considerable decrease in diastolic pressure.[17,39,61] The fall in blood pressure starts in the first trimester, with a peak decrease in midpregnancy and a return toward the nonpregnant level before term. The magnitude of the change varies from study to study.

Both age and parity were observed to have significant effects on blood pressure during pregnancy. Christianson has analyzed his data from white women under the age of 25, between the ages of 25 and 34, and over 35, and has shown that as parity increases in a given age group, both the systolic and the diastolic blood pressures decrease. The greatest difference has been shown between primiparas and nulliparas. Within each parity level, mean systolic arterial pressures were similar for gravidas under 25 and those aged 25 to 34, but increased for gravidas age 35 and over. The mean diastolic pressure increased gradually as age increased within each parity classification.[61] An earlier study by MacGillivray resulted in somewhat different data and showed that in primigravidas the diastolic pressure first began to rise steadily at age 30 (being unchanged in younger women) and that the systolic pressure rose fairly steadily with age.[21] The differences in the results can be explained by variables not being considered in these two analyses such as ethnic background and smoking habits of the gravidas. These factors have been observed to affect mean blood pressure during pregnancy.[62,63] In summary, it seems that increasing age and parity are associated with a rise in both systolic and diastolic blood pressure.

G. Systemic Vascular Resistance

A significant fall in systemic vascular resistance occurs during pregnancy and results in a fall in blood pressure, mainly the diastolic component, and a widening of pulse pressure. The mechanism for this phenomenon is not entirely understood. Metcalfe and Ueland attribute the fall in systemic vascular resistance mainly to the creation of a low resistance circulation in the pregnant uterus.[44] The decline in vascular resistance, however, is not limited to the uterine vascular bed and seems to involve other systems.

The administration of oral contraceptives containing both estrogen and progestational compounds results in a fall in systemic vascular resistance.[64] Both estrogen and prolactin administration to animals have also been shown to have a significant effect on vascular resistance.[65,66] On the basis of these observations, it seems likely that there is an important relationship between the changes in systemic vascular resistance during pregnancy and hormonal activity. In addition, increased heat production by the developing fetus is probably the reason for vasodilation, especially in such heat-losing areas as the hands of the pregnant female, and may also contribute to the decrease in systemic vascular resistance.

TABLE M.I.2. Changes in Regional Blood Flow During Normal Pregnancy

Organ	Change
Uterus	↑
Kidneys	↑ (returns to nonpregnant state at term)
Extremities	↑
Skin	↑
Liver	No change
Brain	No change
Breast	Probably ↑
Coronary arteries	?

H. Regional Blood Flow (Table M.I.2)

1. Uterine blood flow

The decline in uterine vascular resistance allows a rise in blood flow to the uterus during gestation. The blood flow to the uterus rises from approximately 50 ml/min at the 10th week of gestation to around 200 ml/min at the 28th week and increases further to 500 ml/min at term.[67–69] Burwell, in his early communication in 1938, suggested that the fall in uterine vascular resistance was a result of erosion of the maternal endometrial vessels due to invasion of trophoblast at the placental site and formation of an arterial-venous fistula.[70] Subsequent studies provided the evidence for a direct arterial-venous anastomosis in the uterus. Heckel and Tobin injected glass spheres with a diameter of about 200 μm into the uterine arterial system and found them later in the veins of 12 of 21 nonpregnant women and in all of four pregnant women.[71] Although this study confirmed the presence of arterial-venous communications in the uterus of at least 200 μm microns in diameter, the hemodynamic importance of this finding is still unknown. The uterine vascular resistance has also been shown to fall dramatically in species where no erosion of the maternal uterine vessels is found.[72] In addition, the facts that uterine venous blood does not have a particularly high oxygen content and that cardiac output increases most rapidly in early pregnancy, when uterine blood flow is trivial, do not support the hypothesis that arterial-venous fistula is the mechanism behind the significant decrease in uterine vascular resistance during pregnancy. The reduction of uterine vascular resistance in nonpregnant sheep following a direct infusion of estrogen into the uterine artery suggests that the vasodilation in the uterus during pregnancy may be related to the ovarian and placental steroid hormone.[73] The work of Greiss and Anderson further supports the relationship between hormonal activity and hemodynamic changes in the uterus. These investigators showed a decrease in uterine blood flow to barely recordable levels following oophorectomy. A single injection or a daily injection of estradiol increased uterine blood flow markedly for one to two days.[65] Intravenous administration of exogenous angiotensin II in animals was followed by increased uterine blood flow.[67,74] These data suggest that the renin-angiotensin system may contribute to changes in uterine blood flow during pregnancy.

2. Renal blood flow

In the early stages of gestation renal blood flow increases significantly and reaches a peak about 30% higher than that in the nonpregnant state.[75,76] With progression of pregnancy, renal blood flow becomes very sensitive to changes in body position.[77] The flow then decreases in magnitude as pregnancy advances, and at term it falls to the nonpregnant level or even below it.

3. Extremities flow

Early studies have resulted in no general agreement in regard to the forearm flow. It has been variously reported as unchanged,[78] decreased,[79] and increased.[80,81] Similarly, the available studies of the circulation in the legs during pregnancy have provided conflicting data.[78,79] More recent studies show a progressive rise of blood flow through the hands from the early weeks of pregnancy until delivery.[82] The flow subsides during the puerperium and returns to nonpregnant levels over several weeks. It can, however, be still significantly elevated above the level of early pregnancy by the sixth week postpartum. The blood flow through the feet shows similar, though less striking, changes. The flow is somewhat higher in twin pregnancies after the 30th week of gestation when compared to single pregnancies.

4. Skin perfusion

In a recent study Katz and Sokal found a significant increase in skin perfusion during pregnancy.[83] The pattern found by these investigators showed a slow but steady rise up to 18–20 weeks of gestation, followed by a sharp, significant rise between the 20th and 30th weeks, and no significant change thereafter. The increase in skin perfusion was maintained at least one week postpartum. The increased blood flow in the skin causes a considerable increase in skin temperature,[79,84] manifested clinically by a typically warm skin and clammy hands.

Microscopic examination of the nail bed revealed capillary dilatation in most of the pregnant women studied.[17] Vascular spiders and palm erythema are seen in about 60% of white women during pregnancy and are an additional sign of vasodilation.[85] Another area in which blood flow increases during pregnancy is the nasal mucous membrane, which explains the common finding of nasal congestion in pregnancy.[86]

5. Flow to other organs

Early studies showed no significant changes in hepatic and cerebral blood flow during pregnancy.[87,88] The mammary blood flow is probably increased during pregnancy, although no studies have been reported. It is evident by the engorgement of the breast, which begins early in pregnancy, and the dilatation of the veins on the surface of the breast, which is usually accompanied by the sensation of heat and tingling.[44] The effect of pregnancy on coronary blood flow is unknown, but it is assumed to be increased owing to the augmentation of cardiac output.[17]

I. Oxygen Consumption

Oxygen consumption is commonly estimated by measurement of oxygen extracted by the lungs over a given time period, and it reflects the rate of body metabolism. In pregnancy, there is a progressive increase in resting oxygen consumption, with a peak increase of 20–30% seen near term.[89,90] The rise in oxygen consumption should be attributed to the increased metabolic needs of the mother and the growing fetus. There is an obvious discrepancy between the dynamics of changes in cardiac output and oxygen consumption during pregnancy. While most of the increment of cardiac output occurs during the early part of pregnancy with the peak increase seen around the 20th week, the oxygen consumption shows a gradual rise throughout pregnancy, reaching its peak near term. It has been suggested that this discrepancy occurs in anticipation of the reproductive needs: The rapid increase in cardiac output, which is proportionally greater than the rise in oxygen consumption, particularly in early pregnancy, results in well-oxygenated blood flowing to the uterus when it is needed for organogenesis, before the fetal–placental circulation is fully developed.[77] The continuous increase in oxygen consumption in the later phases of pregnancy, when cardiac output increase is slow and small, results in a widening of the arterial venous oxygen difference to the nonpregnant level. The arterial venous oxygen difference is therefore small in early pregnancy and increases gradually throughout pregnancy, reaching the nonpregnant level in the last part of gestation.[29,30,33]

III. CARDIAC FUNCTION DURING PREGNANCY

The techniques that have been used to evaluate the physiological changes in cardiac function during normal pregnancy include cardiac catheterization, circulation time, systolic time intervals, and echocardiography.

A. Cardiac Catheterization

Bader et al have performed right heart catheterization in women with normal pregnancy.[33] The level of right ventricular end-diastolic pressure was found to be related to the period of gestation. The pressure was within the limits of normal in early pregnancy and was found to be elevated in six of 27 patients between the 20th and 35th weeks of gestation. Pulmonary artery pressure showed a slight increase without significant elevation above normal.

B. Circulation Time

Circulation time correlates directly with the velocity of blood flow and, inversely, with the volume of blood in which the indicator is diluted. Therefore, pulmonary and/or systemic venous congestion, as well as reduced cardiac output, tend to cause prolongation of this parameter. Early studies of circulation time during pregnancy resulted in contradictory findings. Greenstein and Clahr reported marked individual variations in circulation time during pregnancy, but their mean value was increased above normal.[91] Other studies showed a decrease or no significant change in the circulation time during pregnancy.[92,93] More recent evaluations, in which circulation time was measured by the photoelectric method, showed a decrease during pregnancy from the nonpregnant values.[42]

In summary, the effect of normal pregnancy on the circulation time is not entirely clear, and the reported data are contradictory. With the advent of more accurate diagnostic methods for the assessment of cardiac function, the clinical importance of circulation time is doubtful.

C. Systolic Time Intervals

The response of the left ventricle to the stress of pregnancy was also evaluated by the technique of systolic time intervals. A review of available data suggests that conclusions should be drawn cautiously, realizing the limitations inherent in the method employed in the determination of the functional status of the left ventricle.[94] The pre-ejection period (PEP) is the period between the electrical stimulation of the ventricle and the onset of ejection of blood through the aortic valve. Serial evaluations of this parameter throughout gestation have provided inconsistent data. While shortening of the PEP during the first trimester of pregnancy and its prolongation at the third trimester were reported by Burg et al,[95] Liebson et al found an increase in PEP throughout pregnancy.[96] According to Burg et al, the left ventricular ejection time (LVET), which reflects the duration of actual ejection of blood from the left ventricle, shows no significant changes during the first and second trimesters and is markedly shortened during late pregnancy. Liebson et al, however, showed a consistent shortening throughout pregnancy. The ratio PEP/LVET was found by Rubler et al to be decreased during the early two-thirds of gestation and increased at the late phase, whereas Liebson et al found that it was increased throughout pregnancy. Although the data obtained by these two studies in early gestation are contradictory, the findings in late pregnancy are consistent.

The duration of LVET correlates well with the magnitude of the stroke volume.[97] Prolongation of LVET when the patient is in the supine position and its reversion toward normal in the lateral position has been seen in late pregnancy and is probably a result of decreased stroke volume secondary to caval compression in the supine position.[96] The prolongation of PEP and the ratio of PEP/LVET in late pregnancy is more difficult to comprehend: The PEP is inversely related to the rate of rise of left ventricular pressure—ie, dP/dT.[98] Prolongation of PEP together with diminished LVET is seen in patients with congestive heart failure because left ventricular function is decreased. Increased peripheral resistance and systemic diastolic blood pressure can also prolong the PEP. In pregnancy, however, systemic vascular resistance has been shown to be decreased rather than increased. In addition, the evaluation of left ventricular performance by both invasive and noninvasive means did not reveal any impairment of myocardial function during pregnancy.[33,38,39]

D. Echocardiography

Katz et al[39] have recently used echocardiography for seriel evaluations of left ventricular response to the chronic volume overload state of pregnancy. In spite of the progressive increase in left ventricular dimensions and volume, no significant change could be found in several indices of left ventricular function, including ejection fraction, percent of fractional shortening, and mean normalized rate of internal diameter shortening. Left ventricular volume overload also did not result in thickening of the left ventricular walls. Increase in left ventricular myocardial contractility measured echocardiographically during pregnancy was reported by Rubler et al.[38] These investigators found an increased velocity of myocardial circumferential fiber shortening and posterior wall slope during pregnancy. Although the discrepency between the results of these two studies is not entirely understandable, it could be related to the difference in study design; serial examinations of the same group of pregnant patients were performed by Katz et al, whereas Rubler et al evaluated separate groups of patients in different stages of pregnancy.

In summary, echocardiographic evaluation during pregnancy indicates that, in spite of volume overload on the left ventricle, myocardial function is well preserved and may even be augmented.

E. Effect of Exercise

The hemodynamic effects of exercise during normal pregnancy have been studied by several investigators. The increase in maternal cardiac output and stroke volume evoked by mild exercise at all stages of pregnancy has been found to be higher than that evoked by the same degree of exercise in the nonpregnant state. Ueland et al showed that the cardiac output increase with exercise is progressively smaller as pregnancy advances.[40,99] These findings are supported by other reports[33,100] and suggest a progressive decline in circulatory reserve as pregnancy advances. Bruce and Johnson suggested that the decline in circulatory reserve is not a result of decreased cardiac function but rather is a consequence of peripheral blood pooling.[101] The exercise-evoked increase in cardiac output during pregnancy is proportionally greater than the increase in oxygen consumption, resulting in a lower arteriovenous oxygen difference.[77] The increase in heart rate during exercise was also found to be higher during pregnancy than that evoked by the same exercise in the postpartum period.[40,99,102,103]

IV. CARDIOCIRCULATORY CHANGES DURING LABOR AND DELIVERY

The significant hemodynamic changes observed during labor and delivery (Table M.I.3) can be attributed in large part to

TABLE M.I.3. The Cardiocirculatory Effects of Uterine Contraction

Central blood volume	↑
Cardiac output	↑
A-V O_2 difference	↑
Blood pressure	↑
Heart rate	↑ ↓
Peripheral resistance	No significant change

pain and anxiety, especially in the primigravida.[104,105] In addition, contraction of the uterus, which is followed by a significant increase in central blood volume (300–500 ml), contributes to the important circulatory changes.[106,107]

In spite of important differences in methodology and technique of determination, significant increases in cardiac output during labor have been consistently reported.[52,106–108] Winner and Romney reported different results and showed variable changes in cardiac output during uterine contractions. The discrepancy between their findings and most other reports may be explained by the limited number of cardiac output determinations performed by these investigators.[109] Henricks and Quilligan, in 1956, used the pulse pressure method to evaluate cardiac output in 47 women in various stages of labor and found a rise in cardiac output of 31% over that during the relaxed state between uterine contractions.[104] Further studies, in which the dye-dilution technique was used for cardiac output determination, have confirmed the results obtained by Henricks and Quilligan.[52,106,108–110] A cumulative increase in cardiac output between contractions was also demonstrated by serial measurements throughout labor. This was most obvious in the late stage of labor or in prolonged labor.

It has been postulated that squeezing the uterus during contraction results in an increase in circulating blood volume and venous return to the heart and is the major mechanism for increasing cardiac output. The increase of pulmonary arterial venous oxygen difference during each uterine contraction also suggests a sudden flow of blood from the maternal uterine vascular bed into the systemic circulation.[30,111] Henricks and Quilligan have clearly shown that pain and anxiety alone have a significant hemodynamic effect associated with a 50–61% increase in cardiac output.[104] Since the increase of cardiac output during contraction was found to be accompanied by a rise in blood pressure and pulse rate, it was suggested by some investigators that increased sympathetic tone due to pain, anxiety, and muscular activity were the major causes for the increased cardiac output during contraction, and that squeezing of blood from the uterus was of only secondary importance.[106]

The reported effect of uterine contraction on heart rate is variable. Adams and Alexander found a tachycardic response to contractions, with a mean increase of 14%.[106] Other investigators also reported an increase in heart rate following uterine contraction; the increase, however, was found to be smaller.[100,112] These data are at variance with the results of Kjeldsen, who showed no significant change in heart rate during contractions,[52] and those of Ueland and Hansen, who showed that uterine contraction was almost invariably accompanied by slowing of the heart rate.[107] A similar decrease in heart rate during uterine contraction was observed by Henricks and was thought to be a result of baroreceptor stimulation.[113] A possible explanation for the discrepancy in the reported heart rate response to uterine contraction may be the different forms of sedation used during labor.[106,109] In addition, the different results have been assumed to reflect the very significant individual variation of heart rate response to uterine contraction.[52]

Both the systolic and the diastolic blood pressure increase during uterine contraction. Winner and Romney found a maximum increase of 35 mm Hg in systolic blood pressure during the first stage of labor, with even a greater increase during the second stage contractions. The diastolic blood pressure increased by more than 25 mm Hg during the first stage and by as much as 65 mm Hg during the second stage. The elevation of blood pressure was shown to precede the uterine contraction by five to eight seconds.[109] The blood pressure returned to the resting level when the contraction subsided. Cunningham confirmed these findings and also showed a progressive increase in blood pressure, with a peak in the second stage of labor.[108] Since the peripheral resistance changes only slightly during labor, the increase in blood pressure is attributed to the rise in cardiac output.[106] The redistribution of the maternal cardiac output to the upper part of the peripheral circulation after compression of the distal aorta and the common iliac artery should also play a role in the elevation of systemic pressure as measured in the arm.[49]

The hemodynamic effect of uterine contraction is less pronounced when the patient is examined in lateral recumbency than when she assumes the supine position.[47,52] The cardiac output effect of an ineffective uterine contraction is unpredictable and inconsistent.[104,107]

Hemodynamic changes during labor are markedly influenced by the form of anesthesia or analgesia employed. Substantial differences were demonstrated by Ueland and Hansen between women receiving local and paracervical block anesthetics and others who received caudal anesthesia.[107] Caudal anesthesia, in general, does not affect the hemodynamic changes caused by uterine contraction. The decrease in pain and apprehension, however, abolishes the progressive rise in cardiac output seen between contractions, and limits the absolute increase of cardiac output at delivery. Both caudal and local anesthesia did not significantly alter the cardiovascular response to uterine contractions. These forms of anesthesia have been shown to be safe in patients with severe heart disease.[114] When the patient was in the supine position contraction of the uterus increased cardiac output approximately 15–20%, regardless of the stage of labor or analgesia.

When local anesthesia is used, tachycardia develops during the second stage of labor and is accentuated by uterine contraction. Both the systolic and the diastolic pressures show a mild gradual rise during the first stage of labor and a significant increase during the second stage. These changes are associated with a progressive increase in stroke volume to a peak immediately post-delivery. In contrast, caudal anesthesia is associated with no significant change in heart rate, and both diastolic and systolic blood pressures are maintained constant throughout labor and delivery. The stroke volume is also maintained throughout labor but rises rapidly after delivery. No difference could be found between local and caudal anesthesia with regard to mean blood volume loss during delivery.[107]

V. HEMODYNAMIC EFFECTS OF CESAREAN SECTION

Cesarean section is often performed to avoid the marked hemodynamic alterations associated with labor. It should be noted, however, that the surgical procedure and some of the anesthetic techniques are also associated with major hemodynamic changes. In 1950 Zimmerman was the first to report the hemodynamic changes of cesarean section under spinal anesthesia in four patients.[31] The delivery of the baby and the placenta was followed by a significant increase in cardiac output (mean increase of 2,434 cc/min). Ueland et al, as a part of an overall investigation of the maternal cardiovascular response to labor and delivery, reported the effect of cesarean section under various anesthetic agents.[115–117] The effect of subarachnoid block anesthesia on maternal cardiodynamics was studied by Ueland et al in 1968 in 12 women undergoing cesarean section for obstetric reasons.[115] Five to ten minutes following the administration of the spinal anesthetic, a significant decrease in stroke volume and cardiac output, associated with a marked increase in heart rate and a decline in blood pressure, was observed. Hemodynamic changes did not correlate with either the dose or the level of anesthesia. The hypotension did not seem to have a deleterious effect on the newborn infant and could be completely reversed by turning the patient on her side. The authors concluded that cesarean section under spinal anesthesia is associated with significant cardiovascular changes, and they recommended not using that form of anesthesia in patients with heart disease.

The hemodynamic fluctuations were found to be significantly smaller when cesarean section was performed under thiopentol, nitrous oxide, and succinyl choline anesthesia.[116] Cardiac output did not change significantly, whereas the heart rate increased slightly and diastolic pressure increased moderately. Delivery was followed by some increase in stroke volume and cardiac output, accompanied by a slight decrease in heart rate and blood pressure.

Stability of the hemodynamics has been seen in normal pregnant women undergoing cesarean section under epidural anesthesia without epinephrine.[117] The administration of anesthesia was followed by only minor hemodynamic changes. Blood pressure showed a moderate decline after induction of anesthesia but then remained constant throughout the surgical procedure. There were no significant changes in heart rate, cardiac output, or stroke volume. Following delivery, cardiac output showed a relatively mild increase (25% above control values), and there was no change in heart rate.

In summary, maternal hemodynamics during cesarean section can be significantly affected by the anesthesia employed. The marked fluctuations seen when subarachnoid block anesthesia is used may not be tolerated by a patient with heart disease. Balanced anesthesia with thiopentol, nitrous oxide, and succinyl choline, and especially with epidural anesthesia without epinephrine, are associated with smaller hemodynamic fluctuations and therefore should be preferred in patients with small cardiac reserves.

TABLE M.I.4. Hemodynamic Changes Postpartum

Blood volume	↓
Cardiac output	↑
Stroke volume	↑
Heart rate	↓
Blood pressure	No significant change
Peripheral vascular resistance	↓

VI. HEMODYNAMIC CHANGES POSTPARTUM (Table M.I.4)

In spite of the external hemorrhage associated with partus, cardiac output is significantly higher one to two hours postpartum than it is prior to the initiation of contractions (Table M.I.4).[14,32,35,48,104,106,107] An increase in cardiac output of 60–80% occurs immediately after delivery, followed by a rapid decrease (within ten minutes) to values approaching those found one hour postpartum. The placental separation per se was not found to cause any further changes. The increase in cardiac output remains almost unchanged for days, and even weeks, postpartum.[107] A 10% loss of blood volume was noted one to ten hours postpartum in patients delivering vaginally.[9,118] Cesarean section was associated with a more significant loss (17–29%). There was, however, no change in the hematocrit in either group. A steady decline in blood volume was then seen after vaginal delivery over the next several days. In the surgically delivered group, blood volume remained stable from one hour to several days after operation. When studied after the third postpartum day, the blood volume was found to be 10% lower than the predelivery values in both groups.[107]

The high cardiac output state following partus is probably a result of both a shift of blood from the emptied uterus into the systemic circulation and a decrease in caval compression, allowing an increased venous return to the heart.[52] The increase in venous return seems also to be the reason for a significantly higher central venous pressure postpartum as compared to before the start of contractions. This occurs despite the bleeding associated with partus.[52] Heart rate decreases shortly after vaginal delivery and cesarean section, with the reported fall in heart rate ranging from 4 to 17 beats per minute.[39,106,107,115] The increase in cardiac output therefore results from an augmented stroke volume.[52,107,110] The arterial blood pressure shows no significant change after delivery.[14,60,100,104,119]

VII. CHANGES IN CARDIAC SIGNS AND SYMPTOMS DURING PREGNANCY

The anatomical and functional changes in the cardiovascular system that occur with normal pregnancy can be associated with the development of physical signs and symptoms that can simulate organic heart disease (Table M.I.5). Obstetric patients are therefore often referred for cardiological opinion because of the development of heart sounds and murmurs that suggest cardiac pathology. The reluctance to use x-rays and invasive diagnostic tools during pregnancy has been a limiting factor in the ability to differentiate between normal physiologic changes and organic heart disease. The development of safe and exact noninvasive tools such as echocardiography and Doppler velocimetry should allow marked improvement in the diagnostic potentials of heart disease during pregnancy.[120]

A. Clinical Features

1. Symptoms

Reduction in exercise tolerance, tiredness, and dyspnea are most commonly found during pregnancy. Lightheadedness or even syncopal episodes can be seen in the late phases of gestation, presumably a result of the mechanical compression of the enlarged uterus on the inferior vena cava, which results in a decrease in venous return to the heart and a fall in cardiac output.[40,45]

2. Physical signs

Hyperventilation is a common phenomenon during pregnancy and can be misinterpreted as dyspnea. Occasional findings of basilar rales may reinforce the impression of heart failure. The pulmonary basilar rales in normal pregnancy are caused by a compression of the basal parts of the lungs and atelactasis secondary to the enlargement of the uterus and increased abdominal pressure. The higher position of the diaphragm during pregnancy displaces the heart toward a more horizontal position. Left ventricular im-

TABLE M.I.5. Cardiac Signs and Symptoms During Normal Pregnancy

Symptoms
- Decreased exercise capacity
- Tiredness
- Dyspnea
- Lightheadedness
- Syncope

Signs
- Hyperventilation
- Peripheral edema
- Distended neck veins with prominent A and V peaks and brisk x and y descents
- Full sharp and collapsing pulse
- Capillary pulsation
- Precordial palpation
  - Brisk, diffuse and displaced left ventricular impulse
  - Palpable right ventricular impulse
  - Palpable pulmonary trunk impulse

Auscultation
- Pulmonary basilar rales
- Increased first heart sound with exaggerated splitting
- Persistent splitting of second heart sound
- Third heart sound
- Early and midsystolic ejection-type murmurs at the lower left sternal edge or over the pulmonic area
- Continuous murmurs (cervical venous hum, mammary souffle)
- Diastolic murmurs

Chest x-ray film
- Straightening of the left upper cardiac border
- Horizontal position of the heart
- Increased lung marking

Electrocardiogram
- QRS axis deviation
- Small Q wave and inverted P wave in lead III (abolished by inspiration)
- ST segment and T wave changes

Echocardiogram
- Slight increase in systolic and diastolic left ventricular dimensions (when patient examined in the lateral position)
- Unchanged or slightly improved left ventricular function
- Slight enlargement of the right ventricular dimension
- Slight enlargement of left atrial size

pulse is usually easily palpated, it is diffuse, brisk and unsustained and may be displaced to the left. A right ventricular impulse at the mid- to lower left sternal border can generally be palpated, as can the pulmonary trunk (at the second left intercostal space). These findings may be obscured because of the increase in breast size associated with pregnancy.

The systemic arterial pulse is usually full; it becomes sharp and jerky between 12 and 15 weeks of gestation and maintains that character until about a week after delivery. The pulse often gives the impression of a high pulse pressure; it is "collapsing" in character and is associated with capillary pulsation simulating the findings in aortic insufficiency, but in pregnancy there is only a slight change in pulse pressure.

The jugular veins appear somewhat distended from about the 20th week of pregnancy and their pulsation is more easily seen than normally.[121,63]

Edema of the ankles and legs is a common finding in late pregnancy,[122] and the incidence of this phenomenon increases with age. The edema can be attributed to a fall in the colloid osmotic pressure of the plasma[123] and a concomitant increase in femoral venous pressure.[124] An increase in capillary permeability during pregnancy has been also suggested as a factor in edema formation, but this could not be convincingly demonstrated.[125]

B. Auscultatory Findings

1. Heart sounds

The first heart sound shows an increased loudness of both components starting at the 12th to the 20th weeks of gestation and remains loud up to about the 32nd week. When the intensity diminishes in some of the cases, the first sound returns to normal two to four weeks postpartum.[121,126] In addition to the increased intensity, the first sound demonstrates an exaggerated splitting, which is maximal in the third to fifth left intercostal spaces, close to the sternum. It is also audible in the pulmonary area, down the left sternal edge, and at the apex. The amplitude of the second or tricuspid element of the first heart sound increases on inspiration and decreases on expiration. The cause for the changes in the quality of the first heart sound in pregnancy is not clear. Cutforth and MacDonald have suggested that increased plasma volume is a major contributing factor.[121] Perloff states that the hyperkinetic circulation during pregnancy results in an accentuation of the intensity of the first heart sound.[63]

There is no change in the character of the second heart sound during the first 30 weeks of pregnancy. In late pregnancy, however, the second sound is also often increased, and when the patient is examined in the lateral position, persistent expiratory splitting of the second sound is exhibited. Compression of the inferior vena cava by the uterus and the lack of good diaphragmatic movement have been suggested as the mechanisms responsible for the normal, or less than normal, splitting of the second sound when patients are examined in the supine position.[121]

A third heart sound is a regular finding during pregnancy and was found in up to 90% of all pregnant women.[121,126] The sound can be heard easily after the 20th week of gestation, and becomes loudest at about the 30th week. In some patients the intensity diminishes two to five weeks before delivery. The third heart sound of pregnancy usually disappears or diminishes significantly within eight days after delivery. A fourth heart sound was found by phonocardiographic study in 16% of pregnant women during early pregnancy (15th–22nd week), but was only rarely detected on auscultation. On the phonocardiogram, the sound was best seen after the beginning of expiration, suggesting its left-sided origin, and in all cases could not be found by the time of delivery.[121,126]

2. Systolic murmurs

As a result of the hyperkinetic circulation during pregnancy, the incidence of innocent systolic murmurs is high, and such murmurs were found in 96% of the

son et al in healthy women during pregnancy showed a progressive decrease in left ventricular ejection time (LVET), a prolongation of the preejection period (PEP), and an increase in the ratio between the preejection period and left ventricular ejection time (PEP/LVET).[96] A similar study by Burg et al resulted in somewhat different data. These investigators showed a significant shortening of the PEP associated with no significant change in LVET during the first and second trimesters of gestation. The LVET was found by these investigators to be significantly shortened at the third trimester, accompanied by a prolonged PEP and an increased PEP/LVET ratio. All changes were more apparent when the patient was supine than when the patient was in the lateral position.[95]

In the postpartum period, LVET returns to baseline values, whereas PEP and the ratio of PEP/LVET remain prolonged.

F. Echocardiography

A slight but significant increase in end-diastolic dimension of the left ventricle is seen with the progression of pregnancy and returns to the baseline values after the postpartum phase.[38,39] This increase is seen when the patient is examined in the lateral position. Examination in the supine position reveals no significant change in the LV diastolic dimensions throughout pregnancy.[39] Left ventricular systolic dimension was reported to increase during systole by Katz et al but was found to be unchanged by Rubler et al.[38,39] Both studies found no significant change in left ventricular wall thickening during pregnancy. Indices of left ventricular function were found to be improved by Rubler et al but unchanged by Katz et al. The E-F slope of the anterior leaflet of the mitral valve is slightly but not significantly decreased during pregnancy. The left atrial size shows a mild increase in dimensions with a return to the baseline at the postpartum period. There is no significant change in the size of the aortic root, and the right ventricular dimension may show a temporary increase during pregnancy.

VIII. ACKNOWLEDGMENTS

We gratefully acknowledge the expert secretarial assistance of Linda Childs and Ellen Mansour in the preparation of this manuscript.

IX. REFERENCES

1. Miller JR, Keith NM, Rownreel LG. Plasma and blood volume in pregnancy. JAMA. 1915; 65:779–782.
2. Dieckmann WJ, Wegner CR. The blood in normal pregnancy. I. Blood and Plasma. Arch Intern Med. 1934; 53:71–86.
3. Berlin NI, Goetsch C, Hyde GM, Parsons RJ. The blood volume in pregnancy as determined by P32 labelled red blood cells. Surg Gynecol Obstet. 1953; 97:173–176.
4. Hytten FE, Paintin DB. Increase in plasma volume during normal pregnancy. J Obstet Gynaecol Br Commonw. 1963; 70:402–407.
5. Rovinsky JJ, Jaffin H. Cardiovascular hemodynamics in pregnancy I. Blood and plasma volumes in multiple pregnancy. Am J Obstet Gynecol. 1965; 93:1–15.
6. Pritchard JA, Rowland RC. Blood volume changes in pregnancy and the puerperium. III. Whole body and large vessel hematocrits in pregnant and non-pregnant women. Am J Obstet Gynecol. 1964; 88:391–395.
7. Lund CJ, Donovan JC. Blood volume during pregnancy. Am J Obstet Gynecol. 1967; 98:393–403.
8. Chesley LC. Plasma and red cell volumes during pregnancy. Am J Obstet Gynecol. 1972; 112:440–450.
9. Ueland K. Maternal cardiovascular dynamics. VII. Intrapartum blood volume changes. Am J Obstet Gynecol. 1976; 126:671–677.
10. Thomson KJ, Hirsheimer A, Gibson JG, Evans WA Jr. Studies on the circulation in pregnancy. III. Blood volume changes in normal pregnant women. Am J Obstet Gynecol. 1938; 36:48–59.
11. Roscoe MH, Donaldson GMM. The blood in pregnancy, Part II. The blood volume, cell volume and haemoglobin mass. J Obstet Gynaecol Br Emp. 1946; 53:527–538.
12. McLennan CE, Thouin LG. Blood volume in pregnancy. A critical review and preliminary report of results with a new technique. Am J Obstet Gynecol. 1948; 55:189–200.
13. Caton WL, Roby CC, Reid DE, Gibson JG. Plasma volume and extravascular fluid volume during pregnancy and the puerperium. Am J Obstet Gynecol. 1949; 57:471–481.

14. Adams JQ. Cardiovascular physiology in normal pregnancy: Studied with the dye dilution technique. Am J Obstet Gynecol. 1954; 67:741–759.
15. Rovinsky JJ. Blood volume and the hemodynamics of pregnancy. In: Philipp EE, Barnes J, Newton M (eds): Scientific Foundation of Obstetrics and Gynaecology. Philadelphia: FA Davis Co. 1970:332–340.
16. Hytten FE, Thomson AM. Maternal physiological adjustments. In: Assali NS (ed): Biology of Gestation. New York: Academic Press, 1968:449.
17. Hytten FE, Leitch I. The Physiology of Human Pregnancy, Ed 2. Oxford: Blackwell Scientific Publications, 1971:1–111.
18. Chisholm M. A controlled clinical trial of prophylactic folic acid and iron in pregnancy. J Obstet Gynecol Br Commonw. 1966; 73:191–196.
19. Butler EB. The effect of iron and folic acid on red cell and plasma volume in pregnancy. J Obstet Gynaecol Br Commonw. 1968; 75:497–510.
20. Pritchard JA. Anemias complicating pregnancy and the puerperium. In Committee on Maternal Nutrition/Food and Nutrition Board. National Research Council (eds): Maternal Nutrition and the Course of Pregnancy. Washington, DC: National Academy of Sciences–National Research Council, 1970:74.
21. MacGillivray I. Hypertension in pregnancy and its consequences. J Obstet Gynaecol Br Commonw. 1961; 68:557–569.
22. Seitchik J. Total body water and total body density of pregnant women. J Obstet Gynecol. 1967; 29:155–166.
23. Tapia HR, Johnson CE, Strong CG. Effect of oral contraceptive therapy on the renin-angiotensin system in normotensive and hypertensive women. J Obstet Gynecol. 1973; 41:643–649.
24. Preedy JRK, Aitken EH. The effect of estrogen on water and electrolyte metabolism I. The normal. J Clin Invest. 1956; 35:423–429.
25. Biglier EG, Forsham PH. Studies on the expanded extracellular fluid and the responses to varis stimuli in primary aldosteronism. Am J Med. 1961; 30:564–576.
26. Pritchard JA. Changes in the blood volume during pregnancy and delivery. Anesthesiology. 1965; 26:393–399.
27. Chesley LC, Duffus GM. Posture and apparent plasma volume in late pregnancy. J Obstet Gynaecol Br Commonw. 1971; 78:406–412.
28. Lindhard J. Ueber das minutenvolumens des herzens bei ruhe und bei muskelarbeit. Pfluegers Arch. 1915; 161:233–383.
29. Hamilton HFH. The cardiac output in normal pregnancy as determined by the Cournand right heart catheterization technique. J Obstet Gynaecol Br Emp. 1949; 56:548–552.
30. Palmer AJ, Walter AHC. The maternal circulation in normal pregnancy. J Obstet Gynaecol Br Emp. 1949; 56:537–547.
31. Zimmerman HA. A preliminary report on intracardiac catheterization studies during pregnancy. J Lab Clin Med. 1950; 36:1007–1008.
32. Werkoe L. Studies in the problems of circulation in pregnancy. In: Toxaemias in Pregnancy. A Ciba Foundation Symposium. London: J.R.A. Churchill, Ltd. 1950:155–160.
33. Bader RA, Bader MG, Rose DJ, Braunwald E. Hemodynamics at rest and during exercise in normal pregnancy as studied by cardiac catheterization. J Clin Invest. 1955; 34:1524–1536.
34. Rovinsky JJ, Jaffin H. Cardiovascular hemodynamics in pregnancy. II: Cardiac output and left ventricular work in multiple pregnancy. Am J Obstet Gynecol. 1966; 95:781–786.
35. Walters WAW, MacGregor WG, Hills M. Cardiac output at rest during pregnancy and the puerperium. Clin Sci. 1966; 30:1–11.
36. Roy BS, Malkani PK, Virik R, Bhatia ML. Circulatory effects of pregnancy. Am J Obstet Gynecol. 1966; 96:221–225.
37. Lees MM, Taylor SH, Scott DB, Kerr MG. A study of cardiac output at rest throughout pregnancy. J Obstet Gynaecol Br Commonw. 1967; 74:319–328.
38. Rubler S, Prabodhkumar MD, Pinto ER. Cardiac size and performance during pregnancy estimated with echocardiography. Clin Obstet Gynecol. 1977; 40:534–540.
39. Katz R, Karliner JS, Resnik R. Effects of a natural volume overload state (pregnancy) on left ventricular performance in normal human subjects. Circulation. 1978; 58:434–441.
40. Ueland K, Novy MJ, Peterson EN, Metcalfe J. Maternal cardiovascular dynamics. IV. The influence of gestational age on the maternal cardiovascular response to posture and exercise. Am J Obstet Gynecol. 1969; 104:856–864.
41. Kerr MG. Cardiovascular dynamics in pregnancy and labour. Br Med Bull. 1968; 24:19–24.
42. Pyorala T. Cardiovascular response to the upright position during pregnancy. Acta Obstet Gynecol Scand. 1966; 45(Suppl 5):1–116.
43. Lees HM, Taylor SH, Scott BD, Kerr MG. The circulatory effect of recumbent postural change in late pregnancy. Clin Sci. 1967; 32:453–465.
44. Metcalfe J, Ueland K. Maternal cardiovascular adjustments to pregnancy. Prog Cardiovasc Dis. 1974; 16:363–374.
45. Kerr MG. The mechanical effects of the gravid uterus in late pregnancy. J Obstet Gynaecol Br Commonw. 1965; 72:513–529.
46. Howard BK, Goodson JH, Mengert WF. Supine hypotensive syndrome in late pregnancy. Obstet Gynecol. 1953; 1:371–377.
47. Kerr MG, Scott DB, Samuel E. Studies of the inferior vena cava in late pregnancy. Br Med J. 1964; 1:532–533.
48. Bieniarz J, Mapueda E, Caldeyro-Barcia R. Compression of aorta by the uterus in late human pregnancy. I. Variations between femoral and brachial artery pressure with changes from hypertension to hypotension. Am J Obstet Gynecol. 1966; 95:795–808.

49. Bieniarz J, Crottongini JJ, Curuchet E, Romero-Salinas G, Yoshida T, Poseiro JJ, Caldeyro-Barcia R. Aortocaval compression by the uterus in late human pregnancy. II. An angiographic study. Am J Obstet Gynecol. 1968; 100:203–217.
50. Holmes F. Incidence of the supine hypotensive syndrome in late pregnancy. A clinical study in 500 subjects. J Obstet Gynaecol Br Emp. 1960; 67:254–258.
51. Kim YI, Chandra P, Marx GF. Successful management of severe aortocaval compression in twin pregnancy. Obstet Gynecol. 1975; 46:362–364.
52. Kjeldsen J. Hemodynamic investigations during labor and delivery. Acta Obstet Gynecol Scand Suppl 89, 1979.
53. Brigden W, Howarth S, Sharpey-Schafer EP. Posture and peripheral blood flow. Clin Sci. 1950; 9:79–91.
54. McRoberts WA, Jr. Postural shock in pregnancy. Am J Obstet Gynecol. 1951; 62:627–631.
55. Quilligan EJ, Tyler C. Postural effects on the cardiovascular status in pregnancy: A comparison of the lateral and supine postures. Am J Obstet Gynecol. 1978; 130:194–198.
56. Abitol MM: Inferior vena cava compression in the pregnant dog. Am J Obstet Gynecol. 1978; 130:194–198.
57. Hansen R. Ohnmacht und schwangershaft. Klin Wochenschr. 1942; 21:241–242.
58. Bieniarz J, Julio H, Grainer L. An angiographic study of blood flow and distribution in late pregnancy. Int J Gynecol Obstet. 1970; 8(Part 2):263.
59. Brehm H, Kindling E. Der kreislauf waehrend schwangerschaft und wochenbett. Arch Gynaekol. 1955; 185:699–712.
60. Gemzell CA, Robbe H, Stern B, Stroem G. Observations on circulatory changes and muscular work in normal labour. Acta Obstet Gynecol Scand. 1957; 36:75–92.
61. Christianson RE. Studies on blood pressure during pregnancy. I. Influence of parity and age. Am J Obstet Gynecol. 1976; 125:509–513.
62. MacGillivray I, Rose GA, Rowe B. Blood pressure survey in pregnancy. Clin Sci. 1969; 37:395–407.
63. Perloff JK. Pregnancy and cardiovascular disease. In: Braumwald (ed), Heart Disease. Philadelphia: W.B. Saunders Company, 1980:1871–1891.
64. Walters WAW, Lim YL. Cardiovascular dynamics in women receiving oral contraceptive therapy. Lancet. 1969; 2:879–881.
65. Greiss FC, Anderson SG. Effect of ovarian hormones on the uterine vascular bed. Am J Obstet Gynecol. 1970; 107:829–836.
66. Bryant EE, Douglas BH, Ashburn AD. Circulatory changes following prolactin administration. Am J Obstet Gynecol. 1973; 115:53–57.
67. Assali NS, Rauramo L, Peltonen T. Measurement of uterine blood flow and uterine metabolism. VIII. Uterine and fetal blood flow and oxygen consumption in early human pregnancy. Am J Obstet Gynecol. 1960; 79:86–98.
68. Metcalfe J, Romney SL, Ramsey LH, Reid DE, Barwell CS. Estimation of uterine blood flow in normal human pregnancy at term. J Clin Invest. 1955; 34:1632–1638.
69. Romney SL, Reid DE, Metcalfe J, Burwell CS. Oxygen utilization by the human fetus in utero. Am J Obstet Gynecol. 1955; 70:791–799.
70. Burwell CS, Strayhorn WD, Flickinger D, Corlette MB, Bowerman EP, Kennedy JA. Circulation during pregnancy. Arch Intern Med. 1938; 62:979–1003.
71. Heckel GP, Tobin CE. Arteriovenous shunts in the myometrium. Am J Obstet Gynecol. 1956; 71:199–205.
72. Metcalfe J, Parer JT. Cardiovascular changes during pregnancy in ewes. Am J Physiol. 1966; 210:821–825.
73. Ueland K, Parer JT. Effects of estrogens on the cardiovascular system of the ewe. Am J Obstet Gynecol. 1966; 96:400–406.
74. Ferris TF, Stein JH, Kauffman J. Uterine blood flow and uterine renin secretion. J Clin Invest. 1972; 51:2827–2833.
75. Little B. Water and electrolyte balance during pregnancy. Anesthesiology. 1965; 26:400–408.
76. Chesley LC. Renal functional changes in normal pregnancy. Clin Obstet Gynecol. 1960; 3:349–363.
77. Metcalfe J, Ueland K. The heart and pregnancy. In: Hurst JW, Logue RB, Schlant RC, Wegner NR (eds). The Heart Arteries and Veins. New York: McGraw-Hill, 1978:1721–1734.
78. Abramson DI, Flacks K, Fierst SM. Peripheral blood flow during gestation. Am J Obstet Gynecol. 45:666–671, 1943.
79. Herbert CM, Banner EA, Wakim KG. Variations in the peripheral circulation during pregnancy. Am J Obstet Gynecol. 1958; 76:742–745.
80. Burt CC. The peripheral circulation in pregnancy. Trans Edinb Obstet Soc Edinb Med J. 1950; 57:18–26.
81. Spetz S. Peripheral circulation during normal pregnancy. Acta Obstet Gynecol Scand. 1944; 43:309–329.
82. Ginsburg J, Duncan SLB. Peripheral blood flow in normal pregnancy. Cardiovascular Res. 1967; 1:132–137.
83. Katz M, Sokal MM. Skin perfusion in pregnancy. Am J Obstet Gynecol. 1980; 137:30–33.
84. Burt CC. Peripheral skin temperature in normal pregnancy. Lancet. 1949: 2:787–790.
85. Bean WB, Dexter MW, Cogswell RC. Vascular changes of skin in pregnancy Surg Gynecol Obstet. 1949; 88:739–752.
86. Fabricant ND. Sexual functions and the nose. Am J Med Sci. 1960; 239:498–502.
87. Munnell EW, Taylor HC Jr. Liver blood flow in pregnancy—Hepatic vein catheterization. J Clin Invest. 1947; 26:952–956.
88. McCall ML. Cerebral blood flow and metabolism in toxemias of pregnancy. Surg Gynecol

Obstet. 1949; 89:715–721.
89. Novy MJ, Edwards MJ. Respiratory problems in pregnancy. Am J Obstet Gynecol. 1967; 99:1024–1045.
90. Prowse CM, Galnslar EA. Respiratory and acid-base changes during pregnancy. Anesthesiology. 1965; 26:381–392.
91. Greenstein NM, Clahr J. Circulation time studies in pregnant women. Am J Obstet Gynecol. 1937; 33:414–421.
92. Spitzer W. The rate of blood flow in normal and disturbed pregnancy. An examination of cardiac function during pregnancy and before birth. Arch Gynaekol. 1933; 154:449–458.
93. Manchester B, Loube SD. Velocity of blood flow in normal pregnant women. Am Heart J. 1946; 32:215–221.
94. Ross J Jr, O'Rourke RA, Peterson KL, Ludbrook P, Crawford M, Leopold GR, Karliner JS, Sobel BE, Ashburn WL. Noninvasive methods for the assessment of cardiac function. Calif Med. 1973; 3:31.
95. Burg JR, Doder A, Kloster FE, Metcalfe J. Alterations of systolic time intervals during pregnancy. Circulation. 1974; 49:560–564.
96. Liebson PR, Mann LI, Evans MI, Duchin S, Arditi L. Cardiac performance during pregnancy, serial evaluation using external systolic time intervals. Am J Obstet Gynecol. 1975; 122:1–8.
97. Weissler AM, Harris WS, Schoenfeld CD. Systolic time intervals in heart failure in man. Circulation. 1968; 37:149–159.
98. Metzger CC, Chough CB, Kroetz FW, Leonard JJ. True isovolumic contraction time: Its correlation with two external indexes of ventricular performance. Am J Cardiol. 1970; 25:434–442.
99. Ueland K, Novy MJ, Metcalfe J. Cardiorespiratory responses to pregnancy and exercise in normal women and patients with heart disease. Am J Obstet Gynecol. 1973; 115:4–10.
100. Rose DJ, Bader ME, Bader RA, Braunwald E. Catheterization studies of cardiac hemodynamics in normal and pregnant women with reference to left ventricular work. Am J Obstet Gynecol. 1956; 72:233–246.
101. Bruce RA, Johnson WP. Exercise tolerance in pregnant cardiac patients. Clin Obstet Gynecol. 1961; 4:665–676.
102. Guzman CA, Caplan R. Cardiorespiratory response to exercise during pregnancy. J Obstet Gynecol. 1970; 108:600–605.
103. Robbe H. Physical working capacity blood volume and heart volume in cardiac patients during and after pregnancy. Acta Obstet Gynecol Scand. 1959; 38:1–61.
104. Henricks CH, Quilligan EJ. Cardiac output during labor. Am J Obstet Gynecol. 1956; 71:953–972.
105. Burch GE. Heart disease and pregnancy. Am Heart J. 1977; 93:104–116.
106. Adams JQ, Alexander AM. Alterations in cardiovascular physiology during labor. Am Obstet Gynecol. 1958; 12:542–549.
107. Ueland K, Hansen JM. Maternal cardiovascular dynamics. III. Labor and delivery under local and caudal analgesia. Am J Obstet Gynecol. 1969; 103:8–18.
108. Cunningham I. Cardiovascular physiology of labor and delivery. J Obstet Gynaecol Br Commonw. 1966; 73:498–503.
109. Winner W, Romney SL. Cardiovascular responses to labor and delivery. Am J Obstet Gynecol. 1966; 95:1104–1114.
110. Hansen JM, Ueland K. The influence of caudal analgesia on cardiovascular dynamics during normal labor and delivery. Acta Anaesthesiol Scand Suppl. 1966; 23:449–452.
111. Hamilton HFH. Blood viscosity in pregnancy. J Obstet Gynaecol Br Emp. 1950; 57:530–538.
112. Goeltner E, Quade C. Intrathorakaler venendruck, pulse und Atmung waehrend der eroeffnungswehen. Gynaecologia. 1967; 163:235–240.
113. Henricks CH. The hemodynamics of uterine contraction. Am J Obstet Gynecol. 1958; 76:969–981.
114. Midwall J, Jaffin H, Herman MB, Kupersmith J. Shunt flow and pulmonary hemodynamics during labor and delivery in Eisenmenger's syndrome. Am J Cardiol. 1978; 42:299–303.
115. Ueland K, Gills RE, Hansen JM. Maternal cardiovascular dynamics. I. Cesarean section under subarachnoid block anesthesia. Am J Obstet Gynecol. 1968; 100:42–54.
116. Ueland K, Hansen J, Eng M, Kalappa R, Parer JT. Maternal cardiovascular dynamics. V. Cesarean section under thiopental, nitrous oxide, and succinylcholine anesthesia. Am J Obstet Gynecol. 1970; 108:615–622.
117. Ueland K, Akamatsu TJ, Eng M, Bonica JJ, Hansen JM. Maternal cardiovascular dynamics. VI. Cesarean section under epidural anesthesia without epinephrine. Am J Obstet Gynecol. 1972; 114:775–780.
118. Pritchard JA. Changes in the blood volume during pregnancy and delivery. Anesthesiology. 1965; 26:393–399.
119. Lees MM, Scott DB, Kerr MG. Haemodynamic changes associated with labour. J Obstet Gynaecol Br Commonw. 1970; 77:29–36.
120. Gleicher N, Knutzen VR, Elkayam U, Loew S, Kerenyi TD. Rheumatic heart disease diagnosed during pregnancy: A 30-year follow up. Int J Gynecol Obstet. 1979; 17:51–57.
121. Cutforth R, MacDonald MB. Heart sounds and murmurs in pregnancy. Am Heart J. 1966; 71:741–747.
122. Hytten EF, Thomson AM, Taggart N. Total body water in normal pregnancy. J Obstet Gynaecol Br Commonw. 1966; 73:553–561.
123. Robertson EG. Increased erythrocyte fragility in association with osmotic changes in pregnancy serum. J Reprod Fertil. 1968; 16:323–324.
124. Bickers W. The placenta: A modified arterio-

TABLE M.II.1. Lung Volumes

	Change	Probable mechanism
Total lung capacity	None or decrease	? Enlarged uterus
Functional residual capacity	Greatly decreased	
Residual volume	Decrease	Reduced chest wall stiffness
Vital capacity	None or decrease	? Enlarged uterus
Closing volume	Increase	Enlarged uterus

movement of the rib cage).[4] In pregnancy, airway closure at the base of the lung occurs at larger lung volumes than normal,[2,5-7] presumably because of congested walls of small airways,[8] which encroach upon airway lumen, and elevated diaphragm,[1] which presses on the lower lung airways at the lung base. Hence, to explain reduced residual volume in pregnancy, it is necessary to invoke a relatively marked reduction of rib cage stiffness.

Therefore, because of decreased stiffness of the rib cage and retention of normal rib cage and diaphragm muscle function, most lung volumes remain in the normal range throughout pregnancy. Functional residual capacity is decreased because of elevated diaphragm, and closing volume is decreased because of airway wall congestion and elevated diaphragm.

B. Airflow

As noted, one of the characteristic changes of pregnancy is capillary engorgement of the airways with subsequent swelling and reddening of both the upper and lower airways.[8] Though nasal stuffiness and voice changes may occur, overall resistance to airflow is actually decreased,[9,10] presumably because of dilatation of such large airways as the trachea and the larger bronchi, where wall congestion would be relatively unimportant. Hence, despite congestion of the walls of the large airways, relaxation of the bronchial smooth muscle produces increased overall airway caliber.

The normal distribution of resistance between large and small airways is disturbed in pregnancy such that a greater than usual proportion of resistance resides in the smaller airways (ie, those less than 2–3 mm in diameter).[10] This phenomenon may be due either to increased large airway caliber (smooth muscle relaxation) or to decreased small airway caliber (small airway wall congestion).

The amount of air that can be forcibly exhaled in one second (FEV_1) is usually normal in pregnancy.[1–3,11] Since this measurement is affected by both large and small airway resistance to flow, the opposite effects are apparently compensatory.

TABLE M.II.2. Airflow

	Change	Probable mechanism
Nasal resistance	Increase	Nasal congestion
Airway resistance	Decrease	Large airway dilatation
Distribution of airway resistance	Dilatation	Large airway dilatation and/or small airway congestion (? Progesterone)
Forced expiratory volume in one second	None	(? Progesterone)

C. Ventilation

Pregnant patients breathe deeper than those in the nonpregnant state.[1–3,12–14] Since respiratory frequency is normal in pregnancy, the product of tidal volume and respiratory frequency, total minute ventilation, is increased. The increase in minute ventilation is considerably greater than the metabolic demands of the products of conception, which produces changes in blood gases.[12–14] The hyperventilation of pregnancy can be shown to be due to increased respiratory drive and sensitivity to carbon dioxide caused by increased progesterone levels.[15] In fact, progesterone has been used in hypoventilation syndromes to increase respiratory drive and lower elevated blood carbon dioxide levels.[16]

Since more energy is required to flatten the diaphragm when the uterus is enlarged, and since the diaphragm must move greater distances in pregnancy, the work that the respiratory muscles must perform (the oxygen cost of breathing) is greatly increased in pregnancy.[13]

D. Gas Exchange

Since total ventilation rises more than the increased metabolic demands of the gravid uterus, carbon dioxide partial pressure is reduced in arterial blood in pregnancy.[14]

The capacity of gases such as oxygen to diffuse through the pulmonary capillaries and combine with hemoglobin is usually assessed by measurement of the diffusing capacity of carbon monoxide, (D_L CO). D_L CO is increased in the first trimester, presumably because of increased pulmonary blood flow and volume and is decreased in the second and third trimesters,[17] presumably because of decreased hemoglobin concentration (due to increased plasma volume).

The partial pressure of oxygen in arterial blood might be expected to be either reduced (low D_L CO during the second and third trimesters and early airway closure at the base of lung leading to potential areas of reduced ventilation) or increased (minute ventilation increased more than metabolic demands) during pregnancy. In

TABLE M.II.3. Ventilation

	Change	Probable mechanism
Tidal volume	Increase	Progesterone
Respiratory frequency	None	
Minute ventilation	Increase	Increased CO_2 sensitivity (progesterone)
Work of breathing	Increase	Enlarged uterus

TABLE M.II.4. Gas Exchange

	Change	Probable mechanism
Diffusing capacity for carbon monoxide	Increase, first trimester	Increased pulmonary blood volume
	Decrease, second and third trimesters	Decreased hemoglobin (plasma volume)
Arterial oxygen pressure	Increase	Hyperventilation
Arterial carbon dioxide pressure	Decrease	Hyperventilation

TABLE M.II.5. Acid/Base

	Change	Probable mechanism
Arterial carbon dioxide pressure	Decrease	Hyperventilation
Base excess	Decrease	Renal base excretion
Arterial pH	None or increase	Matching of above processes

fact, arterial oxygen partial pressure is increased in normal pregnancy, indicating that the effects of early basal airway closure and reduced D_L CO in mid and late pregnancy are not usually physiologically significant.[14,18]

E. Acid/Base

As noted, pregnancy produces increased ventilation with consequent reduction in arterial partial pressure of carbon dioxide. However, arterial pH tends to remain in the normal range because of increased renal excretion of bicarbonate, thereby producing a normal ratio of bicarbonate to partial pressure of carbon dioxide in the blood.[12,14] Other measures of fixed blood base (besides bicarbonate), such as base excess, whole blood buffer base, etc, are also decreased. Therefore, the respiratory alkalosis caused by hyperventilation is compensated by metabolic acidosis due to renal base excretion.[12,14]

F. Summary of Respiratory Physiologic Changes

Pregnancy produces a number of marked and interesting pulmonary physiologic changes, including uterine enlargement, airway wall congestion, and hyperventilation. However, because of reduction of chest wall stiffness, large airway dilatation, and renal base excretion, overall pulmonary function remains very similar to that in the nonpregnant state.

G. Labor

During labor there is often a marked tendency for hyperventilation, particularly during contractions.[19,20] This hyperventilation usually produces decreased arterial carbon dioxide and increased oxygen partial pressures, as well as increased pH (alkalosis). However, on occasion, breathing becomes shallow and atelectasis with attendant hypoxemia

TABLE M.II.6. Factors Potentially Improving Asthma During Pregnancy

Factor	Mechanism	Comments
Corticosteroids	Bronchodilation	2.5 × control during third trimester
Progesterone	Smooth muscle relaxation	See Table M.II.2
Serum, cyclic AMP	Mast cell stabilization smooth muscle relaxation	Small increase only
Decreased cell-mediated immunity	T cells cooperate in production of IgE by B cells	Decreased mediator release
Increased serum histaminase	Histamine increase	Decreased bronchoconstriction
Emotions	Central	Unpredictable

may develop.[21,22] Pain relief, either in the form of narcotics, sedatives, or extradural anaesthesia usually prevents marked hyperventilation.[22]

II. PATIENTS WITH PULMONARY DISEASE

Though the usual changes in pulmonary function are largely compensated in normal pregnancy, patients with pulmonary disease may have special problems. In particular, asthma, pulmonary embolism, tuberculosis, and chronic respiratory insufficiency are common diseases which may present clinical problems during pregnancy.

A. Asthma

The course of asthma during pregnancy is highly variable, with substantial numbers of patients becoming either worse or better.[23,24] Some of the factors that may lead to improvement (Table M.II.6) or worsening (Table M.II.7) are considered in the discussion that follows.

Factors potentially alleviating asthma in pregnancy include increased amounts of several substances in the blood: corticosteroids,[25] progesterone,[26] cyclic adenomonophosphate (c'AMP),[27] and histaminase.[28] Corticosteroids act as bronchodilators by two mechanisms: potentiation of the activity of beta-adrenergic compounds, which is rapid,[29] and a slower process, which presumably involves protein synthesis. In the third trimester, circulating corticosteroids increase considerably.[25]

Progesterone may be one of the substances that produces large airway dilatation Table M.II.2), and cyclic AMP has been shown to be one of the major mediators of the intracellular events that lead to bronchial smooth muscle relaxation.[30] Histaminase accelerates the breakdown of histamines,[28] one of several substances that are mediators of bronchoconstriction. Another potentially beneficial factor is decrease in cell-mediated immunity,[31] which might eventually lead to reduction of IgE production by B cells[24] (Table M.II.6); asthmatic patients with falling IgE levels frequently have diminished symptoms.[32] Finally, the emotional state associated with pregnancy can have unpredictable effects.

There are also a number of factors associated with pregnancy that might aggravate asthma (Table M.II.7). These include the (antigenically foreign) fetus, nasal turbinate congestion,[8] and decreased functional residual capacity.[1–3] Increased progesterone, decreased cell-mediated immunity, and emotions, all cited above as potential ameliorating factors, may, from another viewpoint, be po-

TABLE M.II.7. Factors Potentially Aggravating Asthma During Pregnancy

Factor	Mechanism	Comments
Antigenically foreign fetus	? Autoantibodies	No direct evidence
Nasal turbinate congestion	Mouth breathing	Stimulation of epithelial receptors
Decreased functional residual capacity	Increased airway resistance	
Decreased cell-mediated immunity	Increased susceptibility to viruses	Stimulation of epithelial receptors
Progesterone	Hyperventilation	? Cause of "normal" dyspnea of pregnancy
Emotions	Central	Unpredictable

tentially harmful in asthma. Turbinate congestion could lead to mouth breathing and consequent possible failure to adequately warm and humidify inspired air; epithelial receptors might be activated by the cool dry air and, in patients with easily irritated airways, might cause reflex bronchospasm.[33] Similarly, progesterone, by causing hyperventilation, may exacerbate this problem; progesterone-induced bronchospasm may be partially responsible for the commonly observed dyspnea reported by many (even normal) pregnant patients.[34] Since functional residual capacity is reduced in pregnancy, airway caliber is also somewhat reduced by the smaller lung volume.[35] This factor is usually not important because of relaxation of bronchial smooth muscle caused by substances such as progesterone. Decreased cellular immunity could lead to viral infection, which has been known to cause increased airway irritability.[33]

Since some of the same factors can cause either improvement or aggravation of asthma in pregnancy, the relative sensitivity of individual factors is important in determining the result. For example, if progesterone produced (via hyperventilation) enough cooling and drying of inspired air in an individual with significant reflex bronchospasm, the potential smooth muscle relaxing effect of progesterone may not have a substantial counterbalancing effect.

In general, asthma in pregnancy can be treated as in the nonpregnant state.[23] Beta-adrenergic drugs, theophylline, corticosteroids, disodium cromoglycate, are all effective and probably safe for both mother and fetus. Many of the newer drugs, however, have not been extensively tested in pregnancy and, therefore, cannot be affirmed to be unequivocally safe. Both beta-adrenergic drugs and theophylline dilate uterine muscle and tend to slow or stop active labor.[23]

B. Pulmonary Embolism

Because of the known occlusive effects of the enlarging uterus upon the vena cava and increase of some clotting factors,[8] a high incidence of deep venous thrombosis in the legs and subsequent pulmonary thromboembolism might be expected. However, surveys show that both deep venous thrombosis and pulmonary embolism are rare during the course of pregnancy, except in the first postpartum month.[36] The higher incidence of thromboembolism during the immediate postpartum period may be related to trauma and bed rest associated with cesarean section and other procedures during delivery, plus an increased tendency to clot caused by estrogens, which are given for suppression of lactation.

C. Tuberculosis

Several interesting issues are associated with tuberculosis and pregnancy. The presence of a high diaphragm during pregnancy, which rapidly descends with delivery, has been thought to be the cause of the observation that tuberculosis tends to be more progressive in the postpartum period.[37] However, since the advent of effective chemotherapy, no significant problems or added risks have been noted following delivery.[38]

Even though cell-mediated immunity is somewhat impaired in pregnancy,[31] it is generally agreed that tuberculin skin testing remains a good guide to exposure to tuberculosis during pregnancy.[39] It is also generally accepted that chest films represent no substantial risk to the fetus and can be performed, if indicated.

D. Chronic Pulmonary Disease

It has been noted that pregnancy proceeds with fewer problems in patients with restrictive pulmonary diseases (such as kyphoscoliosis and previous resectional lung surgery) than in patients with airway obstruction (such as bronchitis, bronchiectasis, and emphysema), or mixed restrictive and obstructive problems (such as cystic fibrosis).[40–43]

The response of patients with chest wall

or other restrictive processes to increased respiratory demands is to increase minute ventilation by increasing respiratory rate rather than tidal volume.[40,41] This physiological adaptation is relatively easy to accomplish, particularly when the diaphragm is simultaneously elevated, as in pregnancy. However, in patients who have airway obstruction, increased ventilation is difficult to achieve because of disease limitation on airflow rate; in these patients tidal volume increase is required. Since the enlarging uterus already has increased the work of breathing (Table M.II.3), obstructed patients must work quite hard to maintain ventilation during pregnancy.

III. REFERENCES

1. Cugell DW, Frank R, Gaensler EA, Badger TL. Pulmonary function in pregnancy. I. Serial observations in normal women. Am Rev Tuberc. 1953; 67:568–597.
2. Baldwin GR, Moorthi DS, Whelton JA, MacDonnell KF. New lung functions and pregnancy. Am J Obstet Gynecol. 1977; 127:235–239.
3. Alaily AB, Carrol KB. Pulmonary ventilation in pregnancy. Br J Obstet Gynaecol. 1978; 85:518–524.
4. Leith DB, Mead J. Mechanisms determining residual volume. J Appl Physiol. 1967; 23:221–227.
5. Bevan DR, Holdcroft A, Loh L, MacGregor WG, O'Sullivan JC, Sykes MK. Closing volume and pregnancy. Br Med J. 1974; 1:13–15.
6. Holdcroft A, Bevan DR, O'Sullivan JC, Sykes MK. Anaesthesiology. 1977; 32:517–523.
7. Garrard GS, Littler WA, Redman CWG. Closing volume during pregnancy. Thorax 1978; 33:488–492.
8. Bonica JJ. Principles and Practices of Obstetric Analgesia and Anesthesia. Philadelphia: F.A. Davis, 1967:21–22.
9. Gee JBL, Packer BS, Millen JE, Robin ED. Pulmonary mechanics during pregnancy. J Clin Invest. 1967; 46:945–952.
10. Tien YK, Littlejohn G. Localization of airway dilatation in pregnancy. Presentation at Annual Meeting of Society for Obstetrical Anesthesia and Physiology. San Diego, California, 1981.
11. Milne JA, Mills RJ, Howie AD, Pack AI. Large airways function during normal pregnancy. Br J Obstet Gynaecol. 1977; 84:448–451.
12. Rowe AW, Gallivan DE, Mathews H. The metabolism in pregnancy. VI. The respiratory metabolism and acid elimination. Am J Physiol. 1931; 96:101–111.
13. Bader RA, Bader ME, Rose DJ. The oxygen cost of breathing in dyspneic subjects as studied in normal pregnant women. Clin Sci. 1959; 18:223–235.
14. MacRae DJ, Palavradji D. Maternal acid-base changes in pregnancy. J Obstet Gynaecol Br Commonw. 1967; 74:11–16.
15. Lyons HA, Antonio R. The sensitivity of the respiratory center in pregnancy and after the administration of progesterone. Trans Assoc Am Phys. 1959; 72:173–180.
16. Lyons HA, Huang CT. The therapeutic use of progesterone in alveolar hypoventilation associated with obesity. Am J Med. 1968; 44:881–888.
17. Milne JA, Mills RJ, Coutts JRT, MacNaughton MC, Moran F, Pack AI. The effect of human pregnancy on the pulmonary transfer factor for carbon monoxide as measured by the single breath method. Clin Sci Mol Med. 1977; 53:271–276.
18. Templeton A, Kelman GR. Maternal blood gases, (PAO_2–PaO_2), physiological shunt and VD/VT in normal pregnancy. Br J Anaesthesiol. 1976; 48:1001–1004.
19. Selwyn-Crawford J, Tunstall ME. Notes on respiratory performance during labour. Br J Anaesthesiol. 1968; 40:612–614.
20. Fisher A, Prys-Roberts C. Maternal pulmonary gas exchange. Anaesthesiology 1968; 23:350–356.
21. Archer GE Jr, Marx GF. Arterial oxygen during apnoea in parturient women. Br J Anaesthesiol. 1974; 46:358–360.
22. Bonica JJ. Maternal respiratory changes during pregnancy and parturition. Clin Anesthesiol. 1974; 10:1–19.
23. Weinstein AM, Dubin BD, Podleski WK, Spector SL, Farr RS. Asthma and pregnancy. JAMA. 1979; 241:1161–1165.
24. Gluck JC, Gluck PA. The effects of pregnancy on asthma: A prospective study. Ann Allergy 1976; 37:164–168.
25. Brien TG, Dalrymple IJ. A longitudinal study of the free cortisol index in pregnancy. Br J Obstet Gynaecol. 1976; 83:361–367.
26. Yannone ME, McCurdy JR, Goldfien A. Plasma progesterone levels in normal pregnancy, labor and the puerperium. Am J Obstet Gynaecol. 1968; 101:1058–1061.
27. Ling WX, Marsh JM, Le Maire WJ. Adenosine—3′,5′-monophosphate in the plasma from human pregnancy. J Clin Endocrinol Metab. 1977; 44:514–519.
28. Resnik R, Levine RJ. Plasma diamine oxidase activity in pregnancy: A reappraisal. Am J Obstet Gynaecol. 1969; 104:1061–1066.
29. Elul-Micallef R, Borthwick RC, McHardy GJR. The time course of response to prednisone in chronic bronchial asthma. Clin Sci Mol Med. 1974; 47:105–117.
30. Schultz G, Hardman JG, Sutherland EW. Cyclic nucleotides and smooth muscle function. In: Austen KF, Lichtenstein LM, eds. Asthma: Physiology, Immunopharmacology and Treat-

ment. New York: Academic Press, 1973:123–138.
31. Purtillo DT, Hallgren HM, Yunis EJ. Depressed maternal lymphocyte responses to phytohemagglutinin in human pregnancy. Lancet. 1972; 1:769–771.
32. Lichtenstein LM. The control of IgE-mediated histamine release: Implications for the study of asthma. In: Austen KF, Lichtenstein LM, eds. Asthma: Physiology, Immunopharmacology and Treatment. New York: Academic Press, 1973:91–110.
33. Gold WM, Cholinergic pharmacology in asthma. In: Austen KF, Lichtenstein LM, eds. Asthma: Physiology, Immunopharmacology and Treatment. New York: Academic Press, 1973:169–184.
34. Editorial. Dyspnoea in normal pregnancy. Lancet. 1978; 2:380–381.
35. Bouhys A. The Physiology of Breathing. New York: Grune & Stratton, 1977:53.
36. Aaro LA, Juergens JL. Thrombophlebitis associated with pregnancy. Am J Obstet Gynaecol. 1971; 109:1128–1136.
37. Giercke HW. Tuberkuloseablaufe kurz nach Schwangerschaftbeendigung. Z Tuberk. 1956; 108:1–8.
38. DeMarch AP. Tuberculosis and pregnancy: Five to ten year review of 215 patients in their fertile age. Chest. 1975; 46:706–715.
39. Present PA, Comstock GW. Tuberculin sensitivity in pregnancy. Am Rev Respir Dis. 1975; 112:413–416.
40. Patton WE, Abelmann WH, Frank R, Badger TL, Gaensler EA. Pulmonary function in pregnancy. II. Comparison of the effects of pneumoperitoneum and pregnancy in young women with functionally normal lungs and serial observation during pregnancy and postpartum pneumoperitoneum. Am Rev Tuberc. 1953; 67:755–778.
41. Gaensler EA, Patton WE, Verstraeten JM, Badger TL. Pulmonary function in pregnancy. III. Serial observations in patients with pulmonary insufficiency. Am Rev Tuberc. 1953; 67:779–797.
42. Gazioglu K, Kaltreider NL, Rosen M, Yu PN. Pulmonary function during pregnancy in normal women and in patients with cardiopulmonary disease. Thorax. 1970; 25:445–450.
43. Grand RJ, Talamo RC, Sant'Agnese PA, Schwartz KH. Pregnancy in cystic fibrosis of the pancreas. JAMA. 1966; 195:117–124.

Cardiac Evaluation of the Pregnant Woman

M.III

Diagnostic Approaches to Maternal Heart Disease During Pregnancy

Julius M. Gardin, MD

I. INTRODUCTION

Pregnancy and the peripartum period are normally characterized by significant cardiovascular developments. These hemodynamic changes are related to the development of the fetal placental unit and gestational changes in other maternal organs.[1] Maternal blood volume increases 40% over blood volume in the normal nonpregnant state. This increase begins as early as the sixth week of gestation and continues to term, but the most rapid expansion of blood volume occurs during the second trimester and coincides with the period of accelerated placental vascular expansion.[1] Cardiac output also increases by 40% during pregnancy; this progressive increase is maximal at term. Both components of cardiac output—ie, stroke volume and heart rate—appear to increase during pregnancy, the latter by approximately 10 beats/min (maximum) at term.[1] In general, the additional burden of the altered hemodynamic state of pregnancy is well tolerated by healthy women and poses minimal risks to mother and fetus. However, in women with clinical or subclinical organic heart disease, the gestational period may be more problematic.

In pragmatic terms, cardiologic management of the obstetric patient with known or suspected organic heart disease requires development of a data base that allows for 1) precise diagnosis of the specific form of cardiac disease, 2) quantification of the physiologic consequences of the cardiac lesion, and 3) management of problems and complications unique to the antepartum, labor, delivery, and postpartum phases of pregnancy.[2] Traditionally, this data base is obtained by utilization of the clinical parameters of history and

Cardiac Problems in Pregnancy, pages 37–58

physical examination, supplemented primarily by the chest roentgenogram and electrocardiogram. When further information is needed regarding localization and quantification of the cardiac lesion, various peculiarities of the pregnant state make cardiac catheterization and angiography less than desirable. Specifically, the utility of cardiac catheterization for the management of the obstetric patient is reduced significantly by 1) the radiation exposure inherent in fluoroscopy and angiography, and 2) the inability to repeat these tests frequently in a patient facing somewhat unpredictable cardiovascular stresses of pregnancy, labor, and delivery.

Often the first encounter with a physician in adult life for a woman of childbearing age is that with an obstetrician after she has become pregnant; the suspicion of organic heart disease is often first raised at this time. The consulting cardiologist is then faced with the problem of attempting to quantify the disease and predict the patient's ability to tolerate the cardiovascular stress of pregnancy, labor, and delivery without benefit of cardiac catheterization. Fortunately, a number of techniques for noninvasive cardiac diagnosis and bedside monitoring of cardiac hemodynamics have significantly reduced the cardiologist's reliance on the catheterization laboratory and have concurrently improved the quality of cardiologic care available to obstetric patients.

II. NONINVASIVE EVALUATION OF CARDIAC FUNCTION

A. Echocardiography

Echocardiography involves the use of reflected ultrasound to evaluate the heart. The use of reflected ultrasound for medical diagnosis is not new to obstetrics and gynecology; ultrasound is routinely used to evaluate fetal size and position. Pulsed sound waves in the frequency range of 1.6–5.0 MHz are emitted from a transducer probe that also acts as a receiver for reflected waves. Since ultrasound is reflected at interfaces having different acoustic impedances, internal structures of the heart possessing different impedance—eg, myocardium and atrial and ventricular chambers and valves—can be readily imaged.

The two basic cardiac ultrasound techniques in clinical use are M-mode and two-dimensional echocardiography. Both techniques have the advantages of being painless, relatively rapid (requiring 15 to 45

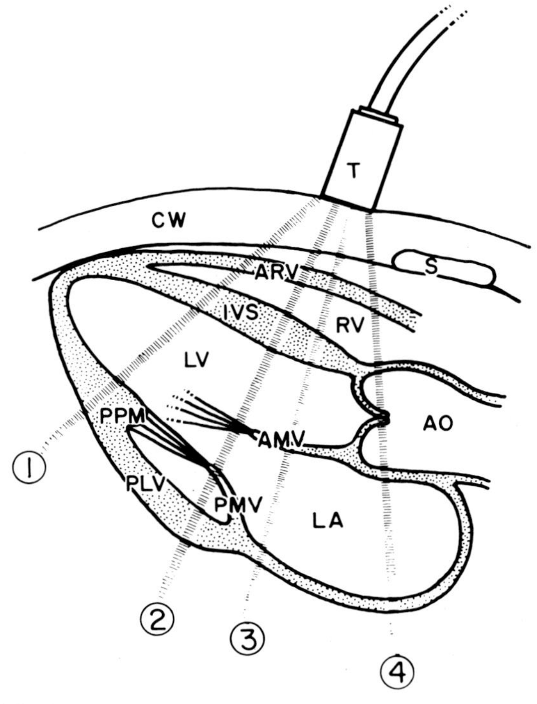

Fig. M.III. 1. Diagrammatic representation of the heart in longitudinal section, depicting structures through which the ultrasound beam passes as it is directed from the apex toward the base of the heart. The numbers (1 through 4) refer to standard positions for recording the M-mode echocardiogram (see Fig. M.III. 2). CW, chest wall; T, transducer; S, sternum; ARV, anterior right ventricular wall; RV, right ventricular cavity; IVS, interventricular septum; LV, left ventricle; PPM, posterior papillary muscle; PLV, posterior left ventricular wall; AMV, anterior mitral valve leaflet; PMV, posterior mitral valve leaflet; AO, aorta; LA, left atrium. (From Feigenbaum H. Clinical applications of echocardiography. Prog Cardiovasc Dis. 1972; 14:531. By permission of the author and Grune & Stratton, Inc.)

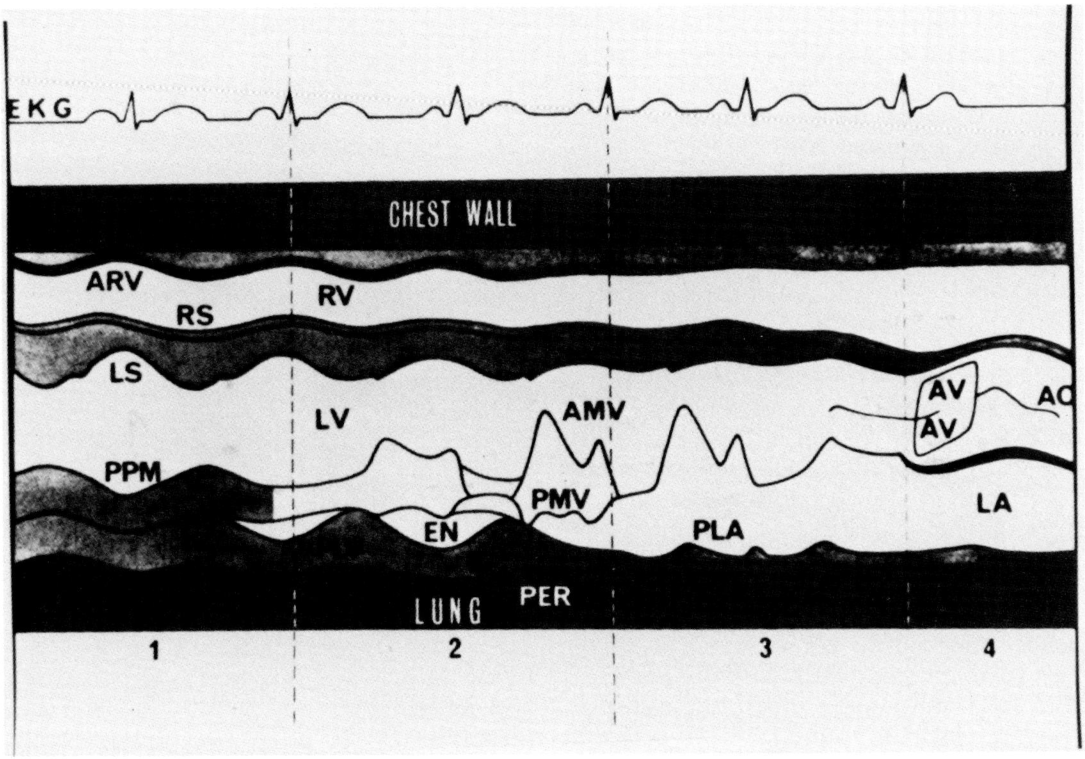

Fig. M.III. 2. Diagrammatic representation of M-mode echocardiogram as transducer is directed from the cardiac apex (position 1) to the base (position 4). Areas between the dotted lines correspond to the transducer positions as depicted in Figure M.III. 1. AV, aortic valve; EN, endocardium of left ventricle; LS, left septum; PER, pericardium; PLA, posterior left atrial wall; RS, right septum; other abbreviations as in Figure M.III. 1. (From Feigenbaum H. Clinical applications of echocardiography. Prog Cardiovasc Dis. 1972; 14:531. By permission of the author and Grune & Stratton, Inc.)

minutes) and, unlike radiation exposure, apparently harmless to the pregnant mother and fetus.[2] Consequently, both techniques can be used repeatedly if necessary for evaluation of a pregnant woman's cardiac function.

The M-mode (time-motion) technique uses a single beam of ultrasound that begins at the chest wall and traverses identifiable cardiac structures at various depths. The reflected ultrasound waves (echoes) are displayed on an oscilloscope in proportion to the depth of the tissues from which they are reflected on the vertical axis and as a function of time on the horizontal axis. Structures are identified by the intensity and motion of the echoes, as well as by the characteristic anatomic relationships of the various structures to one another. The transducer is usually placed in the second to fourth intercostal spaces to the left of the sternum, and a "sweep" is made from the region of the ventricles to the interface of the left atrium and the aorta[3,4] (Figs. M.III. 1 and M.III. 2). Additional views of the heart may be obtained from the apical and subxyphoid positions.

Two-dimensional echocardiography provides a two-dimensional image rather than the single dimension (over time) afforded by the M-mode technique. Various methods have been developed to produce a continuous (real-time) oscilloscopic display of cardiac function in up to a 90° arc (sector). The two most popular cross-sectional methods are the mechanical and the electronic sector scanners. In mechanical sector scanners, a single (or multiple) ultrasound crystal(s) is (are) rotated through a 30-degree to a 90-degree sector on the chest wall, with simultaneous oscilloscopic display of echoes from each position in the arc. In electronic ("phased array") sector scanners, a small multicrystal transducer is held stationary on the chest wall while the echo beam is swept back and forth electronically over an arc of up to 90 degrees.[4] Sweeps are generally performed in long and short axis views, which allows visualization of most areas of the heart (Fig. M.III. 3).

In the absence of localized disorders of left ventricular function (such as those seen in coronary artery disease), M-mode echocardiographic measurements correlate with left ventricular volume and ejection fraction as determined angiographically.[3,5] Although the left ventricular ejection fraction does not perfectly characterize the functional state of this chamber, this measurement is accepted as providing an overall assessment of systolic pump performance. The ejection fraction, defined as the ratio of ventricular stroke volume to end-diastolic volume, is thought to be a more sensitive measure of myocardial contractile state than is cardiac output or left ventricular end-diastolic pressure. The ability to obtain this value by a noninvasive technique represents a significant aid in the evaluation of numerous cardiac disorders.

The approach to volume determination by echocardiography relies on the assumption that the left ventricle is a uniformly contracting, prolate ellipsoid and that its volume in systole and diastole approximates the cube of the left ventricular internal dimension (LVID) in systole and diastole, respectively. Left ventricular internal dimensions are measured from the left ventricular septal surface to the endocardium of the posterior left ventricular wall (Fig. M.III. 2). Left ventricular ejection fraction, it follows, equals

$$\frac{LVID_D^3 - LVID_S^3}{LVID_D^3}$$

$LVID_S$ and $LVID_D$ are the left ventricular internal dimensions in systole and diastole, respectively.[5] Stroke volume is obtained by multiplication of left ventricular ejection fraction by $LIVD_D$, and left ventricular (or cardiac) output is approximated by multiplication of stroke volume by the heart rate (determined from the ECG recorded with the echocardiogram). Conditions such as coronary artery disease, by giving rise to segmental zones of ischemia, scarring, and abnormal contractility, invalidate the above geometric assumptions regarding calculation of left ventricular volume. Since such conditions are rare in the pregnant woman, M-mode echocardiography provides a rapid, safe, and reliable means of monitoring ventricular function on either a one-time or a sequential basis. Two-dimensional echocardiography can be used to evaluate left ventricular function where there is a question of localized wall motion abnormalities.

Another cardiac ultrasound technique that is the subject of much current research and promises to have numerous clinical applications is known as Doppler echocardiography. According to the Doppler principle, ultrasound reflected from a moving target(s)—eg, red blood cells flowing in a cardiac chamber or in the great arteries—will have its frequency shifted to a degree that is directly proportional to the velocity of the target (blood cells). The clinical utility of the Doppler technique has been enhanced by combining it with two-dimensional echocardiography for imaging the cardiac structures and by using a range-gate to allow sampling of the flow velocity in various portions of the heart and great arteries.[6–8] Thus, Doppler flow velocity signals may provide information about the presence of flow disturbances—eg, regurgitant le-

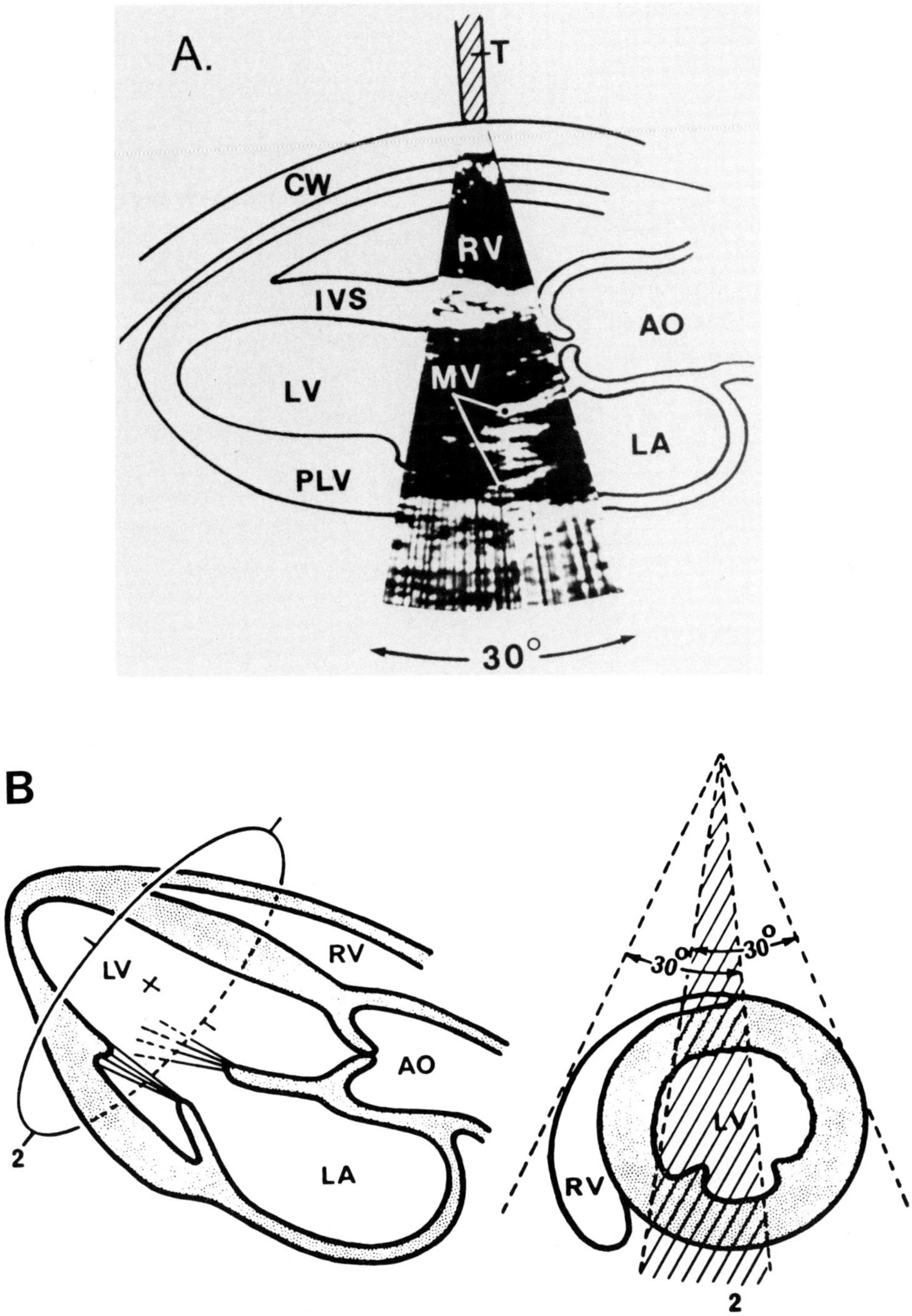

Fig. M.III. 3. Two-dimensional echocardiography. **A.** Diagrammatic representation of the heart in the parasternal long axis view with photograph of a 30-degree sector. **B.** Diagrammatic representation of the heart as viewed in a parasternal short axis view by two-dimensional echocardiography. MV, mitral valve; other abbreviations as in Figure M.III. 1. (Panel B from Feigenbaum H. Echocardiography, Ed 2. Philadelphia: Lea & Febiger, 1976. By permission of the author and the publisher.)

sions or septal defects—about the rate of acceleration and deceleration in peak flow velocity in the ascending aorta or main pulmonary artery and, at least in a semiquantitative fashion, about ventricular stroke volume.[6–8]

B. Systolic Time Intervals

The sequential phases of left ventricular systole can be measured indirectly from simultaneous rapid (paper speed 75–200 mm/sec) recordings of the ECG, phonocardiogram, and carotid arterial pulse tracings. (The latter two are recorded by an appropriate microphone or pressure transducer placed over the base of the heart and the common carotid artery, respectively.) In clinical practice, three basic systolic time intervals are determined[9] (Fig. M.III. 4). Since these intervals are inversely related to heart rate, a correction factor must be applied in order to compare the measured intervals with predicted normal values. Total electromechanical systole (QA_2) is measured from the onset of the QRS complex on the ECG to the first high-frequency aortic component of the second sound and encompasses the interval from the onset of electrical activity to the termination of left ventricular ejection. Left ventricular ejection time (LVET) is directly related to stroke volume and is taken from the initial rapid rise of the carotid pulse upstroke to the trough of the incisura (dicrotic notch). This interval measures the dura-

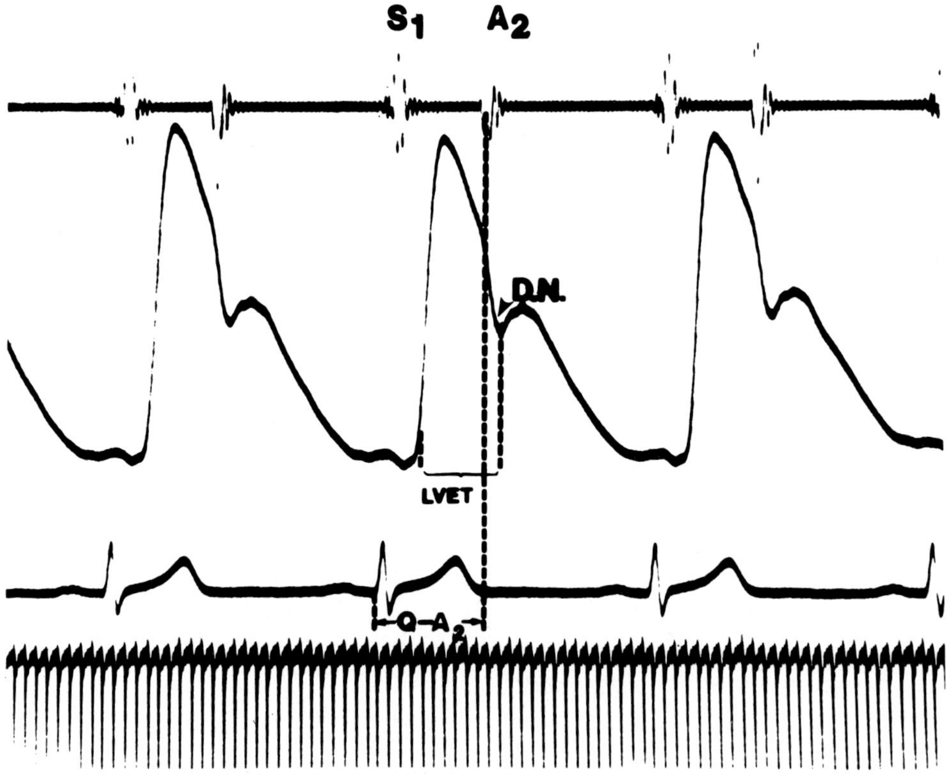

Fig. M.III. 4. Measurement of systolic time intervals from simultaneous ECG, phonocardiogram, and carotid arterial pulse tracing. S_1, first heart sound; A_2, aortic component of second heart sound; D.N., dicrotic notch; Q-A_2, total electromechanical systole; LVET, left ventricular ejection time. (From Gardin et al.[2] This and all subsequent figures, except Figure M.III. 9, are reprinted by permission of Harper & Row, Inc.)

tion of actual ejection of the left ventricle. The preejection period (PEP) sums the electrical-mechanical delay [or QS_1 (onset of Q wave to first heart sound)] and mechanical (isovolumetric contraction) periods that precede aortic valve opening and the onset of ejection. PEP is calculated by subtracting the LVET from QA_2. This method of calculation corrects for the time required for cardiac events to be transmitted to the carotid pulse.[9] In the presence of normal left ventricular conduction (with a normal QS_1 interval), PEP is inversely related to the rate of rise of left ventricular pressure (ie, dp/dt, where dp is the change in pressure and dt is the change in time). Consequently, a patient with congestive heart failure often exhibits a prolonged PEP (slow rate of rise of left ventricular pressure) and diminished LVET (decreased stroke volume). The ratio of PEP to LVET is useful in evaluating ventricular function in many conditions; the use of this ratio eliminates the need to correct the intervals for heart rate. However, with the rise in popularity of ultrasound and radionuclide imaging, systolic time intervals, which do not give a visual image of the heart, have been used less frequently in the assessment of cardiac function.

C. Radionuclide Evaluation of Cardiac Function

In the past decade we have witnessed the development of numerous "nuclear medicine" techniques for the assessment of cardiac function and physiology.[10] Two situations in which radionuclide cardiac imaging may be of value in the obstetric patient are 1) in the quantitative evaluation of left ventricular function—ie, left ventricular ejection fraction—in patients with suspected heart failure and 2) in confirmation of the presence and quantification of the degree of intracardiac shunting in patients with known or suspected atrial or ventricular septal defect or patent ductus arteriosus.

When radioisotope imaging is used during pregnancy, the attendant radiation exposure to the fetus and, therefore, the stage of pregnancy must be considered. Nonetheless, the information that can be gained through radioisotope imaging is generally of high quality and is obtained at relatively low risk to mother and fetus when compared with the risk of standard cardiac catheterization and angiography. For doses of less than 5 rad received at the period critical for the induction of any specific type of maldevelopment (generally during the first trimester), it is unlikely that an increase in this type of malformation could be measurable in human populations.[11] The dose estimated to the embryo from the radiopharmaceuticals generally used for radionuclide cardiac blood flow imaging is less than or equal to 0.8 rad.[12] Consequently, although there is some radiation exposure to the fetus from radionuclide cardiac imaging, this risk is generally low (especially after the first trimester) and can be further minimized by proper attention to technical factors. Radionuclide imaging may be useful in cases such as the evaluation of left ventricular function and intracardiac shunts if sufficient information is not available from echocardiography.

Two radionuclide techniques are available for the determination of left ventricular ejection fraction: the "first-pass technique and the "equilibrium" method.[13] Both employ external monitoring of the cardiac blood pool with a gamma camera, but in the first-pass technique, the initial transit of radioactive tracer is monitored, whereas in the equilibrium method, images are obtained only after the isotope has equilibrated within the blood pool.

In the first-pass technique, counts over the left ventricle are measured with a gamma camera as the intravenously injected bolus of radionuclide traverses the central circulation. The number of counts emanating from the left ventricle is proportional to the quantity of isotope in the ventricle and this, in turn, is related to the volume in the ventricle. Thus, a plot of radioactivity in the ventricle vs time during the first minute after injection re-

1. Mitral stenosis

M-mode echocardiography may give additional information in the determination of the presence and relative severity of mitral stenosis in patients in whom the physical examination is not conclusive. Figure M.III. 8A is an echocardiogram showing a normal mitral valve. Note that in diastole the anterior leaflet of the mitral valve exhibits an M-shaped pattern, whereas the posterior leaflet exhibits a W shape. The two leaflets separate relatively widely and abruptly, reflecting normal trans-mitral flow during ventricular filling. After partial closure during mid-diastole, the leaflets move apart again (at ventricular end-diastole). During ventricular systole, the anterior and posterior leaflets are seen to approximate and remain together in a neutral position or to move slightly anteriorly. In mitral stenosis, M-mode echocardiography usually reveals a number of characteristic findings (Fig. M.III. 8B). There are dense echoes from the mitral leaflets, reflecting fibrosis and/or calcification. There is a diminished opening excursion and a diminished rate of early diastolic closure (E-to-F slope) of the anterior leaflet.[3,4] Because of fusion of the mitral leaflets, the posterior leaflet moves parallel to the anterior leaflet in 90% of cases.[4] Whereas the degree of diminution of the E-to-F slope and of maximal

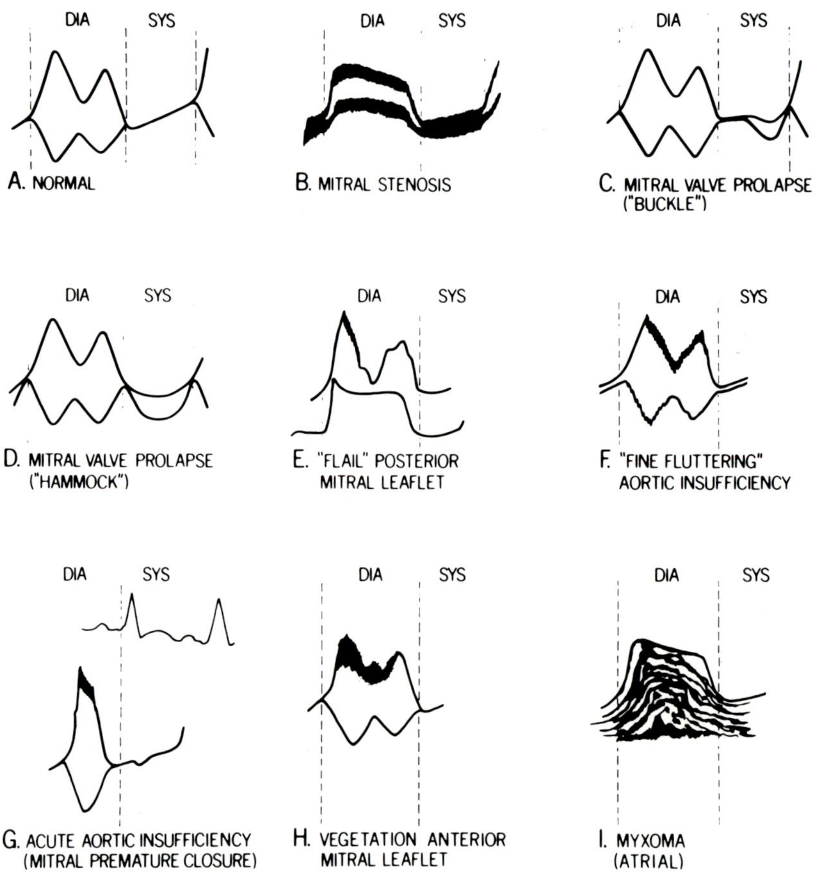

Fig. M.III. 8. Composite of mitral valve echocardiograms seen in various normal and abnormal states. DIA, diastole; SYS, systole. (Reprinted from Gardin et al.[2])

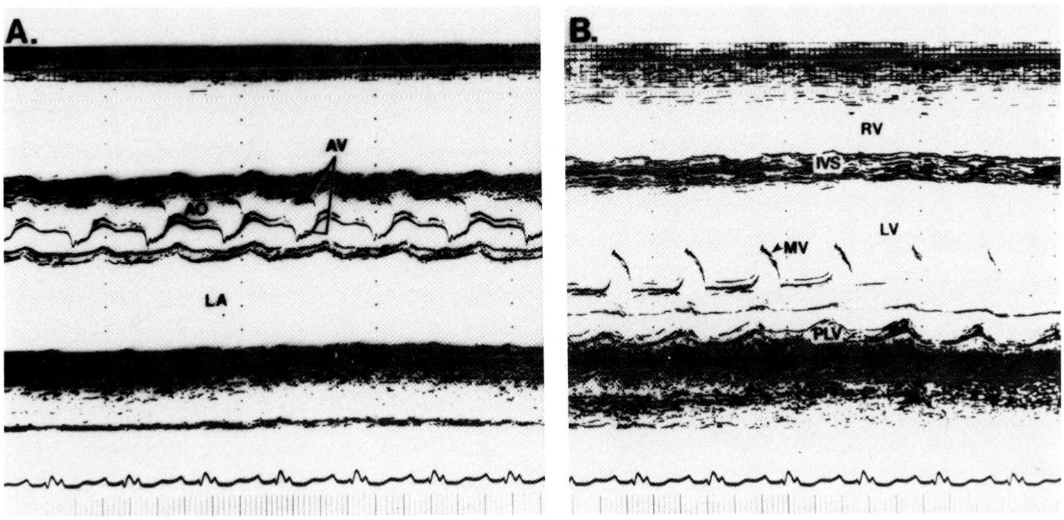

Fig. M.III. 13. Typical echocardiographic findings in congestive cardiomyopathy. **A.** View of left atrium (LA) and aortic root, demonstrating enlarged left atrium, poor aortic root motion, and partial apposition of aortic leaflets prior to end-systole, reflecting diminished ventricular output. AV = aortic valve. **B.** View of right (RV) and left (LV) ventricles, revealing enlarged (dilated) right and left ventricular dimensions, diminished ventricular septal motion, and decreased opening (excursion) of mitral valve (MV). (Reprinted from Gardin et al.[2])

On echocardiography, the separation of a relatively immobile posterior (parietal) pericardium from a moving adjacent epicardium by a relatively "echo-free" space (representing fluid) can be detected in the presence of effusions as small as 50 cc. The degree of separation of the epicardium and pericardium has been shown to correlate roughly with the size of the effusion (Fig. M.III. 12A and B).[28]

Radionuclide imaging techniques are less sensitive than ultrasound in the detection of pericardial effusion. Nonetheless, large effusions can be detected by comparison of the extent of the radiolabeled intracardiac blood pool with the size of the roentgenographic cardiac silhouette.

Dilated (congestive) cardiomyopathy, especially the postpartum variety, may present a diagnostic problem clinically. Echocardiography (M-mode and two-dimensional) is extremely helpful in establishing this as the cause of a large cardiac shadow. Typical M-mode findings in dilated cardiomyopathy include enlarged left ventricular internal dimension, poor motion of the ventricular septum and left ventricular posterior wall, enlarged left atrium and right ventricle, poor aortic root motion, and partial apposition of the aortic leaflets prior to the end of systole (Fig. M.III. 13).[3]

Doppler echocardiography has recently been shown to be of use in differentiating patients with dilated cardiomyopathy from those with normal ventricular function.[8] Peak aortic flow velocity proved to be an excellent Doppler parameter for differentiating the cardiomyopathy patients from the normal subjects. Radionuclide techniques are also of value in the diagnosis of cardiomyopathy.

14. Hypertrophic obstructive cardiomyopathy

Hypertrophic obstructive cardiomyopathy, or idiopathic hypertrophic subaortic stenosis (IHSS), may provide special prob-

TABLE M.III.1. Comparative Usefulness* of Methods for Evaluation of Cardiac Function in the Obstetric Patient

	Echocardiography		Radionuclide imaging	Systolic time intervals
	M-mode	Cross-sectional		
Mitral stenosis	+ + +	+ + +	+	–
Mitral valve prolapse	+ + +	+ + +	–	–
Aortic stenosis	+ +	+ + +	–	+ +
Bicuspid aortic valve	+ +	+ +	–	+
Aortic insufficiency	+ + +	+ + +	+	+
Marfan syndrome	+ +	+ +	–	–
Subacute bacterial endocarditis	+	+ +	–	–
Atrial myxoma	+ +	+ +	+	–
Atrial septal defect	+ +	+ +	+ + +	–
Ventricular septal defect	+	+ +	+ + +	+/–
Tetralogy of Fallot	+ +	+ +	+	–
Patent ductus arteriosus	+	+ +	+ + +	–
Pericardial effusion	+ + +	+ + +	+ +	–
Cardiomyopathy	+ + +	+ + +	+ + +	+
Idiopathic hypertrophic subaortic stenosis	+ + +	+ + +	+ +	+

*Usefulness graded from – (not useful) to + + + (extremely useful)
Reprinted from Gardin et al,[2] with permission.

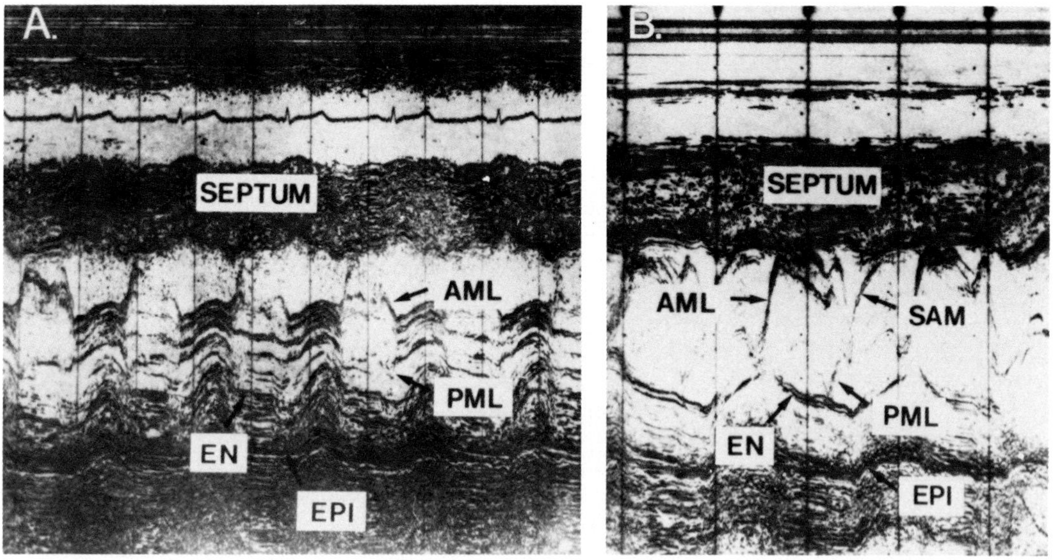

Fig. M.III. 14. Echocardiographic spectrum of asymmetric septal hypertrophy (ASH). **A.** Nonobstructive ASH, in which the septum is thicker than the left ventricular posterior wall by a ratio of more than 1.3:1. **B.** Obstructive ASH (idiopathic hypertrophic subaortic stenosis), in which systolic anterior motion of anterior mitral leaflet (SAM) is also present and reflects a subaortic gradient. Abbreviations as in Figure M.III. 11. (Reprinted from Gardin et al.[2])

lems in the management of pregnancy, labor, and delivery. The availability of noninvasive methods for evaluation of patients with systolic murmurs for this condition has helped considerably in diagnosis. M-mode echocardiography has been the most widely employed technique in this evaluation. The spectrum of IHSS begins with asymmetric septal hypertrophy, in which the interventricular septum is thicker than the left ventricular posterior free wall by a ratio of at least 1.3:1 (Fig. M.III. 14A). The presence, in addition, of systolic anterior motion of the anterior mitral leaflet (Fig. M.III. 14B) is usually associated with a subvalvular gradient (obstruction) at rest.[3,4]

IHSS has also been demonstrated by two-dimensional echocardiography and by radionuclide imaging techniques in which perfusion agents such as thallium are used to outline the thickened ventricular septum and the posterior left ventricular wall.

Table M.III. 1 summarizes the relative utility of M-mode and two-dimensional echocardiography, systolic time intervals, and radionuclide imaging in the diagnosis of specific cardiac problems encountered during pregnancy and delivery. In most conditions, application of a number of noninvasive techniques renders helpful diagnostic information.

III. ACKNOWLEDGMENTS

The author is grateful to Drs. Joseph Askenazi, Michael Lesch, and Philip Braunstein for their contributions to this manuscript, to Kascot Medi-Media of Chicago for their assistance with original artwork and photography, and to Ms Peggy Trigg and Ellen Mansour for assistance in typing the manuscript.

IV. REFERENCES

1. Brinkman CR III, Woods JR Jr. Effects of cardiovascular drugs during pregnancy. Cardiovasc Med. 1976; 1:231–251.
2. Gardin JM, Askenazi J, Lesch M. Assessment of cardiovascular function. In: Sciarra J, Depp R, eds. "Maternal and Fetal Medicine," Vol. III, Gynecology and Obstetrics. Hagerstown, Maryland: Harper & Row, 1979:1–19.
3. Feigenbaum H. Echocardiography, Ed. 2. Philadelphia: Lea & Febiger, 1976.
4. Parisi AF, Tow DE, Felix WR, Sasahara AA. Noninvasive cardiac diagnosis. N Engl J Med. 1977; 296:316,368,427.
5. Pombo JF, Troy BL, Russell RO Jr. Left ventricular volumes and ejection fraction by echocardiography. Circulation. 1971; 43:480–490.
6. Griffith JM, Henry WL. An ultrasound system for combined cardiac imaging and Doppler blood flow measurement in man. Circulation. 1978; 57:925–930.
7. Baker DW. The present role of Doppler techniques in cardiac diagnosis. Prog Cardiovasc Dis. 1978; 21:79–91.
8. Gardin JM, Iseri LT, Elkayam U, Tobis J, Child W, Burn CS, Henry WL. Use of Doppler echocardiography in the non-invasive assessment of left ventricular dysfunction of patients with dilated cardiomyopathy. Circulation. 1980; 62(Suppl III):200 (abstr).
9. Weissler AM. Current concepts in cardiology: Systolic-time intervals. N Engl J Med. 1977; 296:321–324.
10. Nuclear Medicine. Prog Cardiovasc Dis. 1977, 1978; 20(1–4).
11. Medical Radiation Exposure of Pregnant and Potentially Pregnant Women. Recommendations of the National Council on Radiation Protection and Measurements. Washington, DC: National Council on Radiation Protection and Measurements, 1977:13.
12. Handbook of Radiation Doses in Nuclear Medicine and Diagnostic X-Ray. Boca Raton, Florida: CRC Press, 1980:170.
13. Ashburn WL, Schelbert HR, Verba JW. Left ventricular ejection fraction: A review of several radionuclide angiographic approaches using the scintillation camera. Prog Cardiovasc Dis. 1978; 20:267–284.
14. Parker JA, Treves S. Radionuclide detection, localization, and quantitation of intracardiac shunts and shunts between the great arteries. Prog Cardiovasc Dis. 1977; 20:121–150.
15. Askenazi J, Ahnberg DS, Korngold E, La Farge LG, Maltz DL, Treves S. Quantitative radionuclide angiography: Detection and quantitation of left to right shunts. Am J Cardiol. 1976; 37:382–387.

16. Cohn JN. Central venous pressure as a guide to volume expansion. Ann Intern Med. 1967; 66:1283–1287.
17. Forrester JS, Diamond G, McHugh TJ, Swan HJ. Filling pressures in the right and left sides of the heart in acute myocardial infarction: A reappraisal of central-venous pressure monitoring. N Engl J Med. 1971; 285:190–193.
18. Swan HJ, Ganz W, Forrester J, Marcus H, Diamond G, Chonette D. Catheterization of the heart in man with use of a flow-directed balloon-tipped catheter. N Engl J Med. 1970; 283:447–451.
19. Henry WL, Griffith JM, Michaelis LL, McIntosh CL, Morrow AG, Epstein SE. Measurement of mitral orifice area in patients with mitral valve disease by real-time, two-dimensional echocardiography. Circulation. 1975; 51:827–831.
20. Procacci PM, Savran SV, Schreiter SL, Bryson AL. Prevalence of clinical mitral-valve prolapse in 1,169 young women. N Engl J Med. 1976; 294:1086–1088.
21. Markiewicz W, Stoner J, London E, Hunt SA, Popp RL. Mitral valve prolapse in one hundred presumably healthy young females. Circulation. 1976; 53:464–473.
22. Weyman AE, Feigenbaum H, Dillon JC, Chang S. Cross-sectional echocardiography in assessing the severity of valvular aortic stenosis. Circulation. 1975; 52:828–834.
23. Nanda NC, Gramiak R, Manning J, Mahoney EB, Lipchik EO, DeWeese JA. Echocardiographic recognition of the congenital bicuspid aortic valve. Circulation. 1974; 49:870–875.
24. Brown OR, DeMots H, Kloster FE, Roberts A, Menashe VD, Beals RK. Aortic root dilatation and mitral valve prolapse in Marfan's syndrome: An echocardiographic study. Circulation. 1975; 52:651–657.
25. Nanda NC, Gramiak R, Shah PM. Diagnosis of aortic root dissection by echocardiography. Circulation. 1973; 48:506–513.
26. Weyman AE, Wann LS, Hurwitz RA, Dillon JC, Feigenbaum H. Negative contrast echocardiography: A new technique for detecting left-to-right shunts. Circulation. 1977; 56:26 (abstr).
27. Sahn DJ, Sobol RG, Allen HD. Non-invasive direct imaging and measurement of the patent ductus arteriosus (PDA) using real-time cross-sectional echocardiography. Circulation. 1977; 56:191 (abstr).
28. Horowitz MS, Schultz LS, Stinson EB, Harrison DC, Popp RL. Sensitivity and specificity of echocardiographic diagnosis of pericardial effusion. Circulation. 1974; 50:239–247.

Cardiovascular Disorders and Pregnancy

M. IV

Congenital Heart Disease and Pregnancy

Tyson Cobb, MD, Norbert Gleicher, MD, and Uri Elkayam, MD

I. INTRODUCTION

Pregnant patients with congenital heart disease (CHD) present special therapeutic problems, because pregnancy imposes an additional burden of increased blood volume, cardiac output, and heart rate on already abnormal hemodynamics (see Chapter M. I).[1] Although many such patients tolerate the additional circulatory load without any problems, in some cases significant complications develop, sometimes leading to death.

Cardiac disease is the most important nonobstetrical cause of maternal death and has been reported to be 18 times more common than any other cause.[2] Congenital heart disease is responsible for 3–10% of organic heart disease in pregnancy and 0.5–1% of maternal deaths.[3] The chance to encounter pregnant females with congenital heart disease in a medical practice has increased significantly over recent years, reflecting advances in medical and surgical care that have allowed children with congenital heart disease to reach childbearing age. Concomitantly with the increase in number of patients with congenital heart disease reaching adulthood, a marked decrease in the incidence of rheumatic heart disease has been noted. Only several decades ago, the ratio of rheumatic heart disease to congenital heart disease in pregnancy was approximately 20:1, whereas recently this ratio has changed to 3:1.[4]

Cardiac Problems in Pregnancy, pages 61–78

Most types of CHD have been seen in pregnancy, but the most commonly reported lesions are patent ductus arteriosus, atrial septal defects, ventricular septal defects, pulmonary stenosis, coarctation of the aorta, and tetralogy of Fallot.[2,5-9]

The recommendation for either prevention of conception or early induced interruption of pregnancy in almost all women with CHD, a common practice until only the very recent past, does not seem to be justified today. The majority of patients with CHD can tolerate pregnancy, labor, and delivery; the latter either by vaginal delivery or by cesarean section. In principle, even patients with such morbid cardiac malformations as Eisenmenger's syndrome may survive pregnancy even though their risks are appreciably high.[10]

In general, most patients with acyanotic congenital heart disease will tolerate pregnancy without significant complications.[7] In fact, the maternal mortality rate for such patients is essentially the same as that of patients without cardiac disease. Coarctation of the aorta, however, has the potential for more problems in pregnancy and should be managed accordingly.

Pregnancy in cyanotic congenital heart disease and/or pulmonary hypertension carries a marked increase in the risk of complications and mortality for both the mother and the fetus.[9-11] Pregnancy in patients with Eisenmenger's syndrome has an unacceptably high incidence of significant problems for both mother and fetus. Most authorities state that pregnancy is strongly contraindicated in this situation.[5,10]

When categorized according to the functional classification of the New York Heart Association, most patients in classes I or II usually have uneventful pregnancies and vaginal deliveries.[6,7,9] Epidural anesthesia seems to be the method of choice when cesarean section is performed for obstetric indication, as "well-managed" epidural anesthesia produces little hemodynamic or respiratory change.[10,12]

Patients in functional classes III and IV may pose difficult problems and should be the target of a multidisciplinary approach by obstetrician, cardiologist, and anesthesiologist experienced with such conditions. Monitoring of the pulmonary and systemic arterial blood pressures is indicated in most, if not all, such patients. In addition, the second stage of labor should be shortened by using outlet forceps.

II. ATRIAL SEPTAL DEFECT

Three types of atrial septal defects (ASD) may be seen in adults: ostium primum, ostium secundum, and sinus venosus. Among those atrial septal defects, the secundum type is by far the most common one. In fact, with the exception of congenital bicuspid aortic valve, it is the most common form of CHD in the adult. The ratio of female to male is approximately 2:1, resulting in it representing the most common defect seen with pregnancy.

The majority of females with ASD in the childbearing age group are asymptomatic and will have an uneventful pregnancy, labor, and delivery. Physical examination will reveal evidence of right ventricular enlargement manifested by a left parasternal systolic lift. Auscultation of the heart usually reveals a grade 2–3/6 systolic ejection murmur that is loudest at the second left intercostal space. The murmur is secondary to increased flow across the pulmonic valve. The second heart sound (S_2) is wide, with fixed splitting caused by prolongation of right ventricular ejection time secondary to volume overload due to left-to-right shunting. The pulmonary component (P_2) of S_2 may be slightly increased, even without pulmonary hypertension. A diastolic filling sound (S_3) may be present along the lower left sternal border or just inside the apex. A diastolic rumbling murmur caused by increased flow across the tricuspid valve is common in children and can also be heard in adults.[13]

The ECG frequently shows right ventricular hypertrophy and incomplete right bundle branch block; vertical or rightward axis is common in an uncomplicated secundum type of defect, but left axis deviation strongly suggests a primum-type defect. Atrial arrhythmias are frequent in patients with ASD, with atrial fibrillation, atrial flutter, and paroxysmal supraventricular tachycardia most commonly seen.[14]

The chest x-ray film usually demonstrates a prominent pulmonary artery, increased pulmonary vascularity, and an enlarged right ventricle and right atrium.[15] The echocardiogram shows an enlarged right ventricle and paradoxical septal motion. These findings are not diagnostic, as they may also be seen in any other states of right ventricular volume overload such as tricuspid insufficiency, pulmonary insufficiency, and anomalous pulmonary venous drainage. The echocardiographic feature, however, is very useful when considered in conjunction with the clinical findings.[16]

ASD is the most common maternal congenital lesion noted.[2,7,17,18] Not infrequently, it is first diagnosed during pregnancy when a murmur is elicited. The left-to-right shunt and the additional volume of pregnancy place a significant load on the right ventricle and increase pulmonary blood flow. This is usually well tolerated, even when pulmonary blood flow is several times higher than the aortic blood flow. The pulmonary artery pressure remains normal owing to easy adaptation of the pulmonary vascular system. Neilson et al[5] reported 24 patients with ASD who had 70 pregnancies without any significant complications. It should be noted, however, that arrhythmias and congestive heart failure which may become fatal have been reported by others[9] and should be treated promptly.

The development of pulmonary hypertension in patients with ASD rarely occurs until the fourth decade of life. During pregnancy, pulmonary hypertension increases the complications significantly, yet some of these patients have been reported to tolerate pregnancy.[1,19]

If congestive heart failure occurs and persists despite good medical therapy during pregnancy, then surgical closure must be strongly considered.[1,20] Normally, the shunting of blood in an uncomplicated ASD is from left-to-right, but the direction may be reversed by sudden events such as pulmonary embolization, leading to development of pulmonary hypertension. If excessive hemorrhage occurs during delivery, systemic hypotension may be the result, causing a reversal of the shunt and producing cyanosis. This can be corrected by restoring volume with colloid or blood infusion and by increasing systemic vascular resistance with vasopressor agents.

Atrial arrhythmias may occur but are unusual prior to the fourth decade of life. Atrial fibrillation is the most common arrhythmia; atrial flutter and supraventricular tachycardia may also occur.[14] The therapeutic approach to arrhythmias during pregnancy is discussed in detail in chapters M.XIV and M. XIX. In general, repeated episodes of supraventricular tachyarrhythmias can be treated with digoxin, the safety of which during pregnancy has been established. Failure to respond to digoxin alone should be an indication for the addition of quinidine or propranolol, both at the lowest possible dose that is required to prevent recurrence of the arrhythmia. Overriding of the arrhythmia by atrial pacing is another option during pregnancy; the pacer can be introduced in most patients without fluoroscopy with the help of intracardiac electrocardiographic recordings. Arrhythmias associated with symptoms or hemodynamic impairment should and can be treated with electrical cardioversion.

Concomitant findings of an endocardial cushion defect can be seen in patients with ASD. These can vary considerably from a primum-type ASD with a cleft mitral valve to a complete endocardial cushion defect, in which the atrial and ventricular septal defects are one and there is a large cleft in the mitral and tricuspid valves, essentially producing a common AV valve. Recommendations concerning pregnancy in these patients must be considered on an individual basis.

Lutembacher's syndrome is the concomitant occurrence of an ASD and mitral stenosis. Although the stenotic mitral valve accentuates left-to-right shunt, atrial hypertension and pulmonary congestion are prevented by an unloading effect of the ASD on the left atrium. Pregnancy generally carries a good prognosis.[21]

III. VENTRICULAR SEPTAL DEFECT

Isolated ventricular septal defect (VSD) is one of the more common cardiac malformations.[22] It frequently occurs in conjunction with transposition of the great arteries, coarctation of the aorta, pulmonary stenosis, and as part of an endocardial cushion defect. A concomitant aortic regurgitation may occur as a result of a prolapse of the right aortic cusp. The female-to-male ratio is essentially equal.

The clinical picture is determined by the size of the defect and the status of the pulmonary vascular resistance. If the VSD is small, there is no significant hemodynamic effect and the added hemodynamic burden of pregnancy is well tolerated. If the ventricular defect is large, the risk of pregnancy is increased; a large defect may be associated with congestive heart failure, especially in patients with aortic regurgitation due to a prolapsed aortic cusp or due to valvular infective endocarditis. When Eisenmenger's syndrome is present the added burden of pregnancy is not well tolerated and the rate of complications is very high.

Physical examination will frequently reveal a holosystolic thrill palpated over the left parasternal area at the third and fourth intercostal spaces. When the shunt is large the left ventricle may be dilated and enlarged to palpation. The first heart sound is usually loud, and a holosystolic murmur is typically heard in the third or fourth left intercostal space. A third heart sound is common at the cardiac apex, and an apical middiastolic rumble is almost the rule in the presence of a large shunt. When pulmonary hypertension develops, the pulmonic component of the second heart sound increases in intensity and may be palpable. A pulmonic ejection sound can then be heard, and the previously described systolic murmur diminishes or even disappears.[13]

The electrocardiogram may be normal in cases with small VSD but can show left ventricular hypertrophy or biventricular hypertrophy. Left ventricular hypertrophy suggests a moderate to large left-to-right shunt with left ventricular volume overload, and right ventricular hypertrophy suggests pulmonary hypertension. Heart blocks are common when corrected transposition of the great vessels coexists.[14]

The chest x-ray film in patients with a significant left-to-right shunt will show an enlargement of the left ventricle and left atrium and increased pulmonary vascularity. The size of the pulmonary artery and the right ventricle depends on the degree of pumonary hypertension.[15]

Echocardiographic findings similarly depend on the hemodynamic profile. When a large left-to-right shunt is present, the echocardiogram reveals an enlargement of the left atrium and left ventricle. Increased pulmonary artery pressure will be associated with enlargement and hypertrophy of the right ventricle. A discontinuity of the echoes reflected from the interventricular septum can identify the septal defects, although the sensitivity and the specificity of this finding are not very high. Contrast echocardiography is helpful in the identification of a shunt. A right-to-left shunt can be easily diagnosed by early appearance of microbubbles in the left ventricle after peripheral injection of saline. A left-to-right shunt can also be diagnosed by the same technique and will cause an echo-free jet that is surrounded by multiple bubbles secondary to saline passing through the right ventricle.[16] The use of the Doppler technique can further improve the ability to noninvasively diagnose ventricular septal defect.[23]

Women with VSD usually tolerate pregnancy very well. In one series, 56 women with VSD had 141 pregnancies with only two maternal deaths; both were patients with Eisenmenger's syndrome.[9] The other pregnancies were essentially uncomplicated, having only infrequent congestive heart failure and rare arrhythmias. Mendleson[24] reported 110 cases with an 8% congestive heart failure rate and a 5.5% mortality rate. Three of six deaths were secondary to circulatory collapse following delivery. The other three were secondary to congestive heart failure, paradoxical embolism, and infective endocarditis, respectively.

Pregnancy following closure of an uncomplicated ventricular septal defect is essentially unremarkable. Several cases of successful closure of ventricular septal defects during pregnancy have been reported.[25] However, the need for closure of the ventricular septal defect during pregnancy should be rare and is indicated only if there is persistent congestive heart failure despite good medical therapy, or if there are problems with bacterial endocarditis.

Postpartum there is the potential risk of shunt reversal if significant hypotension occurs. Prompt replacement of volume and the use of vasopressor agents to restore blood pressure to normal will prevent catastrophic complications.

IV. PATENT DUCTUS ARTERIOSUS

Patent ductus arteriosus (PDA) is one of the most common congenital cardiovascular anomalies,[26] and it occurs predominantly in women (2:1 ratio). It used to be the most common congenital lesion seen in pregnancy with the exception of an atrial septal defect. It has, however, become a rare finding in pregnancy, as virtually all PDA cases are diagnosed and surgically corrected in early childhood.[1,26]

Most patients with PDA are asymptomatic, but exertional dyspnea and fatigue occur in patients with increased pulmonary vascular resistance. Systolic blood pressure may be elevated and the diastolic blood pressure is usually decreased, resulting in a wide pulse pressure. The precordium may be normal to palpation or exhibit a hyperdynamic left ventricle. A continuous murmur, which is the hallmark of this malformation, is maximally heard in the second left intercostal space and is described as a "machinery murmur." The murmur is continuous without interruption through the second heart sound but does not always persist throughout the cardiac cycle. A third heart sound is occasionally heard at the apex. If pulmonary hypertension develops, right ventricular heave and palpable P_2 are often present, and the diastolic part of the continuous murmur diminishes. A further increase in pulmonary hypertension will result in a disappearance of the murmur, development of a load pulmonic valve closure sound, and occasionally, a diastolic murmur of pulmonary insufficiency.[13] If reversed shunting occurs, one may see cyanosis and clubbing in the lower extremities.

The electrocardiogram may be normal but can show left ventricular or biventricular hypertrophy.[14] The chest x-ray film shows increased vascularity and enlargement of the pulmonary artery, ascending aorta, left ventricle, and left atrium.[15]

The echocardiogram can reveal an enlarged left atrium and left ventricle, and occasionally the actual PDA may be visualized by two-dimensional echocardiography.[16]

Most patients with patent ductus arteriosus tolerate pregnancy without any difficulties.[27]; however, an occasional patient may develop congestive heart failure during pregnancy.[5] If pulmonary hypertension is present and shunt reversal occurs (Eisenmenger's syndrome), then pregnancy carries a significantly higher complication rate, both for the mother and for the fetus.[10,22,27]

V. AORTIC STENOSIS

Congenital obstruction of left ventricular outflow can be valvular, supravalvular, or subvalvular.[28] These defects make up approximately 4–5% of all congenital heart malformations. Aortic stenosis is three to four times more common in males than in females; hence, the incidence in pregnancy is very low.[29] Three-fourths of all congenital obstructions of the left ventricle are valvular and can be unicuspid, bicuspid, or tricuspid. Bicuspid aortic valve is the most common congenital cardiac malformation, occurring in 1–2% of the population, and it is not uncommonly associated with other congenital anomalies such as coarctation of the aorta, bicuspid pulmonic valve, patent ductus arteriosus, or ventricular septal defect. The fewer the number of cusps and commissures of the congenitally malformed aortic valve, the greater the likelihood that it will be stenotic at birth. The bicuspid aortic valve is usually not stenotic at birth but will become so with increasing frequency as the patient grows older.

The natural course of congenital aortic stenosis is highly variable, and sudden death is always a threat, even in asymptomatic patients. When congestive heart failure, angina, or syncope occur in a patient with aortic stenosis, the prognosis becomes poor. Easy fatigability can also suggest that the aortic stenosis is severe, although it is a hard symptom to evaluate. When significant symptoms develop, life expectancy does not exceed five years in the majority of patients.[28] Careful history taking is extremely important in a patient with aortic stenosis, especially in a so-called asymptomatic patient.

On physical examination, the arterial pulse reveals a slow rate of rise that is best felt in the carotid arteries, and thrills or shudders are commonly felt.[13] The pulse pressure is usually reduced and a distinct presystolic apical pulsation is frequently palpable. An aortic ejection click, usually loudest at the cardiac apex, may also be heard. There is a systolic ejection murmur that is low pitched and somewhat harsh and/or rough sounding that is loudest in the second right intercostal space and may radiate to the neck. Occasionally the murmur is very loud at the apex. The murmur is usually short and peaks in early systole in patients with mild aortic stenosis; it encompasses most of systole, with a late peak in severe aortic stenosis. These findings, however, are not always diagnostic, as an unimpressive murmur is sometimes heard in far-advanced tight stenosis. Paradoxical splitting of the second heart sound (S_2) may occur in cases of severe stenosis due to prolongation of left ventricular ejection. The aortic component of S_2 is soft because of reduced mobility of the thickened stiff aortic cusps. A fourth heart sound (S_4) in the absence of a prolonged PR interval on the electrocardiogram suggests significant stenosis and reflects left ventricular hypertrophy and diastolic stiffness. A third heart sound (S_3) is not present unless there is concomitant heart failure.

The chest x-ray film shows a normal or only slightly enlarged left ventricle. Although ventricular mass increases, it results in concentric hypertrophy without dilatation. Significant left ventricular enlargement is seen when aortic stenosis is accompanied by some other valvular problems, simultaneous arteriosclerotic heart disease, or in later stages, when ventricular failure occurs. Poststenotic dilatation of the ascending aorta is a common finding, and left atrial enlargement is present in cases with severe stenosis of the aortic valve. Calcification of the aortic valve may be seen in the lateral or oblique views.[15]

The M-mode echocardiogram offers somewhat limited diagnostic value in valvular aortic stenosis.[16] The presence of a thickened valve is manifested by multiple dense echoes coming from the leaflets. There is restricted motion of the leaflets and the opening in systole is reduced, but frequently the distance between the leaflets cannot be determined because multiple echoes fill the aortic root. Two-dimensional echocardiography has improved on the diagnosis of valvular aortic stenosis especially in congenital aortic stenosis in the young patient where significant thickening or calcification are absent. Besides visualization of thickened aortic valve leaflet, there is doming of the valve, which is the most important two-dimensional echocardiographic finding in stenosis of any valve. Left ventricular hypertrophy can also be evaluated by echocardiography and may help in determining the severity of aortic stenosis.

There are few reports concerning pregnancy in women with congenital aortic stenosis. Those reports that are devoted to the subject suggest that, although pregnancy can be uncomplicated even in cases with severe stenosis (gradient over 100 mg Hg), maternal and fetal mortality can be high. Left ventricular failure and sudden death are the major complications[1]; infective endocarditis is also a potential problem. The absence of symptoms does not always predict an uncomplicated pregnancy. The patient should avoid moderate to severe physical exertion during pregnancy at all costs. Neilson et al[5] reported on four patients with aortic stenosis who had 10 pregnancies with no serious maternal complications; however, one neonatal death occurred following a difficult delivery. In addition, one pregnancy resulted in a spontaneous abortion, and one hysterectomy was performed during the eighteenth week of gestation for nonmedical reasons. Arias and Pineda[29] reviewed the English literature and found 23 patients with 38 pregnancies with a maternal mortality of 17.4% and a fetal mortality of 31.6%. They felt that there were not enough cases to draw any specific conclusions concerning management.

VI. COARCTATION OF THE AORTA

Coarctation of the aorta is a severe narrowing that produces high resistance to aortic flow and results in arterial hypertension.[30] Coarctation can occur at any site along the aorta, but in at least 95% of cases it is located just distal to the left subclavian artery in the region of the ductus arteriosus or ligamentum arteriosum. This malformation accounts for 7–8% of congenital heart disease. The male-female ratio is 3:1, yet the ratio is essentially equal in so-called complicated coarctation, which is associated with other congenital cardiovascular anomalies. Approximately half of the patients with complicated coarctation will have a bicuspid aortic valve, and not infrequently cerebral aneurysms will be found. Life expectancy in uncorrected coarctation of the aorta is severely shortened, with an average of 35 years[18] and almost 90% mortality by the age of 50. The most common causes of death in patients with coarctation of the aorta are congestive heart failure, aortic rupture, dissection of the aorta, infective endocarditis of a congenital bicuspid aortic valve, endarteritis at the site of the coarctation, and intracranial hemorrhage due to rupture of a saccular aneurysm in the circle of Willis.[29]

It has been suggested that the incidence of aortic dissection or rupture is increased during pregnancy. Today, however, coarctation of the aorta in pregnancy is found less and less as diagnosis and surgical correction are accomplished prior to the childbearing years.

Significant symptoms such as congestive heart failure occur either during infancy or in the third decade of life. Not infrequently the disease is diagnosed in late childhood or early adult life in an asymptomatic patient who is found to have hypertension or an abnormal routine chest x-ray film. Rupture or dissection of the aorta in nonpregnant patients occurs most commonly during the third or fourth decade of life.

On physical examination a systolic blood pressure that is higher in the arms than in the legs is essentially diagnostic of coarctation of the aorta.[13] The diastolic blood pressure in the arms may be higher than that in the legs, but not infrequently they are equal and play no part in the diagnosis. In comparing the radial arteries to the femoral arteries simultaneously, the femoral pulses will be diminished and delayed and are occasionally absent. If there is a difference in the systolic blood pressure between the upper arms, then one of the subclavian arteries originates at or below the coarctation. A forceful pulsation and occasionally a thrill may be felt in the suprasternal notch due to dilatation of the aorta proximal to the coarctation. The left ventricular impulse is forceful and sustained secondary to left ventricular hypertrophy. Auscultation reveals an ejection click secondary to dilatation of the ascending aorta or a bicuspid aortic valve. A systolic murmur is usually present as a result of turbulent flow across the coarctation, significant collateral flow, or flow across a bicuspid aortic valve. Auscultation over the coarctation in the interscapular area may reveal a continuous murmur. S_4 is frequently present, as one would expect in a patient with hypertension and decreased left ventricular compliance, and S_3 is heard if congestive heart failure occurs.

The electrocardiogram may be normal but exhibits frequently left ventricular hypertrophy and left atrial enlargement.[14] The chest x-ray film does not show enlargement of the left ventricle until heart failure or aortic regurgitation occurs.[15] The ascending aorta can be dilated. There may be a "3" sign along the left mediastinal area formed by the aorta with the midindentation of the "3" being secondary to the actual coarctation. The "E" sign is the mirror image of the "3" seen on a barium swallow. Rib notching is an erosive defect on the inferior edge of the ribs secondary to dilated intercostal vessels and is almost diagnostic of coarctation. In addition, it indicates that the coarctation involves the thoracic aorta and that it is hemodynamically significant.

The echocardiogram will show left ventricular hypertrophy and can identify a bicuspid aortic valve if present. Examination of the aortic arch and the descending aorta by two-dimensional echocardiography may show the actual narrowing produced by the coarctation and poststenotic dilatation.[16] Marked pulsations of the aorta proximal to the obstruction may also be noted.

In uncomplicated coarctation of the aorta, pregnancy is usually safe to the mother, but fetal development can be impaired because of decreased blood flow distal to the aortic narrowing. In complicated coarctation, there is an increased risk to the mother.[31] Snaith and Szekely in 1974[32] reviewed all published cases of coarctation of the aorta in pregnancy and showed a 3.5% maternal mortality. Fetal mortality has been much higher and has been quoted from 13% to 25%.[33,34] In spite of high blood pressure measured proximal to the coarctation, the incidence of toxemia of pregnancy is not significantly increased.[1,35] The increased fetal loss in patients with unoperated coarctation is felt to be secondary to reduced blood flow to the uterus and placenta because of inadequate collateral circulation.

Previously it was thought that the stress of labor and delivery will produce increased maternal mortality due to rupture of the aorta; and therefore, cesarean section was recommended as the mode of delivery. Recently, however, vaginal delivery has been exonerated, as it has been shown that approximately 80% of all aortic ruptures during pregnancy occur prior to labor and delivery. Contrarily, death during or immediately after labor and delivery is rare.[35]

Surgical correction of coarctation has been successful during pregnancy[36,37] but is not recommended unless major complications develop such as aortic dissection, uncontrollable increased systolic blood pressure over 200 mm Hg, or severe heart failure that does not respond to medical therapy.[1,9,34]

In a review of 136 cases of coarctation and pregnancy by Goodwin in 1958 13 maternal deaths were reported in 354 pregnancies (3.7%). Three patients died of rupture of the aorta, three from rupture of aortic dissection, three from cardiac failure, two from cerebrovascular accidents, one from infective endocarditis of the aortic valve and one from an unknown cause.[37] Even though aortic rupture and dissection do occur during pregnancy it is not as common as previously suspected.

The mainstays of treatment during pregnancy are limitation of physical activity and control of blood pressure, as rupture of the aorta or cerebral aneurysm are less likely to occur in the absence of significant hypertension. Prophylatic treatment with broad spectrum antibiotics should be instituted in situations where bacteremia is highly predictable.

Surgical correction of significant coarctation of the aorta should be performed before pregnancy and childbirth as the maternal mortality in pregnant patients who have undergone previous correction is negligible.

VII. PULMONARY STENOSIS

Pulmonary valvular stenosis is a relatively common congenital cardiac defect with equal occurrence among males and females. Most patients with pulmonary stenosis are diagnosed during their first year of life. Usually mild pulmonary stenosis in a child will remain mild but occasionally may become progressively more severe in adulthood. Patients who have undergone valvulotomy in childhood because of significant stenosis have excellent and lasting results.[38]

Congenital obstruction to the outflow tract of the right ventricle is most commonly at the valvular level but can also be supravalvular or subvalvular (infundibular). The majority of patients with pulmonic valvular stenosis are asymptomatic, and not infrequently, moderate pulmonary valvular stenosis can be found in a patient who is leading a normal life. Symptoms of fatigue and exertional dyspnea are seen in cases with significant stenosis and are a consequence of decreased cardiac output.

Physical examination reveals a prominent "a" wave in the jugular venous pulse, reflecting contraction of the right atrium against a hypertrophied, poorly compliant right ventricle. Right ventricular parasternal lift is palpable and is a result of right ventricular hypertrophy. A systolic thrill may be felt in the upper left sternal border and the left infraclavicular area. A pulmonary ejection click heard louder on expiration may be present early in systole. When the disease progresses and the obstruction becomes more severe, the pulmonic component of the second heart sound becomes softer and delayed. A right-sided fourth heart sound is another sign of significant obstruction and poor compliance of the right ventricle. There is a midsystolic murmur that is somewhat harsh and diamond-shaped, it is loudest in the upper left parasternal area, usually in the second left intercostal space. The murmur radiates upward and leftward to the left infraclavicular area. As the stenosis becomes worse, the murmur peaks later and becomes longer, encompassing more of systole and eventually extending past the aortic component of the second heart sound.[38]

The electrocardiogram may be normal in cases of mild pulmonic stenosis. In significant pulmonic stenosis there will be evidence of right ventricular hypertrophy, and if the stenosis is severe a right axis deviation and right atrial enlargement will be also found.

The chest x-ray film reveals a normal or slightly enlarged heart size with prominent pulmonary arteries secondary to poststenotic dilatation. The pulmonary vascularity will be normal or reduced. In the adult the pulmonic valve may become calcified.[38]

The echocardiogram is frequently not of much help in the diagnosis or evaluation of pulmonary stenosis. It usually allows the visualization of the posterior leaflet of the pulmonic valve only, making a quantitative analysis difficult. The M-mode echocardiogram of the pulmonic valve may show an exaggerated "a" wave, and the two-dimensional echocardiogram may show doming of the pulmonic valve. The finding of right ventricular wall thickening can predict an elevated right ventricular systolic pressure and significant pulmonary stenosis.[16]

Schaefer et al[9] reported on nine patients with pulmonic stenosis who had 21 pregnancies. Six of these had congestive heart failure during 11 pregnancies. There were six abortions, one premature delivery of a stillborn infant and one ectopic pregnancy. Mendelson[39] reported on 59 cases of unoperated isolated pulmonary stenosis in pregnancy. There were only five cases of congestive heart failure and no maternal deaths. Neilson et al[5] reported on 11 patients with pulmonic stenosis with 26 pregnancies. There were four spontaneous abortions and one patient who had severe stenosis had right heart failure during her first pregnancy but following valvotomy, she had three uneventful pregnancies.

It appears that the additional load on the heart during pregnancy in patients with pulmonic stenosis is tolerated fairly well as indicated by the relatively low incidence of cardiac failure. Most of the pregnancies complicated by pulmonic stenosis described in the literature were reported ten to 20 years ago. With today's improvements in medical therapy, the incidence of heart failure should be smaller. If heart failure persists despite good medical therapy, then valvotomy should be performed.

VIII. TETRALOGY OF FALLOT

Tetralogy of Fallot is the most common cyanotic congenital heart disease in children and adults today.[18,40] Its distribution between the sexes is almost equal. This is also the most common cyanotic congenital lesion in pregnancy. As more children with this defect receive palliative or definitive surgical repair of the lesion, more will survive to childbearing age. Therefore, more pregnancies in women with tetralogy of Fallot should be expected.[41] Approximately half of all children with surgically untreated cases of tetralogy of Fallot will die before five years of age,[41,42] and only 5% will be alive by age 25. Garson et al[40] state that the most common causes of death are hypoxia, cerebrovascular accidents (including brain abscess), bacterial endocarditis, and, less often, pneumonia and congestive heart failure. If congestive failure occurs, other causes should be sought such as anemia, endocarditis, systemic hypertension, rheumatic fever, or occult glomerulonephritis. Dysrhythmias may cause sudden death in the uncorrected cases and may even be a cause for late death in a surgically corrected patient. Patients with repaired tetralogy of Fallot, in general, do well, with at least 75% of them being alive and active on long-term follow-up.

Classically, tetralogy of Fallot has four anatomic abnormalities. 1) Pulmonic stenosis, which usually is infundibular but can be valvular, supravalvular, in the level of the pulmonary artery trunk or its branches or subinfundibular. (Frequently a combination of valvular and infundibular stenosis is found.) 2) Ventricular septal defect. 3) Dextroposition of the aorta or the aorta overriding the ventricular septal defect. 4) Right ventricular hypertrophy. From a physiologic standpoint, the pulmonic stenosis and the ventricular septal defect are the important anatomic deformities. The right ventricular hypertrophy is a consequence of the stenotic pulmonic valve. The clinical spectrum can vary widely as the ventricular septal defect can be small or large and the pulmonic stenosis can be mild to severe.

Dyspnea of exertion is a common complaint, and squatting for relief of dyspnea and faintness is essentially pathognomonic of this disease entity. Why squatting relieves symptoms is not totally known, the most probable explanation is that increasing peripheral vascular resistance mediated by squatting results in increasing blood flow through the ventricular septal defect from the left ventricle to the right ventricle and to the lungs. Other symptoms are hypoxic or syncopal episodes, but these are usually seen only in infants. Congestive heart failure (right or left) in tetralogy of Fallot is rare. Cerebrovascular accidents due to venous sinus thrombosis emoblism, or brain abscess are not uncommon.

Physical examination reveals symmetrical cyanosis and not infrequently some physical underdevelopment. There is clubbing of the fingers and toes. The cardiac apex is faint, but there is a left parasternal heave secondary to right ventricular hypertrophy, and one-half of all patients will have a systolic thrill in the third left intercostal space. On auscultation there is a loud ejection murmur due to right ventricular outflow tract obstruction. The murmur is heard along the left sternal border and radiates upward and to the left. The second heart sound is single and loud and may be palpable, as the aorta is closer to the chest wall than usual and the pulmonary trunk is hypoplastic (or atretic). If pulmonic stenosis is severe, collateral circulation through bronchial vessels or other aortic pulmonary communications will develop and produce a continuous murmur heard anywhere over the chest and frequently over the back.[13]

The electrocardiogram usually shows right ventricular hypertrophy; only rarely is there any evidence of right atrial enlargement.[14]

The chest x-ray film reveals right ventricular enlargement especially on the lateral view. The aorta is enlarged and one-fourth of the cases exhibit a right aortic arch.[15] The pulmonary artery is small and concave and the lung fields show diminished vascularity. The left atrium and left ventricle are normal is size and the left ventricular apex is slightly elevated giving the classic "boot-shaped heart" or "coeur en sabot" appearance.

The M-mode echocardiogram shows dilatation and dextroposition of the aorta. Because of the ventricular septal defect, there is a loss of the usual continuity between the aorta and the interventricular septum, and the anterior wall of the aorta is seen closer to the chest wall than the septum. The right ventricular cavity is enlarged and the walls are thickened. Septal motion is normal and the right ventricular outflow tract is narrowed. Two-dimensional echocardiography confirms the M-mode findings and gives a better look at the narrowed right ventricular outflow tract. It is an excellent means of evaluating the size of the pulmonary artery,[19] especially if surgical correction is contemplated.[16]

The natural history of the disease shows a gradual increase in the severity of the pulmonic stenosis with worsening of symptoms and cyanosis. The long-term prognosis is poor, and most patients do not pass the fourth decade of life without surgical correction.

Pregnancy in surgically untreated women with tetralogy of Fallot was reported to have maternal mortality of more than 4%[43] and a rather high perinatal mortality.[44] The fall in peripheral vascular resistance during pregnancy (Chapter M.I) can result in the development or worsening of right-to-left blood shunting and cyanosis. Labor and the time immediately following delivery are critical. Hypotension due to blood loss or a fall in peripheral vascular resistance can cause more right-to-left shunting and thus, more cyanosis and hypoxia with possible death due to circulatory collapse.[45] Obviously, close hemodynamic monitoring and frequent studies of blood gas during labor and delivery are necessary for early recognition and correction of circulatory deterioration. Despite the high risk to mother and fetus, successful pregnancies have been reported in women with tetralogy of Fallot.[2,5,46,47] A maternal hematocrit of over 60%, peripheral arterial oxygen saturation of less than 80%, right ventricular hypertension, and syncopal attacks are poor prognostic signs. Tetralogy of Fallot has been totally corrected surgically during pregnancy[25]; however, surgical intervention in these patients should be performed prior to childbearing years. Patients who have only palliative procedures such as anastomosis of the subclavian artery to the pulmonary artery (Blalock-Taussig), descending aorta to left pulmonary artery (Potts), or ascending aorta to right pulmonary artery (Waterston-Cooley) are still subjected to a significantly higher risk during pregnancy. The incidence of pregnancy in patients who have had a total correction is increasing because of the increased total surgical correction rate over the recent years. These patients should tolerate pregnancy well without any undue risk.[48,49]

IX. EBSTEIN'S ANOMALY

This is a relatively rare entity and it represents less than 1% of all congenital heart defects. Here the tricuspid valve is deformed and the septal and posterior leaflets are displaced downward into the right ventricle.[50] The large anterior leaflet is usually the least affected of the three leaflets. Part of the right ventricle therefore, is cephalic to the tricuspid valve and becomes "atrialized." Hence, the effective right ventricle is smaller, and forward flow is reduced. Clinical symptoms usually reflect reduced cardiac output, right-to-left shunting at the atrial level, which occurs through a frequently found patent foramen ovale or atrial septal defect, and also commonly, supraventricular tachyarrhythmias.

Many patients may have right-sided heart failure and cyanosis in infancy or childhood, but approximately one-half may be asymptomatic until adolescence or adulthood. A woman of childbearing age with Ebstein's anomaly therefore may or may not be cyanotic. The clinical presentation of this malformation varies considerably according to the variation of the anatomy. Venous pressure is usually elevated resulting in a distension of neck veins and hepatomegaly. An increased V-wave is common because of the frequently found tricuspid insufficiency. Palpation of the precordium will often reveal a parasternal heave over the atrialized right ventricle. Cardiac auscultation occasionally reveals a characteristic triple or quadruple rhythm composed of S_1, S_2, S_3, and S_4. A murmur of tricuspid regurgitation is frequently present, but the murmur does not increase in intensity during inspiration because of the inability of the inadequate right ventricle to increase its stroke volume.[50]

In most instances, the electrocardiogram shows normal sinus rhythm. The P waves will, in general, be giant because of right atrial enlargement. A prolonged PR interval and right bundle branch block are usually present. Ten to twenty percent of all patients will show the Wolff-Parkinson-White (WPW) syndrome type B, which has the preexcitation tract going to the right side of the heart. Recurrent supraventricular tachyarrhythmias are common and not only in patients with a concomitant WPW syndrome. Simultaneous recordings of intracardiac electrocardiogram and right heart pressures show atrial pressures in the atrialized part of the ventricle and at the same time a ventricular electrocardiogram.[50]

The chest x-ray film may be essentially normal or will reveal an enlarged and globular cardiac silhouette. Pulmonary vasculature is decreased (low cardiac output) or normal. The M-mode echocardiogram shows a delayed closure of the tricuspid valve compared to the mitral valve of approximately 50 msec. The two-dimensional echocardiogram shows a tricuspid valve displaced into the right ventricle.[50]

Several successful pregnancies have been reported in women with Ebstein anomaly. Neilson et al[5] reported one patient with Ebstein anomaly and cyanosis who had three uncomplicated pregnancies. Kahler reported five patients who had 10 pregnancies with no maternal mortality, but two fetal losses.[46] Serious maternal complications do occur, such as right ventricular failure, infective endocarditis, and paradoxical embolization. Each case should be evaluated on an individual basis, but significant right-to-left shunting at the atrial level with cyanosis seems to be associated with a higher fetal loss and may increase the chance for maternal complications in the patient with Ebstein anomaly.

X. MISCELLANEOUS DEFECTS

Most children with complicated congenital cardiac abnormalities do not reach childbearing age.[50] Most of these defects, in fact, cause death in infancy. Very few cases of tricuspid atresia have been reported in association with pregnancy. Of the two reported by Burwell and Metcalf, one patient had three spontaneous abortions and one died in late pregnancy secondary to hemoptysis during pregnancy.[51] Collins and associates described the only case with tricuspid atresia and relatively normal pregnancy, which led to the delivery of a surviving small infant who subsequently developed normally.[52] The next pregnancy in the same patient resulted in miscarriage at two months of gestation. Spontaneous abortion at two months was the result of a third pregnancy, which was complicated by the development of a stroke with transient hemiplegia. A fourth pregnancy led to severe complications, which included congestive heart failure, multiple pulmonary emboli, arterial embolization with grand mal seizure, and premature labor. The infant, who weighed 590 gm, succumbed to prematurity at three days of age. Because of the great maternal hazard, pregnancy should be prevented in patients with tricuspid atresia, and early therapeutic abortion is indicated should pregnancy occur.

Neilson et al[5] reported one patient who had transposition of the great vessels. She had two spontaneous abortions and one neonatal death of a premature infant. Simon and Lustberg described a patient with truncus arteriosus who had a successful pregnancy and full-term delivery of a normal infant. The mother, however, died suddenly on the third day post partum. The cause of death was thought to be a pulmonary infarction.[53] We have recently seen a 20-year-old patient with truncus arteriosus who had a successful pregnancy and delivered a normal infant without complications.[54] Yuzpe et al[49] reported a successful pregnancy in a patient with a single ventricle, and Seeds and Cefalo[55] reported a patient with a two-chambered heart and a single atrioventricular valve who had one spontaneous abortion and an episode of severe hemoptysis during a second pregnancy. These cases are rare and should be considered for early therapeutic abortion only on an individual basis, as no hard-and-fast rules can be set. Under certain circumstances, these patients should also be considered for sterilization.

XI. EISENMENGER'S SYNDROME

Eisenmenger's syndrome (ES) is a general term used to describe pulmonary hypertension and right-to-left blood shunting as a result of any communication between the systemic and pulmonary circulation.

Clinical experience with Eisenmenger's syndrome in pregnancy has remained limited. No single institution has been able to amass a large enough experience to report statistically significant data based on its own experience only. Furthermore, a large proportion of published cases are either unsatisfactorily or incompletely documented. Recognizing the drawbacks of a retrospective study, Gleicher et al recently presented the most comprehensive review of ES in pregnancy.[10] This review, published in 1979, was based on 115 reported cases; however, only 44, including two of the authors' cases, were felt to be adequately documented by either cardiac catheterization or autopsy. These 44 patients had an obstetric experience of 70 pregnancies, which represented the basis for the retrospective analysis.

Fifty-two percent of all patients with ES and pregnancy died in connection with one of their pregnancies. Thirty and three-tenths percent of all pregnancies resulted in death of the mother. No statistically significant difference in maternal mortality among first, second, and third pregnancies could be identified. This observation led to the conclusion that the successful conclusion of pregnancies in patients with ES could not be taken as a positive indication for further pregnancies. An especially high incidence of maternal death was associated with hypovolemia, thromboembolic phenomena, and preeclampsia/eclampsia (EPH-gestosis). However, the total mortality in preeclamptic/eclamptic pregnancies was not statistically higher than in the nontoxemic group. Cesarean sections and other surgical procedures were found to be associated with extremely high maternal mortality. Nevertheless, it was stressed by the authors that patients who require cesarean section may represent a biased study group, indicating an already severely compromised situation. The widely cited belief that patients with ES should, under almost any circumstances, be delivered vaginally rather than by cesarean section may therefore be based on relatively poor data. A similar suggestion was recently made by Spinnato et al.[12] When maternal mortality was investigated in more detail by Gleicher et al, one of three vaginal deliveries, three of four cesarean sections, and one of 14 pregnancy interruptions (only one by hysterotomy) led to maternal death. The maternal probability of death was found to be significantly higher when any kind of delivery was compared to elective termination of pregnancy. This observation led the authors to suggest that termination of pregnancy was indicated in patients with ES.[10]

Among underlying malformations, causing Eisenmenger's syndrome, ventricular septal defect (VSD) was found to be the most frequent cause of shunt. Maternal mortality in cases with VSD was also found to be the highest (60%). Maternal mortality with atrial septal defect was 44%, followed by a 41.7% mortality in association with patent ductus arteriosus. The vast majority of all maternal deaths occurred during or within the first week after delivery.

In addition to the unfavorable maternal effect, pregnancy in women with Eisenmenger's syndrome also is associated with extremely poor fetal outcome. Only 25.6% of all pregnancies were reported to have reached term. At least 54.9% of all deliveries were clearly premature, and at least 30.2% of all delivered infants showed evidence of intrauterine growth retardation. This number represented almost half of all newborns for whom available information allowed valid clinical evaluation. The total perinatal mortality for this group reached 28.3% and was found to be highly significantly associated with prematurity. Based upon these data, we recommend the following: 1) Pregnancy is contraindicated in patients with ES. 2) Abortion is the treatment of choice once pregnancy has occurred. 3) If interruption of pregnancy is refused by the patient, utmost care should be taken to assure maternal and fetal survival.

The clinical management of a patient who has decided to carry despite advice to the contrary should include the following: 1) The patient should be hospitalized not later than 20 weeks gestational age. 2) Cooperation of all involved medical services is essential to obtain maximum results. 3) Anticoagulation is usually suggested at approximately 20 weeks gestational age, even though the value of anticoagulation during pregnancy is based on theoretical grounds and remains to be proved. Prophylactic anticoagulant therapy in the post partum period has been recommended by some authors[56] but was found not to prevent deterioration or even to possibly compound it by causing significant bleeding.[57] 4) The day-to-day medical management will be dependent on the patient's functional capacity. In general, prolonged bed rest should be encouraged. 5) With an increase in episodes of exertional dyspnea with advancing gestational age, the beneficial effect of oxygen on pulmonary vascular resistance and shunt flow[58,59] should be utilized. 6) Blood gases should be checked regularly to detect a possible shunt increase. 7) Congestive heart failure, if it develops should be treated in a routine way with digitalis and diuretics. 8) Fetal well-being should be followed throughout pregnancy with routine antepartum testing such as the measurement of fetal growth by ultrasound, oxytocin challenge tests, and biochemical evaluations. 9) Premature delivery should be anticipated. 10) Spontaneous labor is preferable to induction. Such a policy should decrease the chance for prematurity and cesarean section delivery. It should, however, be recognized that in some smaller institutions the risk of a night delivery with incomplete or diminished medical staff might outweigh the risk of an induction. In cases of an elective induction, previous evaluation of fetal lung maturity is requisite. 11) Labor and delivery should occur in an intensive care set-up next to an immediately available operating room. 12) No patient with ES should go through labor, delivery, and puerperium without a Swan-Ganz catheter in place. In addition, cardiac monitoring of the mother is essential in order to recognize life-threatening arrhythmias. 13) Anticoagulation with heparin should be stopped with the onset of labor and reinstituted as soon as feasible after delivery. 14) Based on the work by Midwall et al,[59] the administration of high concentrations of oxygen is recommended. Epidural anesthesia represents the best method of anesthesia for these patients.[59] The repeated determination of blood gases during labor, delivery, and the puerperium is essential to detect changes in shunt flow. Elective low forceps delivery seems preferable to normal spontaneous vaginal delivery in order to shorten the second stage of labor. Vaginal delivery seems preferable to cesarean section delivery; however, cesarean section does not seem contraindicated. 15) A postpartum hospitalization of at least two weeks is suggested.

Since the report by Gleicher et al,[10] only very limited additional information has been published. Jewett[60] reported an additional case of pregnancy in a woman with ES that resulted in maternal death. Jewett stated in his report that the responsibility for the mother's death could be assigned to the patient and her husband, who declined good medical advice and decided to accept the risk of pregnancy, a conclusion not necessarily shared by Gleicher and Jaffin.[61] Spinnato et al[12] recently reported the successful management of a pregnant patient with ES delivered by elective cesarean section conducted under continuous epidural anesthesia. This case represented the first elective cesarean section delivery in a patient with ES successfully conducted under such anesthesia. The authors' conclusion that an elective cesarean delivery may represent an acceptable method of delivery for patients with ES at risk for protracted labor remains to be confirmed. Their experience, however, further confirms the relative safety of epidural anesthesia in patients with ES.

With the exception of primary pulmonary hypertension, ES represents the condition with the single most awkward maternal prognosis in association with pregnancy. Even though pregnancy in these patients does seem clearly contraindicated, retrospective studies, which form the basis for such recommendations, have obvious limitations. It remains to be seen how modern medical hemodynamic management of the patient with ES will alter her prognosis. Because no single institution is able to accumulate satisfactory numbers for a prospective study, a large collaborative effort seems indicated.

XII. PREVENTION OF INFECTIVE ENDOCARDITIS IN PATIENTS WITH CHD

Despite excellent advances in antimicrobial therapy and cardiovascular surgery, infective endocarditis is still a serious complication with significant morbidity and mortality. Even though there is no proof that prophylactic antibiotics prevent infective endocarditis in humans, it seems prudent to administer antibiotics prophylactically to patients with congenital heart disease or acquired valvular defects in situations where bacteremia is highly predictable. Congenital cardiac anomalies, with the exception of secundum-type atrial septal defect, are susceptible to endocarditis. Patients with CHD who are at high risk of developing infective endocardits should take measures to avoid or minimize potential sources of bacteremia. As poor dental hygiene and dental disease could induce bacteremia, the highest level of oral health should be maintained; however, the use of oral irrigation devices should be avoided as this procedure can also cause bacteremia. Orotracheal intubation should be preferred to nasotracheal intubation in patients with high susceptibility to bacterial endocarditis. If bronchoscopy must be performed, the fiberoptic rather than the rigid bronchoscope should be used. As the incidence of bacteremia is largely determined by the presence or absence of urinary infection, urine should be made sterile prior to urologic procedures.[62] The American Heart Association, in its most recent committee report,[63] recommends antibiotic prophylaxis with all dental procedures that are likely to cause gingival bleeding, including routine professional cleaning. In addition, prophylactic treatment was recommended before certain procedures on the upper respiratory tract, including tonsillectomy or adenoidectomy, bronchoscopy, and surgical procedures involving the respiratory tract. Prophylactic therapy is also recommended before surgery or instrumentation of the genitourinary tract, the lower gastrointestinal tract, the gallbladder and in cases of obstetrical infections such as septic abortion or peripartum infection. Infective endocarditis in an uncomplicated vaginal delivery is extremely rare. Sugrue et al[64] have recently reported an incidence of 0.09% in 2,165 women with rheumatic or congenital heart disease, and Marquis found no case of endocarditis after normal delivery in over 1,750 cardiac patients during a 25-year period.[65] Considering the low incidence of endocarditis and the fact that routine antibiotic prophylaxis may be harmful, as antibiotic resistance can occur enhancing the risk of antibiotic-resistant endocarditis,[66,67] the American Heart Association has not recommended prophylactic antibiotic therapy before uncomplicated vaginal delivery unless the patient has a prosthetic valve, in which case the incidence of endocarditis is higher and the consequences can be devastating.[65] Despite the American Heart Association's recommendation against routine prophylaxis, antibiotic prophylaxis at time of normal uncomplicated labor and delivery is not an uncommon practice in many hospitals. Furthermore, McNulty et al, in a recent communication, have suggested the use of prophylaxis at the start of uncomplicated labor with continuation of the regimen for two days after delivery in all patients who are susceptible to endocarditis. These authors feel that the relatively low risk and expense of antibiotic proplylaxis and the poor prognosis associated with endocarditis justify their recommendations.[68]

Increased risks for endocarditis have been suggested after manual removal of the placenta, and antibiotic prophylaxis seems therefore indicated in this situation.[65,69]

XIII. SUMMARY

Most patients with mild to moderate congenital heart disease tolerate pregnancy, labor, and delivery well. The management of these patients can be almost routine. Patients with more severe problems require frequent assessment and reassurance by the obstetrician and cardiologist, who should work as a team. Therapy consists of limitation of physical activity, avoidance of excessive weight gain, reduced salt intake, immediate treatment of infection, diuretics for fluid retention, close observation for signs or symptoms of latent congestive heart failure with prompt treatment, and control of dysrhythmias with digitialis, quinidine, or propranolol.

Induction of labor and cesarean sections are indicated only for obstetrical reasons and not for cardiac reasons. The second stage of labor should be as short as possible. Patients with uncorrected cyanotic congenital heart disease or with Eisenmenger's syndrome constitute a high-risk group and should be advised against pregnancy or considered for therapeutic abortion if pregnancy has occurred. It is critical that the patient understand the maternal and fetal risk associated with pregnancy.

If total surgical correction has been performed without significant residual, then the tolerance to pregnancy is essentially normal.

Sterilization is recommended only in patients with severe cardiac disability who cannot be controlled by medical or surgical therapy. Cardiovascular surgery during pregnancy should rarely be indicated. Only in a patient who refuses therapeutic abortion and has severe cardiac disability not responding to optimal medical therapy should cardiovascular surgery even be considered.

Prophylactic antibiotics should be employed at the time of delivery if indicated. Hemodynamic and electrocardiographic monitoring should be used in high-risk patients for early identification and correction of hemodynamic or electrical instability.

XIV. ACKNOWLEDGMENTS

We gratefully acknowledge the expert secretarial assistance of Ellen Mansour and Lyndsay Atchison in the preparation of this manuscript.

XV. REFERENCES

1. Szekely P, Julian DG. Heart disease and pregnancy. Current Problems Cardiol. 1979; 4:1–74.
2. Rush RW, Verjans M, Spracklen FH. Incidence of heart disease in pregnancy. S Afr Med J. 1979; 55:808–810.
3. Naeye RL, Hagstrom JW, Talmadge BA. Postpartum death with maternal congenital heart disease. Circulation. 1967; 36:304–312.
4. Szekely P, Snaith L. Heart disease and pregnancy. Edinburgh and London: Churchill-Livingston, 1974:29–39.
5. Neilson G, Galea EG, Blunt A. Congenital heart disease and pregnancy. Med J Aust. 1970; 30:1086–1088.
6. Chew PC, Chew SC, Lee YK, et al. Congenital heart disease in pregnancy. Singapore Med J. 1975; 16:97–99.
7. Etheridge MJ, Pepperell RJ. Heart disease and pregnancy at the Royal Women's Hospital. Med J Aust. 1971; 2:277–281.
8. Ong HC, Puraviappan AP, Sinnathuray TA, et al. Pattern of heart disease and pregnancy seen in a Malaysian hospital. Singapore Med J. 1978; 19:93–97.
9. Schaefer G, Arditi LI, Solomon HA, et al. Congenital heart disease and pregnancy. Clin Obstet Gynecol. 1968; 11:1048–1063.
10. Gleicher N, Midwall J, Hochberger D, Jaffin H. Eisenmenger's syndrome in pregnancy. Obstet Gynecol Surv. 1979; 34:721–741.
11. Talwar KK, Wahi PL. Pregnancy with heart disease. J Assoc Physicians India. 1979; 27:995–1002.
12. Spinnato JA, Kraynack BJ, Cooper MW. Eisenmenger's syndrome in pregnancy: Epidural anesthesia for elective cesarean section. N Engl J Med. 1981; 304:1215–1217.
13. Harvey WP. Auscultatory features of congenital heart disease. In: Roberts WC, ed. Congenital Heart Disease in Adults. Philadelphia: F.A. Davis Co., 1979:53–90.
14. Ellison CR, Sloss CJ. Electrocardiographic features of congenital heart disease in the adult. In Roberts WC, ed. Congenital Heart Disease in Adults. Philadelphia: F.A. Davis Co., 1979:119–138.
15. Elliott LP. Radiologic differentiation of the common congenital malformations of the heart and great vessels. In: Roberts WC, ed. Congenital Heart Disease in Adults. Philadelphia: F.A. Davis Co., 1979:91–118.
16. Henry WL. Evaluation of older children and adults with congenital heart disease by M-mode and cross-sectional echocardiography. In: Roberts WC, ed. Congenital Heart Disease in Adults. Philadelphia: F.A. Davis Co., 1979:139–171.
17. Veray FX, Cibes-Hernandez JJ, Pelegrina I. Heart disease in pregnancy. Obstet Gynecol. 1968; 32:424–431.
18. Etheridge MJ. Heart disease and pregnancy. Med J Aust. 1968; 2:1172–1174.
19. Espino-Vela J, Alvarado-Toroa. A natural history of atrial septal defect. Cardiovasc Clin. 1971; 2:103–125.
20. Szekely P, Snaith. L. Heart disease and pregnancy. Edinburgh and London: Churchill Livingstone, 1974:155.
21. Mendelson CL. Cardiac Disease in Pregnancy. Philadelphia: F.A. Davis, Co., 1960:150–151.
22. Angle MA, Kline SA. Ventricular septal defect in the adult. In: Roberts WC, ed. Congenital Heart Disease in Adults. Philadelphia: F.A. Davis, Co., 1979:279–305.
23. Stevenson JG, Kawabori I, Guntheroth WG. Differentiation of ventricular septal defects from mitral regurgitation by pulsed Doppler echocardiography. Circulation. 1977; 50:14–18.
24. Mendelson CL. Cardiac Disease in Pregnancy. Philadelphia: F.A. Davis, Co., 1960:151–154.
25. Zitnik RS, Brandenburg RO, Sheldon R, Wallace KB. Pregnancy and open heart surgery. Circulation. 1969; 39(Suppl):257–262.
26. Kelly DT. Patent ductus arteriosus in adults. In Roberts WC, ed. Congenital Heart Disease in Adults. Philadelphia: F.A. Davis, Co., 1979:321–326.
27. Knapp RC, Arditi LI. Pregnancy complicated by patent ductus arteriosus with reversal of flow. NY J Med. 1967; 67:573–577.
28. Friedman WF, Novak V, Johnson AD. Congenital aortic stenosis. In: Roberts WC, ed. Congenital Heart Disease in Adults. Philadelphia: F.A. Davis, Co., 1979:235–251.
29. Arias F, Pineda J. Aortic stenosis and pregnancy. J Reprod Med. 1978; 4:229–232.
30. Maron BJ. Coarctation of the aorta in the adult. In: Roberts WC, ed. Congenital Heart Disease in Adults. Philadelphia: F.A. Davis, Co., 1979:311–319.
31. Ueland K. Cardiovascular diseases complicating pregnancy. Clin Obstet Gynecol. 1978; 21:429–442.
32. Szekely P, Snaith L. Heart disease and pregnancy. Edinburgh and London: Churchill Livingstone, 1974:167–169.
33. Deal K, Wooley CF. Coarctation of the aorta and pregnancy. Ann Intern Med. 1973; 78:706–710.
34. Shanahan WR, Romney SL, Currens JH. Coarc-

tation of the aorta and pregnancy; Report of ten cases with twenty-four pregnancies. JAMA. 1958; 167:275–280.
35. Barash PG, Hobbins JC, Hook R, Stansel HC Jr, Whittemore R, Hehre FW. Management of coarctation of the aorta during pregnancy. J Thorac Cardiovasc Surg. 1975; 69:781–784.
36. Wachtel HL, Czarnecki SW. Coarctation of the aorta and pregnancy. Am Heart J. 1966; 72:251–254.
37. Goodwin JF. Pregnancy and coarctation of the aorta. Lancet. 1958; 1:16–20.
38. Kaplan S, Adolph RO. Pulmonic valve stenosis in adults. In: Roberts WC, ed. Congenital Heart Disease in Adults. Philadelphia: F.A. Davis, Co., 1979:327–339.
39. Mendelson CL. Cardiac Disease in Pregnancy. Philadelphia: F.A. Davis, Co., 1960; 132–135.
40. Garson H, McNamara DG, Cooley DA. Tetralogy of Fallot in adults. In: Roberts WC, ed. Congenital Heart Disease in Adults. Philadelphia: F.A. Davis, Co., 1979:341–364.
41. Campbell M. Natural history of cyanotic malformations and comparison of all common cardiac malformation. Br Heart J. 1972; 34:3–8.
42. Ikeda M, Hirosawa K. Tetralogy of Fallot. Circulation. 1968; 38(Suppl V):21.
43. Szekely P, Snaith L. Heart disease and pregnancy. Edinburgh and London: Churchill Livingstone, 1974:159.
44. Mendelson CL: Cardiac Disease in Pregnancy. Philadelphia: F.A. Davis, Co., 1960:154–159.
45. Shrestha NK, Arora R, Padmavati S. Multiple pregnancies in a patient of Fallot's tetralogy. Indian Heart J. 1979; 31:58–60.
46. Kahler RL: Cardiac disease. In: Burrow GN, Ferris TF, eds. Medical Complications During Pregnancy. Philadelphia: W.B. Saunders, 1975; 105–145.
47. Loh TF, Tan NC. Fallot's tetralogy and pregnancy: A report of a successful pregnancy after complete correction. Med J Aust. 1971; 2:141–145.
48. Lewis BS, Rogers NMA, Gotsman MS. Successful pregnancy after repair of Fallot's tetralogy. S Afr Med J. 1970; 46:934–936.
49. Yuzpe AA, Sanghvi VR, Johnson FL, Robinson JG. Successful pregnancy in a patient with single ventricle and other congenital cardiac anomalies. Can Med Assoc J. 1970; 103:1073–1075.
50. Graham TP, Friesinger GC. Complex cyanotic congenital heart disease in adults. In: Roberts WC, ed. Congenital Heart Disease in Adults. Philadelphia. F.A. Davis, Co., 1979:383–405.
51. Burwell CS, Metcalfe J. Heart Disease and Pregnancy. Boston: Little Brown Co., 1958:222–224.
52. Collins ML, Leal J, Thompson NJ. Tricuspid atresia and pregnancy. Obstet Gynecol. 1977; 50:72–73.
53. Simon DL, Lustberg A. A case of truncus arteriosus communis compatible with full-term pregnancy. Am Heart J. 1951; 42:617–623.
54. Johnston DW, Elkayam U. Personal communication.
55. Seeds JW, Cefalo RC. Pregnancy with congenital heart disease: A two-chambered heart. Am J Obstet Gynecol. 1977; 127:213–214.
56. Neilson G, Galea EG, Blunt A. Eisenmenger syndrome in pregnancy. Med J Aust. 1971; 1:431–434.
57. Pitts JA, Crosby WM, Bosta LL. Eisenmerger's syndrome in pregnancy: Does heparin prophylaxis improve the maternal mortality rate? Am Heart J. 1977; 93:321–326.
58. Coffer FD. Eisenmenger's complex and pregnancy. Obstet Gynecol. 1967; 29:235–240.
59. Midwall J, Jaffin H, Herman MV, Kupersmith J. Shunt flow and pulmonary hemodynamics during labor and delivery in the Eisenmenger's syndrome. Am J Cardiol. 1978; 42:299–303.
60. Jewett JF. Committee on maternal welfare. Pulmonary hypertension and pre-eclampsia. N Engl J Med. 1979; 301:1063–1064.
61. Gleicher N, Jaffin H. Eisenmenger's syndrome and pregnancy. N Engl J Med. 1980; 302:751–752.
62. Everett ED, Hirschmann JV. Transient bacteremia and endocarditis prophylaxis. A review. Medicine. 1977; 56:61–77.
63. Kaplan EL, Anthony BF, Bisno A, Durack D, Houser H, Millard D, Sanford J, Shulman ST, Stillerman M, Taranta A, Wenger N. Prevention of bacterial endocarditis. Circulation. 1977; 56:139A–143A.
64. Sugrue D, Blake S, Troy P, McDonald D. Antibiotic prophylaxis against infective endocarditis in normal delivery is it necessary? Br. Heart J. 1980; 44:499–502.
65. Marquis RM. Bacterial endocarditis following delivery in women with heart disease. In Anguissola AB, Puddu V, eds. Cardiologia d'Oggi. Turin: C.G. Edizioni Medico Scientifiche, 1975:278.
66. Garrod LP, Waterworth P. The risk of dental extraction during penicillin treatment. Br Heart J. 1962; 24:39–46.
67. Sprunt K, Redman W, Leidy G. Penicillin resistant alpha streptococci in pharynx of patients given oral penicillin. Pediatrics. 1968; 42:957–968.
68. McAnulty JH, Metcalfe J, Ueland K. General guidelines in the management of cardiac disease. Clin Obstet Gynecol. 1981; 24:773–788.
69. Lein JN, Stander RW. Subacute bacterial endocarditis following obstetric and gynecologic procedures. Report of 8 cases. Obstet Gynecol. 1959; 13:568–573.

M.V

Rheumatic Heart Disease and Pregnancy

Kent Ueland, MD

I. INTRODUCTION

During the last three decades the incidence of heart disease complicating pregnancy has declined from 2.5% to 3.5% in the 1940s and 1950s to the present rate of 0.5–1.5%. Although rheumatic heart disease continues to be the most common form reported by most centers, congenital heart disease is now being encountered with increasing frequency. The reduction in rheumatic heart disease is illustrated by the report of Szekely et al in 1973[1]; they showed a decline in incidence from 3.5% in 1942–1947 to 0.7% in 1966–1969. There is reason to assume that this trend is characteristic for this country as well, as active rheumatic fever is disappearing in the United States.[2–4] In all likelihood, these logical trends derive from multiple factors, including 1) early and more effective treatment of streptococcal infections, 2) generally improved nutrition and general living conditions, 3) better rheumatic fever prophylaxis, 4) a decrease in the prevalence and severity of acute rheu-

Cardiac Problems in Pregnancy, pages 79–86

matic fever in the Western Hemisphere, and 5) advances in medical and surgical management of the more severe forms of congenital cardiovascular diseases allowing affected women to reach childbearing age. Nonetheless, heart disease, when placed in perspective, continues to be the leading nonobstetric cause of maternal death.[5]

II. ACUTE RHEUMATIC FEVER

Active rheumatic fever is a rare but serious complication of pregnancy. It remains a problem throughout much of the world but, as mentioned earlier, it is disappearing in the United States.[4] The low incidence of active rheumatic fever in pregnancy may be influenced by the difficulties encountered in making the diagnosis. It appears that the endocrine changes of pregnancy modify the symptoms and signs of the disease, and some of the laboratory criteria ordinarily used to assess rheumatic activity are not reliable because of pregnancy-induced changes in the expected normal values. However, the diagnosis of rheumatic fever should be considered when a pregnant woman develops unexplained fever, joint and chest pains, and/or congestive failure.

There is evidence in the literature that rheumatic fever is encountered more frequently during pregnancy.[5–10] The serious nature of active rheumatic fever with myocarditis must be emphasized, because it can be associated with fetal and maternal mortality.[11] If congestive failure occurs, the disease is almost universally fatal in pregnancy.[12]

Chorea gravidarum also seems to be more prevalent during pregnancy and may be especially severe, resulting in spontaneous abortion, preterm labor, intrauterine fetal death, and maternal death.[6,7]

The treatment of rheumatic activity in pregnancy is similar to that in the nonpregnant patient. In patients with severe rheumatic carditis steroids appear to be indicated. Antibiotic prophylaxis against rheumatic fever should be used in all women with rheumatic heart disease, and this should be continued throughout pregnancy.

III. CHRONIC RHEUMATIC HEART DISEASE

A. Mitral Stenosis

The most common rheumatic valvular lesion in pregnant women continues to be mitral stenosis. Historically, this is also the most hazardous during pregnancy because of the unique interaction between the effects of the lesion on pulmonary hemodynamics and those related to pregnancy, especially during labor and delivery. The primary hemodynamic defect is obstruction to blood flow from the left atrium to the left ventricle during diastole. The specific dangerous cardiovascular changes accompanying pregnancy include 1) an increase in cardiac output, 2) an increase in heart rate, 3) an increase in blood volume, and 4) an increase in left atrial irritability. In addition, patients with mitral valve disease have also been shown to have an increase in pulmonary capillary blood volume. The combination of the latter and the normally expected hypervolemia of pregnancy can produce a disproportionate rise in pulmonary vascular pressure and result in acute pulmonary edema.[13] This rise in pulmonary capillary blood volume does not occur in normal pregnant women or in those with aortic valvular disease.

The times of maximum risk for these women are late pregnancy, labor, and the early puerperium. This seems entirely logical when considering the fact that the hypervolemia accompanying pregnancy is progressive to term, the heart rate continues to rise to term, and the cardiac output is maintained at essentially peak levels during the last trimester. During labor and immediately following delivery significant increased demands are placed on the heart, and the risks of pulmonary edema are even greater. The data in the literature support the contention that this is the most dangerous time. In the large series of patients with rheumatic heart disease reported by Szekely et al,[1] 75% of the 225 women who developed "heart failure" did so in the third trimester of pregnancy and in the early puerperium. Forty percent of such cases occurred after 36 weeks of gestation and during the puerperium. In maternal mortality data from California, reported by Hibbard in 1975,[5] 21 of 28 deaths from rheumatic heart disease occurred in the last trimester of pregnancy or postpartum. Of the 20 patients with either pure mitral stenosis or mixed mitral stenosis–mitral regurgitation, 14 died in the third trimester or postpartum. Finally, in two large series of patients reported with pregnancies following mitral valvotomy,[14,15] five of 15 deaths occurred in the third trimester, and nine occurred in the early puerperium. The remaining death occurred at the time of a therapeutic abortion.

Overall, the risk of dying in all patients with mitral stenosis, regardless of functional classification, approximates 1%.[11] If one considers the more severe cases (class III and class IV, New York Heart Association Functional Classification) the maternal mortality reaches 4–5%. If atrial fibrillation is present, this figure reaches 14–17%, and if fibrillation begins during pregnancy, 72% of patients develop heart failure.[16] Even in patients who have had mitral commissurotomy prior to pregnancy the chance of dying during pregnancy is as high as 2–3%.[14,15]

The more recent data reported by Szekely et al[1] are encouraging, as these authors show a much more favorable outcome in patients with rheumatic heart disease treated in the 1960s than in those treated in the 1940s and 1950s. They concluded that the reason for this trend was a change in the natural course of the disease, improved medical management of the more severe cases, and the introduction of cardiac surgery in selected cases.

In patients with mitral stenosis who are severely compromised (N.Y. Heart Association classes III and IV), digitalis therapy is recommended for two reasons. First, it effects a slowing of heart rate, and patients with mitral stenosis depend on diastolic time for flow of blood through the tight mitral valve. Second, pregnant women appear to be more susceptible to cardiac arrhythmias, particularly atrial tachyarrhythmias.[8] Compromised patients with either mitral stenosis or regurgitation are susceptible to atrial fibrillation. A fully digitalized patient who develops atrial fibrillation will usually not exhibit a rapid ventricular response, and hence the danger of congestive failure is circumvented. If cardioversion is necessary, it can be employed without apparent danger to the mother or fetus.[17]

In general, thiazide diuretics should be withheld in patients with rheumatic heart disease during pregnancy. This recommendation is based on the fact that these agents may have potential harmful effects on the fetus and neonate. Severe electrolyte imbalance, thrombocytopenia, liver damage, and death have all been reported with the prolonged use of these drugs.[17] However, diuretics should not be withheld when they are indicated for treatment of pulmonary congestion.

With a more thorough understanding of cardiopulmonary physiology as it pertains to pregnancy, labor, and delivery, management of the patient with mitral stenosis can be more appropriately directed.

B. Mitral Regurgitation

Rheumatic fever is but one of many causes of mitral regurgitation, and in the United States it is most likely not the most common etiology in young adults. If it is found in association with mitral stenosis, the regurgitant lesion is almost certainly a result of rheumatic fever. Echocardiography may help determine the etiology by showing evidence of bacterial endocarditis, rheumatic mitral stenosis, prolapse of the mitral valve, or idiopathic hypertrophic subaortic stenosis.

Patients with mitral regurgitation often remain asymptomatic for years, and it is rare for this lesion to produce problems during pregnancy. However, when the mitral regurgitation becomes severe and there is significant left atrial enlargement and an elevated left atrial pressure, pulmonary vascular congestion may develop. Pregnant women with severe mitral regurgitation are at risk of developing atrial fibrillation and subsequently the formation of atrial thrombi. Since the risk of developing atrial fibrillation in pregnancy is high, prophylactic digitalis therapy is recommended to decrease the risk of a rapid ventricular response should fibrillation occur. When there is evidence that the mitral regurgitation is due to rheumatic fever, antibiotic prophylaxis is indicated to prevent streptococcal infection.

C. Aortic Stenosis

Aortic stenosis is encountered infrequently during pregnancy. It is more common in men than in women. Pulmonary congestion does not appear to be a major problem during pregnancy, but hypovolemia, especially in association with interruption of pregnancy, may pose a real threat to maternal life.[18] In 1970 Arias and Pineda[18] reported a maternal mortality of 17% and a fetal mortality as high as 32% in a small series of pregnant women with aortic stenosis. The highest maternal mortality (40%) occurred in patients undergoing therapeutic abortion.

If severe aortic stenosis is diagnosed prior to pregnancy, surgical correction is recommended. In most instances a commissurotomy will be sufficient. If a prosthesis is required, a heterograft valve rather than a mechanical prosthesis is favored in a woman contemplating pregnancy, as this may circumvent the need for long-term anticoagulation.

If a woman with severe aortic stenosis conceives a child, early therapeutic abortion should be offered as a therapeutic alternative. If undesirable, for whatever reasons, medical therapy should be promptly directed at limitation of physical activity. Since the critical problem in patients with severe aortic stenosis is the inability of the heart to maintain an adequate cardiac output, physical rest becomes crucial in order to meet some of the increased demands placed on the heart by pregnancy. If symptoms persist and are not controlled by restricted physical activity, aortic valve surgery should be considered during pregnancy as, perhaps, a safer alternative than a late therapeutic abortion, which is associated with a high maternal mortality.

In patients with severe aortic stenosis the maintenance of venous return is imperative. Any significant reduction may result in a dramatic drop in cardiac output and cause cerebral and cardiac ischemia. This places the patient at particular risk from such factors as "postural hypotension" late in pregnancy and in the early puerperium, blood loss during a therapeutic abortion or at delivery, and hypotension from anesthesia.

Prophylaxis against bacterial endocarditis at the time of labor and delivery is important in these susceptible women.

D. Aortic Regurgitation

Aortic regurgitation is a more common lesion in women of childbearing age than aortic stenosis. When it is due to rheumatic fever it is invariably associated with mitral valve damage. As with mitral regurgitation, aortic regurgitation is well tolerated during pregnancy. The increase in heart rate associated with pregnancy decreases the diastolic time for the regurgitant flow to the left ventricle and hence increases forward flow.

In the unusual circumstance where pulmonary congestion develops, restriction of physical activity becomes essential and therapy with sodium restriction, digitalis, and diuretics is indicated. Antibiotic prophylaxis during labor and delivery is advised.

IV. GENERAL GUIDELINES TO MEDICAL MANAGEMENT DURING PREGNANCY

A. Restriction of Physical Activity

Since cardiac demands are increased by pregnancy and cardiac capacity is diminished by the diseased heart, a favorable balance must be maintained between the work required of the heart and that which it is capable of performing. If this is not achieved, complications such as pulmonary edema (especially in patients with mitral stenosis) and heart failure may occur.

Cardiac performance in the failing heart may be improved by the cardiac glycosides. Cardiac surgery can also increase cardiac capacity. Although it has been shown that the maternal risks of valvotomy during pregnancy in patients with severe mitral stenosis are no greater than in those performed in the nonpregnant state,[18] in the author's experience, this procedure is seldom necessary during pregnancy. It should be limited to those few patients who have severe cardiac disability that is unresponsive to intensive medical management and who refuse therapeutic abortion or in the occasional patient with debilitating disease who is beyond the point during gestation when safe vaginal evacuation of the uterus is possible. This reasoning is based on the fact that, even though surgery is safe for the mother, the risks to the fetus are considerable, especially if open heart surgery becomes necessary. The best reported maternal and perinatal statistics are found in the series when medical management is primarily used and cardiovascular surgery is reserved for a small number of patients.[1,19]

B. Reassurance

The hemodynamic changes from fear and anxiety can be considerable. Therefore, it becomes important to counsel the patient and provide her with consistent and supportive medical information and emotional support. The cooperative efforts of both the cardiologist and the obstetrician are important so that she is given nonconflicting information and reassurance. Frequent visits to both throughout pregnancy are helpful.

C. Elastic Support

During pregnancy, especially during the last trimester, large fluctuations in maternal hemodynamics occur with changes in maternal position. Inferior vena caval occlusion occurs in most women lying supine in late pregnancy. Venous pooling in the legs occurs upon standing and sitting, and it is not unusual for a woman in the last few months of pregnancy to feel dizzy or at times become lightheaded and even faint when rapidly assuming the upright position. These large rapid fluctuations in cardiodynamics could have serious consequences in the patient with severe mitral or aortic stenosis.

To maintain venous return and to prevent pooling of large amounts of blood in the lower limbs, elastic support is recommended, preferably in the form of pressure-graded pantyhose. These should be used throughout pregnancy whenever the patient is ambulatory. Their use in the early puerperium is important because the veins of the legs are very distensible at that time.

D. Rheumatic Fever Prophylaxis

In patients with rheumatic heart disease antibiotic prophylaxis against streptococcal infection is recommended during pregnancy and during the childbearing years. The most effective prophylaxis is 1.2 million units of benzathine penicillin G intramuscularly every four weeks.[20] If the patient is allergic to penicillin, 1 gm daily of oral sulfadiazine is recommended. A recent report by Baskin and co-workers[21] showed that sulfadiazine can be safely used for rheumatic fever prophylaxis during pregnancy. They reviewed the hospital records of 94 infants born to mothers receiving sulfadiazine prophylaxis during pregnancy and found no increase in prematurity, hyperbilirubinemia, or kernicterus when compared with control infants in the same newborn nursery.

E. Bacterial Endocarditis Prophylaxis

When dental procedures and certain surgical procedures are anticipated in patients with rheumatic heart disease, short-term antibiotic prophylaxis is recommended to prevent bacterial endocarditis.[22] The issue of whether antibiotic prophylaxis should be given during labor and delivery is not entirely settled; however, in my opinion, since bacteremia has been reported following vaginal delivery and a rate in excess of 20% can occur with cesarean section,[23] it is recommended. The antibiotic combination of choice is ampicillin and gentamycin given intravenously or intramuscularly for three doses eight hours apart, beginning 30–60 minutes prior to delivery. This combination of antibiotics offers the broadest coverage for enterococci.

F. Prompt Antibiotic Treatment of All Infections

Infections of any kind that cause pyrexia, and a resultant tachycardia, can place a significant additional burden on the diseased heart. Therefore, appropriate antibiotics should be used early and in instances of upper respiratory infection as prophylaxis against lower respiratory complications.

G. Sodium Restriction

A modest limitation to 2 gm of sodium daily is suggested. Rarely should there be a need for further restriction. Besides, the sodium needs of pregnancy are substantial, and a further long-term restriction may prove harmful. More stringent limitation would also make it difficult for the pregnant woman to maintain an adequate protein intake. The recommended daily sodium intake is basically one that can be met by no added salt at the table and by avoiding extremely salty foods.

H. Iron Supplementation

All pregnant women require some form of iron supplementation to meet the increased iron needs of pregnancy. These requirements cannot be met by diet alone; a minimum daily supplement of 60 mg of elemental iron should be provided. If taken regularly and utilized appropriately, this will maintain a normal hemoglobin level throughout pregnancy and prevent the "physiological anemia of pregnancy."

V. MANAGEMENT DURING LABOR AND DELIVERY

It appears safest to allow patients with rheumatic heart disease to go into labor spontaneously at term. During labor it is important to maintain patient comfort. Intravenous analgesia can be used in early labor, and a lumbar epidural is recommended once the active phase of the first stage of labor has been entered. Epinephrine should not be added to the local anesthetic solution, as this may have a direct inhibiting effect on uterine contractions and can cause significant problems with hypotension.[24] To allow for a complete block, the local anesthetic can be injected while the patient is on her side, after which she should rotate from side to side.

The entire labor should be conducted with the patient on her side. This position, combined with epidural anesthesia, will result in the most stable maternal hemodynamic state.[24] In the second stage of labor, maternal bearing-down efforts should be avoided because they produce large fluctuations in maternal hemodynamics. When deemed safe obstetrically, the judicious use of forceps is indicated.

Maternal hemodynamic monitoring during labor should include a continuous ECG, frequent blood pressure determinations, and, depending on the severity of the disease, a central venous pressure catheter or a Swan-Ganz catheter, together with continuous intraarterial pressure measurements.

In the patient with severely compromised disease or with pulmonary edema, there is some evidence that delivery by cesarean section under balanced general anesthesia may be safest.[25] Since this allows for a planned daytime procedure with maximum utilization of equipment and personnel, this would seem to be a reasonable approach. Maternal hemodynamic stability is reasonably well maintained during surgery with this anesthetic technique.[26] Similar results can be achieved with epidural anesthesia without epinephrine.[27]

During the early puerperium early ambulation is encouraged, but only under close supervision and with appropriate elastic support for the legs.

Following delivery, oxytocin must not be given by bolus injection because of its significant cardiovascular effects.[28] Also, the ergot alkaloids should only be used with caution, as they have been shown to cause hypertension, as well as an elevation in central venous pressure.[28]

VI. PERINATAL MORBIDITY AND MORTALITY

In the large series of patients with chronic rheumatic heart disease presented recently by Szekely and Snaith[29] there has been a progressive decline in perinatal mortality. At the Newcastle General Hospital the mortality rate has fallen from 8.8% between 1942 and 1951 to 3.5% between 1962 and 1971. Improved medical and surgical care accounts for a great deal of this improved outcome, but the changing pattern of the disease itself is also responsible, as there are now very few serious complications from rheumatic heart disease during pregnancy.

Infants born at term to mothers with asymptomatic or mildly symptomatic heart disease are smaller than those born to mothers with normal hearts.[30] The incidence of prematurity, as determined by both gestational age and by weight, is also increased. It appears that, even with mild disease, the heart is incapable of meeting the increased demands of pregnancy, and the uterine circulation suffers. This is particularly true for patients with mitral stenosis. These women seem incapable of increasing cardiac output significantly at rest during pregnancy, and values well below those normally expected are found. Furthermore, with exercise this disparity increases.[30] Thus, limitation of maternal physical activity to decrease the demand on the heart may be most beneficial for fetal growth and development.

VII. THE EFFECT OF PREGNANCY ON THE NATURAL HISTORY OF RHEUMATIC HEART DISEASE

Pregnancy, if survived, does not appear to shorten the life expectancy of women with rheumatic heart disease, and it does not appear to exert any permanent deleterious effects. In 1980 Chesley[31] reported on the long-term follow-up (from 1931 to 1943) of 134 women who were classified as having functionally severe rheumatic cardiac disease and surviving pregnancies. These women were traced to 1975. Ninety-three percent had died at the time of follow-up, a yearly exponential rate of 6.3%. Thorough analysis of the data failed to show any evidence of a delayed adverse effect of pregnancy. But Chesley issues a word of caution: "provided that the patient survives the gestation." Similar conclusions were reached by Handjani et al,[32] who studied 55 women with rheumatic heart disease who had five or more pregnancies. There was no maternal mortality. Their conclusion was that grand multiparity does not seem to alter the remote prognosis in patients with rheumatic heart disease if adequate medical care is administered.

VIII. REFERENCES

1. Szekely P, Turner R, Snaith L. Pregnancy and the changing pattern of rheumatic heart disease. Br Heart J. 1973; 35:1293.
2. Bland EF. Declining severity of rheumatic fever: A comparative study of the past few decades. N Engl J Med. 1960; 262:599.
3. Krause RM. The influence of infection on the geography of heart disease. Circulation. 1979; 60:972.
4. Wilson MG, Lim WN, Birch AM. The decline of rheumatic fever. Recurrence rates of rheumatic fever among 782 children for twenty-one consecutive calendar years (1936–1956). J Chronic Dis. 1958; 7:183.
5. Hibbard LT. Maternal mortality due to cardiac disease. Clin Obstet Gynecol. 1975; 18:27.
6. Clinch J. Chorea gravidarum. Hosp Med. 1967; 2:317.
7. Lewis BV, Parsons M. Chorea gravidarum. Lancet. 1966; 1:284.
8. Mendelson CL. Cardiac Disease in Pregnancy. Philadelphia: F.A. Davis, 1960:114.
9. Ueland K, Metcalfe J. Acute rheumatic fever in pregnancy. Am J Obstet Gynecol. 1966; 95:586.
10. Beresford OD, Ram AN. Chorea gravidarum. J Obstet Gynecol Br Empire. 1950; 57:66.
11. Szekely P, Snaith L. In: Heart Disease in Pregnancy. Edinburgh: Churchill Livingstone, 1974:48.
12. Roess TJ. Acute rheumatic fever with carditis in pregnancy. Report of a case and review of the literature. N Engl J Med. 1958; 258:605.
13. Gazioglu K, Kaltreider NL, Rosen M, and Yu PN. Pulmonary function during pregnancy in normal women and in patients with cardiopulmonary disease. Thorax. 1970; 25:455.
14. Schenker JG, Polishuk WZ. Pregnancy following mitral valvotomy; a survey of 182 patients. Obstet Gynecol. 1968; 32:214.
15. Wallace WA, Harken DE, Ellis LB. Pregnancy following closed mitral valvuloplasty; a long-term study with remarks covering the necessity for careful cardiac management. JAMA 1971; 217:297.
16. Szekely P. Snaith L. Atrial fibrillation and pregnancy. Br Med J. 1961; 1407.
17. Ueland K, McAnulty JH, Ueland FR, Metcalfe J. Special consideration in the use of cardiovascular drugs. Clin Obstet Gynecol. 1981: (in press).
18. Arias F, Pineda J. Aortic stenosis in pregnancy. J Reprod Med. 1970; 20:239.
19. Gilchrist AR. Cardiological problems in younger women: Including those of pregnancy and the puerperium. Br Med J. 1963; 1:209.
20. Kaplan EL, Bisno A, Facklam R, Gordis L, Houser GB, Jackson WH, Millard HD, Shulman ST, Taranta AV, Wannamaker LW. Prevention of rheumatic fever. Circulation. 1977; 55:1.
21. Baskin CG, Law S, Wenger NK. Sulfadiazine rheumatic fever prophylaxis during pregnancy: Does it increase the risk of kernicterus in the newborn? Cardiology. 1980; 65:222.
22. Kaplan EL, Anthony BF, Bisno A, Durack D, Houser H, Millard HD, Sanford J, Shulman ST, Stillerman M, Taranta A, Wenger N. Prevention of bacterial endocarditis. Circulation. 1977; 56:139A.
23. Eschenbach D, Ueland K. Unpublished data, 1981.
24. Ueland K. Intrapartum management of the cardiac patient. Clin Perinatol. 1981; 8:155.
25. Ferraris G, Gambotto C: Cesarean section as the method of choice for patients with cardiac decompensation. Minerva Gynecol. 1962; 14:198.
26. Ueland K, Hansen J, Eng M, Kalappa R, Parer JT. Maternal cardiovascular dynamics V. Cesarean section under thiopental nitrous oxide and succinylcholine anesthesia. Am J Obstet Gynecol. 1970; 108:615.
27. Ueland K, Akamatsu TF, Eng M, Bonica JJ, Hansen JM. Maternal cardiovascular dynamics VI. Cesarean section under epiduran anesthesia without epinephrine. Am J Obstet Gynecol. 1972; 114:775.
28. Hendricks CH, Brenner WE. Cardiovascular effects of oxytocic drugs used postpartum. Am J Obstet Gynecol. 1970; 108:751.
29. Szekely P. Snaith L. Cardiac disorders. Clin Obstet Gynecol. 1977; 4:265.
30. Ueland K, Nova MJ, Metcalfe J. Cardiorespiratory responses to pregnancy and exercise in normal women and patients with heart disease. Am J Obstet Gynecol. 1973; 115:4.
31. Chesley LC. Severe rheumatic cardiac disease and pregnancy; the ultimate prognosis. Am J Obstet Gynecol. 1980; 136:552.
32. Handjani AM, Bolandgray A, Eghtedari A. Grand multiparity and rheumatic heart disease. Obstet Gynecol. 1968; 32:210.

M.VI

Myocarditis and Pregnancy

Thomas C. Cesario, MD

I. VIRAL MYOCARDITIS IN PREGNANCY

Viral myocarditis is a relatively uncommon disorder. In 1947 Gore and Saphir[1] reviewed 40,000 autopsies and found 1,402 cases of myocarditis, 70 of which were associated with viral illnesses and 84 with possible viral illnesses. It was therefore concluded that, by the greatest possible estimate, viral myocarditis accounted for 0.38% of deaths. Since the criteria used in the study of Gore and Saphir were histological, doubts have been expressed about the validity of this estimate. Furthermore, even studies that have used such criteria as electrocardiograms or clinical status to estimate the incidence of myocarditis must be read with caution, as such indices may reflect processes that are not the direct result of viral myocardial invasion.[2] The only accurate means of establishing the diagnosis of viral myocarditis is to perform histological and virological studies directly on myocardial tissue. Because these restrictive criteria have seldom been met, the true incidence of viral myocarditis is not known.

Similar problems are encountered when specific viruses are suggested as causes for myocarditis. In his comprehensive review of this subject in 1971, Abelman[3] noted that fifteen true viruses have been associated with inflammatory myocardial disease. Table M.VI.1 lists the agents known to cause myocarditis in individuals other than neonates.

Abelman himself, however, stressed that only influenza, coxsackievirus, and polioviruses have been isolated from the heart with regularity. Burch et al[4] have also suggested that viruses may affect endocardium as well as myocardium.

The characteristic histologic changes of viral myocarditis consist of necrosis and cellular infiltrations, which may be associated with edema.[1,2,3] Inflammatory exudates are usually interstitial and probably represent the most characteristic lesions; however, viruses have been isolated from animal hearts without any microscopic abnormalities.[5] Pathological changes similar to those noted earlier have been described in "postpartum heart disease,"[6] where the predominant lesion has been described as myocardial degeneration with or without cellular infiltration.

Postpartum heart disease is a clinicopathological entity without a clear-cut single etiological association, and undoubtedly it includes at least some cases of viral infections of the heart. Postpartum heart disease generally refers to a syndrome of myocardial failure with onset

Cardiac Problems in Pregnancy, pages 87–91

TABLE M.VI.1. Viruses Implicated as Causes of Viral Myocarditis

Rubeola	Echovirus
Rubella	Hepatitis
Variola	Epstein-Barr virus
Vaccinia	Poliomyelitis
Varicella zoster	Arboviruses
Mumps	Yellow fever
Influenza	Rabies
Coxsackievirus	Adenoviruses

in the peripartum period, usually coming within six weeks of delivery.[6] In their monograph on the subject, Benchimol et al[7] refer to five categories of postpartum heart disease:

A) cases undoubtedly related to toxemia of pregnancy
B) cases probably related to toxemia of pregnancy
C) cases due to nonspecific myocarditis
D) cases with preexisting hypertension
E) cases due to specific myocarditis

With this classification, viral myocarditis occurring in pregnancy would best be categorized in the last group, but if the etiologic relationship to a specific virus were not recognized, the diagnostic classification might well be the third group.

In a series of comprehensive investigations of factors influencing the localization of viruses in the heart, Pearce[8] found that procedures reducing the myocardial oxygen supply were associated with a higher incidence and increased severity of viral cardiac lesions. Pearce mainly used pharmacological manipulations of the heart in his studies.

Subsequent studies have shown other factors predisposing to viral myocarditis. Kilbourne et al[9] in 1956 found that cortisone administration to mice infected with a strain of coxsackie B virus resulted in myocardial necrosis, whereas infection in the absence of the steroid produced only minimal focal lesions. Tilles et al,[5] using coxsackie A virus in mice, demonstrated that exercise (ie, swimming) resulted in a higher frequency of viral cardiac localization. Furthermore, viral titers were higher in the exercised heart muscles than in unexercised controls.

Finally, Farber et al[10] found that pregnant mice infected with encephalomyocarditis virus had higher titers of cardiac virus than did nonpregnant controls. This was of special interest in light of the fact that brain titers were equal between the two groups.

In summarizing the factors known to influence the cardiac localization of viruses, it is apparent that during pregnancy at least two factors may be operative to enhance the development of viral myocarditis. Thus the increased physiological stresses of pregnancy might lead to some myocardial hypoxia, and the increased activity of endocrine tissues might lead to excessive amounts of circulating steroids, factors acting in concert to enhance myocardial susceptibility. The studies of Farber et al provide evidence that pregnancy is more than a mere theoretical threat to provide circumstances conducive to the development of viral myocarditis.

Little information is available on the specific manifestations of myocarditis in pregnancy, so we review here the usual findings in the general population.

Clinically, myocarditis generally manifests itself either as rhythm disturbances or as cardiac failure.[3] Arrhythmias of either atrial or ventricular types can occur. These may range from a few ectopic beats to fatal tachycardias. Generally tachyarrhythmias predominate; however, conduction disturbances, including heart block, have been reported.[1] Enlargement of the heart, usually due to ventricular dilatation, may occur, and physical findings suggestive of heart failure such as gallop rhythms may be present. Furthermore, pericarditis may be signaled either by pericardial friction rubs or effusions.[3]

Abelmann,[3] in reviewing myocarditis, noted that when mice were infected with Trypanosoma cruzi, with the subsequent occurrence of parasitic myocarditis, the major physiological alteration appeared to be biventricular failure.[3] This was manifest as significant increases in end-diastolic pressures in both the right and the left ventricles. Abelmann noted that these observations were compatible with the available information from humans.

Laboratory support for a diagnosis of viral myocarditis can come from several procedures. Perhaps electrocardiographic changes are among the more common. In addition to rhythm disturbances already noted, the more common abnormalities include ST-T wave changes.[12] Sainani et al,[11] for example, noted such changes in all but one of their patients. Such ST-T wave changes would have to be considered nonspecific. On rare occasions ECG changes similar to those encountered in acute myocardial infarction have been described.[2]

Other useful laboratory procedures include determination of serum enzymes. Such enzymes as serum glutamic oxaloacetic transaminase (SGOT), serum glutamic pyruvic transaminase (SGPT), creatine phosphokinase (CPK), and lactic dehydrogenase (LDH) may be abnormal.

Noninvasive procedures, including echocardiography or radionuclide scintiscanning, may also be useful in the diagnosis of myocarditis, but more information is needed. Furthermore, because of potential hazards to the fetus, radioisotopes should generally be withheld in pregnancy.

Virologic confirmation of cardiac involvement can come only in a limited number of ways, as noted earlier. Lerner and Wilson[12] have recently reviewed the implications of these methods. They point out that high-order associations between viruses and myocarditis exist if a virus is isolated directly from myocardium, pericardium, or endocardium, or if virus is demonstrated at sites of pathological change by such techniques as fluorescent antibody staining. Moderate-order associations include clinical myocarditis associated with viral isolation from remote sites such as pharynx or stool with a concomitant fourfold increase in antibody titer. Low-order associations occur if the myocarditis is associated with a) virus isolations from pharynx or feces, b) a fourfold rise in antibody titer or, c) a single high titer (1:32 or greater) of specific IgM antibodies demonstrated against a given virus.

The prognosis of myocarditis may be somewhat variable. Bengtsson and Lamberger,[13] in reviewing a five-year follow-up study of patients with acute myocarditis, found that approximately 25% had some persistent subjective symptoms, whereas this was true for only 5% of the controls. Although their group included many forms of nonviral myocardial inflammatory disease, it also included a number of patients with aseptic meningitis and poliomyelitis who had evidence of myocarditis presumably due to viruses. The percentage of patients with persistent symptoms in this group of patients with presumptive viral myocarditis was the same as for the group as a whole.

Furthermore, Sainani et al[11] found that five of their 22 patients with coxsackie myocarditis had persisting signs and symptoms of heart failure during follow-up. All five, as well as two others, had electrocardiographic abnormalities during this period.

That myocarditis may have devastating consequences is illustrated by the fact that a number of autopsy series surveying sudden death have been reviewed by Abelmann[14] and have been found to include patients with myocarditis.

Whether chronic myocardiopathies in any way relate to acute myocarditis remains speculative in the majority of cases.

The treatment of viral myocarditis, whether in pregnancy or not, is generally supportive. The usefulness of bed rest has generally been agreed upon since the studies of Tilles.[5] The use of digitalis, vasodilator agents to reduce left ventricular afterload, or anticoagulants must be individualized. The role of steroids remains controversial[2,12]; there has not yet been a carefully controlled study to determine the value of these agents, and thus their use in myocarditis remains empiric.

Finally, we would like to turn specifically to the reported cases of viral myocarditis known to have occurred in pregnancy. In the review of Sainani et al[11] four patients of 22 had myocarditis in the postpartum period. This number seems to represent a relatively high incidence and might support some of the theoretical risks of viral myocarditis during gestation; however, as no denominators are provided, it is impossible to calculate incidence rates from that study. Further data on myocarditis in pregnancy are provided by Sutton et al,[15] who reviewed their experience with 25 consecutive myocardial biopsies. Of six cases of postpartum heart disease biopsied in this series, two had serologic changes suggestive of current viral infections.

Thus viral myocarditis does occur during human pregnancy. Yet to be determined, however, is whether the available data in animals have a human correlate and whether gestational myocarditis in humans is both more frequent and more severe than nongestational myocarditis. Furthermore, future research must establish the relationship of viruses to cases of postpartum heart disease that do not show signs of inflammation or that are not associated with specific viral infections.

II. NONVIRAL MYOCARDITIS IN PREGNANCY

In addition to viruses, other infectious agents[16] are known to cause myocarditis. Table M.VI.2 lists some of these organisms. Any or all of these agents may produce myocardial disease during pregnancy; however, none is known to produce myocarditis during gestation with any frequency or regularity. Two forms of specific myocarditis have been reported in the English literature to occur in pregnancy. These include luetic myocarditis[17] and rheumatic fever.[18] The latter has received some attention in the literature and is discussed elsewhere in this book.

More recently Gumes and Cates[19] have noted a unique myocarditis associated with abortion. All four cases they described ended fatally and had autopsy evidence of myocardial inflammation. All patients died within several days of procedures to evacuate the uterine contents, and no specific etiology was ever established.

TABLE M.VI.2. Nonviral Causes of Myocarditis

Mycoplasma	Fungi
Mycoplasma pneumoniae	Blastomyces dermatitidis
Chlamydia	Cryptococcus neoformans
Chlamydia psittaci	Coccidioides immitis
Rickettsia	Histoplasma capsulatum
R. tsutsugamushi	Parasitic agents
R. burnettii	Trypanosoma cruzi
R. rickettsii	Trypanosoma rhodesiense
Bacteria	Trypanosoma gambiense
Corynebacterium diphtheria	Toxoplasma gondii
Salmonella cholerasuis	Plasmodium falciparum
Mycobacterium tuberculosis	Taenia solium
Streptococcus pyogenes	Echinococcus granulosus
Neisseria meningitides	Toxocara canis
Brucella abortus	Trichinella spiralis
Clostridium perfringens	Noninfectious myocarditis
Borrelia recurrentis	Rheumatoid arthritis
Leptospira (various species)	Systemic lupus erythematosus
	Sarcoidosis

Modified from Wynne and Braunwald.[16]

III. REFERENCES

1. Gore I, Saphir D. Myocarditis: A classification of 1402 cases. Am Heart J. 1947; 34:827–830.
2. Levine H. Virus myocarditis: A critique of the literature from clinical electrocardiographic and pathologic standpoints. Am J Med Sci. 1979; 277:132–143.
3. Abelmann W. Viruses and the heart. Circulation. 1971; 44:950–956.
4. Burch GE, Sun SC, Colcolough H, Schal R, De Pasquale N. Coxsackie B viral myocarditis and valvulitis identified in routine autopsy specimens by immunofluorescent techniques. Am Heart J. 1967; 74:13–23.
5. Tilles J, Elson S, Shaka J, Abelmann W, Lerner A, Finland M. Effects of exercise on coxsackie A9 myocarditis in adult mice. Proc Soc Exp Biol Med. 1964; 117:777–782.
6. Meadows W. Postpartum heart disease. Am J Cardiol. 1960; 6:788–802.
7. Benchimol A, Carnero R, Schlesinger P. Postpartum heart disease. Br Heart J. 1959; 21:89–100.
8. Pearce J. Heart disease and filterable viruses. Circulation. 1960; 21:448–455.
9. Kilbourne E, Wilson C, Perrier D. The induction of gross myocardial lesions by coxsackie (pleurodynia) virus and cortisone. J Clin Invest. 1956; 35:362–370.
10. Farber P, Glasgow L. Viral myocarditis during pregnancy: Encephalomyocarditis virus infection in mice. Am Heart J. 1970; 80:96–102.
11. Sainani G, Krompotic E, Slodki S. Adult heart disease due to the coxsackie virus B infection. Medicine. 1968; 47:133–147.
12. Lerner A, Wilson F. Virus myocardiopathy. Prog Med Virol. 1973; 15:63–91.
13. Bengtsson E, Lamberger B. Five year followup study of cases suggestive of acute myocarditis. Am Heart J. 1966; 72:751–763.
14. Abelmann W. Viral myocarditis and its sequelae. Annu Rev Med. 1973; 14:145–152.
15. Sutton G, Driscoll J, Gunnar R, Tobin J. Exploratory mediastinotomy in primary myocardial disease. Prog Cardiovasc Dis. 1964; 7:83–97.
16. Wynne J, Braunwald E. The cardiomyopathies and myocardites. In: Braunwald E, ed. Heart Disease: A Textbook of Cardiovascular Medicine. Philadelphia: W.B. Saunders, 1980.
17. Perloff J. Pregnancy and cardiovascular disease. In: Braunwald E, ed. Heart Disease: A Textbook of Cardiovascular Medicine. Philadelphia: W.B. Saunders, 1980.
18. Ueland K, Metcalfe J. Acute rheumatic fever in pregnancy. Am J Obstet Gynecol. 1966; 95:586–587.
19. Gumes D, Cates C. Fatal myocarditis associated with abortion in early pregnancy. South Med J. 1980; 73:236–238.

M.VII

Peripartal Cardiomyopathy

Ralph I. Silverman, MD, and Hillel S. Ribner, MD

I. INTRODUCTION

Cardiomyopathy means "disease of heart muscle," and the cardiomyopathies represent a large and varied group of disorders affecting the myocardium. Many of them become manifest as the clinical syndrome of congestive heart failure. Awareness of myocardial diseases dates back to the late 1800s, but the clinical recognition of their importance has developed largely within the last three decades.

Although several different schemes have been proposed for the classification of the cardiomyopathies, two particular approaches appear to have the most clinical relevance. The first classification is a physiologic or functional one, based on the pathophysiologic expression of the particular disease. There are three basic categories within this classification: 1) The first, hypertrophic cardiomyopathy, involves concentric hypertrophy of the left ventricular free wall and septum or asymmetric septal hypertrophy (ASH). The latter entity may sometimes be associated with outflow obstruction of the left ventricle. Sudden death and familial incidence are characteristic of this category, and cardiac dilatation with heart failure is a late and unusual feature. 2) The second is congestive cardiomyopathy (myocardiosis), marked by cardiac dilatation, with congestive heart failure and emboli (peripheral and pulmonary) being key clinical features. 3) The third category is restrictive cardiomyopathy, which is characterized by increased wall stiffness and decreased left ventricular compliance, resulting in impedance of inflow of blood into the heart in diastole. Systolic function is often maintained. The findings may mimic constrictive pericarditis, which must always be considered in the differential diagnosis. Infiltrative diseases of the heart, most notably amyloidosis, may sometimes be present as restrictive cardiomyopathy.

The other mode of classification is etiologic, in which the specific pathologic process responsible for the myocardial disease is the basis for categorization. "Primary" (or idiopathic) cardiomyopathies refer to conditions in which the heart disease is not part of a systemic illness, and

Cardiac Problems in Pregnancy, pages 93–104

in which the pathogenetic mechanism is unknown. "Secondary" cardiomyopathies may be used to refer to conditions in which the myocardial disease is the result of direct toxic, inflammatory, or neoplastic involvement of the heart (eg, "toxic" myocarditis, viral myocarditis, metastatic involvement of the myocardium, "rejection" of a transplanted heart), or is a manifestation of a systemic disease process (connective tissue diseases, sarcoidosis, amyloidosis, neuromuscular diseases, etc). When the myocardial disease is secondary to an underlying cardiovascular abnormality (eg, hypertension, coronary artery disease, etc), the cardiomyopathy is designated accordingly (eg, hypertensive cardiomyopathy, ischemic cardiomyopathy, etc).

Peripartal cardiomyopathy may be considered a primary congestive cardiomyopathy.

II. DEFINITION

Heart failure in association with pregnancy was first recognized by Ritchie in Glasgow in 1849,[1] and a primary heart muscle disease related to late pregnancy and the puerperium was described by Virchow in 1870.[2] Thereafter, little was heard of the disease until the 1930s, when it was again described by Hull and Hafkesbring[3,4] (who suggested the possible etiologic importance of "puerperal factors") and Gouley.[5] Since then many cases have been reported from all parts of the world.

Demakis and Rahimtoola[6] established the following criteria for defining peripartal cardiomyopathy (PPCM):

1) Development of heart failure in the last month of pregnancy or within the first five postpartum months
2) Absence of another determinable etiology of the cardiac failure
3) Absence of demonstrable heart disease prior to the last month of pregnancy

Other authors[7–11] insist that this syndrome be limited to heart failure whose onset is in the postpartal period, to exclude occult or preexistent heart disease that was unmasked by the stress of pregnancy. Thus, the syndrome may also appear in the literature as "*post* partum cardiomyopathy".

Although PPCM appears to be an established clinical syndrome related to pregnancy, controversy remains regarding the specificity of the underlying cardiac lesion, the precise etiologic role of pregnancy, and whether, in fact, this is a distinct clinical entity.

III. INCIDENCE

The true incidence of PPCM is unknown, but it is not rare. Estimates range from one in 1,300[12] to one in 4,000[13] live births. In some parts of the world, 80–83% of premenopausal women with idiopathic heart failure can relate the onset of their symptoms to childbearing.[14,15] Burch[11] reports that of 123 cardiomyopathy patients randomly selected for a bed rest treatment program, 34 were classified as having peripartal cardiomyopathy.

Clearly, PPCM is a disorder of the childbearing years, and most patients develop the disease during the second and third decades of life.[7,12,14,16] Although reported from all over the world, the highest percentage of reported patients are black, especially from warm climates.[6,7,9,11,14] Although early reports in the literature suggested that the incidence of PPCM was highest in primagravidas,[3] more recent reports indicate that it occurs with higher frequency in multiparous women.[9,14,15,17]

Toxemia complicates 15–30% of the pregnancies that are associated with PPCM.[6,11,17] In one study of 27 women with PPCM, twins occurred in 7% of the patients, an incidence several times higher than the general population.[6] Although some authors feel that malnutrition is a significant factor in the development of this disorder,[7] there are many reports of patients with PPCM who have been well nourished.[14,15,17] Pierce[18] has suggested a familial tendency, but this has not been established in other studies.

IV. CLINICAL MANIFESTATIONS

The patient with peripartal cardiomyopathy has clinical evidence of congestive heart failure with a history of orthopnea, paroxysmal nocturnal dyspnea, edema, exertional dyspnea and weakness (Table M. VII.1). In Demakis' series,[6,17] 82% of women with PPCM developed cardiac symptoms in the first three postpartal months, 93% within the first five postpartal months, and only 7% in the last months of pregnancy. Many patients complain of vague abdominal and/or chest discomfort. Palpitations, often secondary to cardiac arrhythmias, are common and may at times be the initial complaint. Up to 25% of patients may have hemoptysis, and a high percentage of these patients will have evidence of pulmonary embolism.[7]

Physical examination generally reveals a young woman in moderate respiratory distress with signs of mild to severe congestive heart failure. Cardiomegaly and a protodiastolic gallop rhythm are almost invariably present. In addition, jugular venous distension, hepatomegaly and peripheral edema, fine basilar pulmonary rales, and an apical holosystolic murmur of mitral incompetence are frequent findings (Table M. VII. 1).

Electrocardiograms are almost always abnormal (Table M. VII. 2). In 15 patients reported by Walsh,[7] all had electrocardiographic changes consistent with left ventricular hypertrophy. Abnormalities of the the T wave and S-T segments are generally the most common abnormalities seen. Other findings may include low voltage QRS complexes or abnormal Q waves. Left bundle branch block occurs only rarely.[19] Rhythm disturbances may occur, particularly ventricular premature contractions, and these may be related to digitalis toxicity. Although atrial fibrillation is a common arrhythmia in congestive cardiomyopathy, it was found in only one of 27 PPCM patients of Demakis.[17]

Chest x-ray films show cardiomegaly in all cases, often with pulmonary venous congestion. Left ventricular, and often left atrial, enlargement is present (Fig. M. VII.1). Echocardiography may be very valuable in excluding valvular or pericardial disease in the patient with unexpected heart failure. The echocardiogram of patients with congestive cardiomyopathy will typically demonstrate a poorly contracting and dilated left ventricle, with decreased motion of both the posterior wall and the septum, and reduced ejection fraction. The left atrium is generally dilated, and an enlarged right ventricular cavity is often seen (Fig. M. VII. 2). It should be noted that these findings are not specific for peripartal cardiomyopathy, but are seen in any type of congestive cardiomyopathy. In addition, serial echocardiographic determinations of left ventricular size and function permit a safe noninvasive means to follow the progress of the disease. Radionuclide ventriculography is another valuable noninvasive technique to confirm the presence of left ventricular dysfunction. Elevated end-diastolic and end-systolic volumes and generalized hypokinesis with reduced ejection fraction are characteristic findings. This

TABLE M.VII.1. Peripartal Cardiomyopathy—Clinical Presentation

Symptoms
Weakness
Exertional dyspnea
Cough
Orthopnea
Paroxysmal nocturnal dyspnea
Chest pain
Palpitations
Abdominal pain
Hemoptysis
Physical findings
Blood pressure normal or slightly reduced
Pulsus alternans
Premature contractions
Jugular venous distension
Right and left ventricular enlargement
Palpable third and fourth heart sounds
First heart sound normal or slightly reduced
Accentuated P_2 of second heart sound when pulmonary hypertension present
Gallop rhythm (third and fourth heart sounds)
Mitral insufficiency and/or tricuspid insufficiency murmurs may be heard
Pulmonary rales
Peripheral edema

TABLE M.VII.2. Peripartal Cardiomyopathy—Laboratory Findings

Chest roentgenogram	Cardiac enlargement with biventricular and often biatrial involvement, moderate to marked pulmonary venous congestion, pleural effusion
Electrocardiogram	Left ventricular hypertrophy or biventricular hypertrophy Atrial arrhythmias Ventricular arrhythmias ST and T wave abnormalities Abnormal Q waves Intraventricular conduction defects Low or high voltage QRS Left atrial or biatrial enlargement
Echocardiogram	Left ventricular dilatation with decreased wall motion and reduced ejection fraction Right ventricular dilatation Left atrial enlargement Right atrial enlargement Possible pericardial effusion
Radionuclide ventriculography	Left ventricular dilatation, diffuse hypokinesis, reduced ejection fraction

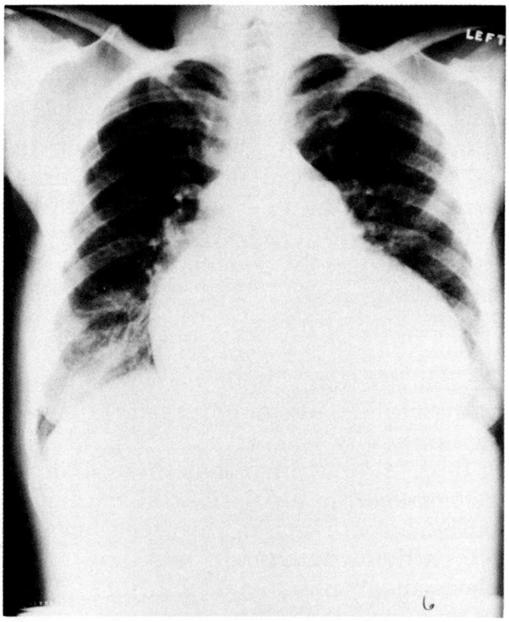

Fig. M. VII. 1. Chest x-ray film from patient with peripartal cardiomyopathy. There is a general cardiomegaly, prominence of the hilar vessels, and pulmonary congestion.

technique is also helpful in following the course of the illness and in evaluating response to therapy.

V. PATHOLOGY

At necropsy, the heart is found to be grossly pale, flabby, dilated, and enlarged, with weights reported in the range of 450–700 gm.[7,11,17] Small amounts of pericardial fluid may be present, but the pericardium is otherwise normal. Endocardial thickening is a frequent finding, often forming permanent areas of gray-white plaques. Mural thrombi are often seen. The heart valves and coronary arteries are generally normal.

Histologically, the myocardium shows varying degrees of muscle fiber hypertrophy, interstitial edema, diffuse focal areas of myocardial degeneration and fibrosis, and scattered areas of perivascular and interstitial infiltration by inflammatory cells, mostly mononuclear. Endocardial thickening may be mild to marked. Histochemical studies of heart muscle were performed by Walsh et al, who found that all patients showed an increase in lipid deposition.[7] They also stained for succinic dehydrogenase activity and found that intensity of reaction was somewhat decreased when compared to normal hearts, with spotty zones of lesser activity of varying degrees. This was strikingly different from their findings in alcoholic cardiomy-

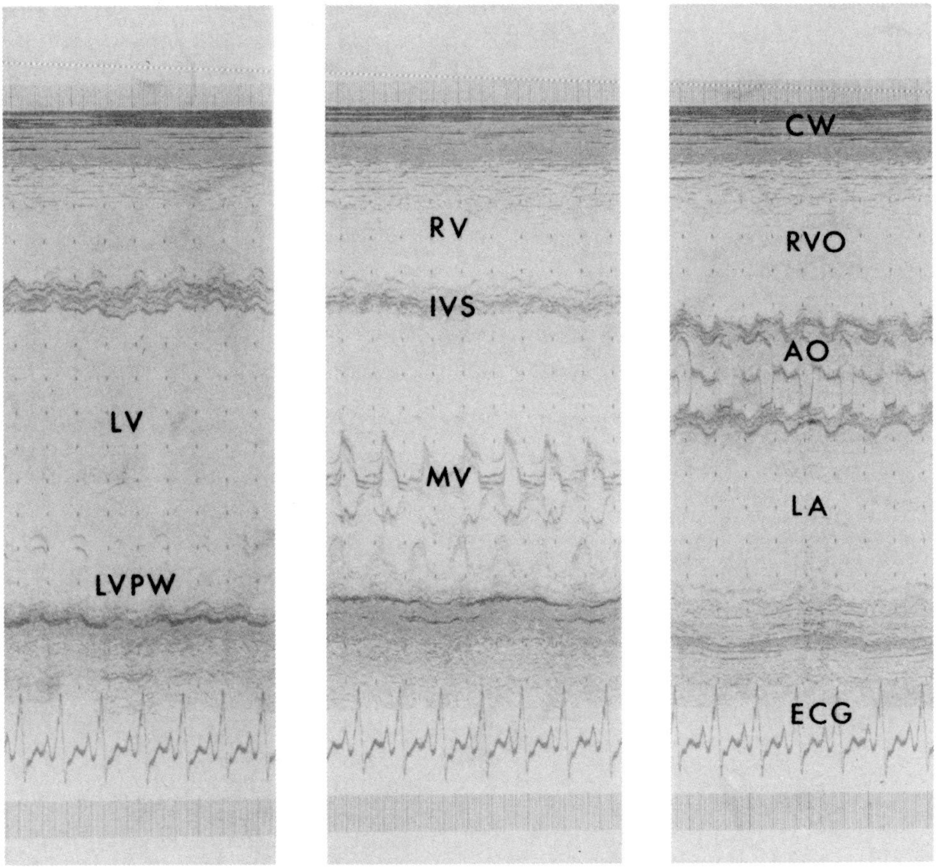

Fig. M. VII. 2. M-mode echocardiogram in patient with peripartal cardiomyopathy. Recording was performed at the level of the aorta (AO) (right), the mitral valve (MV) (middle), and the left ventricle (LV) below the level of the MV (left). There is a marked increase in the dimensions of the left atrium (LA) and both ventricles. The left ventricular posterior wall (LVPW) and the interventricular septum (IVS) show decreased motion. CW = chest wall; ECG = electrocardiogram; RVO = right ventricular outflow tract; RV = right ventricle.

opathy, in which there is a pronounced reduction in activity throughout.[7] It should be noted that, on routine histologic examination, patients with alcoholic cardiomyopathy are indistinguishable from patients with PPCM.

VI. ETIOLOGY

Although it was originally described as "toxic,"[3] no cause for PPCM has as yet been identified. This difficulty stems, in part, from the lack of a universally accepted definition for the syndrome. Heart failure due to exacerbations of preexisting rheumatic disease or to specific infections with tuberculosis or parasites[20] may coincide with the puerperium but clearly should not be classified as PPCM. However, some authors have excluded from consideration patients with any possible identifiable cause such as toxemia or hypertension.[8,21] The danger of this rigorous approach is that it may mask a potentially etiologic relationship. A "middle course" would appear to be the most appropriate approach to classifying this condition.

The contention has been advanced that PPCM represents the expression in young, peripartal women of an idiopathic congestive cardiomyopathy differing in no substantial way from that observed in patients of other age groups, both male and female. In some parts of the world, both congestive cardiomyopathy and PPCM are common causes of heart failure,[14,15,21] and it is possible that a decade or two later PPCM patients would have developed primary myocardial disease were it not for childbirth.[14] The pathologic findings in PPCM and other congestive cardiomyopathies are virtually indistinguishable.[12,14] Furthermore, apart from the temporal association of PPCM with pregnancy, the clinical presentations of these syndromes are quite similar. Indeed, in clinical practice it is occasionally impossible to exclude a preexisting asymptomatic cardiac disorder, and the role of pregnancy in some cases may merely be to unmask such an underlying abnormality.[22,23]

Nevertheless, there is strong circumstantial evidence that PPCM defines a unique syndrome. Even in those areas where idiopathic congestive cardiomyopathy is prevalent, it is unusual to find an afflicted patient below middle age.[8,14] In contrast, the vast majority of premenopausal women who do develop primary myocardial disease relate the onset of symptoms to childbearing.[14,15] Heart failure due to preexisting cardiomyopathy might be expected to appear during pregnancy at the time of the greatest hemodynamic stress—ie, during the second and third trimesters[14,24]—yet most patients with PPCM usually encounter no difficulty until well after delivery.[15,24,25] A feature unique to PPCM is the propensity of the heart failure to recur with subsequent pregnancies.[15] Moreover, complete recovery may occur in PPCM but is distinctly exceptional in idiopathic cardiomyopathy.[6,15]

Even if PPCM constitutes a distinct clinical entity, the question of its etiology remains. Excessive alcohol intake has not been an important association,[6,17] and, as already noted, the histochemical findings are in sharp contrast to those of alcoholic cardiomyopathy.[7] A separate syndrome of postpartal myocardial infarction has been described,[26] but coronary artery disease and ischemic necrosis have been absent in cases of PPCM, despite complaints of chest pain. The pathologic picture also appears to negate the possibility of chronic or intermittent vascular spasm.[21] A relationship of PPCM to lactation has been noted[15] but is not a constant feature of the disease.[27] Meadows drew attention to a superficial similarity between PPCM and congestive heart failure produced by excessive amounts of desoxycorticosterone,[12] but subsequent studies have failed to provide proof of an underlying endocrinologic disorder.

The role of toxemia is somewhat controversial. Demakis et al noted a fourfold greater incidence of toxemia in PPCM patients than in the overall obstetric population,[17] but in other studies the number of PPCM cases with antecedent toxemia appears to be quite small.[7,9,12,15] This discrepancy may be due in part to the rigor with which the diagnosis of toxemia is made. Burch et al were able to objectively confirm only one case of toxemia among 22 patients who reported a history of "preeclampsia/eclampsia."[7,9]

PPCM has been reported most frequently from tropical climates and among blacks. An entirely racial origin is excluded, however, by its occurrence in European whites[27,28] and Asiatics of Korean[29] and Japanese[21] extraction. Pierce et al found a family history of peripartal heart failure in three of 17 patients with PPCM.[18] Others have noted a strong family history of nonpuerperal atherosclerotic and hypertensive heart disease in PPCM patients, but they did not evaluate a control group.[9] A Danish report documents the occurrence of fatal congestive cardiomyopathy in the brother of a 23-year-old woman with PPCM.[30]

A number of authors have postulated an immunologic origin for PPCM.[31,32] Sulfonamide hypersensitivity has been the apparent cause in two cases of puerperal heart disease[33,34]; aside from these rare cases, no specific drugs have been implicated. The higher incidence of PPCM among multiparous women and with twin pregnancies raises the possibility of a reaction to the products of conception.[31] Trophoblastic tissue has indeed been shown to enter the maternal circulation during pregnancy,[35] but how hypersensitivity to this material might affect the heart of the mother has not been explained. Serum antibodies to cardiac muscle have been found in idiopathic cardiomyopathy (including PPCM), but they are considered to be secondary phenomena rather than etiologic.[27,36] Lupus erythematosus tests in PPCM have been uniformly negative.[7,9,30] Aside from a single case demonstrating granulomas in myocardium,[37] pathologic studies have failed to provide confirmatory evidence of a hypersensitivity disorder. A report of improvement in PPCM with steroid therapy has appeared,[38] but in other cases, steroids were ineffective.[37,39,40]

As with other cardiomyopathies of unknown cause, attempts have been made to ascribe PPCM to a prior viral infection.[41] This hypothesis is particularly attractive in PPCM, since viral multiplication in the mouse heart is enhanced by pregnancy, and damage to cardiac tissues can result from even relatively mild infections.[42] PPCM following viral parotitis[43] and epidemic influenza infection[33] have been reported; in other studies of PPCM no evidence of viremia was observed.[17] Sainani et al found four cases of puerperal heart failure among 22 adults with heart disease and a diagnostic antibody response to coxsackievirus B infection; in one case, the virus was also isolated from the stool.[44] Others have failed to demonstrate a rise in serum viral antibody titers.[17,30,40,45] Complement fixation tests for toxoplasmosis have also yielded negative results.[8,9,27] The histologic pattern of PPCM is one of myocardial fiber degeneration,[17,45] in contrast to the widespread inflammatory infiltration characteristically found in diffuse infectious processes.

PPCM is primarily a disease of lower socioeconomic groups, and a number of authorities have suspected a role for nutritional disorders in its genesis.[4,7,15] Blegen found a very high incidence of thiamine deficiency in 28 Korean women with PPCM and noted a reduction in heart size with thiamine therapy.[29] Most authors, however, have been unable to elicit a history of gross malnutrition or to demonstrate stigmata of vitamin deficiency.[12,14,15,17,46] Patients with PPCM usually have reduced cardiac output,[8,18,38,40,43] which contrasts with the elevated values seen in wet beri-beri.[14] Therapy with thiamine has failed to affect the course of the disease in severely ill patients.[8,13,14,40] Conversely, mild cases of PPCM frequently improve without vitamin repletion.[12,15,25] By leading to anemia or general debility, malnutrition may exacerbate heart failure of whatever cause. However, there is little evidence at present that nutritional deficiencies are actually responsible for the initial cardiac deterioration in PPCM.

Mild to moderate arterial hypertension is present on admission in most women with PPCM,[4,12,15,16,25] imposing the burden of increased afterload onto the weakened myocardium. Brockington has gone so far as to call the disease "postpartum hypertensive heart failure," postulating that an acute rise in blood pressure may suddenly overwhelm an unhypertrophied left ventricle.[16] Some patients remain persistently hypertensive following treatment of PPCM[12,16,18,47] and may represent true cases of hypertensive cardiovascular disease.[18] There are strong arguments against a primary etiologic role for hypertension in most instances, however. The majority of patients with PPCM have no history of hypertension prior to the pregnancy[4] and no evidence of end-organ damage to the kidney or retina. In addition, the pathologic manifestations in the heart do not resemble those of patients dying from malignant or essential hypertension.[5,12,13] The blood pressure elevation in PPCM is usually transient, responding rapidly to bed rest and treatment of the heart failure.[12,15,16,18,25] In this respect, PPCM appears to differ little from other idiopathic cardiomyopathies.[48] In many cases the degree of hypertension is too mild to explain the severity of the heart failure.[14,25] Moreover, PPCM clearly can occur[13,25,27,46,47] and progress[47] in the presence of normal blood pressures; even in Brockington's series one-quarter of the patients were normotensive.[16] Hypertension is thus unlikely to be the sole cause of the cardiac lesion. Nevertheless, its presence may well contribute to the hemodynamic disability. Indeed, there is evidence to suggest that hypertension is much more common in PPCM patients who develop *recurrent* heart failure than in those who remain well after initial treatment.[25]

Hypertension may also play a prominent etiologic role in the recently defined syndrome of peripartal heart failure occurring in the Hausa-Fulani people of northern Nigeria. For 40 days following delivery, women of this tribe lie on baked mud beds over a fire twice daily, splash themselves with hot water, and eat large amounts of kanwa, a dried lake-salt.[25] Postpartum hypertension is also prevalent in this group, and the combination of volume overload and pressure overload may be responsible for the very high incidence of peripartal heart failure reported from this region.[49] This entity appears to differ in some respects from the PPCM described from other geographical areas where these postpartum customs are not observed. Gross edema of the extremities and face is almost invariable among the Hausa women,[25] and large amounts of fluid are lost with treatment, reflecting the massive volume overload. These characteristics are less prominent in the United States.[7] In addition, the immediate prognosis in the Hausa appears markedly better than that of the previously described cases of PPCM, and there are very few relapses. In many of the patients, noninvasive and direct hemodynamic measurements have indicated elevated cardiac outputs and relative preservation of ventricular function,[50] rather than the hypokinetic ventricular wall motion and low cardiac outputs documented in prior reports.[7,18,51] The clinical picture in northern Nigeria thus resembles in many respects the state of circulatory congestion seen in acute glomerulonephritis which, while simulating true myocardial failure, is due primarily to volume overload.[50] It is unknown, however, why the syndrome develops in only a small minority of Hausa women when the postpartal practices are universal in this population. It is possible that, in the symptomatic cases, the added stresses of the Hausa customs may be unmasking a subtle myocardial defect common to women with PPCM in all parts of the world.[52] Further research may yet reveal the "postpartal cardiac factor" postulated by Musser et al 43 years ago.[53]

VII. COMPLICATIONS

The important complications of PPCM include those one would expect in any congestive cardiomyopathy.

a) Digitalis toxicity. Although digitalis is an important part of the therapeutic regimen of patients with congestive heart failure, it should be kept in mind that patients with cardiomyopathy are very sensitive to the toxic effects of digitalis glycosides. Walsh noted that all 15 patients in his series of PPCM demonstrated unusual susceptibility to digitalis, marked by frequent multifocal ventricular premature contractions.[32] In many instances it may be difficult to differentiate arrhythmias caused by the underlying cardiac disease from those induced by digitalis. Clearly, the daily dosage of digitalis must be individualized for each patient, and serum potassium must be maintained in the normal range, particularly if diuretics are being administered as well.

b) Thromboembolism. Embolic events, both pulmonary and systemic, are such frequent complications of cardiomyopathy that they may be considered an integral part of the disease process. Embolism occurs particularly commonly in PPCM. Hull reported emboli in 25% of his patients.[4] In Walsh's series six of 15 patients developed pulmonary embolism, and two of the six had associated cerebral emboli.[7] Embolism was the immediate cause of death in the majority of cases reported by Gouley in 1937.[5] It has been suggested that the "hypercoagulable" state that exists in pregnancy may account for the especially high incidence of thromboembolism in PPCM.[14]

c) Arrhythmias. Rhythm disturbances are common in cardiomyopathy in general. In a group of 100 patients with primary cardiomyopathy studied by Hamby, 63% had rhythm disturbances, the most common being ventricular premature beats (43%) and sustained or paroxysmal atrial fibrillation (20%).[54] Similar arrhythmias have been reported in PPCM,[7,17] but they appear to occur less commonly than in other cardiomyopathies.

d) Other complications. Bronchopneumonia may occur and can be a terminal complication in patients with advanced heart failure. Acute pyelonephritis was a complication in three of Walsh's 15 patients with PPCM, one of whom died in uremia.[7]

VIII. THERAPY

Once the diagnosis of peripartal cardiomyopathy is made, intensive medical therapy should be started as early as possible, as this appears to have an important influence on prognosis (see below). Adequate nutrition is an important part of the treatment of these patients, especially if there is evidence of malnutrition during pregnancy.

The mainstay of management of patients with PPCM is the treatment of heart failure and its complications. Digitalis should be administered, but with caution since, as has been mentioned previously, these patients are very sensitive to the drug and may develop dangerous arrhythmias. Diuretics will generally be required, but care must be taken to avoid hypokalemia, which would increase further the sensitivity to digitalis glycosides. Some authors have advocated the use of mercurial diuretics instead of the more potassium-wasting thiazides.[7,11] Because of the high incidence of thromboembolic events in PPCM patients, the institution of anticoagulant therapy must be strongly considered. It has been recommended that anticoagulants be continued as long as cardiomegaly persists.[6]

Burch, Walsh, and their co-workers have stressed the importance of prolonged, complete bed rest in the management of patients with PPCM.[7,9,11] They advocate bed rest for three months after heart size has returned to normal, but if cardiac enlargement persists, prolonged bed rest will be necessary. If no further reduction in heart size is achieved after a six- to 12-month period, then bed rest should be discontinued. Burch reported on 34 patients with PPCM treated with prolonged bed rest (in addition to conventional therapy for heart failure).[9] In 50% of these patients the heart size returned to normal, and in another 25%, heart size diminished. Patients ill for a long time before seeking medical attention were less likely to respond to this therapy. However, other authors[6,15] have also reported a 50% incidence of return of heart size to normal within one year with conventional therapy without prolonged bed rest, suggesting that prolonged bed rest is not always necessary. In addition, it is often difficult, from a practical point of view, to maintain prolonged bed rest in many of these patients.

In patients who fail to respond to conventional therapy for heart failure, additional modalities of treatment should be tried. Ghosh[38] reported marked improvement in two patients following the addition of steroid therapy to the conventional regimen, but other authors[37,39,40] have failed to show a similar effect. Vasodilators affect the peripheral arterial and venous systems by decreasing arteriolar vascular resistance and increasing venous capacitance, thereby reducing cardiac work load. Vasodilator therapy therefore has a definite place in the treatment of the congestive heart failure of cardiomyopathy.[55,56] Nitrates, hydralazine, and prazosin are among the agents that have been demonstrated to improve cardiac output and reduce pulmonary congestion.[55,56] Vasodilator therapy should be employed in those patients with PPCM who fail to respond to conventional therapy. Brantigan et al[57] reported significant transient physiologic benefit in a patient with PPCM during seven weeks of mechanical "unloading" with intraaortic balloon counterpulsation, although the patient died shortly after hospital discharge of intractable congestive heart failure.

It has been observed that women who have had one episode of PPCM are at risk of having recurrences in subsequent pregnancies. Walsh et al[7] reported on six of their patients who, subsequent to their initial episode of PPCM, went on to have six full-term pregnancies, two of which were complicated by congestive heart failure. Cardiac insufficiency became worse postpartum in all six patients. Demakis and Rahimtoola[6] found that only the patients with persistent cardiac enlargement suffered significant cardiac deterioration in subsequent pregnancies, and the authors suggested that only those patients should avoid further pregnancies. Burch et al[9] found that bed rest during subsequent pregnancies was effective in reducing congestive heart failure. Nevertheless, they consider peripartal cardiomyopathy to be a medical contraindication to further pregnancies and recommend sterilization procedures in these patients. Thus, patients with PPCM, particularly those with persistent cardiac enlargement, should be advised to avoid subsequent pregnancies. Oral contraceptives, because of their risk of associated thrombosis, should not be used in these patients, who are already at high risk for thromboembolic events. Should a subsequent pregnancy occur in a patient with PPCM whose heart remains enlarged, it should be interrupted.

IX. NATURAL COURSE AND PROGNOSIS

The immediate prognosis in PPCM patients must be guarded, particularly if the patient is in severe heart failure. In Walsh's series of 15 patients,[7] four died within one month of diagnosis; three of them were admitted with severe congestive heart failure. There were five additional late deaths in that series. Four of those who died were continuously hospitalized for over a year without significant reduction in heart size. Of the six survivors, three became asymptomatic and had return of heart size to normal, and three had marked clinical improvement and reduction (but not normalization) of heart size.

Burch et al[9] reported that of 28 patients with PPCM treated with prolonged bed rest, 14 experienced a return to normal heart size. All 14 patients entered the therapeutic program within six months of onset of their disease. In nine patients in whom therapy was initiated six months or more after the onset of disease, none regained normal heart size. Of the 12 deaths reported in their series of a total of 34 patients, nine occurred in patients whose hearts remained enlarged. Thus, duration of disease prior to institution of therapy and the return of heart size to normal had obvious effects on long-term prognosis.

Demakis and Rahimtoola[6,17] studied 27 patients with PPCM and had similar findings. Their patients were treated with conventional therapy, but without prolonged bed rest. They found that initial clinical manifestations do not predict which patients will have a return to normal heart size and which will maintain cardiomegaly. Fifty percent (14) of their patients had a return of heart size to normal within six months of the onset of disease, and they had a favorable course. Of the 14 patients in this group, followed for an average of 10.7 years, two had pulmonary emboli, nine had return of the electrocardiogram to normal, 12 were in functional class I or II (New York Heart Association Classification), and there were two deaths, or a 14% mortality. In contrast, there were 13 patients who continued to have cardiomegaly and gallop rhythms at the end of six months, and those patients represent a group with an extremely poor prognosis. Of the 13 patients, followed for an average of 5.4 years, six had pulmonary emboli, all 13 had abnormal electrocardiograms, only two were in functional class I or II, and 11 (85%) died of cardiac failure, seven within the first five years. Subsequent pregnancies were well tolerated in the group that had a favorable course, but not in the 13 who did poorly. In fact, three of the eleven deaths occurred in relation to a subsequent pregnancy.

Thus, the long-term prognosis of patients with peripartal cardiomyopathy cannot be predicted at the time of diagnosis. Clearly, the sooner appropriate therapy is instituted, the more likely it is that the heart will return to normal size and the better the prognosis. Patients in whom cardiomegaly persists will require longer periods of close observation and management, which may include prolonged bed rest, and have a much poorer prognosis. Subsequent pregnancies must certainly be avoided in this group of patients.

X. REFERENCES

1. Ritchie C. Clinical contribution to the pathology, diagnosis and treatment of certain chronic diseases of the heart. Edinb Med Surg J. 1849; 2:333.
2. Virchow R. S.B. der Berliner Geburtshueflicher Gesellschaft, 1870.
3. Hull E, Hafkesbring E. "Toxic" postpartal heart disease. N Orleans Med Surg J. 1937; 89:550–557.
4. Hull E, Hidden E. Postpartal heart failure. South Med J. 1938; 31:265–270.
5. Gouley BA, McMillan TM, Bellet S. Idiopathic myocardial degeneration associated with pregnancy and especially the puerperium. Am J Med Sci. 1937; 194:185–199.
6. Demakis JG, Rahimtoola SH. Peripartum cardiomyopathy. Circulation. 1971; 44:964–968.
7. Walsh JJ, Burch GE, Black WC, Ferrans VJ, Hibbs RG. Idiopathic myocardiopathy of the puerperium (post partal heart disease). Circulation. 1965; 32:19–31.
8. Reid JVO. Postpartal cardiomyopathy. S Afr Med J. 1961; 35:165–168.
9. Burch GE, McDonald CD, Walsh JJ. The effect of prolonged bed rest on postpartal cardiomyopathy. Am Heart J. 1971; 81:186–201.
10. Meadows WR. Postpartum heart disease. Am J Cardiol. 1960; 6:788–797.
11. Burch GE, Giles TD, Tsui C-Y. Postpartal cardiomyopathy. Cardiovasc Clin. 1972; 4:270–282.
12. Meadows WR. Idiopathic myocardial failure in the last trimester of pregnancy and the puerperium. Circulation. 1957; 15:903–914.
13. Woolford RM. Postpartum myocardosis. Ohio State Med J. 1952; 48:924–930.
14. Stuart KL. Cardiomyopathy of pregnancy and the puerperium. Q J Med. 1968; 37:463–477.
15. Seftel H, Susser M. Maternity and myocardial failure in African women. Br Heart J. 1961; 23:43–52.
16. Brockington IF. Postpartum hypertensive heart failure. Am J Cardiol. 1971; 27:650–658.
17. Demakis JF, Rahimtoola SH, Sutton GC, Meadows WR, Szanto PB, Tobin JR, Gunnar RM. Natural course of peripartum cardiomyopathy. Circulation. 1971; 44:1053–1061.
18. Pierce JA, Price BO, Joyce JW. Familial occurrence of postpartal heart failure. Arch Intern Med. 1963; 111:651–655.
19. Goodwin JF. Peripartal heart disease. Clin Obstet Gynecol. 1975; 18:125–131.
20. Benchimol AB, Carneiro RD, Schlesinger P. Post-partum heart disease. Br Heart J. 1959; 21:89–100.
21. Koide T, Saito Y, Sakamoto T, Murao S. Peripartal cardiomyopathy in Japan: A critical reappraisal of the concept. Jpn Heart J. 1972; 13:488–501.
22. Boda JL. Idiopathic cardiomyopathy: With particular reference to findings in Africa. S Afr Med J. 1973; 47:570–575.
23. Peripartum cardiac failure (editorial). Br Med J. 1976; 1:302–303.
24. Quash JA. Peripartum myocardiopathy: report of three cases. J Natl Med Assoc. 1974; 66:281–283.
25. Davidson N, Parry EHO. Peri-partum cardiac failure. Q J Med. 1978; 47:431–461.
26. Beary JF, Summer WR, Bulkley BH. Postpartum acute myocardial infarction: A rare occurrence of uncertain etiology. Am J Cardiol. 1979; 43:158–161.
27. Fritz VU, Lakier JB, Klugman LH, Zion MM, Barlow JB. Peri-partum cardiomyopathy in white women. Recent Adv Stud Cardiac Struct Metab. 1973; 2:645–653.
28. Barrillon A, Batiste M, Grand A, Gay J, Gerbaux A. Myocardiopathie de la grossesse chez la femme blanche. Arch Mal Coeur. 1978; 71:406–413.
29. Blegen SD. Post-partum congestive heart failure: Beri-beri heart disease. Acta Med Scand. 1965; 178:515–524.
30. Strunge P. Familiaer kardiomyopati. Ugeskr Laeg. 1976; 138/42:2567–2569.
31. Becker FF, Taube H. Myocarditis of obscure etiology associated with pregnancy. N Engl J Med. 1962; 266:62–67.
32. Walsh JJ, Burch GE. Postpartal heart disease. Arch Intern Med. 1961; 108:817–822.
33. Bashour F, Winchell P. "Post partal" heart disease—a syndrome? Ann Intern Med. 1954; 40:803–808.
34. Parsons V, Porter A, Dische F. Cardiomyopathy and renal failure occurring in the puerperium. J Obstet Gynaecol Br Commonw. 1971;

78:564–569.
35. Douglas GW, Thomas L, Carr M, Cullen NM, Morris R. Trophoblast in the circulating blood during pregnancy. Am J Obstet Gynecol. 1959; 78:960–973.
36. Kirsner AB, Hess EV, Fowler NO. Immunologic findings in idiopathic cardiomyopathy: A prospective serial study. Am Heart J 1973; 86:625–630.
37. Rodriguez RC, Cordero JN, Pereira CB, Mora OM, Isunza JMR. Gravido-puerperal myocardiopathy: Myocardiopathy of hypersensitivity. Arch Inst Cardiol Mex. 1972; 42:164–168.
38. Ghosh JC, Neelakantan C, Chhetri MK. Peripartal cardiomyopathy: A clinical and haemodynamic study. Indian Heart J. 1974; 26:213–218.
39. Goldberg WM. Idiopathic myocarditis of pregnancy. Can Med Assoc J. 1963; 88:1247–1250.
40. Hughes RAC, Kapur P, Sutton GC, Honey M. A case of fatal peri-partum cardiomyopathy. Br Heart J. 1970; 32:272–276.
41. Faruque AA. Acute fulminating puerperal myocarditis. Br Heart J. 1965; 27:139–143.
42. Farber PA, Glasgow LA. Viral myocarditis during pregnancy: Encephalo-myocarditis virus infection in mice. Am Heart J. 1970; 80:96–102.
43. Sangiorgi M, Iacoboni M, Rapisarda R. A case of gravidic myocardiopathy after epidemic parotiditis. Boll Soc Ital Cardiol. 1974; 19:39–48.
44. Sainani GS, Krompotic E, Slodki SJ. Adult heart disease due to Coxsackie virus B infection. Medicine (Balt). 1968; 47:133–147.
45. Sutton GC, Driscoll JF, Gunnar RM, Tobin JR Jr. Exploratory mediastinotomy in primary myocardial disease. Prog Cardiovasc Dis. 1964; 7:83–97.
46. Talwalkar PG, Narulla DV, Mistry CJ, Wagholikar UL. Paripartum cardiomyopathy—A clinico-pathological study. J Assoc Physicians India. 1978; 26:793–798.
47. Fillmore SJ, Parry EHO. The evolution of peripartal heart failure in Zaria, Nigeria. Some etiologic factors. Circulation. 1977; 56:1058–1061.
48. Goodwin J. Congestive and hypertrophic cardiomyopathies: A decade of study. Lancet. 1970; 1:731–739.
49. Davidson N McD, Parry EHO. The etiology of peripartum cardiac failure. Am Heart J. 1979; 97:535–536.
50. Sanderson JE, Adesanya CO, Anjarin FI, Parry EHO. Postpartum cardiac failure—Heart failure die to volume overload? Am Heart J. 1979; 97:613–621.
51. Bertrand F, Langlois J, Renambot J, Chauvet J, Ekra A. La myocardopathie du post-partum: A propos de 25 cas. Arch Mal Coeur. 1977; 70:169–178.
52. Postpartum fluid retention (editorial). Lancet. 1979; 1:960–961.
53. Musser JH, Sodeman WA, Turner RH. Heart failure or acute nephritis with onset about three weeks after delivery. Ann Intern Med. 1938; 12:739–753.
54. Hamby RI. Primary myocardial disease—A prospective clinical and hemodynamic evaluation in 100 patients. Medicine (Balt). 1970; 49:55–78.
55. Cohn JN, Franciosa JA. Vasodilator therapy of cardiac failure. N Engl J Med. 1977; 297:27–37, 254–258.
56. Chatterjee K, Parmley WW. The role of vasodilator therapy in heart failure. Prog Cardiovasc Dis. 1977; 19:301–325.
57. Brantigan CO, Grow JB Sr, Schoonmaker FW. Extended use of intraaortic balloon pumping in peripartum cardiomyopathy. Ann Surg. 1976; 183:1–4.

M. VIII

Hypertrophic Cardiomyopathy and Pregnancy

Celia M. Oakley, MD

I. DEFINITION

Hypertrophic cardiomyopathy (HOCM) is a condition in which there is hypertrophy of the left ventricle and occasionally also of the right ventricle, which is unexplained.[1] The hypertrophy typically involves the septum more than the free wall of the left ventricle (although this is not invariable) and, occasionally, the right ventricle as well. The left ventricular volume is normal or reduced, and the diastolic pressure is usually raised.

Systolic gradients are common, particularly on the left side, but their significance remains controversial. On this account the word "obstructive" has been dropped from the designation.

Inheritance is usually by an autosomal dominant gene but many seemingly sporadic cases occur. Although some of the sporadic cases may represent new mutations, evidence of the disease is frequently found in family studies of asymptomatic first-degree relatives. There is no single diagnostic marker of the disorder, and the clinical expression may vary greatly so that gene-carrying individuals do not necessarily manifest evidence of abnormality. Conversely, with growing awareness of the disorder and the use of echocardiography on which to base a diagnosis, over-diagnosis is now almost as great a problem as missing the condition was a few years ago.

II. NATURAL HISTORY AND PROGNOSIS

The natural history of HOCM is only just beginning to emerge and is still not fully known.[2,3] This is because the disorder was first recognised clinically only in 1958, and then only a narrow spectrum in the most florid of its many guises. Since then the diverse nature of the clinical signs and prognosis has gradually emerged.[4–6]

Although childhood cases are common and HOCM has been recognised in the

Cardiac Problems in Pregnancy, pages 105–114

neonate, the majority of cases are not seen until the second or third decades. We do not even know whether hereditary disease is developmental or whether it is actually congenital, and so we do not know whether the hearts of those who are first seen with HOCM in later decades were abnormal at birth or even in childhood. Patients with undeniable HOCM in middle or even old age have similar features to those who manifest the disease earlier in life. It is not known whether this is because they have milder disease, later onset of disease, or nonprogressive disease. Although the clinical features may not seem to change during many years of observation in some patients who had grossly abnormal hearts at the time of diagnosis, other patients change remarkably over the years. Serial electrocardiographic observations have suggested that hypertrophy progresses in many cases.

Although some patients with pathologically severe HOCM may die as octogenarians,[7] others die at a young age and by far the commonest mode of dying is suddenly. Death is totally unexpected and unassociated with any known preceding change of symptoms.[3,8,9] This tragic frequency of sudden death in otherwise vigorous and often entirely asymptomatic individuals has led to a search for occult arrhythmia in this disorder, and such arrhythmias have been found to be common.[10] In other patients symptoms are caused by the haemodynamic abnormality,[2,4,6] and in these patients the circulatory malfunction may progress over the years to the stage of atrial fibrillation and heart failure.[6] Maybe these patients have an inherently greater electrical stability than those who die suddenly.

During the years of accumulation of experience a clinical folklore grew up, as it seemed that certain features were associated with a poor prognosis in HOCM. These were a bad family history, diagnosis in childhood, symptoms of syncope or dizziness, and a large or enlarging heart on x-ray. Retrospective analysis has now been carried out at the Royal Postgraduate Medical School to assess the prognostic value of all the clinical electrocardiographic, echocardiographic, and haemodynamic features that have been documented in 216 patients with HOCM who had been fully investigated and followed-up by us for up to 23 years.[3,11] Forty-nine of these patients died, 24 of them suddenly. The study indeed confirmed some of our beliefs. A family history of sudden death or blackouts or diagnosis in childhood were all of ill omen but, surprisingly, neither angina, shortness of breath, nor palpitations was found to be associated with a poor prognosis. No feature in the resting electrocardiogram was of prognostic importance and, very surprisingly indeed, no haemodynamic features were found to be helpful. Importantly, neither a resting nor a provokable left ventricular outflow tract gradient was predictive of early mortality. This is of particular interest because a high outflow tract gradient provided the conventional indication for surgical treatment. No clinical or electrocardiographic, echocardiographic, or haemodynamic feature analysed either separately or together revealed any significant difference between the patients who had died and the survivors.

Having said this, very few of the patients studied in this retrospective way by computer-aided analysis had received antiarrhythmic drugs, except for propranolol, which was taken by nearly all of them. It was therefore impossible to assess the effect of this beta-blocker on prognosis, except to say that it had not prevented sudden death in those who had been taking it. Since then a routine search for arrhythmias by us and by others has shown the high incidence of ventricular and supraventricular arrhythmias in HOCM and their relationship to sudden death in those in whom the arrhythmias had not been successfully suppressed by appropriate antiarrhythmic treatment.

Numerically the annual mortality for a patient diagnosed as having HOCM varies between 2% and 8% per annum according to the prognostic features mentioned. The highest annual mortality has been found in young people whose diagnosis has been made in childhood and who had a family history of sudden death as well as personal features of severe disease, including cardiomegaly. The lowest mortality has been found in patients without a family history of sudden death and who had not had syncopal attacks.

III. DIAGNOSIS

The diagnosis of HOCM is most commonly first made in the second and third decades, and it is therefore one of the cardiac disorders that may be first noticed during pregnancy.[12,13]

The first manifestation may be with symptoms or because of a murmur or an abnormality found on an ECG or chest radiograph carried out as routine checks or for life assurance purposes.

Shortness of breath results from a raised left atrial pressure consequent upon the noncompliant left ventricle. Exercise- or emotion-induced tachycardia may further reduce the efficiency of left atrial emptying or increase mitral regurgitation in some cases. In other patients arrhythmias may be provoked during exercise.

Angina pectoris is often an early symptom, but mild, and worsening of this or development of a new symptom may lead to the diagnosis of HOCM. This entity should be considered when a young person describes apparent angina that is of long standing and is sometimes rather atypical.

Syncope, dizzy spells, or palpitations are commonly the result of tachyarrhythmias, although syncope in some patients can have a haemodynamic origin due to fall in stroke volume, blood pressure, and coronary flow during tachycardia. Syncope can sometimes be postural like an ordinary vasovagal attack, except that it tends to occur on standing from sitting rather than during prolonged standing, and it is caused by a sudden reduction in central and left ventricular volume.

Infective endocarditis may occur and lead to the diagnosis of HOCM, with symptoms of fever or because of embolism. Atrial arrhythmias occur, and atrial fibrillation eventually develops in patients with chronically elevated left atrial pressures, but these are usually in the older age group.

The physical signs are teasingly diverse. In the most typical cases, however, a positive diagnosis can be made from the clinical signs alone. In others a clinical diagnosis can be made, but it is one of exclusion and needs the aid of the ECG and chest radiograph. In a few cases, although the diagnosis may be suspected, confirmation comes from the combination of echocardiographic, angiographic, and intracardiac pressure evidence. In all, the clinical diagnosis should be confirmed and amplified by full invasive study, postponed of course until after delivery in the case of pregnant women.

The typical signs that allow the "positive diagnosis of recognition" are those by which the disorder was first recognised and described. The patient is a young adult. The heart is in sinus rhythm, the arterial pulses are jerky and ill-sustained, the venous pulse in the neck shows a small dominant *a* wave. The left ventricular impulse is prominent and quite characteristic, having a palpable atrial beat preceding the systolic impulse and, in some cases, also a second systolic beat providing three elements and a shuddering sensation to the finger. Such an impulse is diagnostic. A loud systolic murmur is placed maximally between the left sternal edge and the apex. It may be heard in the axilla but is poorly relayed to the base or the carotids. The murmur is delayed after the first heart sound and usually ceases before the second. It starts louder and is placed later than the symmetrical, diamond-shaped murmur of aortic stenosis, and there is no click (Fig. M.VIII.1). There is sometimes a soft mid-diastolic murmur at the apex but no opening snap. The palpable atrial beat is usually of too low frequency to be audible, although the first heart sound is often mistaken for an atrial

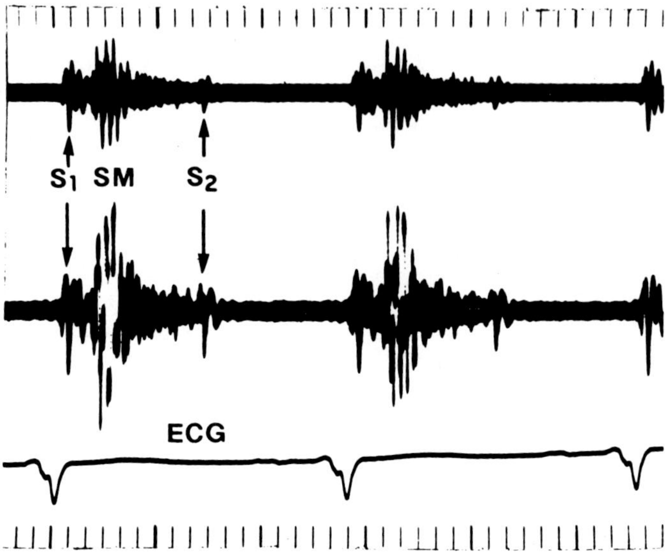

Fig. M.VIII.1. The typical systolic murmur (SM) in HOCM, late of onset and often decrescendo. The main differential diagnosis is from nonrheumatic mitral regurgitation (mitral leaflet prolapse), but echocardiography rapidly differentiates. S_1: first heart sound. S_2: second heart sound.

sound because of its separation from the onset of the murmur. Third heart sounds are occasionally present, especially in the young. Early diastolic murmurs are not heard, and the second heart sound is usually normal, though occasionally there may be a reversed split.

Loud systolic murmurs are usually associated with turbulence and outflow tract gradients. These systolic murmurs may be varied greatly by manoeuvres that alter left ventricular volume. A systolic murmur may often be abolished in the first few beats after squatting from standing and conversely is intensified by the Valsalva manoeuvre, in the post ectopic beat, and after inhalation of amyl nitrite.

Other patients are murmur-free but usually still have a palpable atrial beat.

In a few patients the murmurs simulate those of rheumatic mitral stenosis, with a prominent mid-diastolic murmur but usually no opening snap.

The electrocardiogram usually shows evidence of left ventricular hypertrophy (Fig. M.VIII.2) but is occasionally within normal limits in the young, though with high voltage. More often the electrocardiogram is very abnormal, with tall and often prolonged P waves of left or biatrial enlargement, often a rather short PR interval, and a very abnormal QRS complex. The axis may be normal or leftward, or there may be left anterior hemiblock; such a sequence tends to be progressive in individual cases. These latter patients often show QS waves in the right and mid-chest leads, and the left chest leads show an R wave with no initial Q. In some patients there may be a seeming delta wave, which with the short PR interval and absent Q wave suggests preexcitation. Although this has been described in HOCM, the association seems to be a chance one, and in most patients showing the features mentioned, which are somewhat suggestive of preexcitation, no evidence of it can be found if electrophysiological studies are undertaken. Apart from left anterior hemiblock, which may be an expression of hypertrophy, bundle branch block is uncommon.

The heart may be normal or enlarged on chest radiography, but the contour is usually chunky with a bulging contour high on the left ventricular border (Fig. M.VIII.3). The right atrium may be prominent. In severe cases the left atrium is enlarged, and the lungs may show pulmonary venous congestion. When heart failure develops the heart may become very big due to dilatation of all chambers except the left ventricle, which only very rarely dilates, even in heart failure. Valve calcification is not seen, except in the elderly, in whom the mitral valve may calcify. Rarely the chest x-ray is within normal limits.

IV. DIAGNOSIS OF HOCM WHEN IT IS FIRST SEEN DURING PREGNANCY

Because HOCM is so often asymptomatic, it may often be discovered at routine examination in pregnancy. In other cases it is diagnosed because pregnancy provokes symptoms that had previously been absent. In addition, since loud systolic murmurs are not uncommon in normal hearts in pregnancy, HOCM is sometimes mistakenly diagnosed when the heart is normal; this error is almost worse than missing heart disease when it is there.

Most often the pregnant patient is entirely asymptomatic, and news of suspected heart disease causes dismay. A firm diagnosis is important and can often be made by echocardiography using M-mode and, if available, two-dimensional echo as well.[14,15] Since confirmatory invasive investigation is contraindicated in pregnancy, the echocardiographic abnormalities must be definite before the diagnosis is made, and when this is so the physical signs and ECG are often well outside normal limits, so no problem is presented. It is when the physical signs are in doubt and the ECG within normal lim-

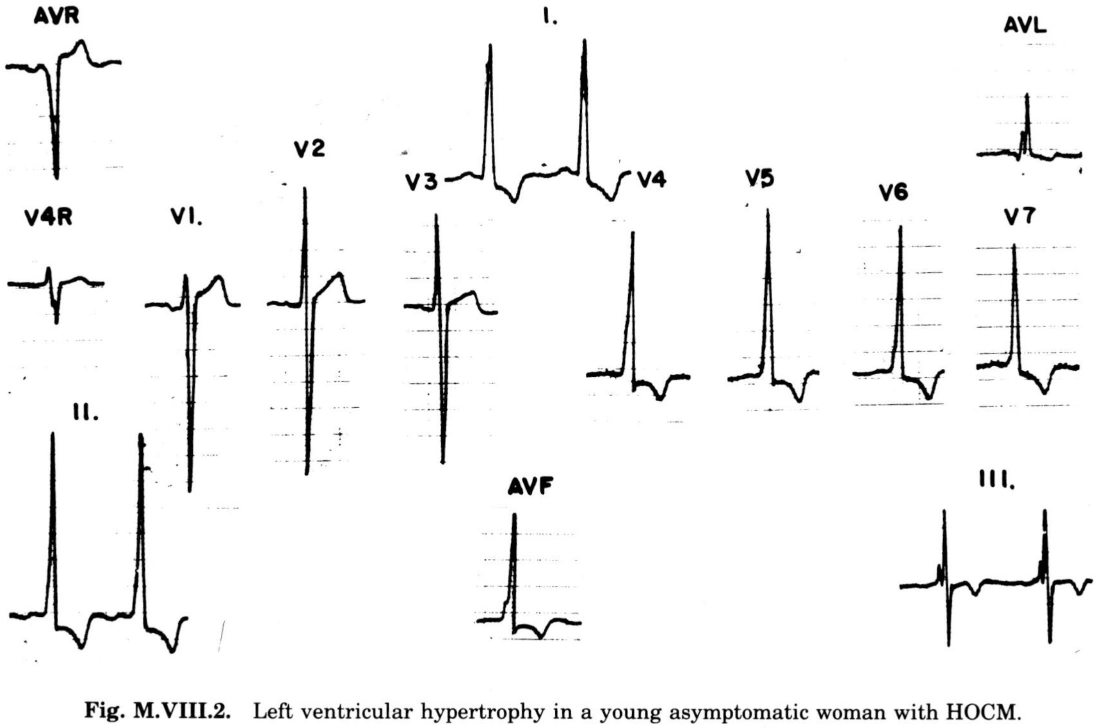

Fig. M.VIII.2. Left ventricular hypertrophy in a young asymptomatic woman with HOCM.

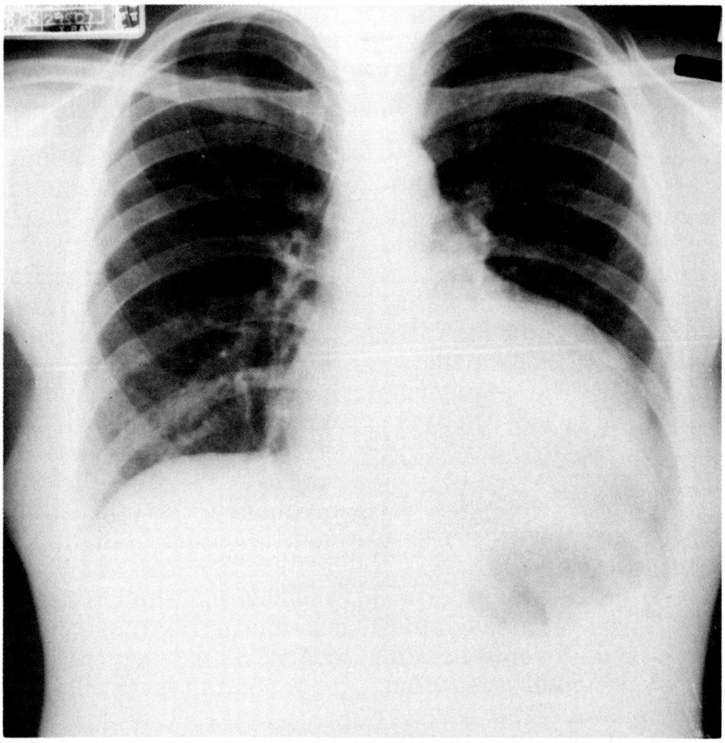

Fig. M.VIII.3. Typical chest radiograph from a young woman with HOCM showing chunky left ventricular outline.

its that the echocardiogram assumes great importance, and then the echocardiographer has a responsibility not to report a firm diagnosis of HOCM on the echo alone, unless most or all of the possible echocardiographic features of HOCM are present (Fig. M.VIII.4, Table M.VIII.1).

In particular, echocardiographic evidence of asymmetric septal hypertrophy (ASH)[14] is not the same thing as the diagnosis of a heart disorder. Asymmetric hypertrophy may be found in normal hearts under some circumstances, and it is easy to "create" through technical error, particularly when elements of the tricuspid valve are unwittingly incorporated into the septal echo, increasing the apparent thickness of the septum. Technique is therefore all important, and for security, ASH should be associated with systolic anterior movement (SAM). SAM can be found in some normal hearts, particularly in hyperkinetic states such as pregnancy, as well as in many other cardiac disorders, and only the full SAM is significant. This is a forward movement of the anterior leaflet of the mitral valve occurring early in systole and carrying the anterior leaflet right onto the septum, where it remains until the end of systole. Usually this is associated with delayed onset of the diastolic closure slope, and the combination results in a diagnostic appearance with the anterior leaflet spending most of the cardiac cycle applied to the septum, apart from the brief early-systolic and late-diastolic closures.

Two-dimensional echo shows the hypertrophy better than M-mode by indicating its asymmetry as well as its extent. Often the hypertrophied muscle gives a hard, sparkling echo, probably due to the large

TABLE M.VIII.1. The M-Mode Echocardiographic Features of HOCM*

1.	Absolute increase in left ventricular wall thickness
2.	Asymmetrical hypertrophy of the septum compared with the posterior free wall of the left ventricle (ratio 1.3:1)
3.	Reduced or low normal absolute left ventricular cavity dimensions
4.	Anterior eccentricity of the mitral valve within the left ventricular cavity
5.	Systolic reopening of the anterior leaflet of the mitral valve on to the septum
6.	Slow and biphasic diastolic closure of the anterior mitral leaflet
7.	Systolic closure of the aortic valve cusps
8.	Reduced septal excursion and systolic thickening compared with the posterior wall

*cf. Figure M.VIII.4.

amount of fibrous tissue that is often present. Two-dimensional echo also shows abnormal mitral valve movement, as well as systolic closure of the aortic valve, which is easier to see on two-dimensional echo than on M-mode.

Investigation in pregnancy should include exercise testing and ambulatory ECG Holter monitoring, both of these with the prime objective of detecting subclinical arrhythmias, particularly ventricular arrhythmias. It cannot be overemphasised that sudden death in HOCM is usually not haemodynamic but electrical, and the detection of arrhythmia identifies the patient who is at risk. Exercise tolerance is sometimes normal but may be surprisingly reduced, and this too is revealed by the test.

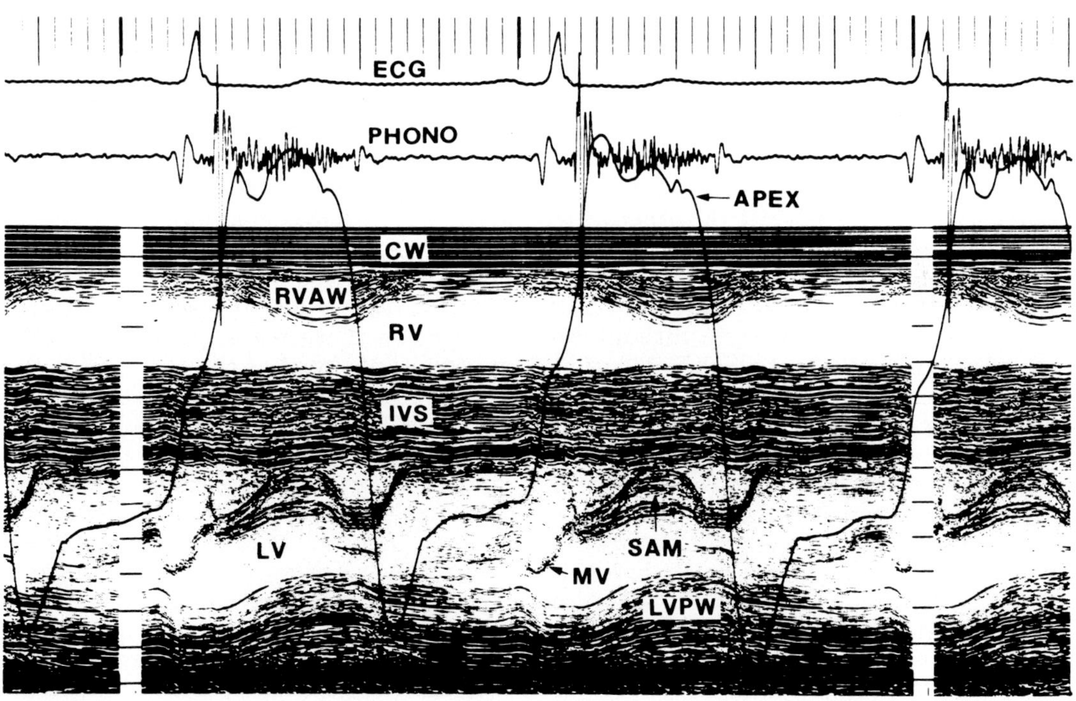

Fig. M.VIII.4. M-mode echocardiography from a patient with HOCM (see Table M.VIII.1). Figure also shows simultaneous recording of phonocardiogram (phono) and apexcardiogram (apex). CW = chest wall; RVAW = right ventricular anterior wall; RV = right ventricle; IVS = interventricular septum; MV = mitral valve; SAM = systolic anterior motion; LV = left ventricle; LVPW = left ventricular posterior wall.

V. MANAGEMENT OF PREGNANCY

Pregnancy and delivery are usually accomplished without difficulty in patients with HOCM, even those with severe disease. Early in our experience elective cesarean section was recommended because we thought that tachycardia, repeated Valsalva manouvres, and the possibility of blood loss would be dangerous during normal delivery. However, after a number of patients had tolerated vaginal delivery without incident, it was learned that, just as in other heart diseases, cesarean section is indicated in HOCM only for obstetric reasons. Also, in our early experience beta-adrenergic blocking drugs (then propranolol) were used routinely throughout pregnancy and continued throughout labour, but recently the use of beta-blocking drugs in pregnancy has caused some concern because of increased numbers of small-for-dates babies, low Apgar scores, neonatal hypoglycaemia, bradycardia, and failure of normal response to anoxic stress. At the same time, the routine use of beta-blockers in HOCM was questioned, and these drugs are now no longer used, except for specific indications. Pregnant patients with HOCM, like others, are now treated individually according to need.

We recently reported the outcome of 43 pregnancies that went to term without the loss of any mothers or babies.[13] Many of these patients had received propranolol, and some had also taken diuretics for pulmonary congestive symptoms. Two infants of mothers who had received propranolol through pregnancy showed a sinus bradycardia for the first 24–36 hours after delivery, but neither developed hypoglycaemia. Three babies were small for dates, but two of the three mothers given propranolol in the same dosage in subsequent pregnancies delivered infants of normal birth weight. We regard epidural anaesthesia for delivery as inadvisable on theoretical grounds in HOCM.

Our experience was representative of a wide range of HOCM from mild to the most severe disease, including two women who had been treated previously by myotomy-myectomy. Three women had had problems in previous pregnancies, which did not recur in the subsequent ones. Deterioration in symptoms was not always predictable by the severity of the disease in any of its features, but patients whose disease was clinically mild never developed congestive features requiring diuretics. Only two patients showed deterioration in angina, and three required diuretics for pulmonary congestive symptoms.

In general terms any factors that would increase left ventricular outflow gradients should probably be avoided, and these include vasodilatation and fall in central blood volume resulting from epidural anaesthesia, hypotension from any cause, violent expulsive effort, and cardiac stimulant drugs. Oxytocic drugs are not contraindicated. As we no longer advocate antibiotic prophylaxis for normal delivery in our patients with heart disease, we do not recommend this for our patients with HOCM, but since patients with HOCM are at risk from endocarditis, instrumental delivery with its greater risk of higher grade bacteraemia should be covered.

A further 58 pregnancies in our patients had been achieved without trouble but were not analysed in detail because of insufficient data; there were no deaths in this group either. Most of the patients in this second group had not received beta-blocking drugs. The indication for the use of these drugs in pregnancy is for the specific indication of angina, sometimes for dyspnoea caused by poor left atrial emptying during tachycardia, or for arrhythmias when beta-blockers have been shown to be effective in suppressing them in the individual patient. In general, beta-blockers are ineffective in suppressing ventricular arrhythmias in HOCM and are not very effective in suppressing supraventricular arrhythmias (although these are slowed). Patients with angina may respond to verapamil, although experience with this drug in pregnancy is less than that with propranolol. We have not been impressed as have others[15] with the symptomatic benefits accruing from the use of verapamil in HOCM.

Clinically important ventricular arrhythmias in pregnancy must be sought and treated with specific antiarrhythmic agents, whose efficacy is subsequently proved by repeat ambulatory monitoring.

If beta-blockers have to be given in pregnancy, it is wise to monitor foetal growth particularly carefully, as well as the heart rate and blood sugar of the neonate for the first 48 hours after birth. Our experience indicates, however, that there should be no fear about giving beta-blockers during pregnancy when they are specifically indicated.

Patients only rarely seek advice about the eugenic aspects of their disease. In a condition like HOCM, with such a variable prognosis, it is very difficult to give wise advice. Our studies have shown that afflicted families tend to run "true to form," so a history of early death from HOCM in a family has predictive value.

VI. OUTCOME OF PREGNANCY

The babies born to mothers with HOCM are usually of normal weight and thrive. It is rare for HOCM to be detectable in the offspring until they are at least five years old, although there are exceptionally severe examples of HOCM showing itself in younger children, even in the neonate. We have deliberately avoided too frequent noninvasive monitoring of the children born to mothers with HOCM unless there is high suspicion of abnormality.

VII. CONCLUSIONS

Pregnancy is safe in most patients with hypertrophic cardiomyopathy. A flexible approach should be adopted towards therapy, based on symptomatic relief and on suppression of arrhythmias. Occult arrhythmias should be sought by ambulatory ECG monitoring and by exercise testing. Many patients need no drug treatment at all. Beta-adrenergic blocking drugs can be used safely when indicated, and although adverse effects on the foetus have been reported, we had no problems associated with the use of these drugs in our patients.

VIII. REFERENCES

1. Report of the WHO/ISFC Task Force on the Definition and Classification of Cardiomyopathies. Br Heart J. 1980; 44:672–673.
2. Swan DA, Bell B, Oakley CM, Goodwin JF. Analysis of the symptomatic course and treatment of hypertrophic obstructive cardiomyopathy. Br Heart J. 1971; 33:671–685.
3. Mckenna WJ, Deanfield JE, Faruqi AM, Oakley CM, Goodwin JF. Prognosis and mortality in hypertrophic cardiomyopathy. Circulation. 1979; 59, 60(Suppl II):154.
4. Braunwald E, Lambrew CT, Rockoff SD, Ross JJN, Morrow AG. Idiopathic hypertrophic subaortic stenosis. Circulation. 1964; 30 (Suppl IV):3.
5. Goodwin JF, Oakley CM. The cardiomyopathies. Br Heart J. 1972; 34:545.
6. Oakley CM. Clinical recognition of the cardiomyopathies. Circ Res. 1974; 34,35 (Suppl II):152–159.
7. Pomerance A, Davies MJ. Pathological features of hypertrophic cardiomyopathy in the elderly. Br Heart J. 1975; 37:305–312.
8. Maron BJ, Roberts WC, Edwards JE, McAllister HA Jr, Foley DD, Epstein SE. Sudden death in patients with hypertrophic cardiomyopathy: Characterization of 26 patients without functional limitation. Am J Cardiol. 1978; 41:803–810.
9. Maron BJ, Lipson LC, Roberts WC, Savage DD, Epstein SE. "Malignant" hypertrophic cardiomyopathy. Identification of a subgroup of families with unusually frequent premature death. Am J Cardiol. 1978; 41:1133–1140.
10. McKenna WJ, Chetty S, Oakley CM, Goodwin JF. Arrhythmias in hypertrophic cardiomyopathy. Exercise and 48 hour ambulatory electrocardiography assessment with and without beta adrenergic blocking therapy. Am J Cardiol. 1980; 45:1–5.
11. McKenna W, Deanfield J, Faruqui A, England D, Oakley C, Goodwin J. Prognosis in hypertrophic cardiomyopathy: Role of age and clinical, electrocardiographic and haemodyanamic features. Am J Cardiol. 1981; 47:532–538.
12. Turner GM, Oakley CM, Dixon HG. Management of pregnancy complicated by hypertrophic obstructive cardiomyopathy. Br Med J. 1968; 4:281–284.
13. Oakley GDG, McGarry K, Limb DG, Oakley CM. Managment of pregnancy in patients with

hypertrophic cardiomyopathy. Br Med J. 1975; 37:305–312.
14. Henry WL, Clark CE, Epstein SE. Asymmetric septal hypertrophy. Echocardiographic identification of the pathognomonic anatomic abnormality of IHSS. Circulation. 1973; 47:225–233.
15. Kaltenbach M, Hopf R, Kober G, Bussman WD, Keller M, Petersen Y. Treatment of hypertrophic obstructive cardiomyopathy with verapamil. Br Heart J. 1979; 42:35–42.
16. Doi YL, McKenna WM, Oakley CM, Goodwin JF. M-mode echocardiography in hypertrophic cardiomyopathy: Diagnostic criteria and prediction of obstruction. Am J Cardiol. 1980; 45:6–14.

M.IX

Pericardial Disorders and Pregnancy

Lawrence Santora, MD, and Uri Elkayam, MD

The pericardium can become involved in every kind of medical and surgical disease process (Table M.IX.1).[1,2] Necropsy involvement is found in 5% of autopsy studies, whereas clinical recognition of involvement is probably less than 1% of hospital admissions. Acute pericarditis is the most important clinical presentation of pericardial disease in women of childbearing age. With pregnancy becoming more commonplace in women in their late thirties and forties, the differential diagnosis will undoubtedly become more difficult as age-related disorders (eg, coronary disease) become more likely. The clinical recognition of pericardial disease will likewise require a higher index of suspicion lest it be overlooked in women in these older age groups.

I. ACUTE PERICARDITIS

Probably no serious disease is so frequently overlooked by the practitioner.[3]

—William Osler

A. General Considerations

Most cases of pericarditis are self-limited and mild. The identification of the subset of patients at risk for serious pericardial involvement guides the initial therapeutic approach and is discussed later. The additional hemodynamic burden of an average blood volume increase of 40–50% during pregnancy, together with the myocarditis that often accompanies pericarditis, may lead to heart failure in the pregnant woman. With the ad-

Cardiac Problems in Pregnancy, pages 115–129

TABLE M.IX.1. Etiology of Acute Pericarditis

Inflammatory
Idiopathic
Infections
Bacterial
Viral
Tubercular
Mycotic
Miscellaneous (protozoal, mycoplasmal, spirochetal)
Associated with acute transmural myocardial infarction
Postmyocardial infarction syndrome (Dressler syndrome)
Postpericardiotomy
Traumatic
Metabolic disorders (uremia, myxedema, gout)
Connective tissue diseases (systemic lupus erythematosus, progressive systemic sclerosis, rheumatoid arthritis, rheumatic fever)
Allergic and hypersensitivity diseases (serum sickness, drugs)
Neoplastic disorders
Postirradiation
Postanticoagulation

vent of improved methods of hemodynamic monitoring and interventions, most complicated cases can safely be brought to term.[4]

B. Etiology

Idiopathic pericarditis is the most common cause of acute pericarditis. Viruses are often implicated in this variety, but they are rarely proved. Coxsackie B is the most common agent. Recently, rubella myopericarditis has been reported during pregnancy.[5] Upper respiratory symptoms will often precede the onset of chest pain and low-grade fever in both the viral and idiopathic varieties. Lymphadenopathy, myalgias, and a rubelliform rash also accompany viral pericarditis. Sporadic exacerbations are not uncommon in either type. Frequently, because of an accompanying myocarditis, fatigue and malaise persist for weeks after the pain has subsided. Bacterial pericarditis usually occurs as a complication of bacterial infection elsewhere, most often from a pneumonia or empyema. The primary source should be vigorously sought. Staphylococci are becoming more common because there are several organisms resistant to antibiotics. Pneumococci are still relatively rare because of their extreme sensitivity to penicillin. In the immunocompromised host, gram-negative organisms and fungi should be sought. Tuberculous (TB) pericarditis requires special consideration because of its often insidious onset and tendency to cause pericardial constriction. One-half of all patients with TB pericarditis have pulmonary or disseminated disease. It is rare before 20 years and after 70 years of age. Even with chemotherapy, 60% of patients with tuberculous effusion will ultimately develop constriction unless pericardiectomy is performed.[6] A presumptive diagnosis should be considered in a patient with recent rapid weight loss, night sweats, anorexia, arthralgias, low-grade fever, positive 5 TU skin test, and a large sanguineous effusion. Precordial pain occurs in less than half of patients with TB pericarditis, but nonproductive cough is an early and prominent feature.[7]

Collagen vascular diseases often involve the pericardium. Most notable among these are systemic lupus erythematosus (Fig. M.IX.1), rheumatoid arthritis, and scleroderma. At some time in the course of systemic lupus erythematosus, 17–50% of the patients will have clinical evidence of pericardial disease; however, only 5% have pericarditis as the cause of their presenting symptoms.[8,9] The disease is often exacerbated in the last trimester of pregnancy and several months postpartum. Treatment with steroids will usually prevent constriction and tamponade. In rheumatoid arthritis, however, only 3% of patients have clinical pericardial disease. Treatment with steroids will not prevent constriction or tamponade, which may occur in up to 10% of those patients with pericardial effusions.[10] Scleroderma will occur in association with clinical pericardial disease in 5–16% of cases. The presence of pericardial involvement in patients with collagen vascular disease will dramatically decrease the five-year sur-

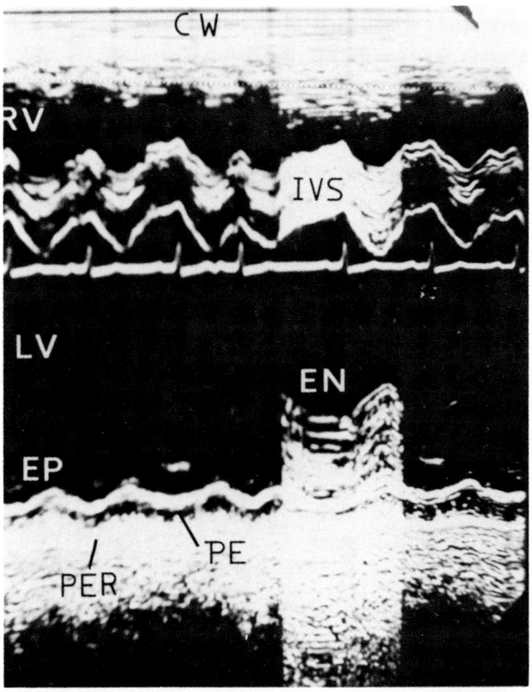

Fig. M.IX.1. Echocardiogram shows a posterior pericardial effusion (PE) in a 31-year-old pregnant woman with systemic lupus erythematosus. CW, chest wall; RV, right ventricle; IVS, interventricular septum; LV, left ventricle; EN, endocardium; EP, epicardium; PER pericardium. (Reprinted with permission from Elkayam et al.[9])

vival rate to 25%, compared to 75% in those without pericardial involvement. Steroids do not seem to alter the prognosis.

C. Clinical Findings

1. Symptoms

Chest pain, often acute, is the hallmark of pericarditis. Usually sharp, stabbing substernal pain radiates to the back, neck, left shoulder, or upper arm. Characteristically it is relieved by leaning forward and is exacerbated by lying supine, swallowing, breathing deeply, or coughing. At times a vague chest heaviness may mimic myocardial infarction. Dyspnea is commonly present when there is a moderate-to-large pericardial effusion; it may result from impaired filling of the ventricles caused by the effusion or by mechanical compression of lung parenchyma and bronchi. This mechanical compression may also cause hoarseness, coughing, and dysphagia. The pregnant patient may incorrectly interpret the physiological hyperventilation of pregnancy as dyspnea.

2. Signs

Friction rubs are characteristic of pericarditis. They are superficial sounding, with a "leathery" or grating quality heard best over the second to fourth left intercostal space in the midclavicular line or at the left sternal border. They are best heard through the diaphragm of the stethoscope while the patient is leaning forward in deep inspiration. A pericardial rub will persist when the breath is held, and therefore it can be distinguished from a pleural rub. Pericardial rubs are often transient, coming and going over short periods of time. They usually have two components: one corresponding to systole and the other presystolic, corresponding to the atrial kick. Occasionally a third component in early diastole may be heard, corresponding to the third heart sound in (S_3) in timing. Since systolic murmurs, split first heart sounds, and an S_3 are very common in pregnancy, differentiation from a rub may be difficult.[11] The following distinctions have been suggested: 1) rubs do not consistently change with respiration like murmurs; 2) rubs do not radiate in a consistent manner as do murmurs; 3) rubs are loudest at the left sternal border rather than at the valve areas; 4) rubs change frequently from one exam to another; 5) a single component rub may develop two or three components after slight exercise.[12]

The chest examination will usually reveal lungs that are clear to auscultation. Dullness may be heard below the left scapula if there is lung compression caused by a large pericardial effusion (Ewart sign); also, heart sounds may be distant if there is a large effusion. Neck veins will not be elevated unless right ventricular diastolic filling is comprised by a large effusion or constriction. The elevated right ventricular diastolic pressure will then cause an elevated right atrial pressure and central venous pressure, which will result in distention of the neck veins. Fever usually occurs and is low grade unless there is an infectious etiology, in which case it may be high (100–103° F). Tachycardia is seen in up to 85% of the cases, and sedimentation rate becomes elevated with the onset of symptoms.

D. Suggested Laboratory Evaluation

1. Electrocardiogram

Electrocardiographic changes occur in up to 80% of patients having an acute attack of pericarditis. The electrocardiographic pattern of pericarditis is characterized by ST segment elevation in several leads, denoting the widespread nature of the disease (Fig. M.IX.2). ST segment changes on the ECG appear as elevations with an upward concavity and initially upright T waves, and they occur within a few hours after the onset of chest pain or fever. The elevations most frequently occur in leads I, II, V_5 and V_6, and they persist for hours to days, followed by T wave flattening and then T inversion, which reverts to normal within weeks to months.[13] Early repolarization changes of normal patients may be impossible to distinguish from pericarditis; however, in the normal patient in early repolarization the ST segment elevation occurs much less frequently in the limb leads than it does in pericarditis. In distinction to acute myocardial infarction, the ECG in pericarditis does not show ST segment depression in leads reciprocal from those in which the elevation occurs, but usually only in leads VR and V_1. The ST segment elevation (usually < 5 mm) in pericarditis is concave upward, as opposed to the convex upward elevation seen in myocardial infarction (Fig. M.IX.3). In addition, there are no pathological Q waves and the T waves usually remain upright in pericarditis as long as there is ST elevation, whereas in myocardial infarction T waves invert while ST segments remain elevated (Fig. M.IX.3). Low voltage and alternation of voltage (electrical alternans) may occur if there is a pericardial effusion. Sinus tachycardia is the most common rhythm, but transient atrial fibrillation occurs in one-third of the patients, and occasionally, atrial flutter and sinus bradycardia occur as a consequence of irritation of the sinus node by the inflamed pericardium.[14] The ECG changes seen in a normal pregnancy without heart disease are described in detail in Chapter M.I. In brief, there is a slight axis shift as a result of altered position of the heart and occasionally T wave inversion and a Q wave in lead III.[16]

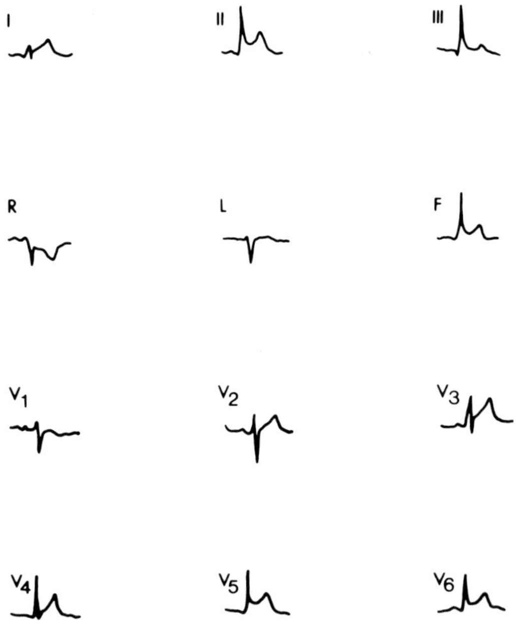

Fig. M.IX.2. Electrocardiogram of a patient with acute pericarditis demonstrating characteristic finding of widespread ST segment elevations (leads: I, II, III, aV_F, V_2–V_6), with upright T waves

2. Chest x-ray film

The chest x-ray film has largely been supplanted by echocardiography in the diagnosis of pericardial effusion. However, it is helpful in determining an underlying lung process (eg, neoplasm, pneumonia, tuberculosis) as an etiology for the peri-

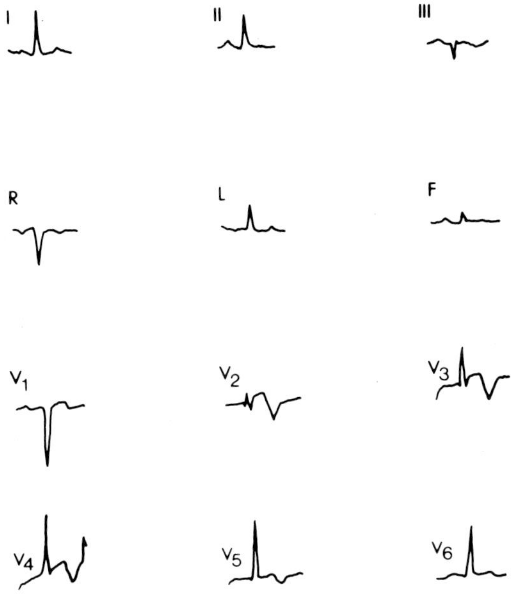

Fig. M.IX.3. Electrocardiogram in a patient with acute anterior-septal myocardial infarction demonstrating convex upward ST segment elevations limited to the anterior chest leads (V_1–V_5) with a concordant T wave inversion

carditis. Pulmonary infiltrates and pleural effusions have been found in up to one-fourth of patients with idiopathic pericarditis. The cardiac shadow will not be enlarged until 250–300 cc of pericardial fluid has accumulated, at which time a rapidly enlarging cardiac size and clear lung fields on serial x-rays will suggest an effusion. At times an epicardial fat line within the border of the cardiac shadow suggests the presence of an effusion.

3. Echocardiogram

The M-mode echocardiogram is very sensitive for detecting pericardial effusion and can reveal as little as 20 cc of fluid (Fig. M.IX.4).[17] It is invaluable in serial quantification of the fluid. Occasionally a loculated effusion will not be detected on the M-mode scan, in which case two-dimensional echocardiography may be helpful. Echocardiography also provides an assessment of valve function and of myocardial function as well. Since peri-

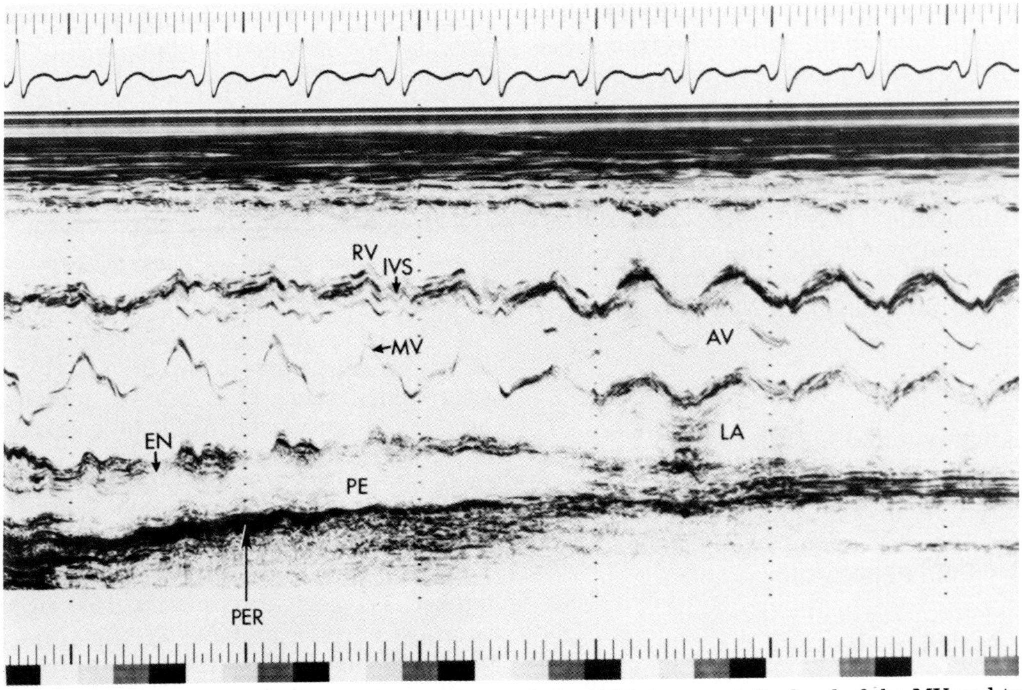

Fig. M.IX.4. M-mode echocardiogram demonstrating a sweep from the level of the mitral valve (MV) to the level of the aorta (Ao). A large posterior effusion (PE) is seen at the level of the MV and typically disappears as scanned behind left atrium (LA). Other abbreviations as in Figure 1.

cardial disease can cause myocarditis with attendant left ventricular dysfunction, the echocardiogram will help to distinguish between these two causes of circulatory impairment. An effusion will usually only affect diastolic filling, so the diastolic dimension of the left ventricle will be normal or small with good systolic contraction of the left ventricle; the left ventricular diastolic dimension may increase and the systolic function will be abnormal as evidenced both by poor contraction of the left ventricular walls in systole and by a low ejection fraction. At times both processes can coexist. Thickening of the pericardium in pericarditis may be present and can often, but not always, be detected by echocardiography.[18] Quantifying a pericardial effusion can be done grossly: an anterior echo-free space as well as a posterior free space denotes a moderate to large effusion; if there is only a posterior free space with separation of the pericardial and epicardial echoes throughout systole and diastole, the effusion is of moderate size; if the separation occurs only in systole, there is a small effusion or no effusion; an isolated anterior echo-free space is mostly a false-positive finding reflecting epicardial fat; in some cases, however, it may be a loculated effusion which can be further evaluated with 2-D echocardiography. In addition to localizing loculated effusions, the 2-D echocardiogram will allow simultaneous viewing of all four cardiac chambers and the assessment of their size and function (Fig. M.IX.5).

E. General Management

1. Bed rest and hospitalization

Bed rest and hospitalization for observation and initial diagnostic work-up are indicated in most pregnant patients suspected of having acute pericarditis.

2. Arrhythmias

Arrhythmias can be treated as in the nonpregnant state. Specific therapy can be found in great detail in Chapter M.XX. In general, sinus tachycardia need not be treated. Atrial fibrillation is usually the most common arrhythmia encountered and in pregnancy it may lead to heart failure because of increased blood volume and the loss of the atrial contribution to cardiac output. If the patient is hemodynamically stable, the ventricular rate can be slowed by digoxin and beta-blocking agents. Quinidine can be used to convert to sinus rhythm, but is rarely necessary since the arrhythmias are usually transient and often convert with digoxin alone. Direct-current cardioversion should be used if there is hemodynamic embarrassment, and it is probably safer than quinidine for elective cardioversion in the pregnant state.[20] Similar regimens apply to atrial flutter and other supraventricular arrhythmias.

3. Analgesia

Analgesia is readily accomplished in most patients with aspirin 650 mg every four hours or other nonsteroidal antiinflammatory agents. If pain is severe and persistent and TB or infectious pericarditis is not suspected, then prednisone may be given in a dosage of 60–100 mg per day. The dosage may be decreased in two to three days, then tapered within two weeks. Exacerbation of symptoms is not uncommon after withdrawing sterioids and they may have to be reinstituted.

4. Pericardiocentesis

Pericardiocentesis can be accomplished in the pregnant patient by the subxiphoid approach if there is at least a moderate amount of pericardial fluid by echocardiogram. The indications for pericardiocentesis are to obtain fluid to identify an organism or malignant cells or to remove fluid if there is hemodynamic compromise. Unfortunately, pericardiocentesis will diagnose TB pericarditis only 15% of the time by culture and 5% of the time by biopsy. If bacterial pericarditis is strongly suspected, most authorities think that early pericardiectomy will reduce the high mortality reported in cases treated

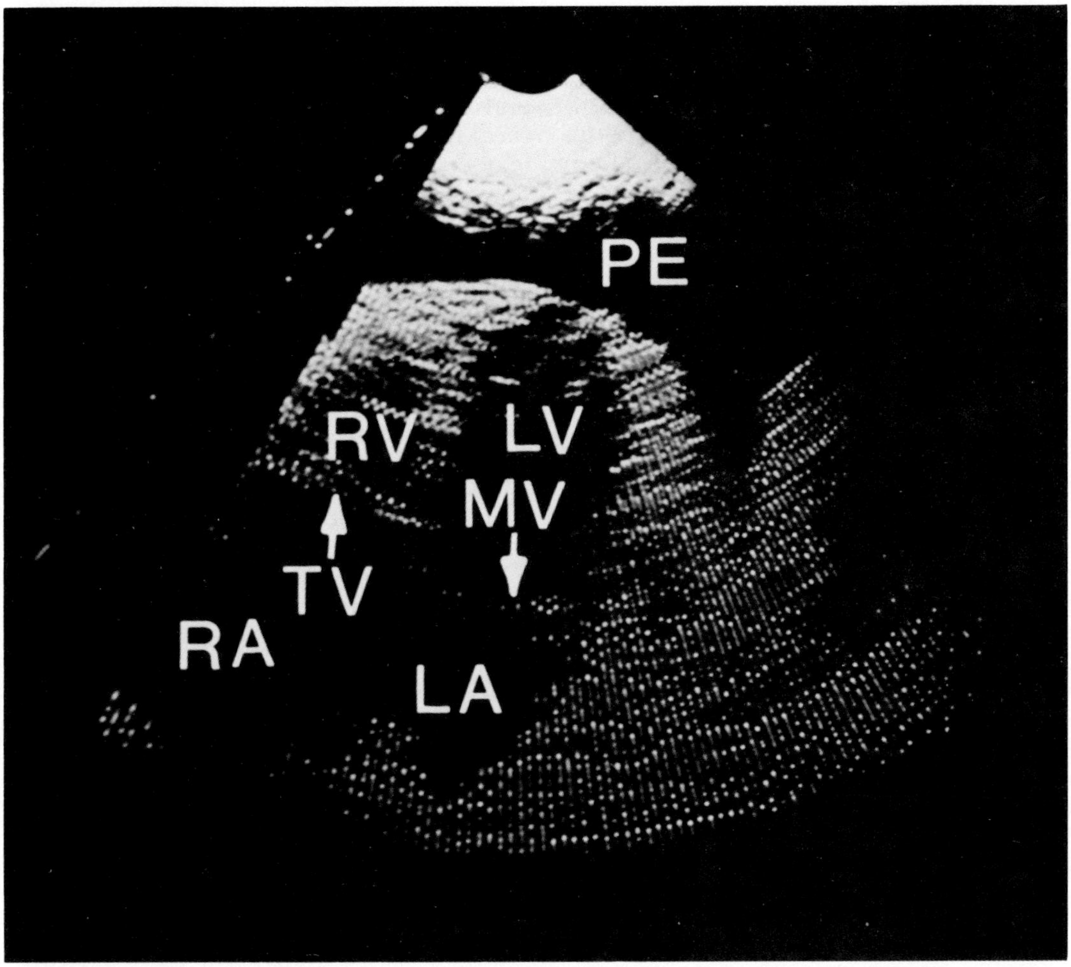

Fig. M.IX.5. 2-D echocardiogram from an apical four-chamber view. All four chambers are visualized surrounded by a large pericardial effusion. TV, tricuspid valve; RA, right atrium; other abbreviations as in Figures M.IX.1 and M.IX.4.

by antibiotics alone.[21] There is controversy about the indications for pericardiectomy in TB pericarditis if there is no pericardial constriction. Some clinicians believe that an early surgical approach can prevent the complications of constriction, whereas others think that operation should be reserved for those patients who manifest signs of persistent increased venous pressure.[22–24] The clear-cut indications for pericardiectomy are bacterial pericarditis, intractable pain despite medical management, and signs of constrictive pericarditis.[21] Pericardiectomy has been done safely during pregnancy for constrictive pericarditis due to TB and radiation.[25,26]

5. Antibiotic therapy

Antibiotic therapy during pregnancy is discussed in great detail in Chapter M.XXV. In general, if pericardial fluid fails to yield an organism on gram stain despite a high index of suspicion of a bacterial agent, antibiotics should be given to cover Staphylococcus and gram-negative organisms. If there is a strong presumptive diagnosis of TB pericarditis when the pericardial fluid and biopsy are nondiagnostic, it is reasonable to start a triple drug regimen and to follow the patient clinically for signs of constriction.[22,27] The antitubercular drugs (ethambutol, streptomycin, para-aminosalicylic acid, and isoniazid) have been shown not to harm the fetus, and the incidence of fetal mortality improves when maternal tuberculosis is treated.[28,29]

6. Prognosis is dependent on underlying disease

Most cases are self-limited idiopathic paricarditis that respond rapidly to aspirin and are uncomplicated except for occasional relapse. Recovery usually occurs from two weeks to several months after onset without residual pericardial thickening or persistent electrocardiographic changes. Occasionally a perimyocarditis will evolve. Some authors have stated that therapeutic abortion is indicated whenever early pregnancy is complicated by active myocarditis.[30] With improved medical management, a great number of patients with this disease are being reported to reach uneventful term deliveries.[4]

7. Differential diagnosis

Differential diagnosis is limited to several conditions usually associated with chest pain, chiefly, pleurisy, acute myocardial infarction, and pulmonary embolism.

a. Pleurisy. Pleurisy often follows an upper respiratory illness and is accompanied by chest pain exacerbated by deep breathing. The rub and pain of pleurisy will usually cease when the breath is held. The chest x-ray film will often show an effusion or infiltrate, and the electrocardiogram will not show the characteristic ST and T wave changes of pericarditis.

b. Acute myocardial infarction. Acute myocardial infarction will show ST segment elevation with a convexity upward, in contrast to the downward concavity in pericarditis (Figs. M.IX.2 and 3). The ST elevation may be accompanied by reciprocal ST segment depression in the other leads. The cardio-isoenzymes creatine phosphokinase (CPK) and lactic dehydrogenase (LDH) will be elevated within 24 hours of an infarction. The pain of infarction is usually a retrosternal pressure or ache and generally is relieved by nitroglycerin. In most cases the pain is not positional unless there is an accompanying pericarditis due to infarction, but the fever, rub, and leukocytosis that may occur with infarction generally will develop 24–72 hours after the onset of pain, rather than with the onset of pain.

c. Pulmonary embolism. Pulmonary embolism requires a high index of suspicion. Sudden onset of dyspnea and tachypnea are the usual hallmarks. Chest pain occurs infrequently, usually only when there is pulmonary infarction (10% of pulmonary embolisms). Often the pain will be pleuritic, sometimes associated with a pleural rub and/or hemoptysis.

F. Acute Pericarditis During Pregnancy

A review of the medical literature has revealed very few reported cases of acute pericarditis during pregnancy. In 1959 Adams reported a case of pericarditis occurring at term; a normal infant was born after induction of labor.[31] The patient's chest pain responded rapidly to steroids and aspirin. Probst and Mier in 1963 reported a similar case occurring in the third trimester; again, a normal term infant was delivered after an otherwise uneventful pregnancy.[32] In 1966 Chrobok et al described a successful delivery after the development of a suppurative pericarditis as a complication of a pleural empyema occurring during pregnancy.[33] One case of chylopericardium diagnosed during the sixth month of pregnancy has also been reported. The term delivery and postpartum course were normal and the pericardial effusion responded to a single pericardiocentesis performed postpartum. Subsequent pregnancies in this patient have not been reported.[34] Fujimoto et al described a case of rubella perimyocarditis occurring at the twenty-third week of pregnancy which resulted in premature delivery at 28 weeks. The 1,000 gm female infant died 12 hours after birth. The mother developed heart failure after delivery but eventually responded to medical therapy. The diagnosis was confirmed by rising anti-rubella antibody titers and a myocardial biopsy.[5] In 1980 Quismorio reported a case of systemic lupus erythematosus pericarditis that resulted in premature delivery at 33 weeks. The patient was initially diagnosed as having preeclampsia/eclampsia. She developed cardiac tamponade on the second postpartum day.[35] In 1978 Krausz et al described three cases of idiopathic pericarditis during pregnancy, each of which resulted in uneventful term deliveries. One of the patients was treated throughout pregnancy with aspirin and steroids for chest pain. A second patient developed symptoms during the sixth month of pregnancy. She was treated with aspirin but required steroids two weeks prior to delivery. During the postpartum period, after the withdrawal of steroids, both patients had relapses of symptoms, but neither had signs of heart failure. One eventually required a pericardiectomy. The third patient was diagnosed as having cardiomegaly one year after her second normal pregnancy. Her third pregnancy was complicated by dyspnea and ankle edema but resulted in a normal term infant and regression of symptoms. Nineteen years later she underwent a successful pericardiectomy for pericardial tamponade. Her heart size then appeared normal, suggesting that her cardiomegaly was due to a chronic pericardial effusion.[4]

In summary, acute pericarditis during pregnancy will usually run a benign course. Symptoms generally respond to aspirin, but at times steroids are required and have been used successfully during pregnancy. Surgical intervention may be required for cardiac tamponade or intractable chest pain. At times an active myocarditis may dominate the clinical picture and result in heart failure and death. Severe myocarditis with heart failure early in pregnancy may be an indication for therapeutic abortion.[30]

II. PERICARDIAL EFFUSION, PERICARDIAL TAMPONADE, AND PERICARDIAL CONSTRICTION

A. General Considerations

Most pericardial effusions do not cause tamponade or any signs of hemodynamic compromise. The size of the effusion and the rapidity of fluid accumulation will determine the degree to which diastolic filling is limited. A large effusion that accumulates slowly may produce no problems, whereas a small effusion rapidly accumulated can cause tamponade. The inability of the right ventricle to expand in diastole causes a rapid rise of left ventricular pressure, which is followed by an increase in right atrial pressure. In addition, the restriction of right ventricular diastolic filling results in a decrease in stroke volume and blood pressure and a compensatory tachycardia. The increasing right atrial pressure is followed by a retrograde elevation of pressures in the venous system. Distension of neck veins is the clinical manifestation of this hemodynamic phenomenon. Paradoxical pulse [systolic BP decrease greater than 15–20 mm Hg (normal < 10) on inspiration] is caused by increased venous return and filling of the right ventricle on inspiration. The right ventricle is then encroaching on the filling of the left ventricle, causing a decrease in stroke volume and thus a decrease in cardiac output and systolic pressure. Constriction occurs when there is scarring of the pericardium that limits diastolic filling of one or both ventricles. Heart size is usually normal or small, but it may appear large on chest x-ray. The presence of an effusion does not rule out pericardial constriction.

B. Etiology

Uremia, collagen vascular disease, TB, malignancy, myxedema, and idiopathic pericarditis are the most common causes of pericardial effusion. Constrictive pericarditis most commonly occurs after TB pericarditis (22–50%); inadequate drainage from a bacterial pericarditis; viral agents (notably Coxsackie B); collagen vascular diseases, especially rheumatoid arthritis and systemic lupus erythematosus (natural or drug induced); chronic uremia; and mediastinal irradiation.

C. Clinical Findings

The clinical symptoms and signs most commonly associated with pericardial tamponade and constriction are listed in Table M.IX.2.

1. Symptoms

The patients complain of weakness, malaise, dyspnea, orthopnea and, at times, chest pain. Paroxysmal nocturnal dyspnea is rarely seen and is helpful in distinguishing heart failure from tamponade. If the rise in right atrial and venous pressure is of gradual onset, hepatomegaly and edema, as well as anorexia, may occur in both constriction and tamponade.

TABLE M.IX.2. Symptoms and Signs of Pericardial Tamponade and Constriction

Signs
Neck vein distention (in tamponade, often prominent X with absence of Y descent; in constriction, prominent X and Y descent)
Tachycardia
Pulsus paradoxus >10 mm
Narrow pulse pressure (<30 mm Hg)
Hypotension (systemic pressure < 100 mm Hg)
Kussmaul's sign (more commonly seen in pericardial constriction)
Pericardial friction rub
Diminished heart sounds
Symptoms
Dyspnea
Chest pain (pleuritic, dull, squeezing)
Chronic
Weakness
Malaise
Anorexia
Weight loss
Diaphoresis

2. Signs

Neck vein distention and clear lungs are the hallmarks of both constriction and tamponade. This presentation should alert the clinician that heart failure is a less likely cause of the patient's dyspnea. Patients usually have tachycardia, a narrowed pulse pressure (< 30 mm Hg), and hypotension. Depending on the duration of impairment, there may also be ascites and hepatomegaly, which may be impossible to detect, especially in the late stages of pregnancy. In cardiac tamponade a pericardial rub may be found in 40% of the patients. The neck veins are distended and show an x but no y descent and usually decrease with inspiration. In the minority of patients, however, the distention of neck veins may increase with inspiration (Kussmaul's sign). In pericardial constriction Kussmaul's sign may be seen in most patients, and inspection of the neck vein pulsations will show a prominent x and y descent. In addition, a prominent diastolic pericardial knock can be heard and may even be felt.

D. Laboratory Findings

1. Chest x-ray film

a. Pericardial effusion with or without tamponade. Pericardial effusion usually causes an enlarged, symmetrical, "water bottle" silhouette of the heart; lung fields are usually clear, and epicardial fat lines can be seen within the cardiac silhouette.

b. Pericardial constriction. Pericardial constriction usually is evidenced by a normal or small heart shadow. Enlargement may occur in up to 10% of cases caused by an effusion or thickened pericardium. Pericardial calcification may be seen in 30–60% of the cases of pericardial constriction.[36] Lung fields are usually clear, except for the not infrequent cases of pleural effusion (40–60%) and superior vena cava engorgement.

2. **Echocardiogram**

a. Pericardial effusion with or without tamponade. An echo-free space between the pericardium and the epicardium is seen in a case of pericardial effusion. The echocardiogram allows a rough quantitation of the amount and extent of the effusion, as discussed earlier in this chapter. It should be noted that pericardial effusion has been recently reported in eight of 40 healthy pregnant women. The condition was clinically silent and was not associated with either precordial pain or pericardial rub. It appeared in late pregnancy and could not be detected two months postpartum.[37] When there is a large effusion, a swinging heart phenomenon may be seen, as well as pseudoprolapse of the mitral and tricuspid valves. Sudden posterior motion of the interventricular septum with an increase in right ventricular and a decrease in left ventricular end-diastolic volume during inspiration may be seen in tamponade. It should be noted that, although the diagnosis of tamponade is based on hemodynamic and clinical findings, the echocardiogram should play an important supportive role.

b. Pericardial constriction. The echocardiogram may show thickened visceral and intense parietal pericardium appearing as two or more parallel intense lines (Fig. M.IX.6).[38,39] Paradoxical septal motion (anterior movement of the septum) is often seen before the onset of systole, and rapid early posterior diastolic motion of the posterior wall with flattened motion occurs through the remainder of diastole.

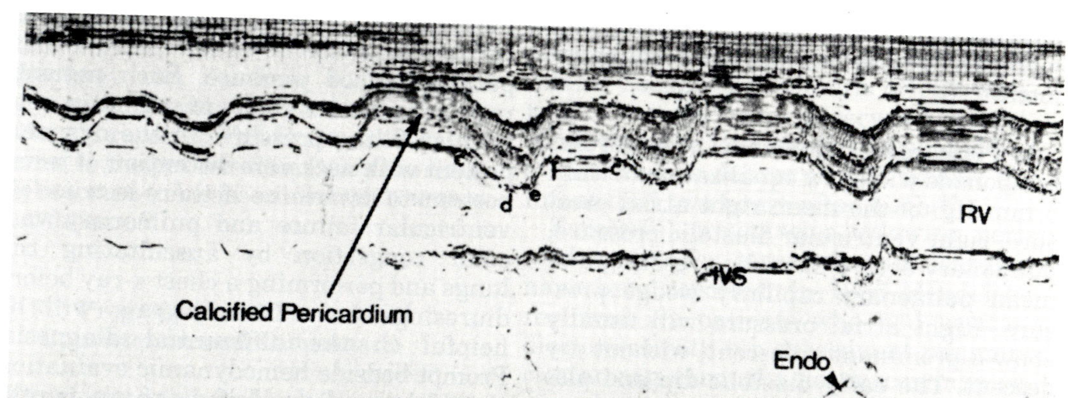

Fig. M.IX.6. Echocardiogram of a patient with constrictive TB pericarditis showing dense band of thickened anterior pericardial echoes, with abnormal flat motion during diastole (f-c). In addition, the right ventricular cavity is slightly enlarged (2.7 cm), and the interventricular septum shows an abnormal flat motion during systole and varying anterior or posterior motion during early diastole, followed by flat motion during the remainder of diastole. Endo, endocardium; ECG, electrocardiogram. (Reprinted with permission from Elkayam et al.[38])

M.X

Infective Endocarditis in Pregnancy

Warren D. Johnston, MD, and Uri Elkayam, MD

I. INTRODUCTION

Infective endocarditis is a rare disease of pregnancy. Crockett et al[1] noted one case of endocarditis occurring in every 200 cases of pregnant women with rheumatic heart disease. Rheumatic heart disease is found in only 1% of pregnant women; thus the approximate incidence of endocarditis in pregnancy is 0.2%. Nazarian et al[2] estimated the incidence of endocarditis in pregnancy as one case in every 8,000 deliveries.

Although endocarditis in pregnancy is extremely uncommon, when it is encountered it presents difficult and perplexing problems. Pregnancy affects the natural history, diagnosis, medical and surgical treatment, and prognosis of endocarditis. Increases in cardiac output, blood volume, and heart rate that occur during pregnancy can complicate the course of endocarditis and cause increased congestive heart failure, refractoriness to medical management, and rapid deterioration in the status of the patient. These hemodynamic changes can also cause problems in the diagnosis and follow-up of patients suspected of having endocarditis. Innocent cardiac murmurs produced by increased blood flow through the heart or through the vessels of the chest wall may falsely suggest the presence of valvular damage. Established murmurs may increase or diminish in intensity as a result of these hemodynamic changes rather than as a result of progression or regression of cardiac disease.[3] Drugs used to treat the infection and its attendant complications must be chosen carefully with due regard to the possible effects on the developing fetus. The surgical treatment of endocarditis in pregnancy must be weighed against the risks of infant mortality and the possible increased risks of maternal mortality.[4] The overall prognosis of women with infective endocarditis may be worsened by the pregnant state. Pedowitz and Hellman[5] reported a mortality of 14.6% in mothers who contracted

Cardiac Problems in Pregnancy, pages 131–139

endocarditis during pregnancy or the puerperium.

Despite the special circumstances posed by pregnancy, the basic disease process in endocarditis is not markedly different in the pregnant and nonpregnant states. Thus most of the general principles and approaches in the diagnosis of endocarditis in the nonpregnant female apply to the pregnant one as well.

II. ETIOLOGY

As in the nonpregnant state, infective endocarditis in pregnancy most often occurs in the presence of underlying heart disease. Lein and Stander,[6] in a series of eight pregnant patients with endocarditis, noted a history of antecedent heart disease in seven of those patients. Friedberg[7] has estimated that 79% of pregnant patients with subacute endocarditis have evidence of rheumatic heart disease. Nazarian et al[2] noted that in a large series of pregnant patients, 84–90% of patients with endocarditis had a prior history of rheumatic heart disease. They stated that the remaining patients in their series had congenital cardiac anomalies. There are, however, occasional reported cases where no antecedent heart disease could be found.[8–10] These cases may be the result of a more virulent type of infection, either because of increased pathogenicity of the organism or because of inadequate host response to the infection. It is also possible that underlying heart disease might not have been recognized, either because of the asymptomatic nature of the patient or because the cardiac findings were relatively subtle. In years past, for instance, it could be speculated that at least some of the patients with "normal" hearts might have had undetected mitral valve prolapse, a recently recognized heart abnormality commonly seen in women.[11] Also, as already mentioned, the changing hemodynamics of pregnancy may cause a pathologic murmur to soften or disappear completely as pregnancy progresses.[12]

The most common organism that causes endocarditis in pregnancy is Streptococcus viridans. This organism most often occurs in the subacute form but occasionally can present a picture of acute endocarditis affecting a previously normal heart and following a rapidly deteriorating course.[13]

The most common organisms involved in acute bacterial endocarditis in pregnancy are Staphylococcus aureus, Pneumococcus, and Streptococcus pyogenes.[10] Acute endocarditis in pregnancy involving group D enterococcus has also been reported.[2]

Bacterial endocarditis in pregnancy has also been reported in association with other organisms such as Haemophilus aphrophilus,[14] Pseudomonas aeruginosa,[6] and Listeria monocytogenes.[15] Any organism capable of causing endocarditis in the nonpregnant state is undoubtedly able to cause it in pregnancy; however, because endocarditis occurs so rarely during pregnancy, it would be expected that the occurrence of unusual organisms would also be extremely rare.

The causal organisms most often reach the site of infection in the heart by way of the bloodstream. Bacteremia may occur in many settings, including dental extractions, surgery, skin or systemic infections, intravenous drug use, and diagnostic procedures, especially those involving the gastrointestinal or genitourinary tracts. The risk of bacteremia after procedures has been recently reviewed by Everett and Hirschman[16] and is summarized in Table M.XXV.1. Many of the organisms that can cause infective endocarditis have been cultured from the normal vagina[17] and postpartum uterus.[18] Lein and Stander[6] reported on eight cases in a series of 31 women with bacterial endocarditis where the infections could be directly attributed to preceding obstetric and gynecological procedures, including criminal abortion, complicated vaginal delivery, and curettage and conization. Obstetric and gynecologic procedures have been thought to be the source of infection in approximately 20% of patients with enterococcal endocarditis.[19] While the incidence of bacteremia in parturition is estimated to be approximately 5%,[16] the occurrence of infective endocarditis directly attributable to normal vaginal delivery is extremely rare.[20,21] Often the underlying cause of the initial bacteremia in cases of endocarditis is unknown.[21]

III. CLINICAL MANIFESTATIONS

Infective endocarditis can become manifest in a variety of fashions, and its onset can either be insidious or fulminant. When endocarditis occurs in the subacute form, its signs and symptoms may suggest a number of other diagnoses, including influenza, tuberculosis, acute rheumatic fever, typhoid fever, malaria, acute meningitis or encephalitis, glomerulonephritis, and acute abdominal crises.[22] When endocarditis is seen in the acute form, it can occur as severe congestive heart failure, stroke, myocardial infarction, peripheral arterial occlusion, pneumonia, or lung abscesses. When it occurs in pregnancy, acute endocarditis can be particularly dangerous to both the mother and the fetus.

Fever is the most common sign of infective endocarditis. It occurs in most cases, but can be absent, especially in elderly patients. During pregnancy absence of fever can be seen in patients who have been given antipyretics for other reasons, or who have been treated with inadequate courses of antibiotics. Fever may also be absent when endocarditis is associated with cardiac failure, uremia, or massive intracerebral or subarachnoid hemorrhage. Other common signs and symptoms include pallor of the skin and mucous membranes, fatigue, malaise, anorexia, weight loss, sleep loss, and loss of sense of well-being.

Cardiac murmurs are another hallmark of the disease. The murmurs that develop are most often murmurs of valvular incompetence, although flow murmurs due to fever or anemia may also be heard. Complicating the diagnosis of endocarditis is the fact that heart murmurs are not always heard. Up to 15% of cases with subacute endocarditis[23] and 33% of cases with acute endocarditis[24] have no detectable murmurs. Murmurs may be absent in approximately one-third of the cases of right-sided endocarditis.[23] The finding of changing murmurs, often considered an important diagnostic feature of endocarditis, is infrequent. Pankey found a change in the character of a murmur in 16.7% of 167 cases.[25] Weinstein, however, has stated that in his personal experience with over 900 cases of subacute endocarditis, he has found changing murmurs to occur much less frequently. He also cautioned that so-called innocent murmurs that have been present for years, especially in elderly patients, may obscure the diagnosis of endocarditis because murmurs may not change in character during the course of the infection. Endocarditis occurring in pregnancy can be particularly difficult to diagnose owing to the common occurrence of cardiac murmurs associated with the changing hemodynamics as pregnancy progresses. New murmurs may develop or established murmurs may become louder, softer, or disappear entirely. A mammary souffle or venous hum may be misinterpreted as a new cardiac murmur. Patients with chronic aortic insufficiency may lose the murmur during pregnancy, only to have it reappear after delivery and be misinterpreted as due to acute valvular damage caused by endocarditis during gestation or delivery.[12]

The presence of bacterial endocarditis may be heralded by the appearance of the peripheral stigmata of the disease. The classic signs include petechiae, Janeway lesions, Osler nodes, and subungual hemorrhages. Petechiae are present in less than half the cases of bacterial endocarditis and are not specific for the disease.[13] They are most commonly seen in the conjunctiva but can also be seen on the skin of the dorsum of the hands and feet, the anterior chest and abdominal wall, the soft palate, and the mucosa of the oral cavity. Janeway lesions, which are small nonpainful macular lesions on the hands and feet, and Osler nodes, which are small, painful nodular lesions, also most often seen on the hands and feet, are valuable clues to the diagnosis of bacterial endocarditis but are no longer seen in the majority of the cases. Subungual hemorrhages occur uncommonly in bacterial endocarditis and, when present, are such a nonspecific finding that they are of little aid in the diagnosis of the disease. Other findings in bacterial endocarditis include Roth spots (small retinal hemorrhages with pale oval centers), splenomegaly, arthralgias, and musculoskeletal complaints, including lumbar, sternal and long bone pain, and clubbing of the fingers, which is especially significant if it develops during observation.

Clinical complications from infective endocarditis are the result of three basic processes: valvular destruction, embolization of vegetations, and the immunologic response of the host to the infection. Congestive heart failure developing as a result of damage done to the aortic valve causing acute aortic regurgitation is the leading cause of death from infective endocarditis.[23] Large vegetations, which occur most commonly in fungal endocarditis, can cause significant valvular obstruction and precipitate cardiac failure. Myocarditis resulting from infective endocarditis can also contribute importantly to the development of congestive heart failure. Embolization of vegetations is the second most common complication of infective endocarditis.[23] While virtually every organ and tissue can be potentially affected by emboli, the more common sites include kidney, spleen, coronary vessels, and brain. Thus the clinical course of infective endocarditis can include such problems as myocardial infarction, stroke, renal failure, abdominal crises, mycotic aneurysms, and abscesses. Pathologic manifestations resulting from the immune response of the host to endocarditis can also complicate the course of the infection. Proliferative glomerulonephritis resulting from deposition of immune complexes in the kidney is an example of an immunologic complication of endocarditis. Sterile pericarditis, myocarditis, arthritis, and the development of Roth spots, Janeway lesions, and Osler nodes are other examples of complications possibly related to immunologic causes.

IV. DIAGNOSIS

The laboratory approach to the diagnosis of endocarditis is similar in pregnant and nonpregnant states. Cultures of the blood remain the most helpful diagnostic procedure confirming the presence of endocarditis. While the majority of cases of patients with endocarditis have positive blood cultures, it has been reported that up to 27% of cases will be blood culture negative.[26] Negative blood cultures may be the result of many factors, such as specific growth requirements of the infecting bacteria, infecting organisms that are nonbacterial, prior antibiotic treatment, and inadequate numbers of blood cultures. Weinstein suggests that blood cultures be drawn every five to ten minutes after one degree Fahrenheit or more of fever is present until six samples of blood are obtained (preferably 10 cc or more of blood per sample).[23] The finding of three or more positive cultures drawn in this fashion is highly suggestive of endocarditis, especially if one or more other factors such as underlying heart disease, new regurgitant murmur, or vascular phenomena are also present. If prior antibiotic treatment confounds the diagnosis of endocarditis, antibiotics should be withheld, if clinically possible, and blood cultures obtained from 24 to 48 hours after termination of therapy until seven days have elapsed. If the cultures are negative during this time course, the diagnosis of infective endocarditis is unlikely.[23]

Examination of blood and urine is often helpful as an aid in the evaluation of possible endocarditis, but the abnormalities found are not pathognomonic for the presence of the disease. Elevation of the sedimentation rate is one of the most common laboratory abnormalities found in endocarditis.[13] The white count may be elevated, especially in the acute form of the disease, but when subacute endocarditis is present, the white count is most often normal. However, a leftward shift to more immature forms of leukocytes is observed in most cases. Anemia is a common but not a universal finding in endocarditis and is often progressive during the course of the disease. Examination of the urine is most often negative in uncomplicated cases; however, the presence of an active sediment may suggest renal involvement due to proliferative glomerulonephritis or renal infarction. Examination of serum electrolytes and liver function tests are most often normal, unless dehydration, renal failure, or hepatic infarction or abscess are present.

The chest x-ray film may reveal heart failure occurring as a result of valvular destruction, or it may show pulmonary infarctions occurring as a result of embolic phenomena from the right side of the heart.

The electrocardiogram is most often normal in uncomplicated endocarditis. However, when the disease is complicated by myocarditis, aneurysm, or cardiac abscess, ST-T segment changes, premature ventricular contractions, and bundle branch blocks can be seen.

In the past several years, echocardiography has become an often helpful tool for diagnosing infective endocarditis. Valvular vegetations can be visualized in 34–55% of cases[27] and are most commonly seen on the aortic and mitral valve. Figure M.X.1 illustrates an example of the echocardiographic appearance of valvular vegetations in a pregnant patient with endocarditis. Alterations in hemodynamics due to valvular destruction and subsequent valvular incompetence can cause specific echocardiographic abnormalities. Thus, findings of left ventricular dilatation, fine fluttering of the anterior leaflet of mitral valve, and premature closure of the mitral valve may suggest acute aortic regurgitation due to endocarditis and may be apparent before the characteristic murmur is clinically appreciated. It is anticipated that Doppler blood flow analysis used in conjunction with the two-dimensional echocardiogram may be helpful in the diagnosis and follow-up of patients with valvular incompetence due to endocarditis.[28]

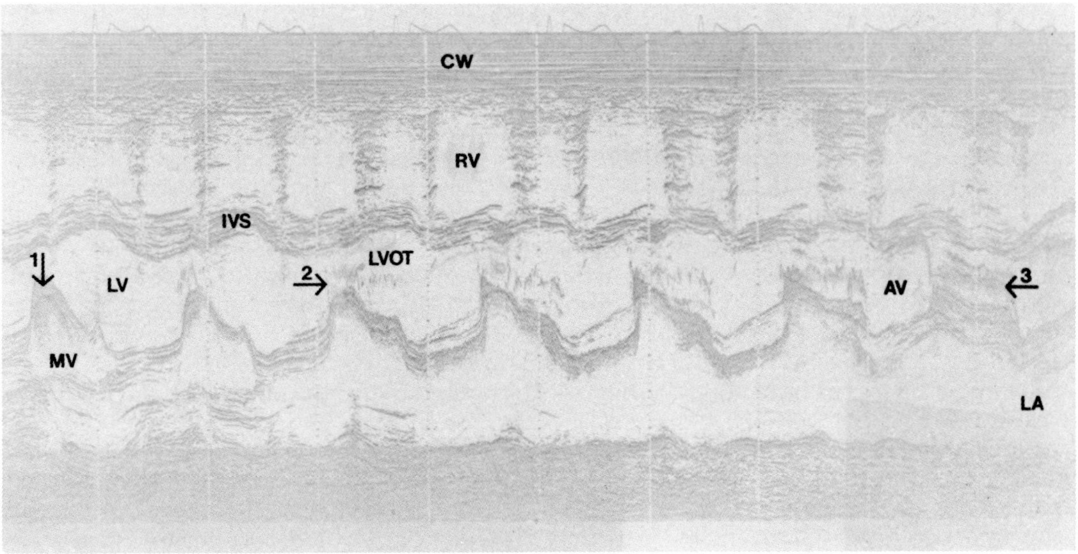

Fig. M.X.1. Echocardiogram demonstrating vegetations on the mitral valve (MV) (1), in the left ventricular outflow tract (LVOT) (2), and on the aortic valve (AV) (3). CW = chest wall; RV = right ventricle; IVS = interventricular septum; LV = left ventricle; LA = left atrium.

Other lab tests or findings that may be helpful in suggesting a diagnosis of endocarditis include Gallium scans of the heart, positive rheumatoid factor, and the presence of circulating immune complexes.

V. MANAGEMENT

Antibiotics remain the mainstay of therapy of infective endocarditis in both the pregnant and the nonpregnant state. In pregnancy, however, the choice of antibiotics must also be tailored to the possibility of adverse effects of these drugs on the fetus. The problems and considerations involved in administering antibiotics to the gravid woman are well detailed in Chapter M.XXV. Specific recommendations for treatment, including antibiotic regimens that are aimed at the most prominent organisms likely to be encountered in endocarditis in pregnancy, are also reviewed in that chapter. Certain principles of antibiotic therapy must be kept in mind if bacterial endocarditis is to be treated effectively. The choice of antibiotics should be dictated by the infecting organism that has been isolated and by the antibiotic sensitivities that are determined for that organism. In general, antibiotics should be administered parenterally in bolus fashion at frequent intervals determined by the drug's half-life in serum. The antibiotic chosen should be bactericidal and should be given in dosages adequate to maintain serum bactericidal levels eight to ten times higher than the level required to kill the organism. Most authors suggest that a minimum of four to six weeks of parenteral antibiotic therapy should be given to minimize the occurrence of relapse of the disease.[19,23,29]

Congestive heart failure complicating endocarditis in pregnancy is treated in the usual fashion, with salt and water restriction and the administration of diuretics and digitalis preparations. The use of diuretics and digitalis in pregnant women is reviewed in Chapters M.XXI and M.XXIV. In general, the use of digitalis preparations in pregnancy is safe for both the mother and the fetus, and dosing schedules need not be changed because of pregnancy. Diuretics can be used in pregnancy to treat congestive heart failure, but care must be taken not to dehydrate the patient, which might lead to compromised uterine blood flow. Furosemide has been shown to cause fetal abnormalities in animal studies and therefore should be used judiciously. The use of preload- and afterload-reducing agents in pregnant patients with intractable congestive heart failure due to mitral or aortic valve incompetence can be helpful in stabilizing the patient for surgery. These drugs can have potent hemodynamic effects on both the mother and the fetus and thus should be used only in conjunction with invasive hemodynamic monitoring of the mother and probably with fetal monitoring as well. Hydralazine has been used safely in pregnancy[30]; however, it has been suggested that intravenous use can be associated with fetal heart rate deceleration and fetal growth retardation.[31] Hydralazine in high dosages has been shown to be teratogenic in mice. Nitroprusside is generally not recommended for use in pregnancy because it crosses the placenta and accumulation of its toxic byproduct, cyanide, may cause fetal death.[32] Prazosin and nitrate preparations have been incompletely studied in pregnancy and should be used only when the potential benefit outweighs potential risk to the mother and fetus.

The intraaortic balloon pump can be useful in stabilizing pregnant patients with acute mitral insufficiency before surgery is performed, but its use is contraindicated in patients with aortic insufficiency.

Cardiac surgery for infective endocarditis in pregnancy should be considered when congestive heart failure has proved intractable to medical therapy, when recurrent embolization of vegetations occurs, or when the infection cannot be eradicated despite optimal antibiotic therapy. The considerations that apply to cardiac surgery performed during pregnancy are reviewed in Chapter M.XVII. Cardiac surgery is best performed after organogenesis of the fetus is complete and before the maximal hemodynamic load of pregnancy is reached. This is, in theory, optimally accomplished between 24 and 28 weeks of gestation.[2] Pregnancy does not seem to increase the risk to the patient of cardiac surgery and, therefore, therapeutic abortion prior to surgery is seldom indicated.[2] The risk to the infant is not extreme if good perfusion of the placenta is maintained by careful attention to the maternal hemodynamics during anesthesia induction and maintenance and during cardiopulmonary bypass. Congenital defects have been reported to be not infrequent in infants exposed in utero to cardiac surgery, again stressing the need to avoid surgery during the early developmental period.[2]

VI. PROGNOSIS

The diagnosis of infective endocarditis in the preantibiotic era almost always carried a terminal prognosis. With the advent of antibiotics, this grim prognosis improved substantially. In most recent series, the overall mortality due to infective endocarditis has been reported as 15–37%. This improvement in the prognosis of the disease over the years has also been the case with endocarditis diagnosed in pregnancy. Ward and Hickman[33] noted that the maternal mortality of infective endocarditis in pregnancy fell from 100% in 1939 to 53% in 1949. Pedowitz and Hellman[5] in 1953 reported a maternal mortality of 14.6% in a series of pregnant women with endocarditis. Factors that portend a more unfavorable prognosis include delays in diagnosis, infection with organisms capable of causing acute valvular damage, aortic valvular involvement, and the development of severe complications, including congestive heart failure, major embolic phenomena, and renal failure. Such factors as improvement in the therapy of congestive heart failure, the availability of maternal and fetal monitoring, and the feasibility of early cardiac surgical intervention, have probably further reduced the risk of endocarditis in pregnancy to both mother and fetus. Thus termination of pregnancy is generally not indicated when the diagnosis of infective endocarditis is made in a pregnant woman. In fact, maternal mortality has been reported to be higher when termination is performed than when pregnancy is allowed to continue.[33]

VII. PREVENTION

Although the treatment and the prognosis of pregnant patients with endocarditis have improved, prevention of this disease remains the primary goal. Thus prophylaxis against endocarditis in pregnant patients with known heart disease is vitally important.[6] This subject is reviewed in detail in Chapter M.XXV, where specific recommendations for prophylaxis are made in accordance with American Heart Association guidelines.[20] In general, it should be noted that pregnant women with prosthetic valves or with a history of rheumatic or congenital heart disease should be given some form of prophylaxis prior to undergoing procedures that carry known risks of bacteremia. Pregnant patients with mitral valve prolapse should also be considered for routine antibiotic prophylaxis[20] (see Chapter M.XVI).

The issue of the need for antibiotic prophylaxis during routine delivery remains somewhat controversial. However, recently Fleming[34] and Sugrue et al[21] have reviewed this subject thoroughly and argued convincingly against the need for routine antibiotic prophylaxis for the normal delivery. The American Heart Association suggests that only patients with prosthetic valves are in need of routine prophylaxis prior to anticipated normal delivery.[20]

VIII. SUMMARY

Although infective endocarditis is a rare disease in pregnancy, the approach to the diagnosis and clinical management of the disease is generally similar in the pregnant and nonpregnant states. The bacteriology and clinical manifestations of endocarditis in pregnancy are also quite similar to those found in the nonpregnant state. Pregnancy can, however, cause difficulty in recognizing the signs and symptoms of endocarditis. The changes in maternal hemodynamics in pregnancy can exacerbate the complications of the disease, especially if congestive heart failure develops. Also, the developing infant must be taken into account in the drug treatment of the disease and its complications. While endocarditis increases the maternal mortality in pregnancy, presence of the disease is not an indication for termination of gestation. With newer medical approaches and earlier surgical intervention, the prognosis of a pregnant woman with endocarditis has been markedly improved. Antibiotic prophylaxis of pregnant patients with known heart disease remains an important measure in the primary prevention of the disease.

IX. ACKNOWLEDGMENTS

We gratefully acknowledge the expert secretarial assistance of Ellen Mansour in the preparation of this manuscript.

X. REFERENCES

1. Crockett EJ, Batchelor TM, Corbeil J. Pregnancy and subacute bacterial endocarditis. Obstet Gynecol. 1960; 16:43–95.
2. Nazarian M, McCullough GH, Fielder DL. Bacterial endocarditis in pregnancy. Successful surgical correction. J Thorac Cardiovasc Surg. 1976; 71:880–883.
3. Marcus FI, Ewy GA, O'Rourke RA, Walsh B, Bletch AC. The effect of pregnancy on the murmurs of mitral and aortic regurgitation. Circulation. 1970; 41:795–805.
4. Zitmik RS, Brandenburg RO, Sheldon R. Pregnancy and open-heart surgery. Circulation. 1969; 39(Suppl):257–262.
5. Pedowitz P, Hellman LM. Pregnancy and healed subacute bacterial endocarditis. Am J Obstet Gynecol. 1953; 66:294–301.
6. Lein JN, Stander RW. Subactue bacterial endocarditis following obstetric and gynecologic procedures. Obstet Gynecol. 1959; 13:568–573.
7. Friedberg CK. Diseases of the Heart. Philadelphia: Saunders, 1956.
8. Gatenby PB, Fitzgibbon H. Subacute bacterial endocarditis in pregnancy. Ir J Med Sci. 1957; 374:66–70.
9. Hanson GC, Phillips J. A fatal case of subacute bacterial endocarditis in pregnancy. J Obstet Gynecol Br Commonw. 1965; 72:781–784.
10. Holt S, Hicks DA, Charges RG, Coulshed N. Acute staphylococcal endocarditis in pregnancy. Practitioner. 1978; 220:619–622.
11. Markiewicz W, Stoner J, London E, Hunt SA, Popp RL. Mitral valve prolapse in one hundred presumably healthy females. Circulation. 1976, 53:464–473.
12. McCans JL, Wenger NK. Problems in management of the pregnant patient with rheumatic heart disease and valve prosthesis. South Med J. 1976; 69:1007–1010.
13. Lerner PI, Weinstein L. Infective endocarditis in the antibiotic era. N Engl J Med. 1966; 274:199–206, 259–265, 323–331, 388–393.
14. Anand CM, MacKay AD, Evans JI. Haemophilus aphrophilus endocarditis in pregnancy. J Clin Pathol. 1976; 29:812–814.
15. Holshouser CA, Ansbacher R, McNitt T, Steele R. Bacterial endocarditis due to listeria monocytogenes in a pregnant diabetic. Obstet Gynecol. 1978; 51(1 Suppl):9s–10s.
16. Everett ED, Hirschman JV. Transient bacteremia and endocarditis prophylaxis: A review. Medicine. 1977; 56:61–77.
17. Hunter CA, Long KR. Study of the microbiological flora of the vagina. Am J Obstet Gynecol. 1958; 75:865–871.
18. Hesseltine HC, Hite KE. Bacteriology of the gynecologic and involuting puerperal uterus. Am J Obstet Gynecol. 1949; 57:143.
19. Freedman LR: Endocarditis updated. DM 1979; 26:1–50.
20. Kaplan EL, Anthony BF, Bisno A, Dukack D, Houser H, Millard HD, Sanford J, Shulman ST, Stillerman M, Taranta A, Wenger N. Prevention of bacterial endocarditis. Circulation. 1977; 56:139A–143A.
21. Sugrue D, Blake S, Troy P, MacDonald D. Antibiotic prophalaxis against infective endocarditis after normal delivery—Is it necessary? Br Heart J. 1980; 44:499–502.
22. Libman E, Friedberk CK. Subacute Bacterial Endocarditis. Ed 2. New York: Ford University Press, 1948.
23. Weinstein L. Infective endocarditis in heart dis-

ease: A textbook of cardiovascular medicine. Braunwald, E (ed). Philadelphia: W.B. Saunders, 1980:1167–1220.

24. Weinstein L. Infective endocarditis: Past, present, future. J R Coll Physicians Lond. 1972; 6:161–174.
25. Pankey GA. Acute bacterial endocarditis at University of Minnesota Hospitals, 1939–1954. Am Heart J. 1962; 64:583–591.
26. Annotation. Culture negative endocarditis. Lancet. 1977; 2:1164–1165.
27. Mintz GS, Kotler MN, Segal BL, Parry WR. Comparison of two-dimensional and M-mode echocardiography in the evaluation of patients with infective endocarditis. Am J Cardiol. 1979; 43:738–744.
28. Johnson SL, Baker DW, Lute RA, Dodge HT. Doppler echocardiography. The localization of cardiac murmurs. Circulation. 1973; 48:810–822.
29. VonReyn CF, Levy BS, Arbeit RD, Friedland G, Crumpacker CS. Infective endocarditis: An analysis based on strict case definitions. Ann Intern Med. 1981, 94:505–518.
30. Bott-Kanner G, Schweitzer A, Reisner SH, Joel-Cotten SJ, Rosenfeld JB. Propranolol and hydralazine in the management of essential hypertension in pregnancy. Br J Obstet Gynaecol. 1980; 87:110–114.
31. Vink GJ, Moodley J, Philpott RH. Effect of dihydralazine on the fetus in the treatment of maternal hypertension. Obstet Gynecol. 1980; 55:519–522.
32. Naulty J, Cefalo RC, Lewis PE. Fetal toxicity of nitroprusside in the pregnant ewe. Am J Obstet Gynecol. 1981; 139:708–711.
33. Ward H, Hickman RC. Bacterial endocarditis in pregnancy. Aust NZ J Obstet Gynaecol. 1971; 11:189–191.
34. Fleming HA. Antibiotic prophylaxis against infective endocarditis after delivery. Lancet. 1977; 1:144–145.

M.XI

Coronary Artery Disease in Pregnancy

Martin E. Goldman, MD, and Jose Meller, MD

I. INTRODUCTION

Coronary artery disease is rare in women of the childbearing age. In the Framingham study not a single case of coronary artery disease was documented in women 30 to 39 years of age, despite 6,726 person years of experience. According to 1977 United States Statistics, there were only 201 deaths from myocardial infarction in women between the ages of 20 and 34 and 1,010 between ages 35 and 44,[1] with a male-to-female ratio of 4.5 to 1.

II. EPIDEMIOLOGY

The incidence of myocardial infarction during pregnancy is estimated to be less than 1 in 10,000 pregnancies.[2] In 1952 Mendelson reported 2,310 cardiac patients out of 64,992 pregnancies (3.6%) at The New York Lying-In Hospital between 1932 and 1950, of which only four were thought to be coronary patients.[3] More recently, Hibbard analyzed maternal mortality in California between 1960 and 1968 and found that myocardial infarction accounted for nine of the 77 maternal deaths in almost 3.2 million reported births.[4]

There have been 62 reported cases of myocardial infarction during pregnancy. Six cases were reported between 1922 and 1950, 45 between 1957 and 1970, and 11 between 1970 and 1980.[4] The first reported case was in 1922 of a 33-year-old woman who died at the onset of labor due to coronary atherosclerosis with acute

Cardiac Problems in Pregnancy, pages 141–152

myocardial infarction.[5] In 1929 a woman survived myocardial infarction at four months of pregnancy and subsequently had an uncomplicated spontaneous delivery.[6] Ginz reported 39 cases of myocardial infarction (literature review and own cases) during pregnancy in 1970. The total maternal mortality was 28%, ranging from nil in the first trimester to 50% in the puerperium.[2] The infant mortality was 29%. No mortalities occurred in the six patients delivered by forceps, while the maternal mortality in spontaneous deliveries was 15%, and that by cesarean section was 37.5%.

In 1971 Husaini accumulated 45 patients (six additional to Ginz' study) and the maternal mortality was similar at 29%.[7] Eleven of the 13 deaths occurred among those who had a myocardial infarction during the last months of pregnancy or during labor.[7] Sixteen of the 45 (36%) had hypertension. Nine additional myocardial infarction-related deaths were accumulated between 1960 and 1968 by Hibbard.[4] Only one patient was younger than 36 years, and only two had a history of prior angina. In 1975 Sasse reported two patients (16 and 26 years old) with myocardial infarctions in the last trimester of pregnancy, and both had normal spontaneous deliveries at term; cardiac catheterization revealed a ventricular aneurysm in one, but both had normal coronary arteries.[8]

III. ETIOLOGY

Though atherosclerosis is the primary cause of progressive coronary artery disease and myocardial infarction, other less common etiologies of ischemic heart disease may be proportionally more prevalent in young women: coronary artery spasm, connective tissue diseases, coronary artery dissection, small vessel coronary disease, impaired hemoglobin–oxygen diffusion, polycythemia, thrombocytosis, homocystinuria, aortic valve disease, hypertrophic cardiomyopathy, metabolic abnormalities, trauma, coronary artery emboli, aortic dissection.

A. Coronary Risk Factors

Epidemiologic studies have identified several coronary risk factors, which include hypercholesterolemia, hypertension, cigarette smoking, age, sex, family history of coronary disease, diabetes, and certain life styles. The first three have the greatest predictive value for coronary atherosclerosis.[9–11]

B. Hypercholesterolemia

There is extensive documentation of the association of serum cholesterol levels with coronary artery disease.[9] Prospective studies have shown a direct correlation between the incidence of coronary disease and serum cholesterol levels[10]; the higher the cholesterol level, the greater the risk of coronary disease.[11] Plasma levels of low density lipoprotein (LDL) are closely correlated to cholesterol levels, as LDL normally transports approximately 70% of total plasma cholesterol. Another lipoprotein, high density lipoprotein (HDL) ordinarily transports 20% of the plasma cholesterol. The LDL level has been directly incriminated in coronary artery disease, whereas HDL has an inverse association with coronary disease.[12,13] It is postulated that HDL may remove cholesterol from the tissues, thereby protecting against the development of atherosclerosis. Studies remain inconclusive regarding the possible role of hypertriglyceridemia in the pathogenesis of coronary artery disease.[10]

C. Oral Contraceptives

Another risk factor for coronary atherosclerosis unique to women is oral contraceptives.[14–21] In women between 30 and 39 years of age taking oral contraceptives there is a reported rate of 2.7 greater risk for myocardial infarction than among women not taking contraceptives; the risk is 5.7 times greater in women 40 to 49.[14] In examining 219 deaths in women less than 50 years of age in 1973, Mann calculated a 2.8 relative risk in women less than 40 years old and 4.7 for women 40 to 44.[15] Of note, oral contraceptives act synergistically with other risk factors to increase the risk of coronary disease.[14] Several mechanisms have been proposed to explain the role of oral contraceptives in coronary disease. One factor may be related to the generalized increase in thromboembolic diseases as evident by the greater incidence of both venous thrombosis and pulmonary emboli by eight- to tenfold and that of cerebral thromboemboli six- to sevenfold.[16] This may be due to increased activity of factors VII and X or induced platelet abnormalities.[17,18]

Oral contraceptives have also been shown to alter blood lipid mechanics. Animal studies performed on birds fed an atherogenic diet followed by estrogens revealed an increasing frequency of ulcerated atheromata in the aorta and coronary arteries.[22] Predictably, the atheromata were limited to those lesions containing a core of lipid covered by a rigid fibro-hyaline cap.[22] It was suggested that estrogens precipitated ulceration of the atheroma by removal of core lipids, thus leading to collapse of the rigid cap under hemodynamic forces. Oral contraceptives have been shown to induce hypertriglyceridemia, probably secondary to elevated very low density lipoproteins (VLDL) stimulated by estrogens. Estrogens may also cause a quantitative alteration in the VLDL with a decreased APO-C2 lipoprotein content.[23,24] Oral contraceptives also raise the total serum cholesterol and LDL levels and decrease HDL lipoprotein.[25] These changes in serum lipids with estrogens can be explained by the increase in molar ratio of insulin:glucagon in portal vein blood together with an estrogen-induced resistance to glucagon effects in the liver.[26]

Oral contraceptives are usually a combination of both estrogen and progesterone compounds in various formulations. In general, the two components have opposite effects on lipids. Ethinyl estradiol results in elevated total phospholipid levels and triglyceride concentration, whereas megestrol acetate decreases the lecithin levels and increases the sphingomyelin. Norethindron decreases total cholesterol levels, triglycerides, and even reverses the effects of ethinyl estradiol.[27] Of importance, HDL levels appear to be directly related to estrogen dose and inversely related to progestin dose.[28]

Another mechanism invoked for the relationship between oral contraceptives and coronary disease is their well-documented association with the development of hypertension.[29,30] A study comparing women using oral contraceptives against those who use mechanical methods of contraception over a four-year period found an increase in mean systolic and diastolic pressures of 14.2 mm Hg and 8.5 mm Hg, respectively. The greatest individual increase was 36 mm Hg in systole and 20 mm Hg in diastole. Similar elevations in systolic and diastolic pressure were found in a British study.[31]

There are reports of women with acute myocardial infarction in the absence of any known major risk factors other than oral contraceptives.[19–21] The pathologic lesion in these cases has been isolated smooth, rounded, long lesions in the proximal portion of the major coronary arteries, which are distinguishable from the irregular and scattered lesions typical of atherosclerosis. The oral contraceptive-related lesion is suggestive of recent thrombi, which may act as a nidus for atheromata formation. Therefore, oral contraceptives may act independently and synergistically with several major atherogenic risk factors to increase the risk of coronary disease.

D. Cigarette Smoking

There is little doubt that cigarette smoking is implicated in the pathogenesis of coronary disease in women. The risk is progressively elevated with increasing numbers of cigarettes smoked. This was illustrated in the study in which the mortality ratio among women aged 40–49 was 1.31, 2.08, 3.62, 3.31 for smokers of 1–9, 10–19, 20–39, 40 or more cigarettes daily, respectively.[32] A British study found that among women aged 30–45 the proportion of smokers in patients who have a myocardial infarction or angina was 4.2 times and 1.3 times greater, respectively, than in nonsmoking women of the same age.[33] Women smokers show the same risk for myocardial infarction as do male smokers.[34] Numerous hypotheses have been invoked for the adverse effects of cigarette smoking on the heart and blood vessels. Both carbon monoxide and nicotine are assumed to be primary culprits. Nicotine raises myocardial oxygen demand and increases platelet adhesiveness, while carboxyhemoglobin interferes with normal oxygen transport and delivery.[35] Smoking has also been implicated in lowering HDL levels.[36] Of note, the elevated risk seems to decline within one to two years following cessation of smoking, but it remains slightly greater than in nonsmokers.[37] According to a recent study, the relative risk of dying from coronary heart disease among persistent smokers was 2.2 times that among quitters.[38]

E. Diabetes

Both insulin-dependent and non-insulin-dependent diabetes mellitus are associated with an elevated risk for the development of coronary artery disease.[39] Diabetes was shown to be an independent risk factor for myocardial infarction in the Coronary Drug Project.[40] The deleterious effect of hyperglycemia may be attributed to several factors. Hyperlipidemia and hypertriglyceridemia are frequently associated with hyperglycemia. Elevated plasma glucose levels are also associated with obesity, which may predispose to hypertension. Controversy still clouds the relationship between modes of therapy of diabetes and their atherogenic potential.[41,42]

F. Blood Pressure

Elevated blood pressure, either systolic or diastolic, is predictive of an increased risk of coronary disease.[43] As with the concentration of plasma cholesterol, there is no clear cutoff at which the risk changes from low to high, but there is a continuum of risk with continued elevated values. The relationship between hypertension and coronary disease is as great in women as it is in men.[43] There has been recent interest regarding the role of renin in hypertension. In 1972 Brunner and Laragh correlated elevated plasma renin levels with the potential for developing hypertension and subsequent myocardial infarction or stroke.[44] The enzyme renin cleaves a substrate protein to liberate angiotension I, which is the inactive precursor of the potent octapeptide hormone angiotensin II. Angiotensin II is a potent vasoconstrictor and is thereby involved in blood pressure control. Elevated levels of angiotensin II, when infused into a rabbit model, produced multiple areas of microscopic myocardial necrosis. Similar lesions were seen in three patients with documented elevated angiotensin II levels.[45] More recently a relationship has been shown between renin levels in the primagravida and diastolic blood pressure.[46] It has also been shown that the chorion is source of renin in human amniotic fluid.[47] Elevated chorionic production of renin may thereby elevate angiotensin II, with subsequent hemodynamic sequelae. As previously mentioned, oral contraceptives may also predispose to hypertension.[29–31]

G. Coronary Artery Spasm

Since first described by Prinzmetal's in 1959 and first documented by Oliva in 1973, coronary artery spasm (also referred to as Prinzmetal's variant or primary angina) has been recognized as playing an important role in angina and myocardial infarction.[48,49] In reviewing 1,000 angiograms of women less than 50 years old with chest pain, Welsh and Proudfit found only 23.6% to have coronary artery disease, in contrast to 49% in young men and 59% in an unselected population.[50] Though most commonly occurring in areas with significant coronary artery narrowing, spasm has been postulated to cause myocardial infarction even in patients with normal vessels.[51] The differentiation of primary or "vasoactive" from secondary or atherosclerotic coronary disease is important, as the management varies significantly. While angina secondary to fixed obstructions is usually exertionally related, the pain of variant angina occurs almost exclusively at rest with pronounced ST elevation on the electrocardiogram, accompanied at times by malignant cardiac arrhythmias and sudden death. The higher incidence of myocardial infarction with normal coronary arteries in pregnancy or the peurperium suggests a role of coronary spasm in these cases. In 1979 Beary reported 11 episodes of postpartum myocardial infarction in patients ranging from 17 to 35 years who developed an acute infarction within ten days postpartum.[52] These patients were generally primagravida and younger than intrapartum infarction patients, who were older and multigravida. Only three of the five patients with subsequently defined anatomy had acute coronary thrombosis, whereas two had normal coronary arteries.

H. Miscellaneous

There are numerous other causes that have been shown to precipitate acute myocardial ischemia and infarction. The connective tissue diseases have been documented to be involved in myocardial infarction, both with severe atherosclerosis and with normal coronary arteries. Meller described a 25-year-old woman with systemic lupus erythematosus who sustained myocardial infarction and succumbed to ventricular fibrillation. Postmortem examination revealed focal, severe atherosclerosis, occlusion by thrombus of the left anterior descending coronary artery, and extensive eccentric intimal fibrosis and dystrophic calcification of the coronary arteries.[53] In another study of nine patients, including six women ranging from 12 to 70 years old, with progressive systemic sclerosis who had myocardial infarction and sudden death, all patients had extensive myocardial fibrosis with widely patent extramural and morphologically normal intramural coronary arteries.[54]

Coronary emboli may lodge in the distal epicardial branches of the left anterior descending coronary artery, leading to infarction. The primary causes are mitral stenosis, atrial fibrillation, bacterial endocarditis, mural thrombi, prosthetic valves, cardiac myxomas, and paradoxical emboli.[55]

Thrombosis of coronary arteries can occur in sickle cell disease, blunt trauma to the chest wall, thrombocytosis, and homocystinuria. The primary vascular abnormality in homocystinuria is altered nonendothelialized arterial surfaces, which predispose to thrombus formation.[56] Syphilic aortitis and Takayasu arteritis can also obstruct the coronary ostia, leading to myocardial damage.

Another rare event, postpartum coronary artery dissection, has been found in 13 patients, 11 by necropsy and two by angiography.[57] The left anterior descending coronary artery has been involved in all 13 cases. Two patients were in the ninth month of gestation, and 11 were between 14 and 120 days postpartum. There were only two survivors.

IV. DIAGNOSIS

The diagnosis of angina and myocardial infarction is primarily clinical, confirmed by electrocardiographic and enzymatic changes, and when necessary by more sophisticated echocardiographic, angiographic, or nuclear studies. It should be remembered that angina and myocardial infarction are different ends of the spectrum of inadequate oxygen supply to myocardial demand. Gorlin described the complex metabolic, neurologic, psychologic, and hormonal factors that contributed to the marked individual variability in the clinical manifestations of coronary arterial disease.[58] The chest pain may be associated with diaphoresis, dyspnea, nausea, vomiting, or syncope. The location is usually precordial, anywhere from the pharynx to the epigastrium, but may be limited to the left shoulder, arm or hand, jaw, teeth, or back; it may radiate to the shoulders, arms, back, or jaw. The chest pain may last from seconds to minutes in angina and several hours if infarction has occurred. Predictably, the episode is precipitated by exertion, cold weather, emotional stress, large meals, or coitus. The differential diagnosis of chest pain is extensive and is beyond the scope of this review. However, in the pregnant patient similar chest pain may be secondary to gastric reflux associated with hiatus hernia, gallbladder disease, costochondritis, mitral valve prolapse, or psychosomatic complaints.

The electrocardiogram is essential in the diagnosis of coronary disease. In 25–50% of patients with chronic stable angina the electrocardiogram is normal.[59] However, the classical ST-T wave changes (and in infarction, Q wave development) will invariably accompany a significant episode of coronary ischemia. Occasionally minor ST segment depression and T wave inversion may be seen in normal pregnancy, and these should be differentiated from myocardial ischemic changes.

Echocardiography is a safe noninvasive test that can be performed during pregnancy and is of value in assessing regional ventricular wall motion and wall thickening. Abnormalities of wall motion in myocardial infarction corresponding to the electrocardiographic site can be detected correctly in the vast majority of patients.[60] Two-dimensional echocardiographic studies are proving more sensitive in the detection of wall motion abnormalities.[61,62]

An exercise tolerance test can be performed for further evaluation of an abnormal electrocardiogram, for elucidation of atypical chest pain, and for prognostic and therapeutic value in coronary disease. The reproducibility of pain with characteristic electrocardiographic ST segment changes can diagnose the presence and severity of coronary disease. Submaximal exercise tests can be performed with minimal risk to the pregnant woman and her fetus. However, false-positive tests may occur, particularly in young women.

In selected cases where a precise diagnosis is necessary, radionuclear or radiographic studies may be required. However, they carry the danger of radiation exposure, expecially to the fetus. Nuclear studies may detect perfusion defects related to abnormal coronary blood flow, as well as wall motion abnormalities. Technetium 99m-labeled albumin distributes in the blood pool and can detect regional abnormalities of right and left ventricular contractility. The estimated fetal radiation per millicurie of ^{99m}Tc human serum albumin administered is 12 millirads.[63] Therefore, for the usual cardiac gated blood pool study requiring 20 mCi, the net fetal dosage is approximately 240 mrads. Thallium 201, a potassium analog, is distributed to areas of normal coronary perfusion and will reveal a "cold spot" in ischemic or infarcted zones. For a myocardial perfusion scan utilizing thallium 201, the approximate fetal exposure would be 780 mrads. It is estimated that for each 200 mrads of dosage to the fetus there is an extra 10% chance of developing cancer.[64] The maximal permissible dose equivalent to the pregnant woman with respect to the fetus is 0.5 mrad during gestation.[63]

As important as the radiation dosage is the time during gestation at which the exam occurs. From experimental data irradiation during the preimplantation period (0–9 days) tends to cause death rather than anomalies; radiation during active organogenesis (9–42 days) causes severe structural anomalies at levels of 25 rads or more of exposure. During the succeeding weeks of pregnancy the resulting anomalies are functional rather than structural.[65] Therefore, the performance of nuclear studies has to be weighted extremely carefully in pregnant women with special consideration to its potential diagnostic benefits and the risks of radiation, particularly to the fetus.

When a myocardial infarction occurs the injured cells release enzymes into the circulation. There are three enzymes of value in the diagnosis of infarction. Serum glutamic oxaloacetic transaminase (SGOT) activity rises above normal within 8–12 hours following the onset of chest pain, peaking 18–36 hours later and returning to normal three to four days later. Serum lactic dehydrogenase (LDH) is elevated within 24–48 hours and peaks in three to six days and normalizes 8–14 days following the infarction. Of the five isoenzymes of LDH, the heart contains primarily LDH1, and can be found elevated in 95% of patients with myocardial infarction. Serum LDH is elevated approximately 18% in the antepartum period and 100% postpartum. Serum creatine kinase (CK) exceeds normal within six to eight hours, peaks at 24 hours, and falls within three to four days and is the most sensitive enzyme for myocardial infarction detection routinely available. Since CK is a function of total muscle mass, its levels in women are about two-thirds those in men. CK also has isoenzymes, of which MB is predominantly myocardial in origin. The measurement of myoglobin levels has recently been evaluated and shown to peak earlier than CK.[66]

V. MANAGEMENT

Pregnancy can create a significant problem when hemodynamic alterations increase myocardial oxygen consumption in a patient with limited coronary reserve. The increase in cardiac output, in resting heart rate, in total blood volume, and the fact that the absolute rise in cardiac output in response to exercise is higher during pregnancy than in the nonpregnant state, make symptoms of myocardial ischemia appear earlier, and it is more difficult to manage.[67–69]

Medical therapy of ischemic heart disease involves modifying the lifestyle and individualizing and titrating specific medications. Avoidance of aggravating factors such as smoking, hot humid environments, and excessive physical activity is mandatory. Known precipitating conditions such as hypertension, anemia, hyperthyroidism, and infections should be sought and promptly treated. Marked restriction of activity may be required in some patients. In some situations, hospitalization and enforcement of strict bed-rest may be mandatory.

The most common medical therapy for angina is the organic nitrate compounds, the use of which was first described by Brunton in 1867.[70] These agents act primarily by relaxing vascular smooth muscle tone, thereby producing a vasodilatory response. A reduction in venous return reduces ventricular filling, which reduces wall tension and afterload—two major determinants of myocardial oxygen consumption. Nitrates may also directly improve regional myocardial blood flow by dilating the coronary arteries. This appears to be essential in the relief of coronary spasm in Prinzmetal's variant angina. Sublingual nitroglycerin (>0.2 to >0.4 mg) is the drug of choice for an acute attack of angina. The response occurs within two to three minutes, and the duration of action is 20 to 30 minutes. Long-acting preparations have a duration of action from two to four hours. Adverse reactions are secondary to the vasodilatory effect—ie, tachycardia, postural hypotension, headache, and flushing. There are no other known adverse effects of nitrate therapy during pregnancy besides the precaution of avoiding excessive postural hypotension.

Beta-adrenergic blocking agents are other important medications for patients with coronary artery disease. They reduce oxygen consumption by decreasing the heart rate, blood pressure, and myocardial contractility. Propranolol, metoprolol, and nadolol are the most common agents of this category presently available in the United States. Propranolol dosage for angina usually ranges from 80 to 320 mg daily; however, as much as 1,000 mg may be necessary. The dosing interval may be every six to eight hours. The dosage of longer acting beta-blocking agents (eg, nadolol) can vary from 80 to 240 mg daily, beginning at 40 mg and titrating thereafter. Because beta blockade can precipitate bronchospasm or hypoglycemia, these drugs are relatively contraindicated in asthmatics and diabetics. Metoprolol, a cardioselective agent in low doses, may be used with caution in patients with bronchospastic disease. Caution is advised in patients with borderline cardiac function, who may develop congestive heart failure with initiation of beta blockade therapy because of its negative inotropic effect. Other side effects include gastrointestinal upset and depression. Propranolol has been shown to have several deleterious effects on the fetus, including bradycardia, fetal depression, hypoglycemia, and delayed neonatal breathing.[71,72] Also embryonal and fetal toxicity has been associated with doses 5–10 times higher than the maximum recommended dosage.[73,74] Since there are no well-controlled studies in pregnant subjects, the risk of using beta-blocking agents during pregnancy should be weighed against their benefits.

The calcium antagonists represent a new class of drugs that have proved effective in the control of angina pectoris, as well as coronary artery spasm. They are potent coronary vasodilators, acting by decreasing the cellular uptake of calcium, thereby inhibiting the contraction of smooth muscle. They are also negatively inotropic and reduce myocardial oxygen consumption by reducing the force of myocardial contractility.

A. Refractory Angina

Most patients with angina pectoris will be controlled with decreased activity, nitrates, and beta-blockade. If the angina remains refractory to intensive medical management the experimental calcium antagonists should be tried. During the first trimester of pregnancy in a woman with angina pectoris not well controlled with maximal medical therapy, consideration should be given to termination of pregnancy. A therapeutic abortion will increase myocardial oxygen consumption and increase the risk of myocardial infarction, but this risk may be lower than the risk of maternal morbidity–mortality if the pregnancy is allowed to continue. Cardiac catheterization can be considered at this point for diagnosis and as a prelude to possible coronary bypass surgery. However, the radiation exposure (5.5 rad per minute for average small field exposure of fluoroscopy with cine angiography) will probably preclude normal fetal development and would warrant termination of pregnancy. Furthermore, all anginal symptoms may decrease dramatically following the termination of pregnancy, thereby making catheterization unnecessary. Between the fourth and eighth months of pregnancy, the patient with refractory angina should be approached like a nonpregnant patient. If coronary artery bypass surgery is a consideration, catheterization and its attendant risks must be weighed. After the eighth month a pregnant patient with refractory angina can be given a trial of labor. If tolerated without clinical or electrocardiographic evidence of significant myocardial ischemia, no other measures are necessary. However, if significant ischemia is detected an intraaortic balloon pump may be inserted to decrease myocardial oxygen consumption, allowing for the successful continuation of labor.

B. Acute Myocardial Infarction

The management of acute myocardial infarction during pregnancy is a function of both its severity and complications. The documentations of successful pregnancy following infarction illustrate that it does not necessarily require termination of the pregnancy. A small myocardial infarction should be well tolerated without special management. The greatest maternal mortality occurs when the infarction occurs during the last months of pregnancy and during labor.[2,7] When indicated, a thermodilution catheter may be advanced, with the use of pressure monitoring for proper positioning to the pulmonary capillary wedge position, for monitoring of both hemodynamic and cardiac output parameters during the different phases of delivery. With careful technique the catheter can be maintained for several days and allows proper titration of fluids and medications. This will facilitate close observation during progression of labor.

Proper anesthesia can mitigate the hemodynamic burden of the cardiac patient. In patients receiving paracervical or pudendal block local anesthesia, there is a progressive increase in cardiac output between contractions. However, when caudal analgesia is employed the increase is attenuated as the pain of contraction is adequately relieved.[75] However, precautions such as cardiac monitors and, when indicated, central venous pressure monitoring should be available when needed.

Delivery by cesarean section prior to the onset of labor will avoid its stresses but introduces the additional risks of general anesthesia and major abdominal surgery. Most general anesthetic agents depress myocardial contractility. Halothane and methoxyflurane cause the greatest depression; diethyl ether and cyclopropane, the least.[76] Newer combinations—ie, droperidol fentanyl, or nitrous oxide–pancuronium bromide—produce very little myocardial depression.[77] Balanced general anesthesia can maintain hemodynamic stability, except for endotracheal intubation, for which thiopental or ketamine may be preferable agents. Epidural anesthesia without epinephrine can also provide a smooth course.[75]

Immediately following labor, venous return to the heart markedly increases. Blood loss accompanies the delivery of the placenta, and there is new cardiovascular risk from the vasoconstricting medications used to control bleeding. Of note, of the pregnant patients who survived a myocardial infarction prior to labor on ly one failed to survive labor and delivery.[7,78]

Most coronary patients can tolerate a natural vaginal delivery, and cesarean section is only indicated for obstetrical purposes. However, there should be full obstetrical, medical, surgical, and anesthesiologic teams readily available in the event of complications. Induction of labor has to be considered when the cervix is mature, after 38 weeks of gestation and after a lecithin/sphingomyelin (L/S) ratio greater than or equal to 2.0 has been documented.[79] A dilute oxytocin solution administered intravenously is used to induce labor, and the amniotomy is performed after a regular labor pattern has been established and progressive cervical effacement and dilatation have begun. Forceps delivery further alleviates stress in a difficult labor.

In the event of maternal death during labor or delivery a post mortem cesarean section should be performed. One hundred and fifty-three cases of successful infant survival under such circumstances were collected by Weber in 1971.[80]

In conclusion, coronary artery disease is rare in the pregnant woman; however, with the trend toward postponement of pregnancy to later in life, the increased use of birth control pills, and the increase in smoking among women, coronary insufficiency may become a much more frequent occurrence. The general management of stable angina and myocardial infarction is similar to that in the nonpregnant patient. However, the increased myocardial oxygen demand during pregnancy and the stress of delivery are particular problems that require careful individual assessment in these patients. With improved methods of diagnosis, treatment, and hemodynamic monitoring, the pregnant patient with coronary disease should be able to anticipate a normal vaginal delivery with a significantly reduced risk of morbidity and mortality more often than in the past.

VI. REFERENCES

1. Vital Statistics of the United States—1977. U.S. Department of Health and Human Services, Hyattsville, Maryland, 1980.
2. Ginz B. Myocardial infarction in pregnancy. J Obstet Gynaecol Br Commonw. 1952; 63: 381–390.
3. Mendelson C. Coronary artery disease in preg-

nancy. Am J Obstet Gynecol. 1952; 63:381–390.
4. Hibbard L. Maternal mortality due to cardiac disease. Clin Obset Gynecol. 1975; 18:27–36.
5. Katz H. About the sudden natural death in pregnancy: During delivery and the puerperium. Arch F Gynakol. 1922; 115:83–85.
6. Carreras F, Cortes C. Crise cardiaque pendant grossesse. Bull Soc Obstet Gynecol. 1929; 18:606–609.
7. Husani MH. Myocardial infarction during pregnancy. Postgrad Med Jl. 1971; 47:660–665.
8. Sasse L, Wagner R, Murray F. Transmural myocardial infarction during pregnancy. Am J Cardiol. 1975; 35:448–451.
9. Kannel WB, Castelli WP, Gordon T. Cholesterol in the prediction of atherosclerotic disease. Ann Intern Med. 1975; 90:85–91.
10. Kannel WB, Castelli WP, Gordon T, McNamara P. Serum cholesterol, lipoproteins and the risk of coronary heart disease. The Framingham Study. Ann Intern Med. 1971; 74:1–8.
11. Stamler J. Lifestyles, major risk factors, proof and public policy. Circulation. 1978; 58:3–5.
12. Stone NJ, Levy RI, Fredrickson DS, Verter J. Coronary artery disease in the 116 kindred with familial type II hyperlipoproteinemia. Circulation. 1974; 49:476–481.
13. Castelli WP, Doyle JT, Gordon T, Haines CG, Hjortland M, Hulley SB, Kagan A, Zukel WJ. HDL cholesterol and other lipids in coronary heart disease. Circulation. 1977; 55:767–773.
14. Mann JI, Vessey MP, Thorogood M, Doll R. MI in young women with special reference to oral contraceptive practice. Br Med J. 1975; 2:241–245.
15. Mann JI, Inman WHW. Oral contraceptives and death from myocardial infarction. Br Med J. 1975; 2:245–248.
16. Vessey MP, Doll R. Investigation of relation between use of oral contraceptives and thromboembolic disease. Br Med J. 1968; 2:199–205.
17. Poller L, Thomson JM. Clotting factors during oral contraceptives, further report. Br Med J. 1966; 2:23.
18. Caspary EA, Peberdy M. Oral contraception and blood platelet adhesiveness. Lancet. 1965; 1:1142.
19. Wexler EB, Kimbiris D, Van Den Broek H, Segal B, Likoff W. Myocardial infarction and oral contraceptive agents. Am J Cardiol. 1971; 28:96–101.
20. Maleki M, Lange R. Coronary thrombosis in young women on oral contraceptives: Report of 2 cases and review of literature. Am Heart J. 1973; 85:749–754.
21. Naysmith JH. Correspondence: Oral contraceptives and coronary thrombosis. Br Med J. 1965; 1:250.
22. Pick R, Katz TN, Century D, Johnson PJ. Production of ulcerated atherosclerotic lesions in cockerels. Circ Res. 1962; 11:811–819.
23. Rossner S, Larson-Cohen N, Carlson LA, Boberg J. Effect of an oral contraceptive agent on plasma lipids, plasma lipoproteins, the intravenous fat tolerance and post heparin lipoprotein lipase activity. Acta Med Scand. 1971; 190:193–197.
24. Glick CJ, Fallat R. Gonadal hormone and triglycerides. Proc R Soc Med. 1974; 67:667–671.
25. Wynn V, Daer JWH, Mills GL. Some effects of contraceptives on serum lipids and lipoprotein levels. Lancet. 1969; 2:761–766.
26. Mandour T, Kissebach AH, Wynn V. Mechanism of estrogen and progesterone in lipids and carbohydrate metabolism: Glucagon moler ratio and hepatic enzyme activity. Eur J Clin Invest. 1977; 7:181–77.
27. Brody S, Kerstell J, Nilsson L, Svenborg A. The effects of some ovulation inhibitors on the different plasma lipid fraction. Acta Med Scand. 1968; 183:1–5.
28. Bradley DV, Wingerd J, Perihi DB, Krauss RM, Ramcharan S. Serum high density lipoprotein cholesterol in women using oral contraceptives, estrogen and progestins. N Engl J Med. 1978; 199:17–23.
29. Crane MG, Harris JJ, Winsor W. Hypertension, oral contraceptive agents and conjugated estrogens. Ann Intern Med. 1971; 74:13–18.
30. Fisch IR, Freedman SH, Myatt AV. Oral contraceptives, pregnancy and blood pressure. JAMA. 1972; 222:1507–1509.
31. Weir RJ, Briggs E, Mack A, Naismith L, Taylor L, Wilson E. Blood pressure in women taking oral contraceptives. Br Med J. 1974; 1:533–535.
32. Hammond EC. Smoking in relation to disease other than cancer. Total death rates. The Second World Conference on Smoking and Health. London: Pitman. 1971.
33. Oliver MF. Ischemic heart disease in young women. Br Med J. 1974; 4:253–259.
34. Slone D, Shapiro S, Rosenberg L, Kaufman DW, Hartz SC, Rossi AC, Stolley PD, Miettinen OS. Relation of cigarette smoking to myocardial infarction in young women. N Engl J Med. 1978; 298:1273–1276.
35. Wald N, Howard S, Smith PW, Kjeldson K. Association between atherosclerotic disease and carboxyhemoglobin levels in tobacco smokers. Br Med J. 1973; 1:761–765.
36. Garrison RJ, Kannel WB, Feinleib M, Casetelli WP, McNamara PM, Padgett SJ. Cigarette smoking and HDL cholesterol. Atherosclerosis. 1978; 30:17–24.
37. Gordon T, Kannel WB, McGee D, Dauber TR. Death and coronary attacks in men after giving up cigarette smoking. Lancet. 1974; 2:1345–1347.
38. Friedman GD, Petitti D, Bansal R, Siegelaub. Mortality in cigarette smokers and quitters. N Engl J Med. 1981; 304:1407–1411.
39. Garcia MJ, McNamara PM, Gordon T, Kannel WB. Morbidity and mortality of diabetes in the Framingham Study. Diabetes. 1976; 23:105–111.
40. Coronary Drug Project Research Group. The

prognostic importance of plasma glucose levels and the use of oral hypoglycemic drugs after myocardial infarction in men. Diabetes. 1977; 26:453–458.

41. University Group Diabetes Program. A study of the effects of hypoglycemic agents vascular complications in patients with adult onset diabetes. II. Mortality results. Diabetes. 1970; 19 (Suppl II):785–789.
42. Carstrom S. Treatment with sulphonylurea drugs and cardiovascular disease. Proc Ninth Congress Int Diabetes Fed. Amsterdam: Exerpta Medica, 1977: 426–433.
43. Kannel WB. Role of blood pressure in cardiovascular disease. The Framingham Study. Angiology. 1975; 26:1–7.
44. Brunner H, Laragh JH, Baer L, Newton M, Goodwin F, Krakoff L, Bard R, Buhler F. Essential hypertension: Renin, aldosterone, heart attack and stroke. N Engl J Med. 1972; 286:441–449.
45. Garras H, Kremer D, Brown J, Gray B, Lever A, MacAdam R, Medina A, Morton J, Robertson J. Angiotensin and norepinephrine induced myocardial lesion. Am Heart J. 1975; 89:321–331.
46. Symonds E, Pipkin F. Pregnancy, hypertension, parity and reinin-angiotensin. Am J Obstet Gynecol. 1978; 132:473–479.
47. Skinner S, Lumbers E, Symonds E. Renin concentration in human and maternal tissue. Am J Obstet Gynecol. 1968; 101:529–533.
48. Prinzmetal M, Kennamer R, Merliss R, Wada T, Bor N. A variant form of angina pectoris. Am J Med. 1959; 27:375–388.
49. Oliva P, Potts D, Pluss R. Coronary artery spasm in Prinzmetal's angina. N Engl J Med. 1973; 288:745–751.
50. Welch C, Proudfit W, Sheldon W. Coronary artery in 1000 females less than 50 years of age. Am J Cardiol. 1975; 35:211–215.
51. Muller JE. Prinzmetal's angina—A model for the role of spasm in ischemic heart disease. J Cardiovasc Med. 1980; 5:19–21.
52. Beary J, Summer W, Bulkley B. Postpartum acute myocardial infarction: Rare occurrence of uncertain etiology. Am J Cardiol. 1979; 43:158–161.
53. Meller J, Conde C, Deppisch L, Donoso E, Dack S. Myocardial infarction due to coronary atherosclerosis in 3 young adults with systemic lupus erythematosus. Am J Cardiol. 1975; 35:309–312.
54. Bulkley B, Klaismann P, Hutchins G. Angina pectoris, myocardial infarction and sudden cardiac death with normal coronary arteries. A clinopathologic study of 9 patients and progressive systemic sclerosis. Am Heart J. 1978; 95:563–569.
55. Perloff JK. Coronary artery disease—Antidote to a stereotype. Am J Cardiol. 1972; 30:437–439.
56. Harker L, Slichter S, Scott C, Ross R. Homocysteinemia. 1974; 291:537–543.
57. Shaver P, Carrig T, Baker W. Postpartum coronary artery dissection. Br Heart J. 1978; 40:83–86.
58. Gorlin R. Pathophysiology of cardiac pain. Circulation. 1965; 32:138–143.
59. Gorlin R. Evaluation of the patient with coronary artery disease In: Gorlin R Ed. Coronary Artery Disease. Philadelphia: W.B. Saunders, 1976:178.
60. Corya BC, Rasmussen S, Knoebel SB, Feigenbaum N. Echocardiography in acute myocardial infarction. Am J Cardiol. 1975; 36:1–7.
61. Weiss JL, Bulkley BH, Hutchins CM, Mason SJ: Two-dimensional echocardiographic recognition of myocardial injury in man: comparison with postmortem studies. Circulation. 1981; 63:401–409.
62. Eaton LW, Weiss JL, Bulkley BH, Garrison JB, Weisfeldt ML. Regional cardiac dilatation after acute myocardial infarction. Recognition by 2-D echocardiography. N Engl J Med. 1979; 300:57–63.
63. NCRP Report # 39. Basic radiation protection criteria. 1980:106.
64. Campbell JA. Antenatal radiation hazards. In: Obstetric Diagnosis by Radiographic, Ultrasonic and Nuclear Methods. Baltimore: Williams and Wilkins Co. 1977.
65. Rugh R. Radiation tetrology in mice and a review of what is known in man. Br J Radiol. 1968; 41:714–717.
66. Kagen L, Scheidt S, Butt A. Serum myoglobin in myocardial infarction. Am J Med. 1977; 62:86–92.
67. Lund CJ, Donovan JC. Blood volume during pregnancy. Am J Obstet Gynecol. 1967; 98:393–398.
68. Adams JQ. Cardiovascular physiology in normal pregnancy: Studies with the dye dilation technique. Am J Obstet Gynecol. 1954; 67:741–750.
69. Ueland K, Navy MJ, Peterson EN, Metcalfe J. Maternal cardiovascular dynamics IV: The influence of gestational age on the maternal cardiovascular response to posture and exercise. Am J Obstet Gynecol. 1969; 104:856–863.
70. Brunton TL. On the use of amyl nitrate in angina pectoris. Lancet. 1967; 2:97–101.
71. Gladstone GL, Hardof A, Gersony W. Propranolol administration during pregnancy. Effects on the fetus. Am J Pediatr. 1975; 86:962–964.
72. Turnstall ME. Effects of propranolol on the onset of breathing at birth. Br J Anaesthesiol. 1969; 41:792.
73. ER Squibb and Sons Inc. March 1981. Medication Insert.
74. Physicians Desk Reference. Oradell, New Jersey: Medical Economics Company, 1981:613–614.
75. Ueland K, Metcalfe J. Circulatory changes in pregnancy. Clin Obstet Gynecol. 1975; 18:41–50.
76. Hillis LD, Cohn PF. Noncardiac surgery in patients with coronary artery disease. Arch Intern Med. 1978; 138:972–978.

77. Wolf M, Braunwald E. General anesthesia and noncardiac surgery in patients with heart disease. In: Heart Disease. Braunwald E, Ed. Philadelphia: W.B. Saunders, 1980:1911–1922.
78. Curry JJ, Quintana FJ. Myocardial infarction with ventricular fibrillation during pregnancy treated with direct current defibrillation. Chest. 1970; 58:82–91.
79. Freeman RK. Intrapartum management of the pregnant patient with heart disease. Clin Obstet Gynecol. 1975; 18:75–79.
80. Weber CE. Postmortem cesarean section: A review of the literature and case reports. Am J Obstet Gynecol. 1971; 110:158–165.

M.XII

Primary Pulmonary Hypertension and Pregnancy

Uri Elkayam, MD, and Norbert Gleicher, MD

Primary pulmonary hypertension (PPH) is an uncommon abnormality that has only rarely been described in association with pregnancy. Early recognition during gestation may be difficult because symptoms of the disease can be attributed to pregnancy itself. The grave prognosis of pregnancy in patients with PPH and the strong recommendations for early abortion in these cases suggest the importance of early recognition of this clinical syndrome. The specifics of pregnancy in patient with PPH are discussed in this chapter, following a brief general review of the disease.

I. PATHOPHYSIOLOGY

Medial constriction of the arteriolar lumen is probably the initiating event leading to an increase in medial thickeness of muscular pulmonary arteries, muscularization of pulmonary arterioles, development of intimal fibrosis and fibroelastosis producing typical "onion skin" configuration, and the development of dilatation lesions, especially plexiform lesions, and in some cases necrotizing arthritis[1] (Fig. M.XII.1).

II. ETIOLOGY

Although the cause of the disease is unknown, numerous etiological factors have been postulated, including occult venous thrombosis and recurrent pulmonary embolism,[2] congenital deficiency of the media of the pulmonary arterial bed resulting in intimal thickening,[3] persistence of fetal pulmonary arterial architecture,[4] increased systemic-to-pulmonary arterial

Cardiac Problems in Pregnancy, pages 153–160

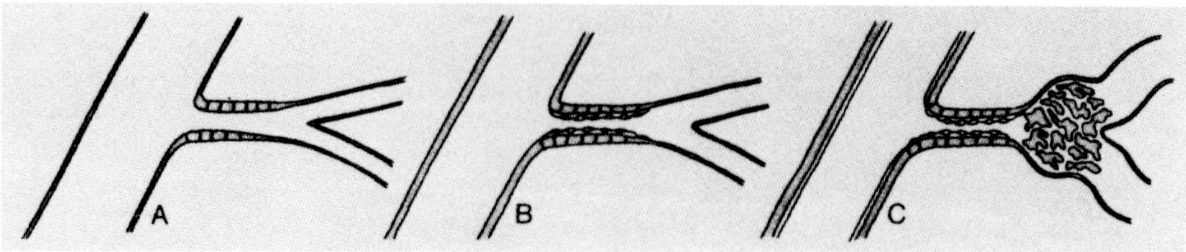

Fig. M.XII.1. Diagram of the probable stages in development of PPH. In **A** there is constriction of the lumen by medial contraction leading to intimal cell proliferation in the constricted segment as shown in **B**. In **C** the glomoid is shown formed distal to the region of constriction produced by intimal cell proliferation. (By permission from Hutchins and Ostrow, American Heart Journal 92:802, 1976)

collaterals,[5] and generalized degenerative pulmonary arteriopathy.[6] The increased incidence of Raynaud's phenomenon seen in patients with PPH may indicate that the disease is a form of collagen vascular disease or an autoimmune disease.[7] Hypersensitivity to various drugs has been suggested, and pulmonary hypertension has recently been reported in patients who ingested the anorexigenic drug aminorex fumarate.[8,9] Increased pulmonary vasoreactivity has also been considered by some investigators as a potential factor in the genesis of PPH[10,11] and familial cases of PPH have been reported with autosomal dominant inheritance.[12,13]

III. CLINICAL PRESENTATION

PPH is a progressive disease, mostly occurring in the young, predominantly in women.[7] Patients usually come to medical attention relatively late in the course of the disease, and death usually occurs a few months to several years after onset of symptoms. The presenting symptoms are most commonly weakness, fatigue, exertional dyspnea, effort syncope, and chest pain. In the later phase of the disease dyspnea at rest, cough, and hemoptysis occasionally develop. A compression of the recurrent nerve by the dilated pulmonary artery may result in hoarseness.[14]

Chest pain is caused either by myocardial ischemia due to increased oxygen demand of the grossly hypertrophied right ventricle or by the distension of the pulmonary artery.[15] Recurrent palpitations are a common complaint in patients with PPH and represent the occurrence of atrial and/or ventricular premature contractions. Ventricular arrhythmias are not uncommon and are probably the cause of the frequent sudden deaths in many of these patients.

IV. PHYSICAL EXAMINATION

The typical physical findings in patients with PPH occur as a result of a substantial pressure increase in the pulmonary circulation and the resulting right ventricular hypertrophy and failure.

Cyanosis, although not commonly seen in the early stages of the disease, can be present later on. The factors contributing to the genesis of this finding are an increased tissue O_2 extraction due to low cardiac output, ventilation perfusion mismatches in the lungs, an increased intrapulmonary right-to-left shunting via vascular anastomoses or, at times, via a patent foramen ovale.[16]

The jugular venous pulse shows an exaggerated A wave, reflecting poor compliance of the right ventricle. The development of tricuspid insufficiency due to right ventricular dilatation is usually accompanied by a high jugular V wave. The carotid arterial pulses have normal rate of rise but low volume, owing to a decreased stroke volume. Palpation of the chest usually reveals right ventricular heave due to hypertrophy and a palpable P_2 reflecting dilatation of the pulmomary artery.

Auscultation of the heart reveals a normal first heart sound (S_1), which often is followed by an ejection sound (click) and a systolic ejection murmur caused by the ejection of blood into a dilated pulmonary artery. Both the click and the murmur are heard maximally over the pulmonic auscultatory area, and the ejection sound usually decreases during inspiration. When tricuspid insufficiency has developed, a pansystolic murmur can be heard maximally at the left lower sternal border or at the apex when this area is being taken over by the enlarged right ventricle. The characteristic inspiratory accentuation of the murmur is lost with the onset of right ventricular failure. The second heart sound (S_2) is characterized by a loud pulmonic component (P_2). The splitting of S_2 is initially normal or narrowed. Failure of the right ventricle in later stages results in a delayed P_2, loss of the characteristic respiratory variation of the second heart sound, and sometimes fixation of splitting of S_2.[17,18] The development of pulmonic valve incompetence due to dilatation of the valvular apparatus is identified by a high-pitched, early diastolic, decrescendo murmur (Graham-Steel murmur) heard loudest at the left sternal border. A right-sided S_4 is usually heard along the lower left sternal border and increases with inspiration, and it is a result of hypertrophied, poorly compliant right venticle. Right ventricular failure is characterized by development of S_3 along the lower left sternal border and peripheral signs, including hepatomegaly, peripheral edema, and ascites.

V. LABORATORY FINDINGS

A. Hematological and Chemical Studies

A decrease in arterial PO_2 and O_2 saturation is often found and can be accompained by polycythemia. Abnormalities in coagulation such as hypercoagulable state, abnormal platelet function, defects in fibrinolysis, and others have been described in patients with PPH.[14]

Pulmonary functions are usually normal. A low Co_2 diffusing capacity has been described in some patients with PPH, probably due to an increase in capillary to alveolar distance secondary to hypertrophy of vascular endothelial cells.

The electrocardiogram (Fig. M.XII.2) commonly reveals normal sinus rhythm or slight sinus tachycardia with signs of right atrial enlargement and right ventricular hypertrophy. Chest x-ray films (Fig. M.XII.3) usually demonstrate enlargement of the heart, with right ventricular and right atrial prominence, and dilatation of the pulmonary trunk and its major divisions. The peripheral pulmonary vasculature is usually decreased.

Echocardiogram often reveals an enlarged, hypertrophied right ventricle with a normal or small left ventricle. The interventricular septum can be thickened and usually shows a paradoxical motion. The

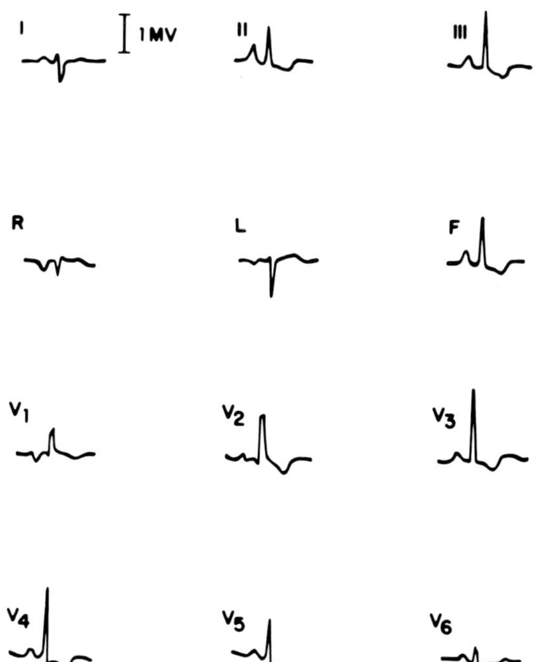

Fig. M.XII.2. Electrocardiogram in a patient with PPH shows right atrial enlargement and right ventricular hypertrophy

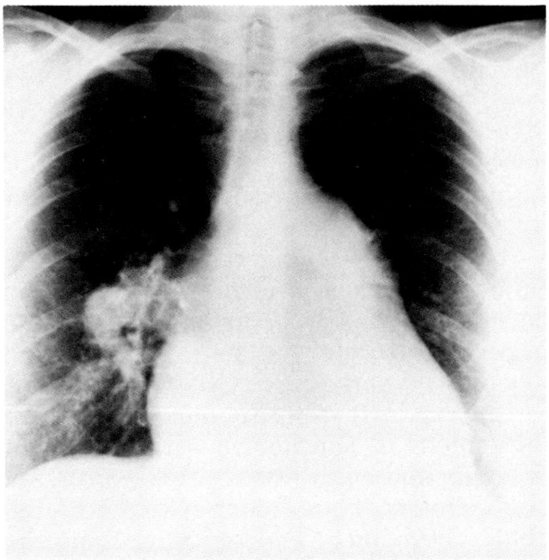

Fig. M.XII.3. A frontal chest roentgenogram in a patient with PPH demonstrates cardiomegaly, enlargement of the main pulmonary artery and its major divisions, and decreased peripheral pulmonary vasculature.

E-F slope of the anterior leaflet of the mitral valve is decreased as a result of decreased flow. In addition, an increased incidence of mitral valve prolapse has been shown in patients with PPH.[19] Bidimensional echocardiography allows visualization of the right atrium, which is enlarged in patients with PPH.

Ventilation-perfusion scan of the lungs is usually within normal limits. It has been suggested that the performance of lung scanning in the late stage of the disease can be hazardous because it leads to further reduction of the luminal area of the pulmonary circulation by macroaggregation of the albumin used for scanning, which can cause a further decrease in pulmonary blood flow.[20]

B. Cardiac Catheterization

A typical hemodynamic profile can be observed in a patient with PPH. A marked increase in pulmonary resistance results in pulmonary hypertension and decreased cardiac output. Right ventricular end-diastolic pressure increases initally because of decreased compliance and later because of failure of the systolic function of the myocardium. Right atrial pressure is elevated and demonstrates an increased A wave and, in the presence of tricuspid valve insufficiency, a tall V wave. Cardiac catheterization is always indicated to exclude correctable cardiac causes of the pulmonary hypertension.

VI. TREATMENT

Supportive treatment with digitalis and diuretics should be instituted in patients with right ventricular failure. Antiarrhythmic therapy is often required to control atrial and/or ventricular arrhythmias.

Anticoagulation has been advocated to prevent pulmonary emboli, a frequent autopsy finding in PPH. There is no evidence, however, that anticoagulation therapy can favorably change the natural history of the disease. Continuous oxygen therapy is sometimes needed to correct hypoxemia.

Numerous recent reports have indicated that the use of vasodilator agents such as isoproterenol, hydralazine, diazoxide, phentolamine, and prazosin can minimize the vasospastic component of PPH and has a beneficial effect on the hemodynamic profile and on symptoms.[20–24] The usefulness of vasodilator therapy in the late stage of the disease is doubtful because of loss of pulmonary vascular reactivity and fixed pulmonary arteriolar resistance. Major side effects such as systemic hypotension and chest pain have been reported and indicate the need for close hemodynamic monitoring when this mode of therapy is initiated.[24,25]

VII. PPH AND PREGNANCY

In an extensive review of the literature we found descriptions of 38 pregnancies in 21 patients with PPH.[26–29] Eleven of those 21 patients (52%) died during pregnancy or in the early postpartum period.[26–30] The duration of symptoms prior to pregnancy did not seem to have a significant influence on the outcome of pregnancy. In general, it seems that gestation is associated with better prognosis in asymptomatic patients or patients with only mild symptoms. It is, however, difficult to predict, on the basis of symptoms before pregnancy, whether a patient will develop right ventricular failure or will die during pregnancy. The incidence of worsening of clinical status and maternal death in asymptomatic and mildly symptomatic women, although lower than in the overall group of patients, is still very high. Maternal mortality in this group has been reported in six of 14 cases or in 42%.[26,28,30,31] Burwell and Metcalfe described a woman with PPH who died during her fifth pregnancy, but had showed significant clinical improvement during each of the preceding four pregnancies. The effect of pregnancy in this case is exceptional, since worsening of symptoms, rather than improvement, is the rule.

McCaffrey and Dunn, in their excellent review of 23 pregnancies in 16 women with PPH, noted that four patients who experienced no adverse effects during pregnancy lived for an average of six years after delivery, whereas the three patients who survived pregnancy but demonstrated clinical deterioration did not live for more than two years after their delivery.[26] These data suggest that pregnancy in the late stage of the disease is associated with higher incidence of complications. The development of cyanosis, chest pain, right ventricular failure, and severe dyspnea during pregnancy represented a grave prognosis.[26] Syncope as an isolated symptom was found in some patients reported by McCaffrey and Dunn and did not seem to have a poor prognostic implication.

Women with PPH usually come to medical attention in the second trimester of pregnancy for symptoms of fatigue, dyspnea, syncope, chest pain, and signs of right ventricular failure. Death can occur at any time from early pregnancy to the puerperium; however, the higher incidence is seen in the last phase of gestation and during the early postpartum period. The cause of maternal death is not entirely clear, as controlled hemodynamic data or electrocardiographic information are unavailable. The high incidence of death during late pregnancy and the early postpartum period suggests a relationship between the increased circulatory burden of pregnancy, labor, and delivery and mortality. The concomitant occurrence of markedly increased blood volume and the anemia of pregnancy can result in increased myocardial work and decreased oxygen availability. Worsening of the balance between myocardial oxygen supply and demand may lead to ischemia and, consequently, to right ventricular failure and fatal arrhythmias.

VIII. EFFECT OF PREGNANCY ON THE NATURAL HISTORY OF PPH

Although it has been suggested by several investigators that pregnancy has a specific effect and serves as a stimulating factor that accelerates the progression of the disease,[9,26,30] this is not established. Giard et al[30] described a 28-year-old woman with PPH who became symptomatic one month after delivering a normal baby by cesarean section after a normal asymptomatic pregnancy. (Cesarean section was necessary because of fetal malposition.) Based upon this clinical presentation of the disease, the authors concluded that pregnancy acted as a trigger in accelerating the evolution of the disease. Jewett and Ober[31] found acute fibrinoid necrosis involving the intima and inner media of the smaller pulmonary arteries, which was superimposed on more chronic vascular changes in a patient with PPH who died during pregnancy. They postulated that these acute changes were attributable to pregnancy and were responsible for the clinical deterioration of the patient. However, the absence of similar findings in other pregnant women and their presence in nonpregnant patients do not support this conclusion.[26] It has also been suggested that the hypercoagulability state, usually associated with pregnancy,[32] may provide a vulnerable basis for the formation of pulmonary thrombi, especially in patients with PPH when the pulmonary vasculature is altered and damaged by the primary disease.[26] Hutchins and Astrow found a correlation between pulmonary artery systolic pressure and the severity of pulmonary arteriolar anatomic damage.[1] The physiological increase in blood volume and cardiac output during pregnancy may result in further rise in pulmonary pressure[25] and, thus, in a progression of pulmonary vascular damage.

IX. FETAL OUTCOME IN PATIENTS WITH PPH

Primary pulmonary hypertension influences fetal outcome as much as it affects maternal outcome.[26] A high incidence of fetal death as a result of spontaneous abortions and intrauterine damage consequent to maternal death has been reported. There is also a high incidence of neonatal death due to congenital cardiac malformations.

X. MANAGEMENT OF THE PREGNANT WOMAN WITH PPH

Pregnancy seems contraindicated in patients with PPH for the following reasons: 1) the high incidence of maternal morbidity and mortality, 2) the inability to predict the course and outcome of pregnancy even in asymptomatic or only mildly symptomatic women with PPH, 3) the high incidence of fetal and neonatal morbidity and mortality, and 4) a possible acceleration of the natural history of the disease during pregnancy.

The physician should make every effort to convince these patients that pregnancy should be avoided. Patients have to be adequately informed about the hazards of pregnancy and the means to prevent it (see Chapter M.XXVI). The selection of the most adequate means of birth control for a patient with PPH may not be easy. Although the relationship between oral contraceptives and primary pulmonary hypertension is not entirely clear, there have been several reports in the literature of pulmonary hypertension secondary to oral contraceptive use.[33,34] Moreover, the development of internal vascular lesions in both veins and arteries, including the pulmonary arteries, has been reported in women using oral contraceptives.[35] The effect of oral contraceptives on the evolution of the disease in women with PPH is unknown. It has been suggested, however, that the development of pulmonary hypertension with oral contraceptive usage may be enhanced in women with predisposing causes such as collagen vascular disease, family history of pulmonary hypertension, and congenital heart disease.[33,35,36]

Tubal ligation was considered inadvisable by McCaffrey and Dunn[26] because of the potential hazard associated with surgery in patients with PPH. Although we agree with the validity of the concern regarding the performance of surgery in patients with known PPH, we think that tubal ligation can be considered a viable option for some of these patients. Other invasive procedures such as cardiac catheterization were also considered to be extremely hazardous to patients with PPH.[37] Improvement of the technique and better understanding of the potential complications of the procedure in these patients resulted in a significant improvement of the results, with only one complication reported during the performance of 92 procedures.[38] For this reason we believe that tubal ligation can be performed in asymptomatic patients or patients with mild symptoms provided the procedure is done under local anesthesia with adequate monitoring of the systemic and pulmonary pressures, as well as the electrocardiogram.[39] Intrauterine devices, which are not recommended in patients with valvular heart disease because of the increased susceptibility to infection and valvular bacterial endocarditis (SBE), can be used in patients with PPH because no increased incidence of SBE has been reported with this disease. The other means of birth control should not be recommended because of the associated high incidence of pregnancy (see Chapter M.XXVI).

If pregnancy occurs, abortion is indicated as early as possible. In additon, we believe that hemodynamic and electrocardiographic monitoring is indicated during the procedure so that irreversible complications can be prevented.

Patients who decide not to terminate the pregnancy should be followed closely. Physical activity should be minimized to avoid a further increase in the circulatory burden. Although death in pregnant women with PPH may occur at any time during pregnancy, it occurs most commonly during the last trimester. To assure restriction of activity and to optimize monitoring, patients should be hospitalized after 20 weeks of gestation, or earlier when there are signs of progression of symptoms or clinical deterioration.

Congestive heart failure should be treated with digoxin and diuretics. The role of anticoagulation in the treatment of PPH has not been established, but the reported hypercoagulability during pregnancy makes it tempting to use anticoagulation. However, significant fetal toxicity has been shown with both heparin and warfarin.[40] It is our opinion that, because of the potential side effects of anticoagulation during pregnancy (Chapter M.XXII), and until further evidence is available regarding the role of thromboembolism in the genesis and progression of PPH, the indication for anticoagulation during pregnancy should be considered questionable. The use of vasodilator therapy has not been described during pregnancy; it is feasible, however, that it would be beneficial, especially during late pregnancy and the time of labor and delivery.

Because of the stress and hemodynamic changes associated with labor and delivery, hemodynamic and electrocardiographic monitoring is indicated in patients with PPH. Pulmonary artery pressure, systemic blood pressure, and cardiac output should be regularly measured during labor and delivery.[39] Every effort should be made to minimize blood loss during delivery, and significant loss should be promptly replaced.

The measurement of blood gases also should be performed repeatedly during labor, delivery, and the puerperium in order to assure adequate oxygenation. Hypoxemia should be prevented by oxygen administration. The significance of appropriate oxygenation during labor and delivery was demonstrated by Slavin, who used hyperbaric oxygenation in two patients with severe symptomatic PPH. Significant improvement of oxygenation and symptoms of dyspnea and cyanosis occurred, which allowed normal delivery.[29]

The experience in normal women and in patients with Eisenmenger's syndrome showed that epidural anesthesia offers hemodynamic stability and represents the best method for cardiac patients.[41,42]

As the incidence of premature delivery is high in women with PPH, this should be anticipated. To decrease the incidence of prematurity and cesarean section deliveries, spontaneous labor is preferable to induction.

Postpartum patients should continue to be monitored hemodynamically and electrocardiographically for three to four days, and a prolonged postpartum hospitalization of ten to 14 days is recommended to assure stability.

XI. ACKNOWLEDGMENTS

We gratefully acknowledge the expert secretarial assistance of Ellen Mansour and Lyndsay Atchison in the preparation of this manuscript.

XII. REFERENCES

1. Hutchins GM, Ostow PT. The pathogenesis of the two forms of hypertensive pulmonary vascular disease. Am Heart J. 1976; 92:797–803.
2. Rosenberg SA. A study of the etiological basis of primary pulmonary hypertension. Am Heart J. 1964; 68:484–489.
3. Evans W, Short DS, Bedford DE. Solitary pulmonary hypertension. Br Heart J. 1957; 19:93–116.
4. Goodale F Jr, Thomas WA. Primary pulmonary arterial disease. Arch Pathol. 1954; 58:568–575.

5. Wade G, Ball J. Unexplained pulmonary hypertension. Q J Med. 1957; 26:83–119.
6. James TN. Degenerative arteriopathy with pulmonary hypertension: A revised concept of so-called primary pulmonary hypertension. Henry Ford Hosp Bull. 1961; 9:271–311.
7. Walcott G, Burcell HB, Brown AL. Primary pulmonary hypertension. Am J Med. 1970; 49:70–77.
8. Trell E. Primary and chronic thormboembolic pulmonary hypertension. Angiology. 1972; 23:558–574.
9. Gurtner HP. Pulmonary hypertension plexogenic pulmonary arteriopathy and the appetite depressant drug Aminorex: Post or propter? Bull Eur Physiopathol Respir. 1979; 15:897–923.
10. Daoud FS, Reeves JT, Kelly DB. Isoproterenol as a potential pulmonary vasodilator in primary pulmonary hypertension. Am J Cardiol. 1978; 42:817–822.
11. Wagenvoort CA, Wagenvoort N. Primary pulmonary hypertension. A pathologic study of the lung vessels in 156 clinically diagnosed cases. Circulation. 1970; 42:1163–1184.
12. Robertson B, Rosenhamer G, Lindberg J. Idiopathic pulmonary hypertension in two siblings. Acta Med Scand. 1969; 186:569–577.
13. Kingdon HS, Cohen LS, Roberts WC, Braunwald E. Familial occurrence of primary pulmonary hypertension. Arch Intern Med. 1966; 118:422–426.
14. Alpert JS, Braunwald E. Primary pulmonary hypertension. In: Braunwald E, (ed.) Heart Disease. Philadelphia: W.B. Saunders Company, 1980:1633–1642.
15. Ross RS. Right ventricular hypertension as a cause of precordial pain. Am Heart J. 1961; 61:134–135.
16. Sleeper JC, Orgain ES, McIntosh HD. Primary pulmonary hypertension. Review of clinical features and pathologic physiology with a report of pulmonary hemodynamics derived from repeated catheterization. Circulation. 1962; 26:1358–1369.
17. Constant J. The second heart sound. In Constant J, ed. Bedside Cardiology, Ed 2. Boston: Little Brown and Company, 1976:175–208.
18. Perloff JR, Harvey WP. Mechanisms of splitting of the second heart sound. Circulation. 1958; 18:998–1009.
19. Goodman DJ, Harrison DC, Popp RL. Echocardiographic features of primary pulmonary hypertension. Am J Cardiol. 1974; 33:438–443.
20. Shettigar UR, Hultgren HN, Specter M, Martin R, Davis DH. Primary pulmonary hypertension: Favorable effect of isoproterenol. N Engl J Med. 1976; 295:1414–1415.
21. Rubin LJ, Peter RH. Oral hydralazine therapy for primary pulmonary hypertension. N Engl J Med. 1980; 302:69–73.
22. Wang SWS, Pohl JEF, Rowlands DJ, Wade EG. Diazoxide in treatment of primary pulmonary hypertension. Br Heart J. 1978; 40:572–574.
23. Ruskin JM, Hutter AM Jr. Primary pulmonary hypertension treated with oral phentolamine. Ann Intern Med. 1979; 90:772–774.
24. Elkayam U. Vasodilator therapy in primary pulmonary hypertension. Chest. 1981; 79:253–254.
25. Elkayam U, Frishman WH, Yoran C, Strorm J, Sonnenslick EH, Cohen MN. Unfavorable hemodynamic and clinical effects of isoproterenol in primary pulmonary hypertension. Cardiovasc Med. 1977; 3:1177–1180.
26. McCaffrey RM, Dunn LJ. Primary pulmonary hypertension in pregnancy. Obstet Gynecol Surv. 1964; 19:567–591.
27. Pomaskin VA, Rosenfeld LI, Osipova SM, Shilova GA. Primary pulmonary hypertension and pregnancy. Vapr Okhr Materin Det. 1968; 13:80–82.
28. Demas NW. Maternal death due to primary pulmonary hypertension. Trans Pac Coast Obstet Gynecol Soc. 1972; 40:64–67.
29. Salvin AG. Importance of hyperbaric oxygenation for a favorable outcome of labor in primary pulmonary hypertension patients. Vopr Okhr Materin Det. 1979; 24:64–66.
30. Giard P, Croccel L, Dutoit A. Idiopathic pulmonary hypertension with severe evolution following pregnancy. J Sci Med Lille. 1967; 85:439–448.
31. Jewett JF, Ober WB. Primary pulmonary hypertension as a cause of maternal death. J Obstet Gynecol. 1956; 71:1335–1341.
32. Fresh JW, Ferguson JH, Lewis JH. Blood clotting studies in parturient women and the newborn. Obstet Gynecol. 1956; 7:117–127.
33. Kleiger RE, Boxer M, Ingham RE, Harrison DC. Pulmonary hypertension in patients using oral contraceptives. A report of six cases. Chest. 1976; 69:143–147.
34. Rivier IL. Hypertension arterielle pulmonaire primitive. Schweiz Med Wochenschr. 1970; 100:143–145.
35. Irey N, Norris H. Intimal vascular lesions associated with female reproductive steroids. Arch Pathol. 1973; 96:227–234.
36. Oakley C, Sommerville J. Oral contraceptives and progressive pulmonary vascular disease. Lancet. 1968; 1:890–893.
37. Caldini P, Gensini GG, Hoffman MS. Primary pulmonary hypertension with death during right heart catheterization. A case report and a survey of reported fatalities. Am J Cardiol. 1959; 4:519–527.
38. Braunwald E, Swan HJC. Cooperative study on cardiac catheterization. Circulation 1968; 37(Suppl 3):1.
39. Rosenthal MH. Intrapartum intensive care management of the cardiac patient. Clin Obstet Gynecol. 1981; 24:789–807.
40. Hall JG, Paull RM, Wilson RM. Maternal and fetal sequelae of anticoagulation during pregnancy. Am J Med. 1980; 68:122–140.
41. Ueland K, Akamatsu TJ, Eng M, Bonica JJ, Hansen JM. Maternal cardiovascular dynamics VI. Cesarean section under epidural anesthesia without epinephrine. Am Obstet Gynecol. 1972; 114:775–780.
42. Midwall J, Jaffin H, Herman MV, Kupersmith J. Shunt flow and pulmonary hemodynamics during labor and delivery in the Eisenmenger's syndrome. Am J Cardiol. 1978; 42:299–303.

M. XIII

Aortic Dissection and Pregnancy

Jonathan M. Tobis, MD

I. INTRODUCTION

One of the more perplexing but, fortunately, rare complications of pregnancy is a dissecting aneurysm. This most often occurs in the aorta, but other arteries may be subject to aneurysm formation or dissection, including cerebral, splenic, ovarian, renal, coronary, or spinal arteries.[1–6] It is difficult to assess the incidence of aortic dissection during pregnancy since most reports consist of isolated case studies.

II. CLINICAL SETTING

The majority of women have no predisposing illness that would make them suspect for this catastrophe. The highest incidence of aortic dissection is from the third trimester to one month post partum.[7] Of note is the low frequency of dissection precipitated during active labor. The majority of case reports describe a woman who is resting comfortably when she is suddenly struck with excruciating pain. The pain typically begins in the chest and is aptly described as a "tearing," "crushing," or "burning," often with radiation to the upper back, into the shoulders, and through the abdomen. Dyspnea and cyanosis may be present and often are misinterpreted as evidence of acute pulmonary embolism. If branch arteries are compromised, then other symptoms may be more prominent, such as cerebral or spinal arteries with neurologic sequelae, or brachial artery with ischemic arm symptoms. If the ascending aorta is involved within a few centimeters of the aortic ring, aortic insufficiency may result from dilation of the annulus. The rapid volume overload raises the left ventricular pressure, which can precipitate acute pulmonary edema. Retrograde dissection through the base of the aorta can rupture through the adventitia into the pericardium with sudden cardiac tamponade. This was the immediate cause of death in 80% of patients in one series.[8] The aortic dissection may also rupture through the adventitia into the pluera or abdomen with associated clinical findings and rapid exsanguination.

Cardiac Problems in Pregnancy, pages 161–165

III. DIAGNOSIS

The most difficult aspect of making a diagnosis of aortic dissection during pregnancy is that one must first consider the possibility in the differential diagnosis. Other events that may produce similarly catastrophic signs and symptoms are acute pulmonary embolism, myocardial infarction, bacterial endocarditis, ruptured aortic or mitral valve, pneumothorax, rupture of the uterus, abruptio placenta, or mesenteric infarction.

Nonspecific laboratory findings may include anemia or fever, which may be an autoimmune phenomenon of dissection and may include pericarditis. The chest x-ray film is helpful in the differential diagnosis since a widened mediastinum is common in thoracic dissections. A radiograph of the abdomen, however, often is unrevealing in abdominal dissections.[9] An echocardiogram may demonstrate a widened aortic root and a false lumen. If aortic insufficiency is present, an echocardiogram will be helpful in demonstrating left ventricular dilatation; early closure of the mitral valve can be seen and is a poor prognostic sign, as it indicates recent, severe insufficiency. An abdominal ultrasound study is useful in outlining the size of the aorta and is a good screening test. Electrocardiograms show nonspecific findings. Computerized tomographic (CT) scans of the chest or abdomen may be diagnostic. However, the definitive study for diagnosis and for proper treatment is an aortic angiogram.

The clinical setting should determine which diagnostic procedure is to be obtained first. If the patient is stable and the diagnosis is unclear, then a noninvasive screening test such as a CT scan, abdominal sonogram, or echocardiogram would be appropriate. However, if the patient's condition is critical or the diagnosis of dissecting aneurysm is suspected, then one should proceed to the definitive angiographic procedure in expectation of surgical intervention. Medical centers that have the capacity to perform digital subtraction angiograms may be able to screen patients for aortic aneurysms with this new, less invasive intravenous approach.

IV. PATHOLOGY

Most pathologic studies reveal medial degeneration with weakened elastic structure and loss of the normal corrugated pattern of elastic tissue.[10] Hirst argues against using the term "cystic medial necrosis," since there is no proof that any cell death has occurred and there may not be any cysts.[11] Gore suggests that the medial degeneration represents a process of wear and repair with generation of new feeding vessels (vasa vasorum) that have deficient vascular support.[12] These vessels rupture and begin an intramural hemorrhage, which then ruptures from the media into the lumen. At this point the false lumen becomes subject to the pressure of the column of arterial blood that flows into it and extends the dissection. This will either clot off or rupture downstream back through the intima, creating two channels of flow.

An alternate theory is that the shearing force comes from within the aortic column of blood, tears into a weakened intima, and then dissects along the plane of the aortic media.

V. ETIOLOGY

The most fascinating aspect of this catastrophic event is the question of why it should occur in pregnancy. Schnitker and Bayer found that in women less than 40 years old with aortic dissection, 50% were pregnant.[8] Clearly, this inappropriate proportion indicates that pregnancy predisposes to aortic dissection. Some early reports noted the association of dissection with the third trimester and suggested that increased blood volume and cardiac output were causative events. This would seem unlikely since many other disease states of the cardiovascular system are associated with excessive volume loads without a predisposition to dissection. Aortic dissection in elderly people is often associated with, and thought to be partially caused by, systemic hypertension. However, only 25–50% of pregnant subjects who developed aortic dissection were hypertensive, and usually this was only of a moderate degree. The fact that aortic dissection is uncommon during labor, when systemic pressure is highest, mitigates against hypertension as the primary factor. A more significant but controversial etiologic factor is the hormonal influence of pregnancy. Manalo-Estrella and Barker studied 16 aortas from pregnant women (15 were in their third trimester) who died from nonvascular causes.[13] They described marked fragmentation of reticulum fibers, a decrease in mucopolysaccharides, disruption of elastic fiber corrugation, and hypertrophy with hyperplasia of smooth muscle cells. However, Cavanzo and Taylor, in their autopsy study of 43 pregnant women, found no difference in aortic histology compared with nonpregnant women.[14]

It is well known that estrogens and relaxin affect connective tissues. The depolymerization of connective tissue ground substance that occurs in the pubic symphysis may be a general phenomenon of connective tissue in pregnancy.[15] However, there is no evidence to suggest an increased incidence of aortic aneurysm in women taking birth control pills.

There are several animal models that indicate that the aorta is an endangered organ during altered nutritional and hormonal conditions. Rats that eat sweet peas (and thereby overdose on beta-aminoproprionitrite) inhibit collagen cross-linkage and develop aortic aneurysms.[16] Aortic aneurysms can also be produced in copper-deficient animals, which suggests that a nutritional etiology may be operational in some cases. Support for a hormonal influence comes from work with turkeys treated with diethylstilbestrol. These animals develop an increased incidence of aortic aneurysm and dissection. Danforth, Manalo-Estrella, and Buckingham treated nonpregnant rabbits with the contraceptive steroids norethynodrel and mestranol.[17] They found the blood vessels developed fragmented reticulum, loss of the corrugated pattern in the elastic tissue, smooth muscle hyperplasia, and a decrease in acid mucopolysaccharides. These histologic alterations were similar to those found in their work on aortas of pregnant women.

Malformations of the aorta predispose to dissection whether the patient is pregnant or not. Schnitker and Bayer found that of 49 women with aortic dissection, 32% had coarctation or hypoplasia of the aorta.[8]

Another controversial area concerns the risk of aortic dissection in people with Marfan's syndrome.[18] Although it is common for these people to suffer aortic dissection or ruptured chordae tendineae, it is unclear whether pregnancy adds any additional risk for these catastrophes. In the past, physicians have cautioned women with Marfan's syndrome against pregnancy since there are reports in the literature of 14 deaths from aortic rupture in 25 women with Marfan's syndrome.[19–21] However, a recent abstract from Johns Hopkins University described their experience in following 26 women with Marfan's syndrome during 106 pregnancies.[22] Only one woman died secondary to endocarditis with mitral regurgitation. They studied three women prospectively through pregnancy with echocardiograms and found no differences compared to pregnant women without Marfan's syndrome. They recommend counseling women against pregnancy if the aortic root is dilated more than 4 cm by echocardiogram; otherwise patients with Marfan's syndrome in their series did not have a significant increase in risk of aortic dissection during pregnancy.

VI. TREATMENT

There is very little information about treatment of acute aortic dissection in pregnancy.[23] Most of the early literature consists of autopsy series. Now that cardiovascular surgery has become more feasible, there is more experience with aortic dissections secondary to atherosclerosis or

Marfan's syndrome.[24] Konishi and coworkers from Japan operated on four women with aortic dissection during pregnancy and there was one operative death.[25] Wolfe and Moran recommend surgery for dissections in the ascending aorta, and medical management is suggested if the dissection occurs distal to the left subclavian artery.[26] Medical therapy consists of altering the shearing force of the column of ejected blood. This is accomplished by lowering the blood pressure with intravenous nitroprusside (0.5–8.0 μg/kg/min) and by reducing the velocity of blood flow with propranolol (1–5 mg intravenously over 20 minutes, followed by 40–80 mg orally every six hours). Surgical intervention is necessary if medical treatment does not control hypertension or if there is persistent pain, expansion of the aneurysm, or vascular compromise of an essential organ.[27] After initial medical control and stabilization, approximately 30% of patients will require surgical repair for an enlarging aneurysm. Therapeutic decisions must vary with the uniqueness of each patient's problem. One must consider the viability of the fetus and the emergent nature of the underlying vascular pathology. The unique considerations of surgical management of the pregnant patient are discussed in detail in Chapter M. XVII. If the diagnosis of aortic dissection in pregnancy is considered, aggressive diagnostic evaluation and therapy, including surgery, may be life-saving.

VII. REFERENCES

1. Robinson JL, Hall CS, Sedzimir CB. Arteriovenous malformations, aneurysms, and pregnancy. J Neurosurg. 1974; 41:63–70.
2. Pollak EW, Michas CA. Massive spontaneous hemoperitoneum due to rupture of visceral branches of the abdominal aorta. Am Surg. 1979; 45:621–630.
3. Burnett RA, Carfrae DC. Spontaneous rupture of ovarian artery aneurysm in the puerpuerium. Br J Obstet Gynecol. 1976; 83:744–750.
4. Cohen SG, Cashdan A, Burger R. Spontaneous rupture of a renal artery aneurysm during pregnancy. Obstet Gynecol. 1972; 39:897–902.
5. Jewett JF. Two dissecting coronary-artery aneurysms post partum. N Engl J Med. 1978; 298:1255–1256.
6. Garcia CA, Dulcey S, Dulcey J. Ruptured aneurysm of the spinal artery of Adamkiewicz during pregnancy. Neurology. 1979; 29:394–398.
7. Pedowitz P, Perell A. Aneurysms complicated by pregnancy. Am J Obstet Gynecol. 1957; 73:720–735.
8. Schnitker MA, Bayer CA. Dissecting aneurysm of the aorta in young individuals, particularly in association with pregnancy. Ann Intern Med. 1944; 20:486–511.
9. Earnest F, Muhm JR, Sheedy PF. Roentgenographic findings in thoracic aortic dissection. Mayo Clin Proc. 1979; 54:43–50.
10. Hirst AE, Johns VJ, Kime SW. Dissecting aneurysm of the aorta: A review of 505 cases. Medicine. 1958; 37:217–273.
11. Hirst AE, Gore I. Is cystic medionecrosis the cause of dissecting aortic aneurysm? Circulation. 1976; 53:915–916.
12. Gore I. Dissecting aneurysms of the aorta in persons under forty years of age. AMA Arch Pathol. 1953; 55:1–13.
13. Manalo-Estrella P, Barker AE. Histopathologic findings in human aortic media associated with pregnancy. Arch Pathol. 1967; 83:336–341.
14. Cavanzo FJ, Taylor HB. Effect of pregnancy on the human aorta and its relationship to dissecting aneurysms. Am J Obstet Gynecol. 1969; 567–568.
15. Perl E, Catchpole HR. Changes induced in the connective tissue of the pubic symphysis of the guinea pig with estrogen and relaxin. Arch Pathol. 1950; 50:233–239.
16. Bonventre MV. Sweet peas, copper, pregnancy, and pills. NY State J Med. 1974; 74:633–637.
17. Danforth DN, Manalo-Estrella P, Buckingham JC: The effect of pregnancy and of Enovid on the rabbit vasculature. Am J Obstet and Gynecol. 1964; 88:952.
18. Husebye KO, Wolff HJ, Friedman LL. Aortic dissection in pregnancy: A case of Marfan's syndrome. Am Heart J. 1958; 55:662–676.
19. Sutinen S, Piiroinen O. Marfan syndrome, pregnancy, and fatal dissection of aorta. Acta Obstet Gynecol Scand. 1971; 50:295–300.
20. Elias S, Berkowitz RL. Marfan syndrome and pregnancy. Obstet Gynecol. 1976; 47:358–361.
21. Donaldson LB, DeAlvarez RR. Marfan syndrome and pregnancy. Am J Obstet Gynecol. 1965; 92:629–640.
22. Pyeritz RE. Risk of aortic complications in the Marfan syndrome during pregnancy. Circulation. 1980; 62:III304.
23. Hume M, Krosnick G. Dissecting aneurysm in pregnancy associated with aortic insufficiency. N Engl J Med. 1961; 268:174–178.
24. Vecht RJ, Bromley LL, Besterman EMM, Eastcott HHG, Kenyon JR. Acute dissection of the aorta: Long-term review and management. Lancet. 1980; 1:109–111.

25. Konishi Y, Tatsuta N, Kumada K, Minami K, Matsuda K, Yamasato A, Usui N, Muraguchi T, Hikasa Y, Okamoto E, Watanabe R. Dissecting aneurysm during pregnancy and the puerperium. Jpn Circ J. 1980; 44:726.
26. Wolfe WG, Moran JF. The evolution of medical and surgical management of acute aortic dissection. Circulation. 1977; 56:503–505.
27. Crawford ES, Palamara AE, Saleh SA, Roehm JOF. Aortic aneurysm: Current status of surgical treatment. Surg Clin North Am. 1979; 59:597–636.

M. XIV

Rhythm Disorders and Pregnancy

Jose Meller, MD, and Martin E. Goldman, MD

I. INTRODUCTION

The approach to arrhythmias occurring during pregnancy is in general similar to that to nonpregnant patients with arrhythmias. When confronting any individual with arrhythmias it is important to determine if there is underlying organic heart disease, if there are any predisposing factors, and most important, if there is risk of death or major morbidity as a consequence of the arrhythmia. If the patient has a life-threatening arrhythmia it is mandatory to treat it even before the diagnostic investigation of its cause is complete and regardless of its electrophysiologic mechanism. A patient with ventricular fibrillation needs emergency defibrillation; a patient with complete heart block and syncope requires medications to increase ventricular rate and/or pacemaker insertion. Once the risk of death has been eliminated, a complete diagnostic work-up can be performed.

Cardiac Problems in Pregnancy, pages 167–178

ease, however, because the rapid heart rate does not allow adequate time for ventricular filling, atrial fibrillation may precipitate heart failure, angina pectoris, dizziness, or syncope. Occasionally, fatigue may be the first manifestation of lower cardiac output. If there is imminent risk of death from hemodynamic decompensation, electric countershock should be performed immediately. In less urgent cases, the ventricular rate can be decreased by increasing AV block with digitalis, beta-adrenergic blockers, or Verapamil, depending on the underlying heart disease. Then, a decision would have to be made regarding the desirability of restoring sinus rhythm, usually by electric countershock. That decision depends on 1) the length of time the patient has been in atrial fibrillation (longer than six months means that it is less likely that sinus rhythm will be maintained after cardioversion); 2) the character of the tachycardia (if it is paroxysmal atrial fibrillation, only drugs should be used); 3) the degree of left atrial enlargement (if it is greater than 4.5 cm by echocardiography, there is less success in keeping sinus rhythm); 4) the presence of associated disease (if there is underlying sick sinus syndrome, then there is risk of severe bradycardia or asystole after cardioversion); and 5) the patient's ability to tolerate antiarrhythmic agents to prevent recurrence of this arrhythmia. Cardioversion, when indicated, should be accomplished with delivery of the energy synchronized with the QRS complexes. When sick sinus syndrome is the underlying condition, a permanent pacemaker may be required to prevent bradycardia, which can be aggravated by drugs used to prevent the tachycardias.

The most difficult decision in pregnant women with atrial fibrillation, paroxysmal or not, relates to the use of anticoagulants. In patients with mitral valve disease, the risk of systemic emboli is high. If the patient was anticoagulated before pregnancy, then the anticoagulation should be continued throughout pregnancy. If the patient was not anticoagulated before pregnancy, a two-dimensional echocardiogram should be performed to determine if thrombi are present in the left atrium. If thrombi are seen, anticoagulation should be given. If thrombi are not seen, the issue remains controversial. In patients with atrial fibrillation, no organic heart disease, and a normal-sized left atrium, anticoagulation usually is not indicated.

IV. VENTRICULAR ARRHYTHMIAS

A. Ventricular Premature Beats

As with atrial premature beats, there seems to be an increased frequency of ventricular premature beats during pregnancy, or again, perhaps the patient is more aware of them during this time. This is a frequently encountered arrhythmia in cardiac patients and in normal individuals. It may be symptomatic, usually as palpitations, or asymptomatic. In the absence of symptoms, pregnant women without organic heart disease do not require therapy. When pregnant women complain of palpitations due to ventricular premature beats, reassurance is often all the therapy that is necessary. If the palpitations produce undue anxiety, then antiarrhythmic therapy may be necessary to eliminate or reduce the symptoms, but it should be understood that the drugs required may be more dangerous than the arrhythmia being treated.

When an apparently healthy woman has frequent premature beats (over 10/min), there is an increased possibility of underlying organic heart disease. In such cases, an echocardiogram may be necessary to diagnose mitral valve prolapse or hypertrophic cardiomyopathy; more rarely an exercise test may be required to detect silent myocardial ischemia due to coronary artery disease.

As in the case of many arrhythmias, ventricular premature beats seem to increase in frequency with the use of stimulants like alcohol or caffeine, and with fatigue and anxiety. Removal of these probable causes or factors should be attempted in every patient with symptomatic ventricular premature beats.

B. Ventricular Tachycardia

Ventricular tachycardia is one of the most serious cardiac arrhythmias because it often is responsible for symptoms of low cardiac output and heart failure, and also it may degenerate into ventricular fibrillation, causing death. It is diagnosed when three or more beats of ventricular origin appear serially in the electrocardiogram. It is more common in patients with frequent ventricular premature beats, especially when they are multiform, or forming couplets. The serious symptoms appear when the tachycardia is sustained, especially at heart rates above 150 beats/min. The differentiation of ventricular tachycardia from supraventricular tachycardia with aberrant QRS complexes is difficult. If the electrocardiogram demonstrates ventricular capture beats or ventricular fusion beats during the tachycardia, the diagnosis of ventricular tachycardia is strongly suggested. However, in some cases His bundle studies are necessary to clarify the diagnosis. If the tachycardia, ventricular or supraventricular, is causing hemodynamic derangement, no time should be lost in trying to make a definite diagnosis, and rapid conversion to sinus rhythm, usually with direct countershock, should be performed.

Ventricular tachycardia is rarely seen during pregnancy. However, even in the absence of organic heart disease, it may cause death during pregnancy or it may recur during consecutive pregnancies.[11] In other cases, the arrhythmia may tend to become less frequent during the last trimester of pregnancy.[12] Ventricular tachycardia is usually associated with organic heart disease and, in the United States, especially with coronary artery disease. However, it may complicate the course of any disease with left ventricular dysfunction, like cardiomyopathy and valvular heart disease. Intoxication with digitalis or antiarrhythmics may also produce this tachycardia. It is assumed to be a cause of sudden death in patients with hypertrophic cardiomyopathy, mitral valve prolapse, and, especially, in the syndrome associated with prolonged Q-T interval.[13]

In patients with ventricular tachycardia hemodynamically well tolerated, antiarrhythmics like intravenous lidocaine can be tried before electric countershock. The latter is especially dangerous in patients with ventricular tachycardia secondary to digitalis intoxication. In these cases, correction of hypokalemia if present, lidocaine, and/or dilantin should be tried if time allows. In emergency situations, intravenous lidocaine followed by electric countershock using low energy is necessary. Bretylium has been used for recurrent ventricular tachycardia and fibrillation.

The energy for conversion of ventricular tachycardia to sinus rhythm is frequently low, and because of this a precordial thump is often effective. If electric counter-shock is being used and if there is no immediate risk of death, 1–10 watt-seconds should be the initial energy used; if there is risk of death, high energy should be used immediately. If the ventricular tachycardia is very rapid, without clear separation of QRS complexes and T waves, synchronized mode of the cardioverter could lead to impulse discharge on the T wave and provoke ventricular fibrillation. In such cases, the chances of firing into the vulnerable period are decreased by using a nonsynchronized mode for cardioversion.

To prevent the recurrence of ventricular tachycardia, the precipitating causes have to be eliminated if possible; then, antiarrhythmic therapy has to be used. Procainamide hydrochloride, quinidine, disopyramide, bretylium, and dilantin are all more or less effective medications. Occasionally, combination of drugs is necessary; in other cases experimental drugs such as amiodorone or mexiletine or combinations with digitalis or beta-blockers are required. In rare cases, electrical mapping with surgical excision of the excitable ventricular area, usually associated with a ventricular aneurysm, is successful in preventing the recurrence of refractory ventricular tachycardias. In patients with the prolonged QT syndrome drugs that provoke further increase of the repolarization time (especially quinidine) are dangerous, usually precipitating ventricular tachycardia. Beta-blockers or permanent ventricular pacing is the preferred therapy in such cases.

C. Ventricular Fibrillation

This is a lethal arrhythmia that usually requires electric countershock. Ventricular fibrillation is the most common cause of death in both the general population and in pregnant women.

V. CONDUCTION DISTURBANCES

A. Bundle Branch Block

Bundle branch blocks are relatively uncommon during pregnancy, having a much higher incidence in older populations. Their presence in the absence of organic heart disease has no clinical importance and requires no special therapy in a pregnant woman. Right bundle branch block is more frequently encountered than left bundle branch block in young people. Occasionally fascicular hemiblocks, especially left anterior hemiblock, are found alone or in combination with a right bundle branch block. When a patient has a history of dizzy spells or syncope, ambulatory electrocardiographic recordings and/or electrophysiologic studies may be required to determine if transient complete heart block is the cause of those symptoms. Bundle branch blocks can be seen in most forms of organic heart disease, especially cardiomyopathies, coronary artery disease, and valvular heart disease. The presence of bundle branch block does not generally affect the way the underlying disease is managed. If transient heart block is suspected or heart block develops, a permanent pacemaker is required.

B. Wolff-Parkinson-White Syndrome

It has been postulated that during pregnancy women with Wolff-Parkinson-White syndrome are predisposed to develop arrhythmias.[14] Because the fetus with Wolff-Parkinson-White syndrome also seems predisposed to the development of cardiac arrhythmias in utero, it has been suggested that the hormonal changes of pregnancy play a role in the development of such arrhythmias.[15]

The electrocardiogram shows a short PR interval and wide QRS complexes with initial slowing (delta wave). The abnormality is due to abnormal muscular bridges with rapid electrical conduction between the atrium and ventricle (bundles of Kent). This avoids the conduction delay at the AV node and is the cause of the short PR interval; also, by having the ventricle depolarized through two pathways, a fusion beat (wide QRS complex) with initial slowing is produced. Some patients have specialized conduction pathways (bypass tracks) in areas of the AV node or between the bundle of His and interventricular septum. The electrocardiographic representation of these variant forms will be a short PR interval with normal QRS complexes (Lown-Ganong-Levine syndrome), or normal PR interval with delta waves in the QRS complexes (Mahaim fibers), respectively.

The finding of an electrocardiographic pattern of Wolff-Parkinson-White syndrome in an asymptomatic pregnant woman without a history of arrhythmias requires no special therapy,[16] except for careful follow-up, because of the higher incidence of arrhythmias during pregnancy. The tachycardias associated with preexcitation of the left ventricle can reach rates of 200–300 beats/min, and they may cause, by themselves, serious hemodynamic derangement, even in patients without organic heart disease. When organic heart disease is associated with this syndrome, the hemodynamic consequences of the rapid tachycardias are even worse.

The therapy of paroxysms of supraventricular tachycardia associated with Wolff-Parkinson-White syndrome is, in general, similar to that of patients without this syndrome. However, digitalis is less effective because it would block conduction of the AV pathway, and rapid conduction over the variant pathway would not be affected. Propranolol and/or procainamide hydrochloride are better choices.

In patients with Wolff-Parkinson-White syndrome and recurrent paroxysmal supraventricular tachycardia refractory to all drugs, surgical interruption of the bypass track has been performed, which will prevent the recurrent tachycardias in most patients.

When a pregnant woman has a very rapid tachycardia due to preexcitation, electric countershock is usually the most rapid and effective way of dealing with the arrhythmia.

C. Heart Block

1. First-degree AV block

First-degree AV block is usually the result of increased time of conduction through the AV junction and is evidenced by a prolonged PR interval on the electrocardiogram. It may be permanent, caused by disease of the AV node, or it may be transitory, the result of increased vagal tone or the effects of drugs like digitalis, beta-adrenergic blockers, or verapamil. This conduction delay does not require therapy, but if it is an effect of drugs, their withdrawal or reduction in dose is suggested in cases of marked PR interval prolongation.

In patients with dilated left atria, a prolonged PR interval will usually precede paroxysmal supraventricular arrhythmias.

2. Second-degree AV block

Second-degree AV block of the Wenckebach type (Mobitz I), will cause progressively longer PR intervals, followed by a dropped ventricular beat. The conduction delay occurs at the level of the AV node junction in these cases. It may be due to an increase in vagal tone or to digitalis excess; it also occurs in patients with acute inferior wall myocardial infarction, myocarditis, after cardiac surgery, and occasionally in normal individuals. When it is a result of digitalis toxicity, the drug has to be withheld; otherwise, this conduction delay does not require therapy. If it is responsible for significant bradycardia, intravenous atropine can be useful. Rarely, a pacemaker is necessary in these cases.

Second-degree AV block of the Mobitz II type is an infrequent and serious arrhythmia. The delay is at a level below the AV junction; it may be progressive and precede complete heart block; the escape ventricular rate is slow and usually causes serious symptoms. Because this arrhythmia can be mimicked in the surface electrocardiogram by junctional premature beats followed by a suddenly dropped ventricular beat, an electrophysiologic study may be required to clarify the diagnosis. These two anomalies require different therapeutic approaches. When the diagnosis of Mobitz II AV block is confirmed, a permanent pacemaker is indicated.

In general, in cases of second-degree AV block with narrow QRS complexes, the block is at the level of the AV junction; with new wide QRS complexes, the block is likely to be below the AV junction.

3. Third-degree AV block

Third-degree AV block at the level of the AV junction will usually have narrow QRS complexes, and, by definition, the atria and the ventricles are totally dissociated. In such cases, the ventricular rate is between 40 and 55 beats/min; thus, this does not often cause hemodynamic abnormalities. Congenital heart block, acute inferior wall myocardial infarction, acute rheumatic fever, and digitalis intoxication are some of the etiologies of this type of heart block. Pacemaker therapy may or may not be required, according to the ecape rate of the ventricle and the presence of symptomatology.

Approximately half of the 21 cases of congenital heart block occurring during pregnancy collected by Mendelson[7] had associated ventricular septal defects. The only death among those cases occurred in a patient who also had toxemia superimposed upon hypertensive disease. Only one of those patients showed an increased tendency to syncopal attacks during pregnancy. Rarely, syncope as the first manifestation of congenital complete heart block will appear during pregnancy.

Third-degree AV block at a level below the AV junction is an extremely grave conduction delay that may cause low cardiac output, or even death, if untreated. This defect is serious because the ventricular escape rate is usually lower than in complete heart block above the AV junction, mostly in the 15–40 beats/min range. The QRS complexes are wide, and during His bundle recording, they are not preceded by His spikes. In the United States coronary artery disease is the most common etiology of this type of AV block. Occasionally, there is disease that involves only the conduction system, without evidence of coronary artery or myocardial disease. In the obstetric age group, rheumatic heart disease accounts for approximately one-half the cases of acquired heart block. Whatever the etiology, ventricular pacemaker is the immediate therapy for this serious arrhythmia. Pacemaker therapy during pregnancy was first reported in 1964[17] and since then, other cases without maternal or fetal mortality have been reported.[18–20]

VI. CARDIOVERSION

The safety of cardioversion in pregnancy has been documented in over a dozen reported cases.[21,22] Only rarely have transient fetal arrhythmia been noted, and those resolved completely after delivery of normal infants.

In an elective cardioversion, as in any other individual, the pregnant woman should be kept fasting for at least six hours. Digitalis (if being used), should be stopped for at least 24 hours, and there should be no electrolyte abnormalities before cardioversion. All the predisposing factors of the arrhythmia should have been corrected—ie, hypoxemia, heart failure, infections, hyperthyroidism. Adequate sedation should be used and an anesthetist should be present during the procedure. A decision regarding the use of anticoagulation before cardioversion (depending on the type of arrhythmia) and on the use of antiarrhythmics before and after cardioversion should be made.

The cardioversion itself, should be performed using a synchronized mode, except in cases of very rapid ventricular tachycardia (ventricular flutter). Low energy levels should be used for ventricular tachycardia (1–10 watt-seconds). With high energy levels there is a greater risk of myocardial damage and postconversion arrhythmias.

After cardioversion, electrocardiographic monitoring of the patient should be continued for at least three to four hours, because of the high incidence of arrhythmias postconversion.

VII. ARRHYTHMIAS AND SUBSEQUENT PREGNANCY

In a society that is medically better educated, it is now common to see women with arrhythmias who request "clearance" for pregnancy. In most cases, this is an easy decision, because no underlying heart disease is present, there is no use of antiarrhythmic therapy, and the arrhythmias are minimally symptomatic. Pregnancy will predispose the woman to a higher frequency of, or to be more aware of, atrial or ventricular premature beats. If she has a history of paroxysmal atrial tachycardias or the Wolff-Parkinson-White syndrome, it is likely that she will have recurrent tachycardias during pregnancy. In the absence of organic heart disease, these arrhythmias are usually easily controllable. On rare occasions, cardioversion will be necessary; more often antiarrhythmic agents may be required to prevent recurrence. In women with paroxysmal ventricular tachycardia there is a definite incidence of sudden death, which seems to be independent of pregnancy.

When organic heart disease is present, any significant tachycardia will easily bring symptoms of heart failure, chest pain, or low cardiac output. In these cases, it is important to be aggressive with medications to prevent the recurrence of the arrhythmias. In some cases, especially in mitral valve disease with paroxysmal atrial fibrillation, anticoagulation therapy may be necessary. When anticoagulation therapy is being used, the mother has to be aware of the teratogenic risk to the fetus. Coumadin, for example, crosses the placenta. The use of heparin throughout pregnancy has not decreased fetal morbidity or mortality, and it has been associated with increased maternal mortality.[23]

When a permanent pacemaker has been inserted for treatment of sick sinus syndrome or complete heart block, there is no higher morbidity during pregnancy unless other problems are also present.

VIII. CONCLUSIONS

A woman with arrhythmias during pregnancy has to be treated, in general, similarly to when she is not pregnant. However, because of the cardiovascular changes during pregnancy, similar arrhythmias are more likely to produce symptoms during pregnancy than in a nonpregnant state. With benign, well-tolerated arrhythmias, the emphasis has to be on reassurance, avoiding the use of medications. If serious arrhythmias complicate pregnancy, they have to be treated in the same way as they would be in a nonpregnant woman. Cardioversion should be used whenever there is a life-threatening arrhythmia. Medications to prevent a serious arrhythmia should be used as they would be used in a nonpregnant patient.

Therefore, the pregnant woman may be more aware of arrhythmias, and arrhythmias may precipitate symptoms more easily during pregnancy; however, the management of the arrhythmias is similar to that in nonpregnant patients. Refractory arrhythmias during pregnancy may occasionally be seen, and these probably are related to the pregnancy because they become easily manageable after the pregnancy is over. Finally, any woman with organic heart disease is exposed to serious and potentially life-threatening arrhythmias during childbirth. Therefore close follow-up and electrocardiographic monitoring of these patients is necessary.[24]

IX. REFERENCES

1. Mendelson CL, Pardee HEB. The pulse and respiratory rate during labor as a guide to the onset of cardiac failure in women with rheumatic heart disease. Am J Obstet Gynecol. 1942; 44:370–383.
2. Pardee HEB, Mendelson CL. The pulse and respiratory variations in normal women during labor. Am J Obstet Gynecol. 1941; 41:36–44.
3. Ferrer MI. Sick sinus syndrome. Circulation. 1973; 27:635–643.
4. Narula OS, Samet P, Javier RP. Significance of the sinus node recovery time. Circulation. 1972; 45:140–146.
5. Jensen J. The Heart in Pregnancy. St. Louis: The C.V. Mosby Company, 1938.
6. Szekely P, Smith L. Paroxysmal tachycardia in pregnancy. Br Heart J. 1953; 15:195–198.
7. Mendelson CL. Disorders of the heartbeat during pregnancy. Am J Obstet Gynecol. 1956; 72:1268–1301.
8. Braunwald E. Heart Disease. Philadelphia: W.B. Saunders, 1980:1885.

9. Robards GJ, Saunders DDM. Refractory supraventricular tachycardia complicating pregnancy. Med J Aust. 1973; 2:278–280.
10. Sussman HF, Duque D, Lesser ME. Atrial flutter with I:I AV conduction. Dis Chest. 1966; 49:99–103.
11. Russell RO. Paroxysmal ventricular tachycardia associated with pregnancy. Alabama J Med Sci. 1969; 6:111–120.
12. Peters M, Penner SL. Orthostatic paroxysmal ventricular tachycardia. Am Heart J. 1946; 32:645–652.
13. Roy PR, Emanuel R, Ismail SA, El Tayib MH: Hereditary prolongation of the QT interval. Am J Cardiol. 1976; 37:237–241.
14. Gleicher N, Meller J, Sandler RZ, Sullum S. Wolff-Parkinson-White syndrome in pregnancy. Am J Obstet Gynecol. 1981; 58:748–752.
15. Kerenyi TD, Gleicher N, Meller J, Brown E, Steinfeld L, Chitkara V, Rancher H. Transplacental cardioversion of intrauterine supraventricular tachycardia with digitalis. Lancet. 1980; 2:393–395.
16. Lichstein E, Goyal S, Chadda K, Gupta PK. Alternating Wolff-Parkinson-White (preexcitation) pattern. J Electrocardiogr. 1978; 11:81–84.
17. Shouse EE, Acker JE. Pregnancy and delivery in a patient with external-internal cardiac pacemaker. Am J Obstet Gynecol. 1964; 24:817–818.
18. Schonbrun M, Rowland W, Quiroz AC. Complete heart block in pregnancy. Am J Obstet Gynecol. 1966; 27:243–246.
19. Ginns HM, Holliurake K. Complete heart block in pregnancy treated with an internal pacemaker. Br J Obstet Gynecol. 1970; 77:710–712.
20. Schatz JW, Fischer JA, Lee RF, Lampe RM. Pacemaker therapy in pregnancy for the management of sinus bradycardia–junctional tachycardia syndrome. Chest. 1974; 65:461.
21. Schroeder JS, Harrison DC. Repeated cardioversion during pregnancy. Am J Cardiol. 1971; 27:445–446.
22. Finlay AY, Edmunds V. DC cardioversion in pregnancy. Br J Clin Pract. 1979; 33:88–94.
23. Hall JG, Pauli RM, Wilson KM. Maternal and fetal sequelae of anticoagulation during pregnancy. Am J Med. 1980; 68:122–140.
24. Spritzer RC, Seldon M, Mattes LM, Donoso E, Friedberg CK. Serious arrhythmias during labor and delivery in women with heart disease. JAMA 1970; 211:1005–1007.

M. XV

Hypertensive Pregnancy

Thomas J. Benedetti, MD

I. INTRODUCTION

Recent observations concerning the pathophysiology of hypertensive pregnancy have stimulated vigorous debate.[1–3] The intent of this chapter is to analyze the known hemodynamic data from hypertensive pregnancy. Summary and synthesis of recently published data has been accomplished wherever possible, and the clinical application of these new observations is suggested when appropriate.

Hypertensive diseases in pregnancy have been classified by the committee on Maternal Health. More recently the term "pregnancy-induced hypertension" (PIH) has been popularized.[4,5] This term, which includes preeclampsia/eclampsia and transient hypertension has helped to simplify the approach to clinical management of these disorders.

In the ideal situation, only nulliparous patients should be included in the study of pregnancy-induced hypertension. Unfortunately, much of the available data on cardiovascular function does not differentiate between multiparous and nulliparous patients. As a consequence, there is no alternative but to generalize from data that are known to include some patients whose hypertensive pathophysiology may be different from that associated with PIH.

Pregnancy-induced hypertension may present a wide spectrum of disease severity. Assessment of cardiovascular function is made more difficult by the fact that patients with severe hypertension may show different hemodynamic status than patients with mild hypertension. Despite these reservations, new information regarding the cardiovascular pathophysiology has increased our understanding of this disease and has provided new insights, even as it has raised many unanswered questions.

Cardiac Problems in Pregnancy, pages 179–190

II. MEASUREMENT OF ARTERIAL BLOOD PRESSURE

Demonstration by Gant et al that there is altered vascular sensitivity to the infused effects of angiotensin early in the pregnancies of patients destined to develop PIH was a major finding.[4] With the hope of finding a clinical tool for predicting the development of PIH, these investigators described their findings with the supine pressor or rollover test.[5] A 20 mm rise in diastolic blood pressure noted with position change from the lateral recumbent to the supine position was advocated as a test with a high sensitivity and specificity in prediction of PIH. Subsequently, other investigators appeared to confirm these initial observations.[6–9]

The usefulness of this test has been questioned recently because of the failure to consider some basic mechanisms of blood pressure measurement and interpretation.[10-14] The initial description of the supine pressor test often did not make reference to whether the superior or inferior arm was used to record a blood pressure. In a 60 kg pregnant woman, a 10–12 mm Hg difference in blood pressure is measureable between the inferior and superior arm in the lateral recumbent position. Thus at least a 10 mm increase in the blood pressure position change can be secondary to hydrostatic forces alone.[10] In addition, duplication errors in blood pressure readings have been shown to be on the order of 5 mm Hg.[13] Two recent carefully conducted studies failed to document significant changes in systolic or diastolic blood pressure in hypertensive or potentially hypertensive patients when corrections were made for the effects of hydrostatic blood pressue.[13,14] One study, however, did show a small decrease in pulse pressure (5 mm Hg), which reached statistical significance ($P = .05$) in patients with PIH.[13]

These studies make one point very clearly: the measurement of blood pressure and the interpretation of the results need to be standardized in hypertensive pregnant patients. The measurement of blood pressure in the upper arm in the lateral recumbent position will give falsely low blood pressure readings and may falsely reassure the clinician that the mean arterial pressure is lower than it really is. Blood pressure is best recorded in the supine position or in the inferior arm in the lateral recumbent position. Even more important is the measurement of the blood pressure in the same position with each observation. Attention to these two factors should help ensure optimal patient care, as well as allow for comparison results from investigators in different institutions. At present, it is my opinion that we still do not have a simple clinical test that will allow the reliable prediction of patients who are destined to develop PIH. This is especially true for those patients destined to develop early-onset PIH. These patients have the highest perinatal mortality secondary to the forced delivery of a premature infant because of altered maternal cardiovascular dynamics.

III. BLOOD VOLUME

The total blood volume is reduced in PIH.[15] This reduction appears to be proportional to the severity of the hypertensive disorder.[15] The observation that the plasma volume is reduced has stimulated a major controversy in the obstetric literature. This controversy revolves around the possible treatment implications of this observation. The major debate centers on whether volume infusion has a beneficial or potentially adverse effect in PIH. Some observers maintain that slightly reduced blood volume has no hemodynamic significance.[1] They feel that reduced volume is "merely fitting a contracted vascular bed. Volume infusion in this instance will result in vascular overload with resultant cardiac failure and pulmonary edema."

A number of recent studies have questioned this traditional concept. A reduction in mean arterial pressure associated with volume infusion in PIH has been shown (Fig. M.XV.1).[16] Another study

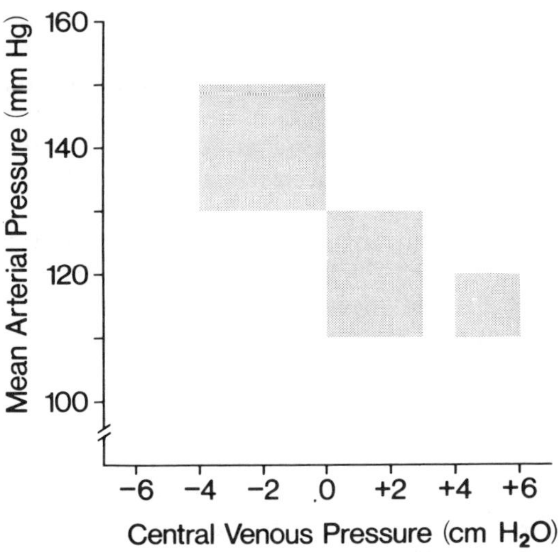

Fig. M.XV.1. Central venous pressure as a function of mean arterial pressure during volume infusion with colloid and crystalloid in a patient with severe preeclampsia/eclampsia. Within each of three groups, as CVP increases mean arterial pressure falls. (Adapted from Joyce, Anesthesiology. S51:297, 1979.)

showed that volume infusion with colloidal fluids was associated with a movement of fluid from the extravascular extracellular space to the intravascular space. Associated with this finding was a reduction in measured mean arterial pressure.[17] These acute volume loads resulted in a pressure reduction for short periods (two to three days).

Expansion of the plasma volume is an important factor for fetal growth.[18] Intravenous volume infusion could not be expected to have an influence on fetal growth unless given repeatedly over a number of weeks. There would appear to be logistic and cost factors that would weigh against this approach. Recently, nonselective beta-blockade with oxyprenolol has been shown to be associated with an increased plasma volume.[19,20] Treatment with alpha-methyldopa was not associated with a similar expansion in plasma volume. However, many of the patients in this study were multiparous and probably had chronic hypertension, not PIH.

From these studies it would appear that pharmacologic control of blood pressure with beta-blockade can allow plasma volume expansion and result in improved fetal growth. Previous reports have alluded to impaired fetal growth with beta-receptor blockade with propranalol.[21,22] Oxyprenolol apparently does not have the adverse effects on fetal growth allegedly associated with propranolol. One would expect therapy with selective beta-1 blockade with a drug such as metoprolol to be even less hazardous to fetal growth. Reports in the literature, as well as our own experience with metoprolol in this instance, point to the safety of administration during pregnancy.[23]

A major unanswered question in this regard involves attempted long-term conservative treatment. Once the syndrome is well established and significant end organ damage has been done, it is difficult to control or reverse PIH with antihypertensive medication. However, a study involving therapy early in gestation associated with fetal immaturity needs to be done to assess whether this form of therapy has any advantage over the traditional treatment, bed rest.

One must ask whether these new observations are consistent with what is known regarding cardiovascular physiology and the control of arterial blood pressure during pregnancy. Arterial pressure is regulated by factors that alter cardiac output and/or peripheral resistance. The renin–angiotensin system, the autonomic nervous system, and the kidneys all play essential roles in blood pressure regulation. These concepts have been adequately discussed elsewhere.[4]

The arteries, arterioles, and capillaries exert a major influence on the total peripheral resistance. They are a low-compliance system. The veins are a high-compliance system and contain 60–70% of the total blood volume at low pressures. Vasomotor tone in the two systems can vary independently, and there can be vasoconstriction in the resistance vessel without affecting the capacitance vessels.[24] It is possible for the venous system to be underfilled at the time the arterial system is vasoconstricted. The traditional concept that the blood volume reduction in PIH reflects a reduced vascular capacity may not be correct.

By what mechanism does the plasma volume become reduced and the extravascular extracellular space become increased? One possibility involves the transport of proteins from the intravascular space to the interstitial space. This would result in an osmotic force drawing fluid to the interstitial space. However, recent evidence using ^{131}I-labeled albumin could demonstrate no increased albumin mass in the extravascular space in PIH when compared to normotensive pregnant women.[25]

Another mechanism might involve altered venous compliance. In nonpregnant hypertensives, a change in the venous compliance was strongly correlated with disturbed partition of extracellular fluid volume.[26] A reduction in venous compliance could account for an increase in interstitial fluid and a reduction in the plasma volume. However, this hypothesis still leaves unexplained the repeated observation of low central venous pressures in established PIH.

From the preceding discussion, it is apparent that no static theory can encompass all the hemodynamic observations made in patients with PIH. This should not surprise us, since it is now thought that PIH develops over a period of weeks or months. Hypertension and proteinuria are a relatively late occurrence. Gant et al has shown an altered response to the pressor effect of angiotensin II infusion long before the mean arterial pressure becomes elevated.[4] In addition, Worley has shown that concomitant with the altered pressure response, there is an increase in the dehydroepiandrosterone sulfate (DHEA-S) clearance.[27] This observation implies an increased placental flow at an early stage in the disease. Increased placental flow could be the result of increased cardiac output, or it could be secondary to some alteration of autoregu-

TABLE M.XV.1. Cardiac Output in Hypertensive Pregnancy

Author (year)	Number of patients /type	Primiparous/ multiparous	Gestation (weeks)	Position
Assali[33] (1980)	10/severe	—	33–40	Left lateral
Benedetti[29] (1980)	10/severe	8/2	29–42	Supine & with hip wedge
Graham[31] (1980)	10/severe	8/2	—	Supine
Goodlin[3] (1979)	2/severe	—	—	Lateral
Hamilton[32] (1950)	17/(15 severe, 2 mild)	14/3	31–40	Supine
Lim[35] (1979)	25/mild	11/14	6–41	Left lateral
Littler[36] (1973)	15/mild	—	18–37	Left lateral
Rafferty[30] (1980)	3/severe	2/1	—	Supine & with hip wedge
Smith[37] (1970)	16/severe	16/0	—	Supine

*Standard deviation.

lation of flow to the uterus and placenta. Increased cardiac output could be secondary to a decrease in venous compliance and would help explain the increase in extravascular water. These postulations remain purely hypothetical in patients with PIH but have been shown to occur in experimentally induced nonpregnant hypertension.[28]

In nonpregnant patients, the hemodynamic alterations associated with hypertension encompass a spectrum. The picture depends on when in the course of the disease the study is performed. It may be that the same will eventually be found to be true in PIH.

IV. CARDIAC OUTPUT

Debate over the conflicting observations is especially frequent where the determination of cardiac output in PIH is concerned. Table M.XV.1 illustrates a summary of studies of cardiac output in PIH. There are many factors that may influence cardiac output. Older methods of indirect measurement without simultaneous confirmation by direct methods are probably of questionable value inasmuch as there have never been confirmatory studies in pregnant patients with the older noninvasive methods. Standard methods, such as thermodilution or Fick oxygen consumption studies or echocardiography are more reliable.

Another problem with interpretation of data regarding cardiac output involves the indexing of values. It is common practice to index the various hemodynamic variables to body surface area, despite the fact that body surface area standards for pregnant patients do not exist. Nevertheless, it is important to have a way to compare data in subjects with vastly different body size, and at present indexing to body surface area is probably the most widely used.

If one disregards the technical considerations of measurement, considerable

Medications	Method of determination	Cardiac output	
		Hypertensive	Controls
—	Cardiogreen dye dilution	110 ml/kg/min	109 ml/kg/min
$MgSO_4$	Thermodilution	5.7–9.3 liters/min	—
$MgSO_4$	Thermodilution	8.8 ± 0.6 liters/min	—
—	Thermodilution	13.4, 13.1 liters/min	—
—	Fick—O_2 consumption	5.0–8.2 liters/min	4.5–6.0 liters/min
Barbiturates	Photoelectric transcutaneous dye dilution	8.8 ± 2.1*liters/min	7.8 ± 1.0*liters/min
Alpha methyl dopa hydralazine	N_2O, plethysmography	5.7 ± 1.2*liters/min	8.5 ± 2.6*liters/min
$MgSO_4$, hydralazine	Thermodilution	14.2,8.6,8.3 liters/min	—
—	RISA	3.3 ± 0.6*liters/min/m^2	4.5 ± 1.4*liters/min/m^2

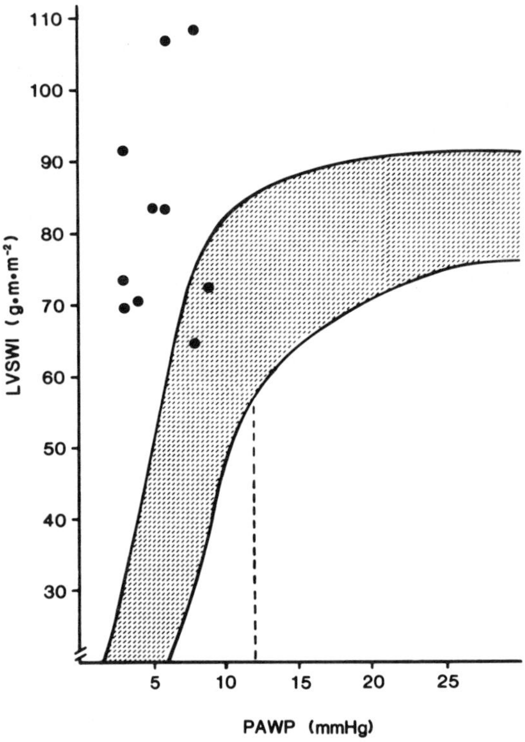

Fig. M.XV.2. Left ventricular function in patients with severe preeclampsia/eclampsia during early labor. Normal LV should fall within the hatched area. Abnormal LV function should lie to the right of the curve. Hatched line represents upper limits of normal for PAWP during pregnancy. Each patient with severe preeclampsia/eclampsia is illustrated with a dot. (Reproduced with permission from Am J Obstet Gynecol. 136:468, 1980.)

problems remain regarding interpretation of data. Most authors have included at least a few multiparous patients in their studies. These patients are known to have a greater chance of having chronic renal diseases and other causes of their hypertension that have been unmasked by pregnancy. Whether the pathophysiology in this circumstance is the same as the nulliparous patient without previous renal disease has never been determined.

Patients with early-onset preeclampsia/eclampsia are at highest risk of having intrauterine growth retardation and they may have a hemodynamic picture different from that of the patient who has mild PIH at term. In light of the cited problems, it is not surprising to find a wide range of reported cardiac outputs in patients with PIH.

Our own studies have shown an apparent increase in the cardiac output of patients with severe PIH.[29] A number of other studies have confirmed this observation[30–32]; however, the best controlled study could find no increase in the cardiac output in comparison with normal pregnant patients.[33] At present it is my belief that cardiac output is elevated above normal nonpregnant levels at some point in the pathogenesis of PIH. It is conceivable that an increase in the cardiac output is one of the early changes in this condition. This could produce an elevation in blood pressure as it does in a nonpregnant

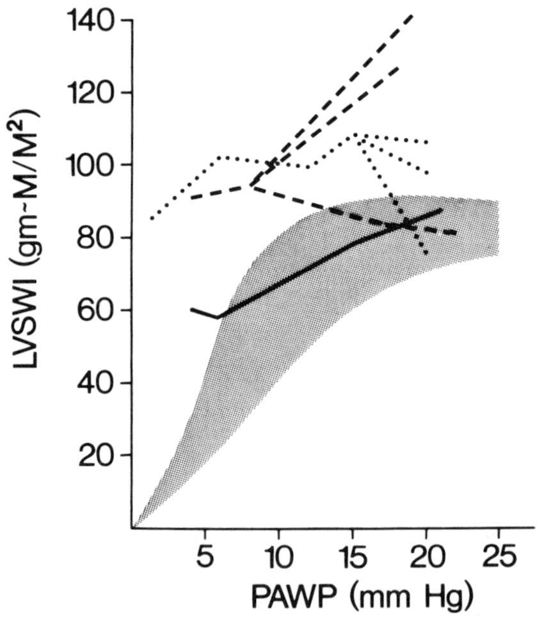

Fig. M.XV.3. Left ventricular function in three patients with severe preeclampsia/eclampsia. Normal or augmented LV function appears to be maintained until PAWP approaches 15–20 mm Hg. However, in two of the three patients multiple readings at the same PAWP show different results. LVSWI = left ventricular stroke work index. Each line (dashed, dotted, solid) represents a single patient. (Adapted from Rafferty, Am J Obstet Gynecol. 138:263, 1980.)

woman with renal hypertension. This hypothesis would help explain the findings of increased DHEA-S clearance in patients with altered vascular sensitivity to angiotensin II. When the arterial pressure finally becomes elevated, cardiac output could have a variable response, depending on a number of factors. These would include drug administration, volume infusion, prolonged treatment with bed rest, and others.

Pulmonary artery pressures in PIH are not increased and the pulmonary vascular resistance is low to low-normal for pregnancy.[27] Pulmonary artery wedge pressure (PAWP) in patients with PIH, when measured, has been found to be low.[27] PAWP increases with uterine contractions[3] and increases transiently, postdelivery.[30] Colloid osmotic pressure is reduced in pregnancy and is further reduced in PIH.[34]

V. VENTRICULAR PERFORMANCE IN PREGNANCY-INDUCED HYPERTENSION

Recent published data document excellent myocardial performance in PIH, despite increased left ventricular afterload.[27] Figure M.XV.2 illustrates ten patients with severe preeclampsia/eclampsia. Even with low PAWP, left ventricular stroke work index is elevated. This indicates hyperdynamic myocardial function. Factors that could account for this observation are positive inotropic effect of endogenous or exogenous substances, or Starling effect resulting from an increased cardiac volume without a significant increase in pressure.

Augmented myocardial performance is maintained until the PAWP reaches 20 mm Hg. Figure M.XV.3 illustrates the ventricular performance curve in three patients reported by Rafferty and Berkowitz.[30] When the filling pressures reached around 20 mm Hg, there appeared to be some disparity in the recorded left ventricular stroke work index. Observations at levels significantly greater than 20 mm Hg in these patients were not made. In other studies, when the PAWP was greater than 20 mm Hg, cardiac decompensation was demonstrated.[38–40] Table M.XV.2 shows patients reported in the literature with pulmonary edema and PIH. In some patients, the wedge pressures ranged from 22 to 33 mm Hg, and were all associated with abnormally low left ventricular stroke work indices. These data would suggest that the downside of the ventricular function curve at PAWP >20 mm Hg may be as steep as the rapid rise in the left ventricular function curve at PAWP as low as 2–5 mm Hg.

Echocardiographic data in patients with PIH have not been frequently recorded. Table M.XV.3 contrasts two stud-

TABLE M.XV.2. Hemodynamic Studies in Patients With Pregnancy-Induced Hypertension and Pulmonary Edema

Author	Age	P	GA	MAP	CO	PAW	CVP	C/NC
Strauss[8]	25	2	32	125	5	33	8	C
Strauss[8]	35	2	37	135	4.7	23	10	C
Strauss[8]	25	5	35	120	4.6	22	18	C
Cotton[9]	38	7	36	110	6.4	24	20	C
Berkowitz[44]	20	1	32	125	—	5	—	NC
Benedetti[34]	23	2	20	130	7.2	16	—	NC
Roberts[45]	23	0	36	123	—	28	8	C
Freund[40]	22	0	34	132	4.6	24	—	C
Andersen[46]	21	0	40	—	—	7	5	NC

P = parity; GA = gestational age; MAP = mean arterial pressure (mm Hg); CO = cardiac output (liters/min); PAW = pulmonary artery wedge pressure (mm Hg); CVP = central venous pressure (mm Hg); C = cardiogenic; NC = noncardiogenic.

TABLE M.XV.3. Echocardiographic Studies in Normotensive and Hypertensive Pregnancy

Study	Position	End-diastolic volume (ml)	End-systolic volume (ml)	Left ventricular mass (gm)	Ejection fraction (%)	Stroke volume (cc)	Cardiac output (liters/m)	Cardiac index (liters/m/m^2)
Katz[41]								
Normotensive	Lateral	132 ± 6	35 ± 4	162 ± 8.3	73 ± 1	97 ± 5	8.6	4.9
3rd Δ n=19	supine	117 ± 6	30 ± 3	—	75 ± 1	87 ± 5	8.1	4.5
Rubler[42]								
Normotensive	Lateral	94 ± 19	24 ± 8	—	74 ± 1	70 ± 8	5.9	3.5
3rd Δ n=12	supine	78 ± 17	24 ± 8	—	69 ± 1	55 ± 15	4.6	—
Larkin[43]								
Mild hyperten-sive	Lateral	77 ± 14	21 ± 6	123 ± 12	72 ± 1	58 ± 14	4.4	2.5
	supine	—	—	—	—	—	—	—
3rd Δ n=11								
Benedetti								
Severe PIH	Lateral	—	—	—	—	—	—	—
3rd Δ n=5	supine	131 ± 10	35 ± 10	—	74 ± 6	96 ± 3	9.3	5.3

ies of normal pregnancy with one preliminary study on hypertensive pregnancy, as well as unpublished data from our institution on five patients with severe PIH. The two studies of normal pregnancy indicate good myocardial performance, with ejection fractions of 70–75%.[40,41] However, there are fairly large differences in the absolute values of end-systolic volume (132 ml vs 94 ml) and cardiac index (4.9 liters/min/m^2 vs 3.5 liters/min/m^2) Data on untreated mild hypertensives at around 32 weeks show a slightly lower cardiac index but a normal ejection fraction.[43] These values are not different from the normal controls in the same study. The five severe preeclamptic/eclamptic patients we studied showed normal or augmented myocardial function, with a mean cardiac index of 5.3 liters/min/m^2 and ejection fraction of 74%. These findings would lend further support to the thesis that myocardial function in mild and severe PIH is not impaired and is probably augmented at some stage in the development of the disease in comparison to normotensive pregnancy.

VI. PULMONARY EDEMA

Pulmonary edema in the pregnant hypertensive patient has been reported to occur by three different mechanisms. Left ventricular dysfunction as a result of increased afterload appears to be the most common mechanism. In this situation, afterload reduction will correct impaired myocardial performance.[38] Intravenous hydralazine has been the traditional drug used in hypertensive episodes in obstetrics. It is probably the drug of choice because of its lack of adverse fetal effects. Nitroprusside has a number of advantages over hydralazine in the postpartum period. Nitroprusside has been reported to cross the placenta in animals with lethal fetal effects.[46] Preliminary human data would suggest that placental transfer may not occur in the human.[47] Until more data become available, nitroprusside is best not given to parturients with fetus in utero.

Clinical differentiation between cardiogenic and noncardiogenic pulmonary edema is difficult, if not impossible, in pregnant patients. Permeability pulmonary edema has been reported in hypertensive pregnant patients.[44,48] This diagnosis can only be made with the use of a pulmonary artery catheter by documentation of normal cardiac filling pressures with normal left ventricular performance. Treatment in this instance should center on supporting cardiac and respiratory function. Supplemental oxygen, positive end-expiratory pressure, and mechanical ventilation are usual essential therapeutic modalities. Volume status in these patients must be monitored very carefully. Over-expansion of the intravascular volume in this instance may contribute to increased pulmonary shunting. In contrast, vigorous diuresis may aggravate hypovolemia and have an adverse effect on cardiac output.

Pulmonary edema has also been reported in hypertensive pregnant patients and is associated with a reduction in the intervascular colloid osmotic pressure (COP).[34] When the COP is reduced to less than 16 mm Hg, a small rise in the PAWP can result in a reversal of the normal Starling forces and result in the accumulation of extrapulmonary lung water. Fluid therapy when the colloid osmotic pressure is significantly less than 16 mm Hg should involve use of colloidal rather than crystalloid fluids.

When the hypertensive pregnancy patient develops respiratory distress, invasive hemodynamic monitoring will be an invaluable tool in establishing a diagnosis and in monitoring the response to therapy. The ability to measure interarterial pressure and pulmonary artery pressure should be present in all institutions caring for these critically ill patients.

Table M.XV.2 illustrates the reported patients with pulmonary edema and PIH. The relationship, if any, between the PAWP and the central venous pressure (CVP) has been investigated.[29] Initially we reported three patients in whom PAWP and the CVP did not correlate in PIH. This poor correlation, however, was within a relatively narrow range with the central venous pressures and pulmonary artery wedge pressures. From Table M.XV.2 it is now apparent that these observations have been extended to include patients with higher wedge pressures. For example, the table shows two patients with a central venous pressure of 8 mm Hg, while the wedge pressures were 28 and 30 mm Hg, respectively. Because of the propensity for some patients with preeclampsia/eclampsia to have discordant function in the right and left heart it would seem important to use a pulmonary artery catheter to monitor filling pressures during volume infusion. This is essential when central venous pressure is greater than 5–6 mm Hg.

VII. ANESTHESIA

As with other aspects of PIH, there is controversy regarding appropriate anesthetic management of affected patients. Pritchard feels that conduction anesthesia is contraindicated because of the fear of maternal hypotension and subsequent fetal compromise.[49] His published experience without any maternal mortalities using general anesthesia for cesarean section and narcotic analgesic for labor in 154 patients with preeclampsia/eclampsia would appear to speak for the safety of this method of anesthesia.[50] However, recent data from our institution, among others, has attested to the safety for both mothers and the fetus of carefully conducted epidural anesthesia in all forms of PIH.[51,52,16]

The hemodynamic consequences of epidural and general anesthesia have been recently reported. During tracheal intubation and extubation there is a significant rise in the mean arterial pressure (45 mm Hg), pulmonary artery pressure (20 mm Hg), and pulmonary artery wedge pressure (20 mm Hg).[51] These elevations may persist for as long as ten minutes before the return to baseline. Such large increases in mean arterial pressure and pulmonary artery pressure may predispose to cerebral hemorrhage and pulmonary edema. We have observed acute decreases in pulmonary compliance associated with general anesthesia and tracheal intubation that may be secondary to these rapid increases in pulmonary artery wedge pressure.[52] These effects could be altered by the use of deeper general anesthesia, but this would probably have adverse fetal effects. Another approach would be to use continuous infusion of a long- or short-acting antihypertensive or to use a bolus of antihypertensive prior to the induction of anesthesia. Hydralazine would appear to be the drug of choice in this instance, and it has been successfully used to limit the hypertensive response in nonpregnant patients during induction before tracheal intubation.[53] Nitroglycerin and nitroprusside need more investigation in pregnant patients before they can be recommended. Propranolol should be avoided since it has been shown to have adverse fetal effects when given intravenously to the mother for blood pressure control just prior to the delivery of the fetus.[54]

Epidural anesthesia preceded by adequate volume expansion is not associated with a significant change in hemodynamic parameters.[16,51] The previous negative experiences of others may have resulted, in part, from the failure to recognize that patients with PIH need a significant volume load prior to the induction of epidural anesthesia. In patients with severe PIH 750 ml of 5% albumin, plus 2,000 cc of saline was needed to provide adequate volume load prior to conduction anesthesia.[16] The same volume load can probably be accomplished with 50–75 gm of salt-poor albumin. We are reluctant to give large saline loads to patients with PIH because of the reported propensity for the saline to exit from the intravascular space and end up in the extravascular space. We have previously reported three patients in whom massive cerebral edema was associated with large volume infusions of crystalloid fluids.[55]

Caution must be used with conduction anesthesia, however, in patients with severe preeclampsia/eclampsia. Thrombocytopenia is a frequent occurrence in the severe forms of the disease. In addition, we have recently observed abnormal bleeding times associated with platelet counts greater than 150,000 mm^3. We routinely perform a bleeding time on all patients with severe preeclampsia/eclampsia prior to the institution of epidural anesthesia.

VIII. IMPLICATIONS FOR TREATMENT

In patients with severe preeclampsia/eclampsia, severe perinatal morbidity and mortality are related, in large part, to the forced delivery of the fetus at high risk for the development of respiratory distress syndrome.[52] Although some authors have reported accelerated pulmonary maturity in patients with PIH,[56] this does not appear to be a consistent observation, especially in patients between 28 and 32 weeks of gestation.[52,57,58] A previous report indicated that glucocorticoid therapy to accelerate fetal pulmonary maturity may have an adverse effect on the fetus and result in an increased incidence of fetal demise.[59] However, subsequent uncontrolled reports suggested that glucocorticoids can be safely administered with intensive and continuous fetal monitoring.[60,61] Maintenance of maternal homeostasis during 48 hours to allow acceleration of fetal pulmonary maturity has involved the use of magnesium sulfate and hydralazine therapy. The recent demonstration that administration of colloidal fluids to the mother may aid in stabilizing blood pressure, and may even transiently improve fetal status, may add another element in the therapeutic armamentarium of the clinician.[16] Pharmacologic and maternal treatment for a period of 48 hours to allow acceleration of pulmonary maturity may reduce the incidence and severity of respiratory distress syndrome in the infant. However, this must be carefully done with the optimum in hemodynamic monitoring for the mother in order to ensure maternal safety during this short period.

Newer hemodynamic observations previously illustrated in this manuscript should provide a basis for the design of new treatment trials. The largest impact on fetal morbidity and mortality would involve studies in the small group of patients with PIH between 28 and 32 weeks of gestation. Carefully designed clinical trials are needed to determine whether departure from traditional concepts of treating patients with preeclampsia/eclampsia is sufficiently safe for both mother and fetus to warrant reconsideration of some traditional treatments.

IX. REFERENCES

1. Assali N, Vaughn R. Blood volume in preeclampsia: Fantasy and reality. Am J Obstet Gynecol. 1977; 129:355–359.
2. Goodlin RC, Cotton DB, Haesslein HC. Severe preeclampsia-edema-hypertension gestosis. Am J Obstet Gynecol. 1978; 132:595–598.
3. Goodlin RC. Letter to the Editor. Am J Obstet Gynecol. 1979; 135:276–278.
4. Gant NF, Daley GL, Chand S, Whalley PJ, MacDonald PC. A study of angiotensin II pressor response throughout primigravid pregnancy. J Clin Invest. 1973; 52:2682–2689.
5. Gant NF, Chand S, Worley RJ, Whalley P, Crosby ND, MacDonald PC. A clinical test useful for predicting the development of acute hypertension of pregnancy. Am J Obstet Gynecol. 1974; 120:1–7.
6. Gusdon JP, Anderson SG, May WJ. A clinical evaluation of the "roll-over test" for pregnancy-induced hypertension. Am J Obstet Gynecol. 1977; 127:1–6.
7. Karbhari D, Harrigan JI, LaMagra R. The supine hypertensive test as a predictor of incipient preeclampsia. Am J Obstet Gynecol. 1977; 127:620–622.
8. Marshall GW, Newman RL. Roll-over test. Am J Obstet Gynecol. 1977; 127:623–626.
9. Phelan JP, Everridge GJ, Wilder TL, Newman C. Is the supine pressor test an adequate means of predicting acute hypertension in pregnancy? Am J Obstet Gynecol. 1977; 128:173–176.
10. Sobel B, Laurent D, Ganguly S, Favro L, Lucas C. Hydrostatic mechanism in the roll-over test. Obstet Gynecol. 1980; 55:285–290.
11. Lassar MS. Aldridge J, Quirk B. Roll-over test. Obstet Gynecol. 1980; 55:411–413.
12. Hovinga G, Aarnoudse JG, Hutsjes HJ. The effect of supine and lateral positions on intra-arterial pressure in hypertensive pregnancies. Am J Obstet Gynecol. 1978; 131:233–238.
13. VanDongen PW, Eskes T, Martin C, Van T, Hof M. Postural blood pressure differences in pregnancy. Am J Obstet Gynecol. 1980; 138:1–5.
14. Benedetti TJ, Read JA, Miller FC. The effect of hydrostatic pressure on interpretation of the supine pressor test. J Reprod Med. (in press).
15. Soffronoff EC, Kauffman DM, Connaughton JF. Intravascular volume determination and fetal outcome in hypertensive disease of pregnancy. Am J Obstet Gynecol. 1978; 127:4–10.
16. Joyce TH, Debnath KS, Baker EA. Preeclampsia—The relationship of CVP and epidural anesthesia. Anesthesiology. 1979; S51:297.
17. Gallery E, Boyce E, Saunders D, Gyory A. The effect of volume expansion on blood pressure, plasma and extracellular fluid volumes in hypertensive pregnancy. Aust NZ J Obstet Gynecol. 1980; 20:189–190.
18. Arias F. Expansion of intravascular volume and fetal outcome in patients with chronic hypertension and pregnancy. Am J Obstet Gynecol. 1975; 123:610–616.
19. Gallery E, Saunders D, Hunyor S, Gyory A. Randomized comparison of methyldopa and oxprenolol for treatment of hypertension in pregnancy. Br Med J. 1979; 1:1591–1594.
20. Gallery ED, Saunders D, Hunyor S, Gyory A. Improvement in fetal growth with treatment of maternal hypertension in pregnancy. Clin Sci Mol Med. 1978; 55:3593–3598.
21. Habib A, McCarthy JS. Effects on the neonate of propranolol administered during pregnancy. J Pediatr. 1971; 91:808–815.
22. Sabom M, Curry C, Wise D. Propranolol therapy during pregnancy in a patient with idiopathic hypertrophic subaortic stenosis: Is it safe? South Med J. 1978; 71:328–331.
23. Sandstrom B. Antihypertensive treatment with adrenergic beta recepter metoprolol during pregnancy. Gynecol Obstet Invest. 1978; 9:195–204.
24. Shepherd JT. Role of the veins in circulation. Circulation. 1966; 33:484–494.
25. Henshall W. Differences in albumin distribution and dynamics between toxemic and non toxemic pregnant women. Br J Obstet Gynaecol. 1979; 86:463–467.
26. London G, Safar M, Simon A, Alexandre J, Levenson J, Weiss Y. Total effective compliance, cardiac output and fluid volumes in essential hypertension. Circulation. 1978; 57:995–1000.
27. Worley RJ, Evertt RB, Madden JD, MacDonald PL, Gant NF. Fetal considerations—Metabolic clearance rate of maternal plasma dehydro iso androsterone sulfate. Semin Perinatal. 1978; 2:15–24.
28. Ferrario C, Page I, McCubbin S. Increased cardiac output as a contributory factor in experimental renal hypertension in dogs. Circ Res. 1970; 27:799–810.
29. Benedetti TJ, Cotton DB, Read JA, Miller FC. Hemodynamic observations in severe preeclampsia using a flow directed pulmonary artery catheter. Am J Obstet Gynecol. 1980; 136:465–470.
30. Rafferty TD, Berkowitz RL. Hemodynamics in patients with severe toxemia during labor and delivery. Am J Obstet Gynecol. 1980; 138:263–271.
31. Graham C, Goldstein A. Epidural anesthesia and cardiac output in severe preeclamptics. Anaesthesia. 1980; 53:709–712.
32. Hamilton HF. Cardiac output in pregnancy. Edinburgh Med J. 1950; 57:1–9.
33. Assali NS, Holm L, Parker H. Systemic and regional hemodynamic alterations in toxemia. Circulation. 1956; 29,30(Suppl II):53–59.
34. Benedetti TJ, Carlson RW. Studies of colloid osmotic pressure in pregnancy induced hypertension. Am J Obstet Gynecol. 1979; 135:308–311.
35. Lim YL, Walters WA. Haemodynamics of mild hypertension in pregnancy. Br J Obstet Gynecol.

1979; 86:198–204.
36. Littler W, Bonnar J, Redman C, Beilin L, Lee G. Reduced pulmonary arterial compliance in hypertensive pregnancy. Lancet. 1973; 2:1274–1275.
37. Smith RU. Cardiovascular alterations in toxemia. Am J Obstet Gynecol. 1970; 107:979–983.
38. Strauss RG, Keefer JR, Burke T, Civetta JM. Hemodynamic monitoring of cardiogenic pulmonary edema complicating toxemia of pregnancy. Obstet Gynecol. 1980; 55:170–174.
39. Cotton DB, Benedetti TJ. Use of the Swan-Ganz catheter in obstetrics and gynecology. Obstet Gynecol. 1980; 56:641–645.
40. Freund U, French W, Carlson R, Weil M, Shubin H. Hemodynamic and metabolic studies of a case of toxemia of pregnancy. Am J Obstet Gynecol. 1977; 127:206–208.
41. Katz R, Karliner J, Resnik R. Effects of a natural volume overload state (pregnancy) on left ventricular performance in normal human subjects. Circulation. 1978; 58:434–441.
42. Rubler S, Damani P, Pinto E. Cardiac size and performance during pregnancy estimated with echocardiography. Am J Cardio. 1977; 40:534–540.
43. Larkin H, Gallery E. Cardiac size and performance in normotensive and hypertensive pregnancy assessed by M-mode echocardiography. Aust NZ J Obstet Gynecol. 1980; 20:190–191.
44. Berkowitz R, Rafferty D. The use of the Swan-Ganz catheter in obstetrics and gynecology. Am J Obstet Gynecol. 1980; 137:127–134.
45. Roberts J. Preeclampsia–eclampsia—Medical Staff Conference Univ of California, San Francisco. West J Med. 1981; 135:34–43.
46. Lewis PE, Cefalo RC, Naulty NS, N'dhay FL. Placental transfer and fetal toxicity of sodium nitropresside. Gynecol Invest. 1977; 8:46–47.
47. Stempel J, O'Grady JP, Morton M, Johnson K. Use of sodium nitropresside in gestational hypertensive emergencies. (in preparation).
48. Andersen FH, Lynch JP, Johnson TRB. Adult respiratory distress syndrome in obstetrics and gynecology. Obstet Gynecol. 1980; 55:291–295.
49. Pritchard J. Management of severe preeclampsia and eclampsia. Semin Perinatol. 1978; 2:83–97.
50. Pritchard JA. Standardized treatment of 154 consecutive cases of eclampsia. Am J Obstet Gynecol. 1975; 123:543–549.
51. Hodgkinson R, Husain J, Hayashi R. Systemic and pulmonary blood pressure during cesarean section in parturients with gestational hypertension. Can Anaesthesiol Soc J. 1980; 27:389–393.
52. Benedetti TJ, Benedetti JK, Stenchever MA. Severe preeclampsia—Maternal and fetal outcome. Clin Exp Hypertension (in press).
53. Davies M, Cronin K, Cowie R. The prevention of hypertension at intubation. Anaesthesia. 1981; 36:147–152.
54. Tunstall ME. The effect of propranolol on the onset of breathing at birth. Br J Anesth. 1969; 51:792.
55. Benedetti TJ, Quilligan EJ. Cerebral edema in severe PIH. Am J Obstet Gynecol. 1980; 137:860–862.
56. Gluck L, Kulovich MV. Lecithin/sphingomyelin ratios in amniotic fluid in normal and abnormal pregnancy. Am J Obstet Gynecol. 1973; 115:539–547.
57. Yoon J, Kohl S, Harper RG. The relationship between maternal hypertensive disease of pregnancy and the incidence of idiopathic respiratory distress syndrome. Pediatrics. 1980; 65:735–745.
58. Skjaerassen J. Amniotic fluid phospholipid concentrations in pregnancies with preeclampsia and/or intrauterine growth retardation. Acta Obstet Gynecol Scand. 1979; 58:191–197.
59. Liggins GC, Howie RN. A controlled trial of antepartum glucocorticoid treatment for prevention of respiratory distress syndrome in premature infants. Pediatrics. 1972; 50:515–526.
60. Nochimson DJ, Petrie RH. Glucocorticoid therapy for the induction of pulmonary maturity in severely hypertensive gravid women. Am J Obstet Gynecol. 1979; 133:449–451.
61. Ricke PS, Elliott JP, Freeman RK. Use of corticosteroids in pregnancy-induced hypertension. Obstet Gynecol. 1980; 55:206–210.

M.XVI

Mitral Valve Prolapse and Pregnancy

William F. Rayburn, MD

Mitral valve prolapse (MVP) has been reported to be the most common congenital heart lesion and is one of the most common cardiac abnormalities.[1] Its reported incidence in the general population is up to 6%.[1,2] Women predominate in most studies, and the diagnosis is frequently made in young women of childbearing age. This chapter reviews the diagnosis and management of MVP, then considers changes to be expected and special precautions to be taken during pregnancy.

I. BACKGROUND

Mitral prolapse is characterized by myxomatous transformation of the mitral valve leaflets, usually the posterior leaflet in those few cases seen at autopsy or surgery.[3] Redundancy of mitral leaflets may produce either localized protrusion or generalized ballooning of leaflet tissue into the left atrium. The chordae tendineae are typically elongated, thin, and attenuated.[3,4] Mitral annular dilatation may be moderate or marked. MVP may be associated with many other cardiac conditions (rheumatic heart disease, congestive cardiomyopathy, Marfan's syndrome, coronary heart disease, atrial septal defect). Infective endocarditis and severe mitral regurgitation are rare complications. Significant coronary artery disease has been found in about 5% of patients with MVP who have undergone coronary arteriography for evaluation of chest pain.[5]

Most nonpregnant patients are asymptomatic and do well. The symptoms of palpitations, anxiety, fatigue, lightheadedness, and chest pain are not often associated with objective findings. One or more midsystolic clicks, with or without a late-systolic murmur, are the auscultatory hallmarks of MVP. The "snapping" click usually occurs during maximal valve pro-

Cardiac Problems in Pregnancy, pages 191–196

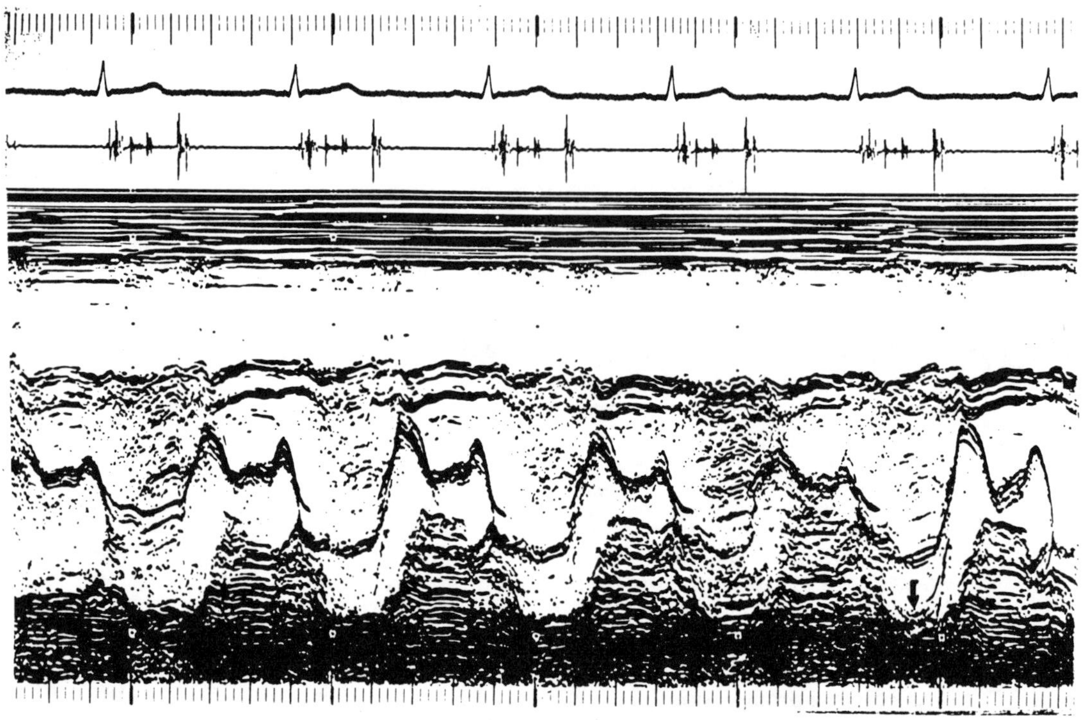

FIG. M.XVI.1. Echocardiogram of mitral valve prolapse in a pregnant woman. An echocardiogram on a pregnant woman at 18 weeks gesation reveals a pansystolic prolapse of the posterior leaflet at the level of the mitral valve (arrow). The phonocardiogram demonstrates a midsystolic click and a systolic murmur, and a normal sinus rhythmn is seen on the electrocardiogram.

lapse and may be absent, single, or multiple at any time.[6] The typical mid- or late-systolic murmur begins with or just follows the click and is usually crescendo in quality. During sitting, standing, or the Valsalva maneuver the click occurs earlier and the murmur becomes longer, although softer. Prompt squatting and isometric exercises may move the click toward the second heart sound and delay the onset of the louder murmur.

Late-systolic prolapse of one or both leaflets can be directly visualized by echocardiography as posterior movement interrupting normal anterior motion (Fig. M.XVI.1).[7] Other echocardiographic abnormalities suggestive of, but not specific for, MVP include exaggerated mitral leaflet mobility producing diastolic contact with the interventricular septum, minimal systolic sagging diminishing normal anterior motion of the mitral leaflets, and a multiplicity of parallel mitral leaflet echoes. Hemodynamic measurements calculated from left ventricular cineangiograms are usually normal in patients with uncomplicated MVP.[3,5] Right ventricular cineangiograms may demonstrate tricuspid prolapse. Care must be taken not to overdiagnose mitral prolapse in the presence of normal radiographic variants.

Electrocardiographic (ECG) abnormalities occur in up to two-thirds of patients with MVP.[3,6] The most typical abnormality consists of a flattened or inverted T wave in leads II, III, and aVf. Less common ECG changes include prolongation of the Q-T interval, premature ventricular contractions, atrial fibrillation, and first-degree AV block. Ambulatory ECG monitoring is the most sensitive method for detecting arrhythmias. Except for the effect of thoracic bony abnormalities, chest x-ray films are normal in patients with uncomplicated mitral prolapse.[8]

The long-term natural history of patients with MVP is unknown, but the outlook is generally favorable. The most feared and rarest complication is sudden death, which may occur after exercise after a prior syncopal episode or without warning.[2,3,9] Endocarditis may occur in individuals with isolated clicks and in those with late-systolic murmurs. The value of antibiotic prophylaxis against infective endocarditis is unknown but doubtful in patients with echocardiographic prolapse unaccompanied by auscultatory signs of regurgitation.[8] Spontaneous rupture of the delicate, attenuated chordae tendineae may suddenly augment mitral regurgitation, causing the murmur to be louder and holosystolic.

People in whom the diagnosis is made accidentally on routine physical examination are usually asymptomatic and require no therapy. Reassurance that symptoms, if present, do not signal cardiac compromise or impending death is usually all that is necessary. Beta-blocking agents such as propranolol may control arrhythmias (premature ventricular contractions, repetitive firing, supraventricular tachycardia) and limit symptoms of chest pain and palpitations. By using these drugs, the increased left ventricular volume and decreased contractility may decrease the valve prolapse and the tension on the chordae and adjacent myocardium. Quinidine has been used in combination with propranolol; however, digitalis, procainamide, or quinidine alone is less effective.[10]

II. EFFECTS OF PREGNANCY ON MVP

Because it was recognized only recently, mitral valve prolapse during pregnancy has not been well studied. Data reported here were gathered from a prior published report at The Ohio State University Hospital[11] and from a review of antepartum and intrapartum charts of any pregnant patient who had MVP and was delivered at The University of Michigan Women's Hospital between 1978 and 1981. To qualify, the diagnosis had to be made clinically by a cardiologist and confirmed by echocardiography before conception. Pregnancy comparisons were made with a control group of patients with no known cardiac disorder and who consecutively delivered during a two-month period in 1981. No differences in patient profiles were found between the study (MVP) and control groups (Table M.XVI.1).

Clinically evident hemodynamic abnormalities were uncommon during pregnancy in women with MVP. Clicks, murmurs, and possibly symptoms were less obvious during pregnancy. This probably related to the expanded intravascular volume and to a reduced peripheral vascular resistance. The increased blood volume may realign the mitral valve complex by increasing left ventricular and end-diastolic volume and by lengthening the long axis of the left ventricle.[12]

No patient required hospitalization for a cardiac complication. Propranolol was used in 13 pregnancies involving nine patients, and the medication was discontinued in all but three pregnancies during early gestation with no apparent adverse effect. Marfan's syndrome was the only

TABLE M.XVI.1. Patient Profiles in Study (Mitral Valve Prolapse) and Control (no Apparent Cardiac Disease) Groups (Mean ± Standard Deviation)

	Study (N = 32)	Control (N = 235)
Age (years)	25 ± 4	25 ± 6
Race (%)	86 white, 14 black	78 white, 22 black
Primiparity (%)	42	39
Gestational age (weeks)	39 ± 6	39 ± 3

TABLE M.XVI.2. Pregnancy Outcomes in the Study and Control Groups

	Study (N = 53)	Control (N = 235)	
Antepartum			
Hospitalization	0	11 (5%)	NS[a]
Other medical illnesses	9 (17%)	24 (10%)	NS
Intrapartum			
Premature delivery	6 (11%)	29 (12%)	NS
Meconium	9 (17%)	38 (16%)	NS
Cesarean section	12 (23%)	42 (18%)	NS

[a]NS = not statistically significant at $\chi^2 < 3.84$, $P > 0.05$.

other accompanying cardiac condition; that pregnancy was also complicated by a premature rupture of the amniotic membranes at 32 weeks gestation. Induced uterine contractions were well tolerated, and the delivery and postpartum courses were uncomplicated. Other illnesses (asthma, seizure disorder, drug addiction) were uncommon and did not influence the heart condition.

III. EFFECTS OF MVP ON PREGNANCY

Most patients should be expected to deliver vaginally at term after an uncomplicated antepartum course. In our experience, the incidence of spontaneous abortion or premature delivery in women with MVP is no higher than in women without an apparent cardiac disorder. The frequency of intrapartum complications is also not significantly greater among patients with MVP when compared to those with no cardiac disorder (Table M.XVI.2). All but five of the 53 patients received prophylactic antibiotics during labor. Local anesthesia was commonly used, but epidural or spinal anesthesia was given in seven patients without signs of hypotension or congestive heart failure. Twelve cesarean sections (23% of total deliveries) were performed because of failure of labor to progress, breech presentation, repeat cesarean section, or suspected fetal distress; all were tolerated well.

Most infants were appropriately sized and delivered without asphyxia (Table M.XVI.3). One case of conjoint twins (xiphopagus) was the only major anomaly recognized at birth. Prolonged neonatal hospitalization for reasons other than prematurity was unnecessary.

IV. SPECIAL CONSIDERATIONS DURING PREGNANCY

A. Genetic Counseling

A familial occurrence has been reported to be uncommon in most large series.[1,3] However, this may be underestimated because of asymptomatic prolapse, and autosomal dominant inheritance with variable expressivity has been suggested in certain studies.[8,13] Examination of other family members is therefore recommended. Otherwise, genetic counseling for MVP alone is not routinely recommended before or during pregnancy.

B. Propranolol Medication

The routine use of propranolol during pregnancy is discouraged because of the reported increased risk of fetal growth retardation and initial neonatal complications such as hypoglycemia, respiratory distress, bradycardia (see Chapter M.XIX).[14] In our experience, the medication is taken infrequently during early pregnancy, and very few patients require continuation of propranolol during the second half of pregnancy. Propranolol should, however, be prescribed if persist-

TABLE M.XVI.3. Neonatal Outcomes in the Study and Control Groups

	Study (N = 53)	Control (N = 235)	
Spontaneous abortion	9 (17%)	24 (10%)	NS
Low birth weight (< 2,500 gm)	6 (11%)	45 (19%)	NS
Five-minute Apgar score ≤ 6	4 (7%)	8 (3%)	NS
Major anomaly	1 (2%)	5 (2%)	NS
Perinatal mortality	1 (2%)	4 (2%)	NS

ent chest pain or cardiac arrhythmias are present.

C. Antibiotic Prophylaxis

The issue of antibiotic prophylaxis for delivery in patients with MVP is not settled. A recent study concluded that antibiotics were not needed for routine vaginal delivery in patients with heart disease.[15] It should, however, be given for any complicated delivery and for dental or surgical procedures. For other than routine vaginal delivery, most authors agree that prophylaxis should be given to women with MVP if a mitral regurgitation murmur is present but not for isolated clicks.

The issue is complicated by the almost inevitable presence of a parasternal systolic ejection murmur during pregnancy in normal women and the variability of the murmur depending on the left ventricular volume and contractility in patients with MVP. Prophylaxis should be given according to the American Heart Association recommendations (Table M.XVI.4),[16] although controversy regarding efficacy continues and revisions will likely occur in the future (see Chapter M.XXV).

TABLE M.XVI.4. Recommended Cardiac Antibiotic Prophylaxis for Gastrointestinal and Genitourinary Tract Surgery and Instrumentation*

Aqueous crystalline penicillin G (2,000,000 units IM or IV)
or
Ampicillin (1 gm IM or IV)
plus
Gentamicin (1.5 mg/kg, not to exceed 80 mg, IM or IV)
or
Streptomycin (1 gm IM)
For penicillin allergy:
Vancomycin (1 gm IV over 30 min)
plus
Streptomycin (1 gm IM)

*Repeat every 12 hours × 1 for penicillin and streptomycin or repeat every 8 hours × 2 for ampicillin and gentamicin. Modified from Kaplan, E.L.: American Heart Association Committee Report: Prevention of bacterial endocarditis, Circulation 56:139a, 1977.

V. SUMMARY

Mitral valve prolapse is the most common congenital heart lesion, and the diagnosis is frequently made in young women of childbearing age. From our experience involving 53 pregnancies among 32 patients with MVP, all patients with no other cardiovascular disorder tolerated pregnancy well and developed no remarkable cardiac complications. Clicks, murmurs, and possibly symptoms became less evident. The incidence of antepartum and intrapartum complications and signs of fetal distress were not more frequent when compared to pregnant patients with no known cardiac disorder. Except for antibiotic prophylaxis in selected cases and monitoring for arrhythmias, no special precautions seem necessary. Each patient should be re-examined in the immediate and late postpartum periods to determine if the midsystolic click and late-systolic murmur remain present.

VI. REFERENCES

1. Schlant RC, Felner JM, Miklozek CL, et al. Mitral valve prolapse. Disease of Month. 1980; 26:1.
2. Barlow JB, Pocock WA. Mitral valve prolapse, the specific billowing mitral valve syndrome, or an insignificant non-ejection systolic click. Am Heart J. 1979; 97:277–285.
3. Jeresaty RM. Mitral valve prolapse-click syndrome. Prog Cardiovasc Dis. 1973; 15:623–652.
4. Marshall CE, Shappell SD. Sudden death and the ballooning posterior leaflet syndrome. Arch Pathol. 1974; 98:134–158.
5. Scampardonis G, Yang SS, Maranhao V, Goldberg H, Gooch AS. Left ventricular abnormalities in prolapsed mitral leaflet syndrome. Circulation. 1973; 48:287–297.
6. Barlow JB, Pocock NA. The problem of non-ejection systolic clicks and associated mitral systolic murmurs: Emphasis on the billowing mitral leaflet syndrome. Am Heart J. 1975; 90:636–655.
7. Dillan JC, Haine CL, Chang S, Feigenbaum H. Use of echocardiography in patients with prolapsed mitral valve. Circulation. 1971; 43:503–507.
8. Devereaux RB, Perloff JK, Reichek N, Josephson M. Mitral valve prolapse. Circulation. 1976; 54:3–14.
9. Shappell SD, Marshall CE, Brown RE, Bruce TA. Sudden death and the familial occurrence of mid-systolic click, late systolic murmur syndrome. Circulation. 1973; 48:1128–1134.
10. Winkle RA, Lopes MG, Fitzgerald J, Goodman D, Schroeder J, Harrison DC. Arrhythmias in patients with mitral valve prolapse. Circulation. 1975; 52:73–81.
11. Rayburn WF, Fontana ME. Mitral valve prolapse and pregnancy. Am J Obstet Gynecol. 1981; 141:9–11.
12. Haas JH. The effect of pregnancy on the midsystolic click and murmur of the prolapsing posterior leaflet of the mitral valve. Am Heart J. 1976; 92:407–408.
13. Kramer R, Devereaux R, Brown W, et al. Inheritance of mitral valve prolapse: Autosomal dominant with variable expression. Abstract 249, p 86a Meeting of the American Society of Human Genetics, Dallas, October 28–31, 1981 (abstr 249).
14. Rubin PC. Beta blockers in pregnancy, N Engl J Med. 1981; 305:1323–1326.
15. Sugrue D, Blake S, Troy P, MacDonald D. Antibiotics against infective endocarditis after normal delivery, Br Heart J. 1980; 44:499–502.
16. Kaplan EL. American Heart Association Committee Report: Prevention of bacterial endocarditis. Circulation 1977; 56:139a–143a.

Cardiac Surgery and Pregnancy

M.XVII

Cardiac Surgery During Pregnancy

Alan Gazzaniga, MD

I. INTRODUCTION

Cardiac surgery during pregnancy is uncommon, and in general, represents more of a threat to the fetus than to the mother. Since the introduction of surgical techniques for the treatment of mitral stenosis in the late 1940s, many patients have undergone cardiac surgery during pregnancy with successful results. While there have been great advances in surgical technique, there remains much to be learned about the response of the fetus and placenta to anesthesia and cardiopulmonary bypass. With advances in fetal monitoring, the status of the fetus can be more appropriately assessed during cardiac surgical procedures.

II. HISTORICAL BACKGROUND

In 1952, Brock,[1] Cooley and Chapman,[2] Logan and Turner,[3] and Mason[4] reported the first cases of cardiac surgery during pregnancy. These surgical procedures were done without the use of cardiopulmonary bypass and were for mitral stenosis. Leyse et al in 1961 reported the first case of cardiac surgery during pregnancy using cardiopulmonary bypass. Their patient subsequently delivered a fullterm fetus who died four months following surgery as a result of congenital defects. Because the mother had undergone surgery during the fourth month of pregnancy, the authors proposed that cardiopulmonary bypass was contraindicated during that phase of fetal development.[5] A subsequent collective review by Zitnik et al showed that cardiac surgery using cardiopulmonary bypass did not expose the mother or fetus to an undue risk. Their conclusions were that cardiac surgery, although preferably done during the twenty-fourth to the twenty-eighth week of pregnancy, when organogenesis is complete, was not contraindicated at any time during pregnancy.[6] Some of the patients had undergone cardiac surgery early in their preg-

Cardiac Problems in Pregnancy, pages 199–206

nancy and had delivered normal infants. Most of the patients in the review by Zitnik underwent surgery for repair of congenital heart defects. Since that review, patients have undergone cardiac valve replacement during pregnancy with excellent results.[7,8] Many patients who have had prior valve replacement have had a successful pregnancy and delivery.[9–11] Recent reports have stressed the importance of fetal monitoring during cardiac procedures in pregnant patients.[8,12,13]

III. PHYSIOLOGIC CHANGES DURING PREGNANCY

The normal cardiovascular response to pregnancy is a gradual and disproportionate increase in cardiac output. Cardiac output rises by 1.0 to 1.5 liters/min during the first 10 weeks of pregnancy to levels of 6.0–7.0 liters/min. This level is maintained until delivery.[14–16] It has been shown that when a woman in late pregnancy assumes the supine position, the inferior vena cava is nearly occluded by the enlarged uterus.[17] This decreases venous return and cardiac output. Ueland and co-workers demonstrated that turning the pregnant woman from the supine to the lateral position increased cardiac output 8% at 20–24 weeks gestation; 13.6% at 28–32 weeks; and 28.5% at term.[18] This information is important in the positioning of the patient at the time of cardiac surgery. With pregnancy there is an increase in oxygen consumption, but not proportionately as great as that of cardiac output. The progressive increase in both cardiac output and oxygen consumption is due to the increase in uterine blood flow and oxygen demands of the fetus. At term it is believed that uterine blood flow may be as great as 500 cc/min. Coinciding with the increased cardiac output is an increase in blood volume, which, at term, may be as great as 40% of the prepregnancy value. This amount represents an increase in both plasma volume[19,20] and red cell mass.[16] The resting pulse in the pregnant patient increases so that at term it is approximately 15 beats above the prepregnancy value.[14,21,22]

IV. SURGICAL PROCEDURES

Surgical procedures during pregnancy are to be discouraged if medical management of the patient is possible. When cardiac disease is discovered prior to or during pregnancy and the possibility of surgical intervention exists, the patient should be followed by both the cardiologist and the surgeon. Inclusion of the cardiac surgeon in the initial management of these patients allows him or her to become familiar with the patient should surgery become necessary.

Since the physiologic response to pregnancy is a gradual increase in cardiac output, oxygen consumption, and blood volume, it is clear that patients will become more symptomatic as pregnancy progresses. This is particularly true for fixed-orifice lesions such as mitral stenosis, for which no type of medical therapy will decrease the orifice size. Obviously, for the fetus, surgery would be safest during the last phase of pregnancy, but it is also more of a risk for the mother.

V. CARDIAC PROCEDURES DURING PREGNANCY

A. Acquired Heart Disease

1. Mitral stenosis

Mitral stenosis occurs in almost all cases as a result of rheumatic fever.[23–25] Previously asymptomatic patients with mitral stenosis can become severely symptomatic during periods of stress, when cardiac output is increased. Symptoms are generally congestive in nature and are manifested by dyspnea on exertion, shortness of breath, and orthopnea. In severe cases there may be acute or chronic interstitial pulmonary edema and/or hemoptysis. If severe symptoms develop in the second trimester of pregnancy and the patient cannot be managed medically, then surgery is indicated. However, there is risk of hypervolemia at the time of delivery, when the uterus is evacuated and suddenly contracts, and hypervolemia can precipitate pulmonary edema.

The original surgical procedures on the mitral valve were reported by Harken et al[26] and Bailey[27] in 1948. Although similar procedures were done earlier than this, for all practical purposes, these two pioneers in cardiac surgery developed this operation, and they did so simultaneously. The procedure involved placing a finger through the left atrial appendage and dilating the mitral valve orifice or physically fracturing the commissures. Harken stressed the importance of freeing the subvalvular mechanism (which included the chordae tendineae) with the finger. He termed this operation "mitral valvuloplasty" rather than commissurotomy.

In the 1950s and early 1960s, closed techniques for the mitral valve were the procedures of choice. The purposes of the procedure were to increase orifice size and to allow for relief of symptoms of pulmonary congestion. Szekely and Turner achieved an overall maternal mortality rate of 1.5% in 761 patients with rheumatic heart disease during pregnancy between 1948 and 1971.[25] Closed mitral valvuloplasty was performed in 29 patients with only one maternal death and two neonatal deaths. The desirable features of the closed operation are that cardiopulmonary bypass is not required and that the operation can be done rapidly with minimal insult to the mother and fetus. However, completeness and overall safety of the closed operation do not compare to the results obtained with open mitral valvuloplasty as recommended by Gerami et al.[28]

2. Cardiac valve replacement

Valve replacement during pregnancy is most common for lesions of the mitral and/or aortic valves. Operations to replace the mitral valve have been performed during pregnancy to improve the patient's deteriorating clinical status and allow the mother to proceed to a fullterm pregnancy.[7,29] Valve replacement is indicated if medical management cannot control congestive heart failure associated with valvular cardiac defects. Valve replacement under normal conditions carries a low mortality and should not be any different during pregnancy. With the use of fetal monitoring, the risk to the fetus has been lessened. For these reasons, the decision for valve replacement should be based on the usual indications if there is potential benefit to the mother.

In general, it is best to replace valves with porcine or tissue valves in order to avoid anticoagulation in the postoperative period.[9] Mechanical prosthetic valves in both the aortic and mitral positions in most cases require anticoagulation. During the first trimester warfarin derivatives (Coumadin) may be teratogenic and throughout pregnancy Coumadin can pass the placental barrier and anticoagulate the fetus.[11] Although the risks are real, a number of pregnant women have gone to fullterm pregnancy on Coumadin.[11] In the usual circumstances, Coumadin is changed to heparin at some time prior to delivery. Under this program many patients have delivered normal infants after prosthetic valve replacement.[9–11]

3. Endocarditis

The occurrence of acute bacterial endocarditis has become a common indication for emergency valve replacement. Surgery is indicated whenever endocarditis becomes refractory to medical management and cardiac failure is progressive.[30] In some cases valve replacement is done when there is known infection on the valve leaflet and in the annulus. The following case illustrates the management of a patient who was at term and underwent emergency cesarean section followed by double valve replacement.

a. Clinical history. This 29-year-old white woman entered the UCI Medical Center with a 30-week intrauterine pregnancy. She presented with anemia, shortness of breath, dry cough, and left-sided pleuritic chest pain. Prior to admission she had been treated at another hospital for anemia with intermittent blood transfusions. On physical examination at admission she was dyspneic, complained of right upper quadrant pain, and had a loud diastolic murmur along the left sternal border. There were rales on auscultation. Pulse pressure was wide. The liver was enlarged and tender. Following admission a Swan-Ganz catheter was placed and the right atrial pressure was 12 mm Hg, right ventricular pressure 60/12 mm Hg, and pulmonary artery pressure 60/30 mm Hg, with a wedge of 28 mm Hg. Her cardiac output was 6.2 liters/min. Blood cultures were drawn, and the patient was started on intravenous nafcillin and gentamicin. Echocardiogram revealed dilatation of the left ventricle with vegetation in the aortic and mitral valves. One week after admission, a cesarean section was performed and a 1,400 gm infant was delivered and subsequently did well.

Postoperatively the patient developed further symptoms of congestive heart failure and underwent emergency double valve replacement two days after cesarean section. The valves were grossly infected and extensively necrotic. Postoperatively, she had a stormy course, but subsequently made a complete recovery and was discharged without signs of congestive heart failure.

b. Comment. This patient was admitted at 30 weeks of pregnancy with a near fullterm infant. Because she was in severe congestive heart failure from her endocarditis, it was thought that she should undergo cesarean section. She tolerated the procedure reasonably well, although clinically her heart failure became worse after the cesarean section. If she had had the same clinical course and was less than 28 weeks pregnant, a double valve replacement would have been done with the use of fetal monitoring during anesthesia and cardiopulmonary bypass.

B. Congenital Heart Disease

1. Cyanotic congenital heart disease

A number of case reports have documented the clinical course of pregnancy in patients with congenital heart defects.[31–34] Congenital defects producing cyanosis, such as tetralogy of Fallot and transposition of the great vessels, will certainly produce greater symptoms during pregnancy. There appears to be a higher incidence of congenital defects in infants born to mothers with cyanotic heart disease.[31] Indications for surgery in the pregnant woman with cyanotic congenital heart disease should be based on the risks to the mother. Progressive shortness of breath, rising hematocrit, cardiac enlargement, and desaturation are all indications for surgery. The increasing hematocrit places the mother at risk for stroke or myocardial infarction. Baker et al reported one patient who underwent closed pulmonary valvotomy and survived her operation and delivered a fullterm infant.[33]

2. Acyanotic congenital heart disease

Successful pregnancy in patients with acyanotic cardiac defects, such as ventricular septal defects and atrial septal defects, have been reported.[6,32] In most cases these patients will not require cardiac surgery. In the immediate postpartum period, the possibility of paradoxical embolism exists in those patients with left-to-right shunts at the atrial level. The presence of an atrial septal defect should be a relative indication for surgery in any patient who has a known history of deep venous thrombosis or pulmonary emboli, and who is planning pregnancy.

The clinical course of women with coarctation of the aorta during pregnancy has been documented.[35,36] Barash stressed the importance of fetal monitoring if coarctation correction is carried out during pregnancy.[35] In general, if the patient has a coarctation, it should be repaired prior to pregnancy because repair during pregnancy presents the risk of harm to the fetus.

3. Pulmonary hypertension

Eisenmenger's syndrome is the result of balanced right-to-left and left-to-right shunts, or right-to-left shunts in patients with pulmonary artery hypertension. Eisenmenger's syndrome is most often associated with ventricular septal defects, atrial septal defects, or patent ductus arteriosus.[37,38] Patients with Eisenmenger's syndrome who become pregnant risk death; the associated mortality has been described at over 60%. A recent report by Spinnato et al emphasized the use of epidural anesthesia and elective cesarean section for these patients.[39] Because they are right ventricle dependent, any decrease in venous return would result in a drop in cardiac output and could produce decreased coronary blood flow and ventricular fibrillation.

Because the outlook for pregnant Eisenmenger's syndrome patients is so poor, any woman with pulmonary hypertension (whether due to intracardiac defects or primary pulmonary hypertension) should be carefully evaluated before becoming pregnant. If a woman is found to be pregnant and to have this syndrome, then cardiac catheterization may be indicated to detect the degree of pulmonary artery hypertension. In general, therapeutic interruption of pregnancy is indicated when pulmonary hypertension is confirmed.[39] (See for more detail, chapters M.IV and M.XII.)

4. Left atrial myxoma

Two cases of removal of left atrial myxoma discovered during pregnancy have been reported.[13,40] In both situations the patients underwent uncomplicated pregnancies despite the use of cardiopulmonary bypass to open the atrium and remove the tumor. Neither patient experienced significant hemodynamic problems due to the presence of the myxoma. In one case the patient did have fatigue and shortness of breath. The patients underwent removal of myxoma to reduce symptoms in one patient and to prevent embolism in both. Fetal heart rates were monitored during cardiopulmonary bypass.[13] Both patients delivered fullterm infants without complication.

5. Other cardiac lesions

Other cardiac lesions that might require surgical intervention during pregnancy include heart block,[41–43] constrictive pericarditis,[44] and dissecting aortic aneurysm.[45,46] In general, indications for surgery are conditions refractory to medical management that present a risk to the mother as well as to the fetus. A survey of the literature and our own experience show that coronary artery bypass has not been performed during pregnancy. Although women in the childbearing years do not usually develop coronary artery disease, it can occur in women who have been on birth control pills or who smoke.

VI. INTRAOPERATIVE MANAGEMENT

The anesthetic management of pregnant patients undergoing cardiac surgery is aimed at safety of the mother and fetus to ensure continuation of pregnancy. Careful planning should be done whenever possible, but in some cases emergency surgery does not allow for orderly planning of the procedure. It is important to have protocols regarding the intraoperative management of the pregnant patient during cardiac procedures.

Preoxygenation and rapid induction of anesthetic agents avoid hypoxia during intubation. Also, intraarterial blood pressure monitoring and blood gas analysis must be performed frequently during operation. Swan-Ganz catheter placement should be a part of the monitoring protocol to permit assessment of left ventricular filling pressures and to treat hypovolemia and/or pulmonary edema. Estafanous and

Buckley prefer the use of pancuronium bromide as a muscle relaxant because of its relative lack of hypotensive effects.[47] Most anesthetic and analgesic agents cross the placenta to the fetus. Therefore, only fully investigated anesthetic/analgesic drugs free from any organogenetic effects on the fetus should be used. The effect and fate of the drugs in the fetus differ from the mother because fetal enzyme systems are immature, fetal serum proteins and pH differ from those of the mother, and the placenta is a site for biotransformation of some drugs.[47]

Most cardiac procedures are done through a median sternotomy. To accomplish this, the pregnant patient is supine, and hypotension may result because the enlarged uterus presses on the vena cava. Devices have been developed that attach to the operating table and can be positioned to push the uterus off the vena cava when the patient is supine.[15]

Closed cardiac techniques include mitral valvuloplasty through the left atrial appendage, repair of coarctation of the aorta through a left lateral thoracotomy, as well as ligation and division of patent ductus arteriosus. For these, the patient can be placed in the right lateral decubitus position, and the uterus will fall away from the vena cava avoiding changes in cardiac output.

When cardiopulmonary bypass is used, the venae cavae are independently cannulated through the right atrium. The aorta is cannulated for arterial return. Operations on the mitral valve are done through the left atrium via the intraatrial groove, or depending upon the surgeon's preference. When cardiopulmonary bypass is begun, there is usually a severe drop in systemic vascular resistance as more blood is diverted from the patient's pulmonary circulation to the pump oxygenator. At the same time systemic vasodilation occurs.[48] This sudden drop in blood pressure and flow is gradually compensated for by volume transfusion from the oxygenator to the patient and endogenous catecholamine response.[48] During this phase of cardiopulmonary bypass fetal monitoring is critical to ensure adequate perfusion of the uterus. Alterations in the rate of blood flow during cardiopulmonary bypass can be gauged by the fetal response with fetal monitoring. Estafanous and Buckley[47] have recommended that high flow bypass be used during cardiopulmonary bypass in pregnant patients. Laboratory studies on uterine blood flow in monkeys during extracorporeal circulation did not show a decrease in blood flow in the nonpregnant uterus. In the pregnant human uterus, however, blood flow probably is reduced. It has been determined that blood flow to the human uterus at term is approximately 500 cc/minute.

For most cardiac procedures, systemic hypothermia is generally used, and this may be of some benefit to the fetus when core temperatures are lowered to 32°–30°C; however, this has not been proved. Other questions regarding the conduct of cardiopulmonary bypass, including use of pulsatile versus nonpulsatile perfusion, as well as the degree of hemodilution instituted, have not been fully studied.

VII. POSTOPERATIVE MANAGEMENT

Postoperative management of pregnant women undergoing cardiac surgery would consist of continued fetal heart monitoring, careful intraoperative hemostasis at the conclusion of the procedure, and early return to normal activated clotting times. Left atrial, pulmonary diastolic, or wedge pressures should be monitored by use of the Swan-Ganz catheter. Endotracheal intubation on the ventilator should be maintained for the first 24 hours after operation. This will allow use of analgesics to control the mother's pain so that an exaggerated or accelerated pain response will not cause the uterus to contract. This will also provide optimal oxygenation to prevent hypoxia for the fetus.

VIII. SUMMARY

Cardiac surgery during pregnancy provides a risk to both mother and infant. Despite this, the mother should undergo operation with careful fetal monitoring in the presence of indications for operative intervention. In general, closed cardiac techniques offer a better result for the fetus than open cardiac techniques. When valve replacement is required, tissue valves should be used to avoid Coumadin anticoagulation. Patients with congenital heart defects usually do not require cardiac surgery unless they have cyanotic heart disease. Pulmonary hypertension due to fixed pulmonary vascular resistance and right-to-left shunting carries with it a high maternal and infant mortality. If a patient is discovered early in pregnancy to have this lesion, cardiac catheterization should be performed. If pulmonary artery hypertension is present and is unreactive to oxygen administration, therapeutic abortion is strongly indicated. Fetal monitoring is essential during any cardiac surgical procedure whether or not cardiopulmonary bypass is used. Blood flow to the uterus can be assessed during cardiopulmonary bypass, and alterations in flow can be made.

IX. REFERENCES

1. Brock RC. Valvulotomy in pregnancy. Proc R Soc Med. 1952; 45:538–543.
2. Cooley DA, Chapman DW. Mitral commissurotomy during pregnancy. JAMA. 1952; 150:1113–1117.
3. Logan A, Turner RWD. Mitral valvulotomy in pregnancy. Lancet. 1952; 1:1286–1290.
4. Mason J. In discussion of Stabler FE, Szekely PJ. Obstet Gynaecol Br Emp. 1952; 59:569–573.
5. Leyse R, Ofstun M, Dillar DH, Merendino KA. Congential aortic stenosis in pregnancy, corrected by extracorporeal circulation. JAMA. 1961; 176:1009–1012.
6. Zitnik RS, Brandenburg RO, Sheldon R, Wallace RB. Pregnancy and open-heart surgery. Circulation. 1969; 39(Suppl. 1):257–262.
7. Miller M, Buchanan N, Cane RD, Kinsley R. Two mitral valve replacements during the course of a single pregnancy. Intensive Care Med. 1978; 4:41–42.
8. Levy DL, Warriner RA, Burgess GE. Fetal response to cardiopulmonary bypass. Obstet Gynecol. 1980; 56:112–115.
9. Limet R, Grodin CM. Cardiac valve prostheses, anticoagulation, and pregnancy. Ann Thorac Surg. 1977; 23:337–341.
10. Szekely P, Snaith L. Mitral valve prosthesis, warfarin anticoagulation and pregnancy. Lancet. 1969; 2:598–601.
11. Tejani N. Anticoagulant therapy with cardiac valve prosthesis during pregnancy. Obstet Gynecol. 1973; 42:785–793.
12. Koh KS, Friesen RM, Livingstone RA, Peddle LJ. Fetal monitoring during maternal cardiac surgery with cardiopulmonary bypass. CMA J. 1975; 112:1102–1104.
13. Trimakas AP, Maxwell KD, Berkay S, Gardner TJ, Achuff SC. Fetal monitoring during cardiopulmonary bypass for removal of a left atrial myxoma during pregnancy. Johns Hopkins Med J. 1979; 144:156–160.
14. Walters WAW, MacGregor WG, Hills M. Cardiac output at rest during pregnancy and the puerperium. Clin Sci. 1966; 30:1–3.
15. Lees MM, Scott DB, Kerr MG, Taylor SH. The circulatory effects of recumbent postural change in late pregnancy. Clin Sci. 1967; 32:453–458.
16. Hytten FE, Lind T. Diagnostic indices in pregnancy. Basle: Ciba-Geigy, Ltd., 1973:44–50.
17. Kerr MG, Scott DB, Samuel E. Studies of the inferior vena cava in late pregnancy. Br Med J. 1964; 1:532–537.
18. Ueland K, Novy MJ, Peterson EN, Metcalfe J. Maternal cardiovascular dynamics. Am J Obstet Gynecol. 1969; 104:856–861.
19. Hytten FE, Paintin DB. Increase in plasma volume during normal pregnancy. J Obstet Gynaecol Br Commonw. 1963; 70:402–409.
20. Hytten FE, Leitch I. The physiology of human pregnancy, 2nd ed. Oxford: Blackwell. 1971:185–191.
21. Schwarz R. Das verhalten des kreislaufs in der normalen schwangerschaft. Arch Gynakol. 1964; 199:663–667.
22. Metcalfe J, Euland K. The heart and pregnancy. In: Hurst JW (ed.) The Heart, 4th ed. New York: McGraw-Hill, 1978:1721–1734.
23. Maynard EP, Grover V. The effect of childbearing on the course of rheumatic heart disease: A 25-year study. Ann Intern Med. 1960; 52:163–171.
24. Besterman E. The changing face of acute rheumatic fever. Br Heart J. 1970; 32:579–582.
25. Szekely P, Turner R, Snaith L. Pregnancy and the changing pattern of rheumatic heart disease. Br Heart J. 1973; 35:1293–1303.
26. Harken DE, Ellis LB, Ware PF, Norman LR. The surgical treatment of mitral stenosis. N Engl J Med. 1948; 239:801–805.
27. Bailey CP. The surgical treatment of mitral stenosis (mitral commissurotomy). Dis Chest. 1949; 15:377–381.
28. Gerami S, Messmer BJ, Hallman GL, Cooley

DA. Open mitral commissurotomy: Results of 100 consecutive cases. J Thorac Cardiovasc Surg. 1971; 62:366–370.

29. Taguchi K. Pregnancy in patients with a prosthetic heart valve. Surg Gynecol Obstet. 1977; 145:206–208.
30. Palafox BA, Gazzaniga AB, Thrupp LD, Iseri LT, Connolly JE. Surgical treatment of infective valvular endocarditis. Arch Surg. 1976; 111:707–710.
31. Jacoby WJ. Pregnancy with tetralogy and pentalogy of Fallot. Am J Cardiol. 1964; 14:866–873.
32. Copeland WE, Wooley CF, Ryan JM, Runco V, Levin HS. Pregnancy and congenital heart disease. Am J Obstet Gynecol. 1963; 86:107–110.
33. Baker JL, Russell CS, Grainger RG, Taylor DG, Thornton JA, Verel D. Closed pulmonary valvotomy in the management of Fallot's tetralogy complicated by pregnancy. J Obstet Gynecol. 1970; 18:154–157.
34. Littler WA. Successful pregnancy in a patient with Ebstein's anomaly. Br Heart J. 1970; 32:711–713.
35. Barash PG, Hobbins JC, Hook R, Stansel HC, Whittemore R, Hehre FW. Management of coarctation of the aorta during pregnancy. J Thorac Cardiovasc Surg. 1975; 69:781–784.
36. Goodwin JF. Pregnancy and coarctation of the aorta. Clin Obstet Gynecol. 1961; 4:645–664.
37. Neilson G, Galea EG, Blunt A. Eisenmenger's syndrome and pregnancy. Med J Aust. 1971; 1:431–434.
38. Pitts JA, Crosby WM, Basta LL. Eisenmenger's syndrome in pregnancy. Am Heart J. 1977; 93:321–326.
39. Gleicher N, Midwall J, Hochberger D, Jaffin H. Eisenmenger's syndrome in pregnancy. Obstet Gynecol Surv. 1979; 34:721–741.
40. Casarotto D, Bortolotti U, Russo R, Betti D, Schivazappa L, Thiene G. Surgical removal of a left atrial myxoma during pregnancy. Chest. 1979; 75:390–392.
41. Schonbrun M, Rowland W, Quiroz AC. Complete heart block in pregnancy. Obstet Gynecol. 1966; 27:243–246.
42. Ginns HM, Hollinrake K. Complete heart block in pregnancy treated with an internal cardiac pacemaker. J Obstet Gynecol Br Commonw. 1970; 77:710–712.
43. Kenmure ACF, Cameron AJV. Congenital complete heart block in pregnancy. Br Heart J. 1967; 29:910–912.
44. Watson PT, Havelda CJ, Sorosky J, Kochenour NK, Sohi GS, Gray L. Irradiation-induced constrictive pericarditis requiring pericardiectomy during pregnancy. J Reprod Med. 1980; 24:127–130.
45. Mandel W, Evans EW, Walford RL. Dissecting aortic aneurysm during pregnancy. N Engl J Med 1954; 251:1059–1061.
46. Hume M, Krosnick G. Dissecting aneurysm in pregnancy associated with aortic insufficiency. N Engl J Med. 1961; 268:174–178.
47. Estafanous FG, Buckley S. Management of anesthesia for open heart surgery during pregnancy. Cleveland Clin Q. 1976; 43:121–124.
48. Bartlett RH, Gazzaniga AB. The physiology and pathophysiology of extracorporeal circulation. In Ionescu MI, Wooler GH (eds.): Current Techniques in Extracorporeal Corporeal Circulation, 2nd ed. London: Butterworth's, 1980:1–56.

M. XVIII

Pregnancy After Cardiac Surgery

Kenneth L. Noller, MD

I. INTRODUCTION

Cardiac disease in pregnancy has changed remarkably during the past 25 years. Older textbooks and articles reviewing this topic deal mostly with the management of pregnant women having severe valvular disease of rheumatic origin. However, earlier treatment for streptococcal infections has reduced the incidence of rheumatic heart disease.[1] Conversely, the developing ability of surgeons to correct many of the congenital cardiovascular defects has enabled more patients with these problems to live to an age when pregnancy is possible.

Since 1952,[2] the implantation of prosthetic heart valves in the human has further changed the nature of cardiac disease in pregnancy. Women with one or more artificial heart valves are now appearing in prenatal clinics. It has been estimated that more than 200,000 valves have been implanted in humans,[3] and more than 150 pregnancies have been reported in women with such valves.[4] As is shown later in this chapter, these women present particular management difficulties during pregnancy. The recently developed glutaraldehyde-treated porcine heart valves[5,6] cause markedly less trouble during pregnancy than do mechanical heart valves.

Cardiac Problems in Pregnancy, pages 207–218

II. MEDICAL ASSESSMENT PRIOR TO PREGNANCY

It has been stated often that the best time to diagnose cardiac disease in pregnancy is prior to conception. With the many methods of improving or correcting organic heart lesions now available, it is unfortunate that some patients enter a prenatal clinic with undiagnosed organic heart disease. However, even when diagnosis and correction have been accomplished prior to pregnancy, many afflicted women fail to seek advice prior to becoming pregnant. Special cardiodynamic problems often remaining in these cases need investigation that is feasible only before pregnancy. Unfortunately, even when information about such needs is sought from a physician, the response frequently is inadequate or inappropriate.[4]

It is important for a couple considering the advisability of pregnancy after cardiac surgery to understand the effect that pregnancy superimposed on cardiac disease may have on the long-term survival of the patient. Chesley[7] and Estafanous and Buckley[8] have shown clearly that long-term survival of women with organic heart disease is the same with and without pregnancy. However, it is important for the couple to realize that long-term survival of patients with significant cardiac lesions is never the same as that of the general population. Despite the best of care, some women with serious valvular disorders will be expected to die from their disease, even if artificial heart valves have been placed. Left ventricular dysfunction, valve dysfunction, cardiac dysrhythmias, and thromboembolic episodes account for the slow but steady attrition in this group of women.

A. Advisability of Pregnancy

Women whose congenital heart lesions have been completely corrected by surgery often have no cardiac problems during pregnancy. The majority of women with small atrial or ventricular septal defects experience no cardiac compromise with the added stresses of pregnancy. If the lesions have been corrected early in life, and if the functional status remains class I (New York Heart Association classification), these women usually proceed through pregnancy without any difficulty, and they should be counseled accordingly. Of course prophylactic antibiotic coverage is desirable to prevent bacterial endocarditis.

Women with congenital heart disease should be advised that there is a small but increased risk of their children also having a congenital heart defect. This tendency is strongest in patients with cyanotic heart disease, and it is not always clear whether the anomaly is due to a genetic defect or to lowered oxygen supply to the fetus.[9]

Major congenital cardiac anomalies—particularly those causing cyanosis—offer their own particular problems. Tetralogy of Fallot is the most common form of congenital cyanotic heart disease. A number of pregnancies subsequent to correction of this condition have been reported, but no large series exists. In general, the patients should be advised that pregnancy may require considerable compromise of their activity. Some form of cardiac stress testing to simulate the increased work load that will be experienced during pregnancy should be performed in a cardiac exercise laboratory prior to conception. The results of such testing will help greatly in determining the likelihood that cardiac compromise will or will not develop during pregnancy.

Some conditions, of course, are never corrected completely; and exercise testing may suggest the effect of a superimposed pregnancy in these cases. It should be noted, however, that women who have pulmonary hypertension as an initial or acquired component of their heart disease do not do well during pregnancy. Even mild pulmonary hypertension carries with it a markedly increased risk of maternal and fetal mortality. These women should be strongly advised of the dangers of pregnancy.

Acquired valvular lesions may be corrected by repair of the mitral valve or by installation of an artificial valve, either biologic or mechanical. In relating the cardiac problem to pregnancy, both the kind of valve present and the general cardiac status must be considered. If the correction was successful—that is, if the patient is presently in functional class I or II—it is unlikely that she will experience deterioration to class III or IV unless some new cardiac insult (such as an arrhythmia) occurs. The type of valvular repair, however, makes a tremendous difference in the fetal prognosis.

It appears now that porcine grafts may be the safest solution to valvular heart disease during pregnancy. Although no large series are available, women with such grafts do not need anticoagulants (unless the graft is in the mitral location and there is atrial fibrillation, left atrial enlargement, or previous thromboembolism[10,11]), and they do very well during pregnancy.[4,12] These patients may be somewhat reassured and told that their pregnancy should be successful.

Mechanical heart valves lead to large numbers of pregnancy losses.[4,13–15] Table M.XVIII.1 shows the outcomes of pregnancy in the two series whose reports include all pregnancy outcomes. Unfortunately, most series of pregnancies following cardiac valve insertion do not include information on the frequency of spontaneous abortion. The difference between spontaneous abortion rates with and without anticoagulant medication is striking.

These data indicate that pregnancy after insertion of mechanical valves is not dangerous to women themselves; but they should be advised that anticoagulants increase the rate of pregnancy loss, most notably in the form of spontaneous abortion. The women should also be counseled that congenital abnormalities are more likely to occur if they are taking coumarin during pregnancy.

A number of reports have described anomalies following in utero exposure to coumarin derivatives.[4,13,16] Although the exact frequency with which this happens is not known, it is common enough that the women should be counseled in early pregnancy. A method of management is discussed below.

B. Assessment of Fertility

Because all pregnancies in women taking anticoagulants should be carefully planned, and because these pregnancies require adaptation of the anticoagulant management, it is very important to establish the degree (or absence) of fertility. A woman who has had several pregnancies prior to the insertion of her mechanical valve is likely to be fertile, and she knows that unprotected intercourse is likely to result in another pregnancy. However, a woman who has never been exposed to the possibility of pregnancy and has a mechanical heart valve, but now desires pregnancy, should have an evaluation of her fertility status prior to

TABLE M.XVIII.1. Outcome of Pregnancy Following Placement of Mechanical Heart Valve

	Lutz et al[4]				Oakley and Doherty[13]			
	Coumarin Rx		No anticoagulant		Coumarin Rx		No anticoagulant	
	N	%	N	%	N	%	N	%
Live birth[a]	12	38	5	63	8	53	23	96
Spontaneous abortion	14	44	2	25	3	20	1	4
Other loss or termination	6	18	1	12	4	27	0	
Total	32		8		15		24	

[a]Includes some with fetal anomalies.

attempting conception. It would be unfortunate to make all the necessary arrangements for a woman to discontinue coumarin drugs for ten or 12 cycles and then discover that some easily diagnosed primary infertility problem was present.

Of course the easiest step in the fertility investigation is establishment of the normality of the patient's husband's semen, and a semen analysis should always be ordered in these cases. The second step is collection of several basal body temperature charts. The woman who has regular cycles with a normal rise of the basal temperature at mid cycle can be assumed to be ovulating. If both the cycle of basal body temperature and the results of semen analysis are normal, no further workup need be done unless the woman has undergone extensive abdominal surgery or has had pelvic inflammatory disease. In those circumstances the addition of hysterosalpingography should be considered. It is not recommended as a routine procedure, because of the possibility of initiating severe bleeding in patients taking anticoagulants and because of the need to use antibiotics to prevent bacterial endocarditis. When the resultant information is necessary, however, hysterosalpingography may be done.

C. Medical Assessment

Five procedures are indispensable for pre-pregnancy evaluation of the woman who has had cardiac surgery, and two others may be needed in some cases. The necessary five require no special equipment.

1. Consultation with cardiologist

Certainly all women who have had cardiac surgery require consultation with a cardiologist before initiating a pregnancy. Although most women who have had complete correction of minor congenital heart defects may proceed to pregnancy without fear of undue complications, cardiologic consultation is needed to rule out subtle changes that may have occurred since the last visit. Women with mechanical or biologic heart valves need to be screened with special care for any evidence of early failure of the valve.

2. Electrocardiography

An electrocardiogram should always be obtained to establish the pre-pregnancy baseline rhythm. This is particularly important in women with mitral stenosis who have had sinus rhythm. It has been shown repeatedly that sudden development of atrial fibrillation during pregnancy is much more threatening to successful outcome of the pregnancy than either having atrial fibrillation before pregnancy or remaining in sinus rhythm during pregnancy.[1,13,17] If the patient is in sinus rhythm, she should be instructed in taking her pulse. The changes she might detect if atrial fibrillation occurs must be carefully explained.

3. Chest roentgenography

Although roentgenography of the chest is not necessary as a routine test in normal prenatal care,[18] it should be done before the beginning of pregnancy in all cases wherein heart disease has been corrected surgically. The roentgenogram will show whether cardiac size has been increased by any subtle deterioration since the cardiac surgery and will provide a baseline if cardiac deterioration occurs subsequently.

4. Hematologic examination

It is important to determine the hematologic status of the patient before pregnancy. Women with heart disease do poorly in pregnancy if anemia is present. If the blood study reveals an anemia, it should be corrected prior to conception. Because some mechanical heart valves (especially older models) may destroy red blood cells, they can cause anemia. Supplementation of the diet with appropriate vitamins and iron preparations will provide a stable hematologic state for the beginning of pregnancy. Additionally, the patient's iron stores may be measured.

This is of particular interest if there is a history of heavy menstruation, for moderate to severe menorrhagia has been found in many women taking oral anticoagulants. The adequacy of the platelets should be established, and also a baseline leukocyte count should be obtained.

5. Echocardiography

This procedure provides accurate information on several aspects of cardiac function and (in two-dimensional mode) the presence or absence of mural thrombus in enlarged cardiac chambers. This is very important in cases where cardiac function is of class I but some slight deterioration of cardiac function is suspected. It should be noted here that this is also a most useful technique for evaluation of cardiac status during pregnancy without exposure to ionizing radiation (especially undesirable in pregnancy) and without invasion.

6. Optional procedures

Recently, exercise testing has been used increasingly in cardiac examinations. Although no large series have been reported in which this modality was employed for pre-pregnancy assessment, it may be a prudent choice if available locally and approved for the purpose by the consulting cardiologist. Objective measurements of exercise capacity often differ from historical assessments, and exercise capacity cannot be estimated from any resting parameter of left ventricular function (especially not from heart size on the chest roentgenogram).

III. MANAGEMENT OF PATIENTS WITH SURGICALLY CORRECTED CONGENITAL HEART DISEASE

A. Prenatal Care

In regard to management during pregnancy, patients with corrected congenital heart defects may be considered in two general categories: those who had small atrial or ventricular septal defects, and all others.

After successful correction of a small septal defect, patients may be considered "noncardiac," except for prophylaxis against bacterial endocarditis at the time of delivery. These patients may maintain normal activity throughout pregnancy. However, they should be advised to avoid the possibility of systemic infections.

Few reported studies have documented pregnancy outcome following surgical correction of serious congenital heart defects,[19] but many have been concerned with pregnancies of women whose congenital heart defects had not been corrected. The latter show rather low maternal mortality but increased fetal mortality. It is likely that the past excellent maternal outcome has been related to minor defects, since only those women who have lived with their condition for many years can achieve pregnancy. The high fetal death rate probably results from relative anoxia in most cases.[20]

Thus it is difficult to arrive at specific recommendations for each form of surgically corrected congenital heart defect. As a rule, it is far better to analyze each case individually and to suggest treatment based on the patient's functional status and known cardiac condition. A judgment must be made about whether the woman's heart can sustain a marked increase in cardiac output in the pregnancy and adapt to the increased work required for labor and delivery. It is important to recognize whether pulmonary hypertension is a part of the residual cardiac disease. As noted earlier, women with such hypertension do not do well in pregnancy.

B. Labor and Delivery

At the onset of labor, all women with surgically corrected congenital heart disease should receive prophylaxis against bacterial endocarditis. For those who have had atrial or ventricular septal defects repaired, no further special arrangements need be made.

Women with corrected defects but with a decrease in functional reserve must be watched very carefully at the onset of labor. Cardiac work is increased by 50% during normal labor and delivery. Also, immediately after delivery of the placenta the marked reduction in size of the uterus adds 500–1,000 ml of volume to the intravascular space, and the cardiac output is transiently increased further.

Efforts should be made to decrease this workload as much as possible. The patient should be maintained in a supportive atmosphere, her anxiety relieved in all possible ways. It is particularly useful for the pregnant cardiac patient to have taken childbirth preparation classes so that she is aware of the general course of labor and delivery.

If the patient begins to perceive significant pain during labor, continuous lumbar epidural anesthesia is perhaps the best choice for pain relief. The only significant side effect of such a procedure is maternal hypotension, and this may be avoided with proper preanesthetic preparation and close observation. A fluid load should be given prior to initiation of the block. The patient's blood pressure and pulse are then carefully monitored every five minutes, preferably by an anesthetist. Should hypotension begin to appear, it can be corrected easily by increasing the intravascular volume. The total fluid load must be watched, and careful intake and output records must be maintained. However, the excellent relaxation and pain relief that can be achieved by lumbar epidural anesthesia will markedly decrease the anxiety and its resultant unnecessary increased cardiac work. This anesthesia is also ideal for delivery, since it is recommended that the second stage of labor be shortened with the use of forceps. Forceps may be applied easily under epidural anesthesia.

IV. MANAGEMENT OF PATIENTS WITH MECHANICAL HEART VALVES

A. Anticoagulant Management

All women who have had mechanical heart valve placement because of rheumatic heart disease will be taking oral anticoagulants. Though some authors have suggested that use of these drugs may be omitted when the aortic valve has been replaced, the majority opinion is that this is unwise.[10,11,21–23] Many authors have suggested that coumarin derivatives are teratogenic in early pregnancy; but such effects are not universally manifest, and most infants exposed to these drugs in early pregnancy will be normal.[4] Still, the abnormalities are serious enough that, whenever possible, coumarin treatment should be withheld during early pregnancy.

If the fertility of the patient has been assessed as described earlier, she should have a thorough medical assessment and then attempt pregnancy. There are two choices for management of early pregnancy. In the first the patient may be maintained with a coumarin derivative while attempting to become pregnant but seek medical attention at the first sign of pregnancy. (She should report to her physician any delay of menses for more than one week.) It is now possible to determine pregnancy quickly by one of the qualitative serum radioimmunoassay pregnancy tests or by determination of the serum concentration of β-hCG (human chorionic gonadotropin). Both of these tests give positive results prior to implantation. The tests may be repeated daily; and at the first slight increase of β-hCG, administration of the coumarin drug can be stopped and heparin substituted.

The second plan is to discontinue maintenance with coumarin derivatives and use heparin during the time the patient is attempting to become pregnant. This avoids any possibility of fetal contact with the drug during the early developmental period. However, exposure of the embryo to coumarin during the first week is unlikely to cause the defects attributed to this drug. Additionally, if this second approach is taken the woman may be without the oral anticoagulant many times without achieving pregnancy.

As soon as conception is known to have occurred, use of all coumarin drugs should be stopped. Heparin is the ideal choice during this period, since its high molecular weight prevents its crossing the placenta. Studies have shown that heparin may be administered successfully by a number of routes.[24,25] In the United States a heparin lock is often used, and the patient is taught to self-administer the drug on a regular schedule. This results in full anticoagulation. The heparin lock must be changed frequently to avoid vasculitis.

An alternative is to give heparin subcutaneously on a rigid schedule.[24,25] This is discussed at length in Chapter M.XXII.

Heparin administration may be stopped and use of oral coumarin derivatives resumed after the first 14 weeks of pregnancy, and the patient may be maintained with these drugs until discontinuance is necessary prior to labor.

B. Prenatal Care

In pregnancy, women with mechanical heart valves are subject to the same general recommendations that apply to all women with organic heart disease in pregnancy[26] (Table M.XVIII.2). The most important part of management is close supervision of their anticoagulant status. Thrombosis of a mechanical valve during pregnancy can result in maternal morbidity and even mortality. The overall hypercoagulability of the blood during pregnancy adds somewhat to this risk, though adequate anticoagulation may carry the patient safely through pregnancy. Women taking oral anticoagulants during pregnancy should have a prothrombin time determination at least biweekly. The amount of coumarin derivative needed to maintain adequate anticoagulation usually increases during the course of a normal pregnancy. Drugs that interfere with or influence the action of the oral anticoagulants should be avoided—and many sedatives, tranquilizers, and antibiotics have such effects.[27]

Careful surveillance of cardiac rhythm must be maintained. With sudden development of atrial fibrillation during pregnancy, thromboembolic episodes are frequent. In most of these cases a predisposition to pulmonary and systemic embolism arises from the presence of mitral stenosis and partial obstruction of venous blood flow by pressure of the fetus on the pelvic veins. Should atrial fibrillation occur during pregnancy, it is very important to assess the anticoagulant status immediately and to provide additional coverage if needed. Cardioversion may be attempted; theoretically, this can induce labor and cause ventricular fibrillation in the fetus, but the procedure has been performed many times without the adverse fetal effects.[28]

TABLE M.XVIII.2. Prenatal Care for Women With Mechanical Heart Valves

Cardiac consultation
Close supervision of anticoagulant status (biweekly prothrombin time)
Adequate rest
Avoidance of strenuous exercise
Avoidance of exposure to systemic infections
Prevention of anemia
Reduction of dietary sodium
Surveillance of heart rhythm

The patient should be instructed carefully in the avoidance of exposure to systemic infections. A woman who is exposed to young children should attempt to reduce or avoid such exposure. Particularly vulnerable to these infections are teachers and others who work in child-care situations. Exposure to β-hemolytic streptococcal and other virulent bacterial infections may lead to development of bacterial endocarditis.

A persistent fever, or fever accompanied by malaise, is a bad sign in these patients. Should this occur, one must search immediately for evidence of cardiac decompensation or bacterial endocarditis; if evidence of such compromise is found, the patient should be hospitalized and stabilized quickly. In severe situations, administration of antibiotics may be started after blood for cultures has been obtained. Careful monitoring for congestive heart failure should be begun, with particular attention to any minimal changes suggestive of pulmonary congestion. In a patient with impaired function of a mechanical valve, pulmonary congestion may lead rapidly to frank pulmonary edema and severe congestive heart failure.

Routine digitalization may not be helpful, since the difficulty often is not one of heart muscle function but rather of some compromise of the mechanical valve. Vegetations on the valve may markedly decrease blood flow.

C. Labor and Delivery

1. Prophylaxis of bacterial endocarditis

During labor, all patients with valvular defects should receive adequate coverage for prevention of bacterial endocarditis. Administration of drugs effective against both gram-negative and gram-positive organisms should be instituted immediately. Also recommended is coverage against anaerobic organisms, because so many of them may contaminate the vaginal tract. In the past a combination of penicillin and an aminoglycoside was considered adequate. At present consideration should be given to including clindamycin or to replacing penicillin with one of the cephalosporins that is effective against anaerobes.

2. Anticoagulant management at term

It is most important that labor not begin while the patient is fully anticoagulated with coumarin derivatives. Therefore it is best to plan to induce delivery and prepare for the date chosen. According to the usual schedule, the patient taking coumarin derivatives is admitted to the hospital at approximately the 37th week of gestation. (For assessment of gestational age, the menstrual history and ultrasonography performed at several points during the pregnancy should provide adequate data.) Upon admission to the hospital the oral administration of anticoagulants is discontinued and heparin is given intravenously.

Although effects of coumarin may disappear rapidly from the maternal circulation, it has been reported that the fetus may exhibit some anticoagulant status for seven to ten days after the last dose. In addition, although anticoagulation in the mother may be reversed quickly by vitamin K preparations, this does not effectively reduce the anticoagulated status of the fetus; and if the birth is vaginal, cerebral hemorrhage may occur. In cases where labor begins spontaneously before adequate reversal, an attempt should be made to stop the labor by use of one of the tocolytic drugs, which are quite effective. This will allow for correction of both the maternal and fetal anticoagulated status. If the patient is refractory to these drugs and labor continues (or spontaneous rupture of membranes occurs) cesarean section should be done to protect the fetus from the trauma of delivery.

3. Delivery

The patient who has been maintained with heparin usually can be delivered with omission of only one or two doses of the drug. Depending on the likely duration of labor, the last dose of heparin may be given and induction begun by intravenous administration of oxytocin (Pitocin). After four to six hours the patient should be in a fairly normal coagulable state, and delivery may occur without undue blood loss. All bleeders present should be sutured with great care. After delivery, Pitocin may be given intravenously to help contract the uterus. Intravenous administration of heparin should be resumed within 12 hours following delivery. The patient should remain in bed the first two days to allow for sealing of the small bleeders in the episiotomy site and on the cervix. It is unusual for heavy bleeding to occur from the uterus. Vaginal and perineal hematomas have been reported, but they are rare when great attention has been paid to achieving adequate hemostasis. Even if a hematoma should occur, it is a much less serious problem than thromboembolism resulting from discontinuance of anticoagulation.

4. Management of labor

Electronic fetal monitoring is absolutely essential during labor of women with mechanical heart valves. If a fetal electrocardiogram can be obtained, that also is desirable. When proper attention has been given to reversing the anticoagulated state of the fetus, abnormalities will not be expected. Electronic fetal monitoring provides continuous surveillance and will show evidence of fetal compromise should it occur. This is particularly important if the mother develops cardiac decompensation.

The mother must be monitored continuously for evidence of cardiac failure. Blood pressure and vital signs must be checked frequently. Cardiac failure is a strong possibility in all of these cases, and one-on-one nursing care is recommended. A single-lead maternal cardiac monitor is recommended for detection of fibrillation should it occur. The change from sinus rhythm to atrial fibrillation during labor is particularly ominous; it may be followed by severe congestive heart failure.

It is important for the patient to remain comfortable with as little anxiety as possible. She and her husband would benefit from attending childbirth education classes before the initiation of labor, so that they will have some knowledge of the mechanism and events of labor and delivery.

Pain management can be a particularly difficult problem during labor in these cases. Although continuous lumbar epidural anesthesia is most reliable for alleviation of the pain due to labor,[29] most anesthesiologists are reluctant to use this procedure on a woman who will be given anticoagulants again shortly after the epidural catheter is removed. Consequently, the safest and most effective form of analgesia remaining is judicious use of small doses of narcotics, with or without addition of mild tranquilizers. For the properly prepared patient, little if any narcotic will be necessary. This regimen should carry the patient to the second stage of labor.

It is beneficial to shorten the second stage of labor as much as possible to limit the workload added to the heart by pushing. However, if a patient has had an entirely normal prenatal course and has experienced no complications during labor, and if she has been properly prepared in the correct method of delivery, she may be allowed to push with careful cardiac monitoring. But if any cardiac compromise has been noted, however slight, it is best to avoid this stage of labor and to take the patient to the delivery room as soon as complete cervical dilatation has occurred.

The presence of an anesthesiologist familiar with and fully trained in obstetric anesthesia is of great benefit at this point. Because it is necessary to use forceps to shorten this stage of labor, cooperation between the two specialties is most important. Although most forceps deliveries may be accomplished with pudendal regional anesthesia, it is not a wise choice for someone who will be receiving anticoagulants again shortly after delivery. Therefore small doses of gaseous anesthetic agents should be used for rapid vaginal delivery with the aid of forceps. This is quite satisfactory in the majority of cases and results in no maternal or fetal compromise. The status of the fetus should be monitored continuously by means of a fetal scalp electrode. Local anesthesia in the area of the episiotomy may be used, since any bleeding wound related to it can be sutured carefully during the episiotomy repair.

Generally, the choice of vaginal or abdominal delivery should be made on the basis of obstetric indications.[26] The one exception is the case of a patient who is taking anticoagulants orally and who presents in active labor that cannot be stopped by tocolytic agents. In this case the danger to the fetus from intercerebral bleeds, should vaginal delivery occur, is significant enough that consideration should be given to performing cesarean section as soon as the mother's anticoagulated status can be corrected. In all other circumstances the decision for vaginal or abdominal delivery depends on the obstetric condition. Cephalopelvic disproportion, fetal distress, and other usual indications for cesarean section apply in these cases. If cesarean section is performed, obviously much care must be taken to maintain hemostasis. One region that must be watched carefully is the area under the bladder flap on the anterior wall of the uterus. Great care should be taken to ensure that no bleeders are left in this space. Anticoagulant therapy must be restarted soon after delivery, even if cesarean section is employed.

D. Postpartum Management

1. Maternal monitoring

After delivery, patients with mechanical valves remain at high risk for cardiac decompensation for 72 hours. If the prenatal course and labor and delivery have been accomplished without any evidence of cardiac compromise, the patient may be followed in the usual postpartum recovery room. But if cardiac compromise has been noted, it is wise to admit the patient to the coronary intensive care unit for observation. Because of the bolus of blood that is delivered to the circulation immediately after delivery, it is not unusual for cardiac decompensation to occur during the next few hours.

2. Postpartum anticoagulation

Intravenous administration of heparin should be resumed four to 12 hours after delivery.[30] The patient should be restricted mostly to bed for the first 48 hours and should avoid bending, stooping, lifting, or any other activity that applies pressure to the area of the episiotomy. Perineal vaginal and vulvar hematomas have occurred after prompt reinstitution of anticoagulants, but they are unusual. Oral anticoagulant therapy may be begun on the third or fourth postpartum day. It is advisable to wait this long in case hemorrhage into the episiotomy site occurs. With either kind of anticoagulant, heavy postpartum uterine bleeding is unusual. Care must be taken to be sure the uterus remains fully contracted. For the first 24 hours, 20 units of Pitocin should be given in each liter of intravenous solution.

3. Breast-feeding

Nearly 80% of women delivering babies prefer to breastfeed their infants, and many women taking oral anticoagulants choose to do likewise. No problem is encountered while the patient is taking heparin, because this does not cross into the milk. The oral coumarin derivatives, however, do pass into breast milk and the infant readily absorbs them from its gastrointestinal tract. No case of resultant serious neonatal bleeding has been reported, but some prolongation of the prothrombin time in the neonate has been described.[22] If the woman chooses to breastfeed her infant, prothrombin determinations should be made on the child, weekly at first and monthly later. Supplementation with vitamin K will easily correct any prolongation that might be noted.

V. MANAGEMENT OF PATIENTS WITH OTHER VALVE IMPLANTS OR REPAIRS

A. Pregnancy Following Biologic Valve Implant

Cardiovascular surgeons have begun to implant glutaraldehyde-preserved porcine heart valves instead of mechanical valves. A recent review of 128 cases[6] in which this type of valve was implanted showed that the five- to eight-year survival of the valves paralleled that expected with mechanical heart valves. The main advantage of the biologic valve is that the patient does not need continuous anticoagulation. The main disadvantage, however, is uncertainty over long-term survival of the valve and the possibility that another replacement will be needed after ten to 15 years.[12] The review by Cohn et al[6] showed good results over a number of years, which makes such valves seem most attractive—particularly for young women who wish to consider pregnancy.

Management of labor and delivery is essentially the same as that described for patients with mechanical heart valves, except that the considerations concerning anticoagulant status do not apply (unless the patient has a mitral biologic valve with previous embolism, atrial fibrillation, or left atrial enlargement). The effects of labor and delivery on the biologic heart valve are less well known than are their effects on mechanical heart valves. It seems prudent, however, to maintain the patient as comfortably as possible so that cardiac output will not be increased unnecessarily. Here again, the second stage of labor should be shortened by the use of forceps. Lumbar epidural anesthesia seems to be the ideal kind for delivery, since anticoagulation is not a factor in most of these cases.

B. Pregnancy Following Valvular Repair (Mitral Commissurotomy)

Prior to the availability of valve replacement, closed mitral commissurotomy was a frequently employed procedure. Large series of cases have been reported in which pregnancy followed it, or it was performed during pregnancy. Maternal mortality when the procedure was done during pregnancy has been approximately 2%, but the fetal mortality was generally reported to be 8–10%.[31]

Now closed mitral commissurotomy has nearly disappeared from surgical practice. The indications have become so strict that it is unlikely to be performed during pregnancy. Most women who have severe enough cardiac compromise to require cardiac surgery will require valve replacement. As already noted, this is best performed before initiation of pregnancy. The preceding section of this chapter reviewed the indications for valve replacement or commissurotomy during pregnancy.

If a woman who has had commissurotomy performed becomes pregnant, she may be expected to experience cardiac compromise if the mitral valve is unable to permit the additional cardiac output that occurs during normal pregnancy. A woman not able to tolerate exercise before pregnancy would be expected to have serious complications during pregnancy, and consideration should be given to valve replacement before conception. Should pregnancy occur first, consideration must be given to placement of an artificial heart valve during its course if it appears that the patient is experiencing cardiac decompensation. The signs of such compromise might occur quite early in pregnancy, since the intravascular volume increases rapidly during the first five months of pregnancy. The patient must have adequate bed rest and must avoid any unnecessary exercise. This is true even if her cardiovascular status has been fairly stable and normal before pregnancy. It must be remembered that in these cases the mitral valve is often quite rigid and the aperture for blood flow very limited.

VI. ACKNOWLEDGMENTS

The author wishes to express his gratitude to James H. Chesebro, MD, Division of Cardiovascular Diseases and Internal Medicine, Mayo Clinic, for his help in the preparation of this chapter.

VII. REFERENCES

1. Szekely P, Turner R, Snaith L. Pregnancy and the changing pattern of rheumatic heart disease. Br Heart J. 1973; 35:1293–1303.
2. Bloomfield DK, Rubinstein LI. Mitral-valve prosthesis, warfarin anticoagulation, and pregnancy. Lancet. 1969; 2:290–291.

3. Harrison EC, Roschke EJ. Pregnancy in patients with cardiac valve prostheses. Clin Obstet Gynecol. 1975; 18:107–123.
4. Lutz DJ, Noller KL, Spittell JA Jr, Danielson GK, Fish CR. Pregnancy and its complications following cardiac valve prostheses. Am J Obstet Gynecol. 1978; 131:460–466.
5. Beadle EM Jr, Luepker RV, Williams PP. Pregnancy in a patient with porcine valve xenografts. Am Heart J. 1979; 98:510–512.
6. Cohn LH, Mudge GH, Pratter F, Collins JJ Jr. Five to eight-year follow-up of patients undergoing porcine heart-valve replacement. N Engl J Med. 1981; 304:258–262.
7. Chesley LC. Severe rheumatic cardiac disease and pregnancy: the ultimate prognosis. Am J Obstet Gynecol. 1980; 136:552–558.
8. Estafanous FG, Buckley S. Management of anesthesia for open heart surgery during pregnancy. Cleve Clin Q. 1976; 43:121–124.
9. Zitnik RS, Brandenburg RO, Sheldon R, Wallace RB. Pregnancy and open-heart surgery. Circulation. 1969; 39(Suppl 1):257–262.
10. Chesebro JH, Fuster V. Thromboembolism in heart valve replacement. In: Kwaan HC, Bowie EJW, eds. Textbook of Thrombosis. Philadelphia: W.B. Saunders Company (in press).
11. Fuster V, Chesebro JH. Series on pharmacology in practice. 10. Antithrombotic therapy: Role of platelet-inhibitor drugs. III. Management of arterial thromboembolic and atherosclerotic disease (third of three parts). Mayo Clin Proc. 1981; 56:265–273.
12. Kirklin JW. The replacement of cardiac valves (editorial). N Engl J Med. 1981; 304:291–292.
13. Oakley C, Doherty P. Pregnancy in patients after valve replacement. Br Heart J. 1976; 38:1140–1148.
14. Limet R, Grondin CM. Cardiac valve prostheses, anticoagulation, and pregnancy. Ann Thorac Surg. 1977; 23:337–341.
15. Casanegra P, Avilés G, Maturana G, Dubernet J. Cardiovascular management of pregnant women with a heart valve prosthesis. Am J Cardiol. 1975; 36:802–806.
16. DiSaia PJ. Pregnancy and delivery of a patient with a Starr-Edwards mitral valve prosthesis: Report of a case. Obstet Gynecol. 1966; 28:469–472.
17. McCans JL, Wenger NK. Problems in management of the pregnant patient with rheumatic heart disease and valve prosthesis. South Med J. 1976; 69:1007–1010.
18. Bonebrake CR, Noller KL, Loehnen CP, Muhm JR, Fish CR. Routine chest roentgenography in pregnancy. JAMA. 1978; 240:2747–2748.
19. Schaefer G, Arditi LI, Solomon HA, Ringland JE. Congenital heart disease and pregnancy. Clin Obstet Gynecol. 1968; 11:1048–1063.
20. Ho PC, Chen TY, Wong V. The effect of maternal cardiac disease and digoxin administration on labour, fetal weight and maturity at birth. Aust NZ J Obstet Gynaecol. 1980; 20:24–27.
21. Editorial. Anticoagulants and heart valve replacement in pregnancy. Br Med J. 1977; 1:1047–1048.
22. Fenech A, Winter JH, Douglas AS. Individualisation of oral anticoagulant therapy. Drugs. 1979; 18:48–57.
23. Laros RK Jr, Hage ML, Hayashi RH. Pregnancy and heart valve prostheses. Obstet Gynecol. 1970; 35:241–247.
24. Spearing G, Fraser I, Turner G, Dixon G. Long-term self-administered subcutaneous heparin in pregnancy. Br Med J. 1978; 1:1457–1458.
25. Kakkar VV. The current status of low-dose heparin in the prophylaxis of thrombophlebitis and pulmonary embolism. World J Surg. 1978; 2:3–18.
26. Ibarra-Perez C, Arevalo-Toledo N, Alvarez-de la Cadena O, Noriega-Guerra L. The course of pregnancy in patients with artificial heart valves. Am J Med. 1976; 61:504–512.
27. Moseley P, Kerstein MD. Pregnancy and thrombophlebitis. Surg Gynecol Obstet. 1980; 150:593–599.
28. DeSilva RA, Graboys TB, Podrid PJ, Lown B. Cardioversion and defibrillation. Am Heart J. 1980; 100:881–895.
29. Pedersen H, Finster M. Anesthetic risk in the pregnant surgical patient. Anesthesiology. 1979; 51:439–451.
30. Gothard JWW. Heart disease in pregnancy: the anaesthetic management of a patient with prosthetic heart valves. Anaesthesia. 1978; 33:523–526.
31. Editorial. Mitral commissurotomy during pregnancy. J Assoc Physicians India. 1978; 26:929–931.

Cardiovascular Drugs in Pregnancy

M.XIX

Use of Beta-Adrenergic Blocking Agents During Pregnancy

Neal A. Klein, MD, and William H. Frishman, MD

I. INTRODUCTION

The therapeutic indications for β-adrenergic blocking drugs are varied. These drugs have proven efficacy in the treatment of hypertension, arrhythmias, hyperthyroidism, atherosclerotic heart disease, migraine headache, and glaucoma.[1] Many of these conditions will manifest themselves during the reproductive years of the female patient. The desire to ensure both maternal health and normal fetal growth and development has led to questions regarding the safety of β-blocker use during pregnancy. In this review, the world experience with β-blocker treatment during pregnancy is assessed. Recommendations concerning β-blocker administration during pregnancy are proposed in light of this world experience.

II. ADRENERGIC INFLUENCE ON MATERNAL–FETAL PHYSIOLOGY

Beta-adrenergic activity during pregnancy assumes physiological importance because of the direct effects the sympathetic nervous system has on umbilical blood flow and uterine tone and contractility (see Table M.XIX.1). Because of the difficulty in studying humans and the need to separate direct from indirect sympathetic effects, most experimental work on umbilical blood flow has been conducted in the pregnant ewe. Oakes et al[2] studied the effects of propranolol and isoproterenol in nonlaboring anesthetized pregnant sheep that were near term. During fetal or maternal infusion of the β-blocker, there was a significant decrease in umbilical blood flow and in the maternal and

Cardiac Problems in Pregnancy, pages 221–225

TABLE M.XIX.1. Effects of Adrenergic Stimulation or Blockade on Maternal–Fetal Physiology

	Stimulation		Blockade
	α-Receptor	β-Receptor	β-receptor
Umbilical blood flow	No effect	↑	↓
Myometrial activity	↑	↓	↑
Fetal heart rate	No effect	↑	No effect or ↓

fetal heart rate. Uterine blood flow and systemic blood pressure remained unchanged. With isoproterenol infusion there was an increase in umbilical blood flow and only a small increment in fetal heart rate. It may therefore be concluded that β-adrenergic tone affects basal umbilical blood flow and a disturbance in sympathetic inputs could be potentially harmful to the developing fetus.

Alpha-agonists influence umbilical blood flow indirectly through their action on uterine blood vessels. When a low dose of norepinephrine was infused directly into a uterine artery, a profound reduction in uteroplacental blood flow developed.[3] A direct action of norepinephrine on the umbilical circulation has not been demonstrated.[4,5]

In the myometrium there are adrenergic receptors of the α and β types. Stimulation of the β-receptor results in myometrial relaxation, whereas increased α-adrenergic stimulation potentiates contractility.[6] In animal studies propranolol has been shown to reverse the myometrial depressant action of β-stimulation.[7] Barden and his associates[8] also demonstrated this effect of propranolol in pregnant humans. In their study, pregnant women at term were selected for elective induction of labor. Maternal and fetal heart rates, maternal blood pressure, and intrauterine pressure were measured in all patients. After an infusion of oxytocin to eight patients, epinephrine was administered and caused a consistent inhibition of uterine activity while accelerating maternal heart rate. These effects were completely reversed by prior propranolol treatment. Norepinephrine infusion potentiated uterine activity while decreasing maternal heart rate and increasing blood pressure. Prior propranolol treatment had no effect, whereas the α-adrenergic blocker phentolamine significantly attenuated the actions of norepinephrine. After these studies, all the subjects had normal term vaginal deliveries.

The influence of the autonomic nervous system on normal fetal circulation has also been studied in the fetal lamb preparation. In a report by Joelson,[9] isoproterenol administered to the fetus caused an increase in heart rate and a decrease in blood pressure, whereas propranolol caused only a slight drop in heart rate. All of the isoproterenol effects could be blocked by previous propranolol administration. When the fetus was stressed by cord occlusions, propranolol completely abolished the normal increased heart rate. It was apparent that the effects of β-adrenergic blockade from the unstressed and undisturbed fetus were minimal. However, when the fetus is stressed, stimulation of the β-receptor may provide an important reserve for neonatal adaptation. Thus, maternal treatment with β-blockers may impair the response to fetal distress.

II. CLINICAL EXPERIENCE

A. Propranolol

Propranolol, the oldest of the available nonselective β-blockers, was the first such agent to have wide application in pregnant patients (see Table M.XIX.2). Since its early use in the late 1960s, many favorable reports have accumulated. The drug has been employed successfully in the treatment of gestational hypertension,[10] thyrotoxicosis,[11] obstructive cardiomyopathy,[12] paroxysmal atrial tachycardia,[13] dysfunctional uterine activity,[14] and fetal tachycardia.[15]

TABLE M.XIX.2. Reported Adverse Reactions of β-Adrenergic Blocking Drugs in Pregnancy and in the Neonate

Intrauterine growth retardation
Maternal and fetal bradycardia
Premature labor
Delayed neonatal breathing
Neonatal hypoglycemia
Neonatal hyperbilirubinemia

Despite this encouraging experience in therapy, many severe adverse reactions have also been reported. The most consistent observation has been intrauterine fetal growth retardation. In a long-term study of 12 human pregnancies during which chronic propranolol was administered, Pruyn et al[16] demonstrated poor intrauterine growth in half of the cases. They suggested that the experimental model of decreased umbilical blood flow in the ewe after propranolol administration could explain their findings. A decrease in umbilical blood flow could deprive the growing fetus of needed nutrients and thus impair growth.

Other reported adverse effects in the fetus include apnea at birth,[17] bradycardia,[18] hypoglycemia,[19] polycythemia,[20] hyperbilirubinemia,[16] and prolonged labor.[18] None of the above reactions was reported consistently in chronic therapy studies. Many of these reactions may represent the consequences of fetal distress occurring in high-risk obstetrical patients. However, these isolated case reports deserve close attention and consideration. In treating any pregnant patients with propranolol, the benefits of this treatment can be weighed against adverse effects upon the fetus.

B. Metoprolol

Metoprolol is a β_1-selective blocking agent. It is similar in its effectiveness to other, nonselective β-adrenoceptor blocking drugs used in the treatment of angina pectoris[21] or essential hypertension.[22] Because of its primary β_1-selective properties, the drug would theoretically not interfere with β_2-mediated peripheral vasodilatation or β_2 effects on uterine tone.

In a large-scale clinical study,[23] 101 pregnant patients with systemic hypertension were treated with metoprolol alone or in combination with hydralazine and a diuretic for a mean period of four weeks during pregnancy. This group was compared to 97 hypertensive gravidae treated with hydralazine. Perinatal mortality was lower in the metoprolol group as was the rate of fetal growth retardation. No significant adverse effects were reported in the fetus. Apparently metoprolol, like propranolol,[19] crosses the placenta; however, the concentration of the drug was relatively low in umbilical blood samples. This low drug level in the umbilical circulation was apparently related to poor maternal drug absorption, as maternal blood levels were also comparatively low. This experience with metoprolol, and a similar experience with the β_1 selective blocking agent atenolol,[24] raises the hope that a selective β-blocker could be used more safely during pregnancy.

C. Labetalol

Labetalol is a recently developed drug which, like propranolol, blocks both β_1 and β_2 adrenoceptors.[25] However, labetalol is unique in that it also has both α-adrenergic blocking properties and direct vasodilatory activity. This drug has been shown to be a potent antihypertensive agent.[26,27]

The use of this drug in the treatment of pregnant patients with hypertension is limited; however, those few reports that are available are favorable. In one study, 25 pregnant women suffering from severe hypertension received labetalol.[28] Effective reductions in blood pressure were achieved in 22. No adverse effects were reported, and it was not necessary to discontinue the drug in any patient. Perinatal mortality was reported to be 3.5 %. When compared to methyldopa, in a separate investigation, labetalol was found to be more effective in reducing blood pressure.[29] Again, no detrimental effects were reported, and all the pregnancies went well without postnatal complications. Further large-scale studies using this unique adrenergic blocking agent are eagerly awaited.

IV. RECOMMENDATIONS

A comprehensive recommendation concerning the use of β-adrenergic blocking drugs for the treatment of complicating medical disorders in pregnancy is extremely difficult to make. This difficulty arises from a lack of any large-scale clinical experience with these agents in pregnant patients. More studies are needed to define drug pharmacokinetics in mother and fetus. Also comparative studies are warranted to assess the safety and efficacy of β-blocking drugs and existing therapies.

At present, the use of β-blockers in pregnancy must be individualized to the needs of each patient. It is probably advisable to offer other effective drugs prior to using β-blocker therapy, if the other agents have been proved safe during pregnancy. If a β-blocker must be used, then the pregnant patient should be considered at risk for developing potential complications. Careful fetal monitoring is required, and the potential risks must be explained to the patient. In some patients, the β-adrenoceptor blocking agents may hold promise as effective therapies for controlling maternal disease states, thereby allowing for normal fetal development (Table M.XIX.3). The use of β-adrenergic blocking agents as antihypertensive drugs is presented in chapter M.XXI.

TABLE M.XIX.3. Clinical Uses of β-Adrenergic Blocking Agents in Pregnancy

Hypertension
Supraventricular arrhythmias
Hypertrophic cardiomyopathy
Maternal thyrotoxicosis
Dysfunctional labor
Fetal tachycardia

V. ACKNOWLEDGMENTS

Dr. Frishman is a Teaching Scholar of The American Heart Association. This work was supported in part by grant HL 00653-1 of the National Heart–Lung Institute.

VI. REFERENCES

1. Frishman W, Silverman R. Clinical pharmacology of the new beta-adrenergic blocking drugs. Part 3. Comparative clinical experience and new therapeutic applications. Am Heart J. 1979; 98:119–131.
2. Oakes GK, Walker AD, Ehrenkranz RA, Chez RA. Effect of propranolol infusion on the umbilical and uterine circulations of pregnant sheep. Am J Obstet Gynecol. 1976; 126: 1038–1042.
3. Ladner E, Brinkman CR, Weston P, Assali NS. Dynamics of uterine circulation in pregnant and non-pregnant sheep. Am J Physiol. 1970; 218:257–263.
4. Adams FH, Assali NS, Cushman M, Westersten A. Interrelationships of maternal and fetal circulations. 1. Flow-pressure responses to vasoactive drugs in sheep. Pediatrics. 1961; 27:627–635.
5. Chez RA, Ehrenkranz RA, Oakes GK, Walke AM, Hamilton LA, Vrennan SC, McLaughlin MK. Effects of adrenergic agents on bovine umbilical and uterine blood flows. In: Longo L, Reneau DD, eds. Fetal and Newborn Cardiovascular Physiology, Vol 2. New York: Garland, 1978.
6. Maughan GB, Shabanah EH, Toth A. Experiments with pharmacologic sympatholysis in the gravid. Am J Obstet Gynecol. 1967; 97:764–776.
7. Wansbrough H, Nakanishi H, Wood C. Effect of epinephrine on human uterine activity in vitro and in vivo. Obstet Gynecol. 1967; 30:779–789.
8. Barden TP, Stander RW. Effects of adrenergic blocking agents and catecholamines in human pregnancy. Am J Obstet Gynecol. 1968; 102: 226–235.
9. Joelson I, Barton MD. The effect of blockade of the beta-receptors of the sympathetic nervous system of the fetus. Acta Obstet Gynecol Scand. 1969; 3(Suppl)48:75–79.
10. Eliahou HE, Silverberg DS, Reisin E, Romem I, Mashiach S, Serr DM. Propranolol for the treatment of hypertension in pregenancy. Br J Obstet Gynaecol. 1978; 85:431–436.
11. Bullock JL, Harris RE, Young R. Treatment of thyrotoxicosis during pregnancy and propranolol. Am J Obstet Gynecol. 1975; 121:242–245.
12. Turner GM, Oakley CM, Dixon HG. Management of pregnancy complicated by hypertrophic obstructive cardiomyopathy. Br Med J. 1968; 4:281–284.

13. Schroeder JS, Harrison DC. Repeated cardioversion during pregnancy: Treatment of refractory paroxysmal atrial tachycardia during three successive pregnancies. Am J Cardiol. 1971; 27:445–446.
14. Mitrani A, Oettinger M, Abinader EG, et al. Use of propranolol in dysfunctional labour. Br J Obstet Gynecol. 1975; 82:651–655.
15. Teuscher A, Bossi E, Imhof P, Erb E, Stocker F, Weber J. Effect of propranolol on fetal tachycardia in diabetic pregnancy. Am J Cardiol. 1978; 42:304–307.
16. Pruyn SC, Phelan JP, Buchanan GC. Long-term propranolol therapy in pregnancy: Maternal and fetal outcome. Am J Obstet Gynecol. 1979; 135:485–489.
17. Turnstall MB. The effect of propranolol on the onset of breathing at birth. Br J Anesthesiol. 1969; 41:792.
18. Habib A, McCarthy JS. Effects on the neonate of propranolol administered during pregnancy. J Pediatr. 1977; 91:808–811.
19. Cottrill CM, McAllister RG, Gettes L, Noonan JA. Propranolol therapy during pregnancy, labor, and delivery: Evidence for transplacental drug transfer and impaired neonatal drug disposition. J Pediatr. 1977; 91:812–814.
20. Gladstone GR, Hordof A, Gersong WM. Propranolol administration during pregnancy: Effects on the fetus. J Pediatr. 1975; 86:962–964.
21. Adolfsson L, Areskog NH, Furberg C, Johnsson G. Effects of single doses of alprenolol and two cardioselective β-blockers (H 87/07 and H93/20) on exercise induced angina pectoris. Eur J Clin Pharmacol. 1974; 7:111–118.
22. Bengtsson C, Johnsson G, Regardth CG. Plasma levels and effects of metoprolol on blood pressure and heart rate after acute dose and between two doses during long-term treatment. Clin Pharmacol Ther. 1975; 17:400–408.
23. Sandström B. Antihypertensive treatment with the adrenergic beta-receptor blocker metoprolol during pregnancy. Gynecol Obstet Invest. 1978; 9:195–204.
24. Lunell NO, Persson B, Aragon G, Fredholm BB, Aström H. Circulatory and metabolic effects of acute beta-1 blockade in severe pre-eclampsia. Acta Obstet Gynecol Scand. 1979; 58:443–445.
25. Frishman W, Halprin S. Clinical pharmacology of the new beta-adrenergic blocking drugs. Part 7. New horizons in beta-adrenoceptor blockade therapy. Am Heart J. 1979; 98:660–665.
26. Mehta J, Cohn JN. Hemodynamic effects of labetalol, an alpha and beta adrenergic blocking agent in hypertensive subject. Circulation. 1977; 55:370–375.
27. Prichard BNC, Boakes AJ. Labetalol in long-term treatment of hypertension. Br J Clin Pharmacol. 1976; 3(Suppl 3):743–750.
28. Michael CA. Use of labetalol in the treatment of severe hypertension during pregnancy. Br J Clin Pharmacol. 1979; 8(Suppl 2):211s–215s.
29. Lamming GD, Symonds EB. Use of labetalol and methyldopa in pregnancy-induced hypertension. Br J Clin Pharmacol. 1979; 8(Suppl 2):217s–222s.

M. XX

Clinical Pharmacology of Antiarrhythmic Drugs in the Pregnant Patient

Heschi H. Rotmensch, MD, Joseph B. Lessing, MD, and Yoel Donchin, MD

I. INTRODUCTION

The pregnant woman with cardiac arrhythmias constitutes a major concern and challenge to the physician, since arrhythmia-related hemodynamic alterations may harm the fetus by decreasing uterine blood flow and may place the mother in jeopardy.

Arrhythmias may occur in an otherwise healthy woman or in those with valvular heart disease, pericardial disease, mitral valve prolapse, myocarditis, cardiomyopathy, endocrine disorders, and coronary artery disease. Therapy should be directed toward the underlying disease, when present, with the goal being improvement of cardiovascular function by termination of symptomatic arrhythmias, prevention of their recurrence, or rate control. Recently, administration of drugs to the mother for the management of arrhythmias in the fetus has been recognized as a reasonable therapeutic intervention. The decision regarding the necessity of antiarrhythmic therapy will be based upon the nature and severity of the maternal or fetal arrhythmia, weighing the benefit of therapy against the risk of adverse effects to both the mother and the fetus.

II. GENERAL CONSIDERATIONS

Recent advances in the detection of drugs in serum and tissue have demonstrated that there are virtually no body

Cardiac Problems in Pregnancy, pages 227–243

tissues, including the placenta and the fetus, that do not receive some fraction of the administered dose.[1] Thus, availability of any pharmacologic agent to the developing fetus within the pregnant woman has become an increasing source of concern. In addition to acting directly on the fetus, the pharmacological agent may affect uteroplacental blood flow. The breastfed neonate is also vulnerable, since a number of potential harmful drugs are excreted in the milk.[2]

The pharmacologic and toxic effect of a drug on the human fetus will depend on a balance between three factors: the dose and disposition in the maternal-placental-fetal unit, the stage of fetal development, and the genetic susceptibility of the fetus.[3]

Early in pregnancy, during the period of embryogenesis, human fetal tissues are highly susceptible to chemical dysmorphogenesis, and drug exposure may result in abortion or malformations. Therefore, in principle, it is advisable to minimize or avoid drug administration during the first trimester of pregnancy. In the second and third trimesters, interference with normal growth and development is the major problem encountered. Subtle and late effects of some agents may be assessed only some time after delivery when neuro-behavioral studies can be performed.[4]

In view of the nature of the physiological and biochemical changes that occur during pregnancy, it is to be anticipated that pharmacokinetic parameters are modified.[5] For example, the reduced gastrointestinal motility that occurs during pregnancy is likely to enhance drug absorption, while metabolism of drugs in the placenta and/or the fetus may account for their increased clearance. Reduction in serum albumin concentrations during pregnancy may increase the amount of free drug reaching the fetus.

Additional factors that may influence the fetal exposure to, and neonatal burden of, drugs administered in childbirth include the mode and interval from maternal drug administration to delivery and fetal pH.[6]

At present little definite information is available to show the pharmacokinetic relevance of prenatal metabolic processes on changes in plasma concentrations of drugs in the maternal or fetal blood of humans.

When pharmacological treatment is necessary, only drugs with a long history of safety during gestation should be considered. Unfortunately, studies on the effects of antiarrhythmic agents on the course of gestation and the human fetus are scant, and treatment continues to be largely empirical. Some of the data available derives from the relatively extensive use of drugs such as lidocaine and phenytoin during pregnancy for reasons unrelated to cardiac disease.

This chapter summarizes the current state-of-knowledge of antiarrhythmic agents, with emphasis on clinical pharmacology and therapeutic use in the pregnant patient. Both established agents and several new or experimental drugs are reviewed.

III. ANTIARRHYTHMIC AGENTS

A. Lidocaine

Lidocaine, a local anesthetic, has gained considerable popularity for the relief of maternal discomfort during labor and delivery. It is also useful in the treatment of arrhythmias, particularly ectopic and reentrant ventricular arrhythmias of many etiologies, including digitalis toxicity. It is of little use in supraventricular arrhythmias.[7,8] Because of its efficacy and rapid action, lidocaine is usually the agent of first choice for terminating acute ventricular arrhythmias. After control of the arrhythmia, administration for 24 to 36 hours is customary to prevent recurrence.

1. Electrophysiological properties

Lidocaine reduces the action potential duration in normal myocardial cells. It also reduces the effective refractory period, but less so, and therefore the ratio of effective refractory period to action potential duration is increased. It has also been shown to depress automaticity in Purkinje fibers by retarding phase 4 depolarization.[9] In therapeutic doses, its effect on conduction velocity in normal fibers is negligible, while it may slow conduction in the His-Purkinje system and the ventricular myocardium in fibers depressed by ischemia.[10]

2. Pharmacokinetics

Lidocaine is administered only parenterally because bioavailability after oral doses is very low. When given intramuscularly, absorption is rapid and complete. Action is immediate after a single intravenous bolus of the drug, and dissipation begins within ten to 20 minutes owing to drug redistribution. Lidocaine is eliminated primarily by hepatic metabolism, and its active metabolites (monoethylglycinexylidide, MEGX; glycinexylidide, GX) may contribute to both therapeutic and toxic effects. The half-life of lidocaine is about 100 minutes,[11] but it may be markedly prolonged in disease states, resulting in decreased hepatic blood flow. The therapeutic range of lidocaine is 2–4 μg/ml, although control of ventricular premature beats can be achieved with levels as low as 0.6–2 μg/ml,[12] which may be reached after the administration of an epidural block for labor pain. Toxic effects are seen at levels of about 6–10 μg/ml.

For a prompt therapeutic effect, an initial loading dose of 1–1.4 mg/kg of lidocaine should be given intravenously; then a continuous infusion of 1–4 mg/min should be started. Half the loading dose may be given as a further bolus after ten minutes if the arrhythmia has not been abolished.

3. Adverse effects

In therapeutic doses, lidocaine exerts no cardiac depressant effects, but rare cases of atrioventricular block[13] and asystole[14] have been reported. Toxic doses can cause myocardial depression, hypotension, and neurological abnormalities such as dizziness, disorientation, respiratory depression, and seizures.

4. Obstetric considerations

Numerous studies have demonstrated the ability of lidocaine to cross the placenta after epidural and intravenous administration to the mother.[15–17] After epidural administration of lidocaine to women in labor, the intrauterine fetal blood concentrations, and the corresponding umbilical vein and artery concentrations, at delivery are approximately 50–60% of the concomitant maternal levels.[18,19] Measurements of lidocaine and its active metabolites (MEGX, GX) in cord plasma and the neonate urine showed that the fetus at term is capable of metabolizing the drug.[20] Recent experiments in pregnant sheep have demonstrated no difference in the total body clearance of lidocaine between pregnant and nonpregnant ewes.[21]

The half-life of lidocaine in neonates who have acquired the drug in utero is approximately three hours,[19] as opposed to about 100 minutes in adults. At therapeutic blood levels there is no evidence of any adverse effects on either the uterus or the uteroplacental circulation.[22] High doses of lidocaine injected directly into the dorsal aorta were found to cause a temporary decrease in uterine blood flow, whereas prolonged exposure with blood levels of 2–4 μg/ml did not significantly alter amniotic fluid pressure and uterine blood flow. No effect on uterine activity during labor was observed at therapeutic levels.[23] Intrauterine injection of lidocaine into the fetus had no influence on fetal heart rate.[24] Even though the incidence of serious adverse effects is generally low, there exists a potential risk of central nervous system and cardiac toxicity in the fetus and neonate when lidocaine is administered in the presence of fetal acidosis. Since lidocaine is a weak base, the lower the fetal pH, the greater the amount of drug that will be ionized. This will lead to ion-trapping in the fetal circulation.[25] Fetal plasma binding of lidocaine may be decreased in the presence of acidosis, and this may exacerbate the trapping of the agent in fetal tissues.[26] There is no evidence to suggest that exposure to lidocaine early in pregnancy is related to an increased risk of any particular malformation.[27] Neurobehavioral studies performed on newborns of mothers given an epidural block with lidocaine demonstrated that subtle changes in the neonatal period may occasionally occur.[28,29]

In conclusion, it appears that the use of lidocaine for the treatment of acute ventricular arrhythmias is safe for both mothers and their fetuses.

Congeners of lidocaine such as tocainide[30] and mexiletine[31] are undergoing clinical evaluation in the United States. These orally effective antiarrhythmic agents have pharmacologic and electrophysiologic properties similar to those of lidocaine. Both agents undergo much less rapid hepatic metabolism and have higher oral bioavailability with longer half-lives. There is virtually no experience with these drugs in the pregnant patient, and for this reason they cannot be recommended at this time.

B. Quinidine

The efficacy of quinidine in suppressing premature extrasystoles and tachycardias of both supraventricular and ventricular origin is well established.[32] Quinidine is used to terminate paroxysmal supraventricular tachycardia, atrial fibrillation, or atrial flutter of recent onset as well as to prevent their recurrence after successful conversion to sinus rhythm. It is a widely used agent against ventricular arrhythmias of various etiologies and against tachyarrhythmias associated with the Wolff-Parkinson-White syndrome.

1. Electrophysiological properties

Quinidine has a direct depressant effect on automaticity, conduction velocity, and contractility in the heart, as well as indirect anticholinergic actions. The effective refractory period is increased in atrial, ventricular, and Purkinje fibers, with a lesser increase in action potential duration, so that the ratio of effective refractory period to action potential duration is increased.[33] By prolonging the conduction in depressed myocardial fibers of a reentrant pathway, quinidine may terminate reentrant ventricular arrhythmias. The direct effect of quinidine on the atrioventricular node is to increase the refractory period, but its anticholinergic action opposes this and usually predominates. Thus, the use of quinidine in supraventricular tachycardia may result in a more rapid atrioventricular nodal conduction, followed by an increase in ventricular rate, and it should therefore be preceded by digitalization.

Quinidine produces peripheral vasodilation, which together with a decreased cardiac output, may lead to hypotension.

2. Pharmacokinetics

Oral quinidine is well absorbed, and systemic bioavailability varies from 70 to 90%.[34] The onset of action with oral administration begins within 30 minutes, and a peak effect is reached in two to three hours. Quinidine is metabolized in the liver to several compounds, some of which have antiarrhythmic properties. Since about 20% of a dose is excreted unchanged in the urine, it is advisable to adjust the dosage according to renal function. The dosage should be reduced in patients with congestive heart failure.

Therapeutic plasma concentrations for prophylactic effect are in the range of 2–5 μg/ml. Higher plasma levels ranging from 4 to 9 μg/ml are usually required for conversion of atrial fibrillation to normal sinus rhythm.[35] These levels may be achieved by 200–400 mg of quinidine given every two hours for five to six doses for loading, followed by 1–2 gm per day. Nonacute therapy may begin with maintenance doses. The administration of quinidine to patients receiving digoxin was found to raise the serum concentration of the latter and to increase the incidence of digitalis intoxication.[36,37] Therefore, serum digoxin concentrations and electrocardiograms should be followed carefully when quinidine is given in digitalized patients.

Quinidine has a relatively short plasma half-life of four to eight hours. For long-term use in the prevention of arrhythmias, sustained-release oral preparations on a twice-daily regime are most useful in maintaining therapeutic levels. Blood levels of quinidine will help the clinician judge how much drug should be given. The intravenous route of administration can lead to severe hypotension and should therefore be avoided.

3. Adverse effects

Side effects of quinidine, including nausea, vomiting, diarrhea, and vertigo are common and may prompt cessation of therapy in up to one-fourth of patients. Hypersensitivity phenomena may occur and be manifested as skin rash, thrombocytopenia, hemolytic anemia, fever, and hepatic granuloma.[38,39] Toxic plasma levels (< 8 μg/ml) may lead to sinoatrial depression, atrioventricular block, marked QRS widening, and bundle branch blocks, as well as prolongation of the QT interval. Paroxysms of atypical ventricular tachycardia of the "torsade de pointes" type in association with QT prolongation may cause syncope and sudden death, even in the absence of toxic plasma levels.[40,41] Quinidine suppresses the synthesis of vitamin K-dependent clotting factors, and concomitant use of anticoagulants may produce profound hypoprothrombinemia and hemorrhage.[42]

4. Obstetric considerations

Quinidine was used in the obstetric population as early as the 1930s,[43,44] and experience with this agent is extensive.[45–53] However, detailed pharmacologic studies in this patient group are scant.

Quinidine readily crosses the placenta,[45,46] and maternal and neonatal plasma concentrations are similar at birth.[46] The amniotic fluid level, however, was found to be elevated, possibly as a result of fetal voiding of neo-metabolized quinidine.[46]

Quinidine has been shown to diffuse freely into breast milk at the concentration similar to that of the serum. Continued exposure to quinidine by breast feeding may result in accumulation of the drug in the immature newborn liver.[46] There is no evidence of teratogenic effects or major obstetric or fetal difficulties in association with quinidine therapy.[52] However, quinidine may occasionally exert a minimal oxytocic effect,[44,50] but usually not until spontaneous uterine contractions have begun.[50] At therapeutic doses it may rarely cause premature labor,[51] while toxic doses may lead to abortion.[54]

Quinidine has been incriminated as a cause of damage to the eighth nerve of the fetus, but this has been with the use of doses much larger than usually required for treating arrhythmias.[49] A rare complication encountered with its use may be transient neonatal thrombocytopenia.[55] The pregnant patient on anticoagulant therapy may occasionally hemorrhage when concomitantly treated with quinidine.[42]

Despite the occasional adverse effects related to its use, in the experience of the majority of authors,[45,46,50,52,53] quinidine, at therapeutic doses, may be used safely throughout pregnancy when antiarrhythmic therapy is considered necessary.

C. Procainamide (Pronestyl)

The clinical use of procainamide is similar to that of quinidine, but its most beneficial results are seen in the termination and prevention of ventricular arrhythmias. Procainamide may also be used to prevent recurrence of atrial flutter or fibrillation following cardioversion when quinidine is not tolerated, and in tachyarrhythmias associated with the Wolff-Parkinson-White syndrome.[56] The electrophysiologic actions of procainamide and its mechanism of action in suppressing arrhythmias are essentially the same as those for quinidine.

1. Pharmacokinetics

Procainamide may be administered orally or parenterally. The drug is 15% bound to plasma proteins[57] and is metabolized in the liver to N-acetylprocainamide (NAPA), which has antiarrhythmic activity. The rate of acetylation is genetically determined. Consequently, when treated with a given dose of the drug, slow acetylators will have higher plasma concentrations than fast acetylators.[58] Thus, in order to interpret plasma levels meaningfully, measurements of both procainamide and NAPA are necessary. About 50% of an oral dose is excreted in the urine unchanged, and 7–24% is recovered as NAPA.[59] The half-life of procainamide varies with the acetylator status of the patient and is approximately four hours. The therapeutic level of the agent is 4–8 μg/ml, and for procainamide plus NAPA it is 8–16 μg/ml. Lower dosages may be required in patients with renal or cardiac failure.

For rapid control of arrhythmia, procainamide is given as a 100 mg intravenous bolus over four minutes under electrocardiographic and blood pressure monitoring. This dose may be repeated every ten minutes until the arrhythmia is abolished or side effects develop or a total dose of 500 mg is reached. The total oral maintenance dose is 40–50 mg/kg per day given in four divided doses.

2. Adverse effects

Serious toxic effects include asystole, ventricular fibrillation, and myocardial depression, and hypotension may occur, particularly with the intravenous use of procainamide. Idiosyncratic reactions may include skin rash, agranulocytosis, hepatic damage, and psychosis.[57,60,61] Long-term therapy may result in high titers of antinuclear antibodies in over 50% of patients, and about 20% may show clinical evidence of a lupus erythematosus-like syndrome.[62]

3. Obstetric considerations

There are no data on maternal–fetal distribution and fetal metabolism of procainamide. However, neither procaine, a local anesthetic, nor procainamide used in the early stages of pregnancy appears to cause teratogenic effects.[27,63] Merx et al[63] recommend procainamide as the drug of choice in the chronic therapy of maternal arrhythmias, and according to the experience of other investigators[44,52,62] it is a relatively safe drug during pregnancy. However, in view of the high incidence of antinuclear antibodies and the lupus-like syndrome, the use of procainamide should be limited to patients who do not tolerate or are unresponsive to quinidine.

D. Phenytoin (Diphenylhydantoin)

The nonbarbiturate anticonvulsant drug phenytoin is recognized as a primary agent for the treatment of supraventricular and ventricular arrhythmias resulting from digitalis excess.[65,66] In the absence of digitalis toxicity, its utility as an antiarrhythmic is rather limited,[67,68] although phenytoin may be of value in ventricular tachyarrhythmias refractory to standard agents.

1. Electrophysiological properties

Phenytoin reduces automaticity in the Purkinje fibers and raises the atrial and ventricular fibrillation thresholds. Unlike quinidine and procainamide, phenytoin may enhance atrioventricular conduction and occasionally increase intraventricular conduction velocity.[67] A possible depressant action of phenytoin on sympathetic centers in the central nervous system may also play a role in its antiarrhythmic properties.

2. Pharmacokinetics

Phenytoin may be administered orally or intravenously. The drug is well absorbed and metabolized by the liver, with less than 5% of a dose appearing unchanged in the urine. To reach antiarrhythmic plasma levels (10–18 μg/ml). an oral loading dose of 1,000 mg is given the first day, and 500 mg the following days. For emergency therapy, intravenous doses of 100 mg are given every five minutes until the arrhythmia is abolished or until adverse effects appear; the total dose should not exceed 1,000 mg per 24 hours. There is a wide range of intersubject variability in plasma concentrations of phenytoin, depending on the individual genetically determined metabolic capacity, for a given administered dose. At therapeutic and toxic plasma concentrations, phenytoin follows nonlinear kinetics,[69] with the mean plasma half-life increasing at higher plasma drug concentrations. Maternal plasma levels of the drug tend to decrease as a result of the enhanced hepatic metabolism during pregnancy. Serial determinations of plasma concentrations are often helpful in view of the complex pharmacokinetics.

3. Adverse effects

Phenytoin toxicity is uncommon when the agent is administered carefully in small incremental doses. However, at toxic levels (above 25 μg/ml), transient hypotension and bradycardia may occur, as well as nystagmus, ataxia, lethargy, and gastrointestinal disturbances. Hepatocellular injury, folate-responsive megaloblastic anemia, peripheral neuropathy, and pseudolymphoma are rare complications.

4. Obstetric considerations

Phenytoin readily crosses the placenta, and maternal and neonatal serum concentrations are roughly equal at birth.[69] Although there do not seem to be any maternal problems peculiar to the obstetric patient, a number of serious fetal side effects are recognized with its use. When phenytoin is taken during the first trimester of pregnancy, a large spectrum of birth defects may result, known as the "fetal hydantoin syndrome".[70–72] The risk is almost 6%, versus 2% for the general population.[73] The most common defect is mental retardation, followed in frequency by growth retardation.[74] Craniofacial malformations consisting of broad low nasal bridge with short upturned nose and cleft palate,[70,71,72,75] genital abnormalities in male infants,[76] and serious cardiopulmonary disorders[77] occur less frequently. Several reports[77–79] have documented the potential for life-threatening bleeding in infants exposed to phenytoin in utero, which is possibly due to the anti-vitamin K effect of phenytoin. Recently, four cases of neuroblastoma,[80] as well as mesenchymoma,[81] in association with the fetal hydantoin syndrome were described. Although some investigators[27] suggested that phenytoin-associated malformations may be due to maternal epilepsy, rather than to its treatment, they probably are caused by toxic metabolites of the chemical.[73] Mothers receiving phenytoin develop only low concentrations of the drug in breast milk, and no adverse responses have been reported in their children following breast feeding.[69]

A joint report of the American Academy of Pediatrics and the American College of Obstetricians and Gynecologists[82] recommended withdrawal of any anticonvulsant therapy; however, its use during pregnancy is not considered an absolute indication for termination of pregnancy.

The only possible obstetric use of phenytoin as an antiarrhythmic is in the patient with digitalis-induced arrhythmias that are unresponsive to conventional safer therapy. In such a case, phenytoin should be used only to control the acute episode.

E. Disopyramide (Norpace)

Disopyramide is a new antiarrhythmic agent that has electrophysiologic properties and indications similar to those of quinidine. It was shown to be as effective as quinidine in the treatment of patients with a variety of supraventricular and ventricular arrhythmias, but it is claimed to have fewer side effects.[83] It may also be useful in selected patients with ventricular tachycardia refractory to other agents.[84]

1. Pharmacokinetics

Disopyramide is well absorbed and has a bioavailability of 70–85%[85]; its half-life is six to seven hours.[86] The drug is metabolized in the liver, with about 50% of an oral dose being eliminated unchanged in the urine.[87] The N-dealkylated metabolite of disopyramide also has mild antiarrhythmic properties. The pharmacokinetics of disopyramide are nonlinear; the percentage that is plasma protein bound decreases with increasing serum concentrations.[88] The therapeutic range for disopyramide in terms of total concentration is 3–7 μg/ml; atrial arrhythmias are controlled at lower levels than those required for ventricular arrhythmias.[89] When administered concomitantly with digoxin, disopyramide does not result in changes in serum digoxin levels.[90]

The oral dosage is 200–300 mg as a loading dose, followed by 100–200 mg every six hours. Lower dosages may be required in patients with renal disease and heart failure.

2. Adverse effects

Disopyramide is usually well tolerated, but it has significant side effects related to its anticholinergic action, such as dry mouth, urinary retention, blurred vision, and constipation. It exerts a potent negative inotropic effect on the myocardium and may cause cardiac decompensation.[91] Occasionally, the drug may cause profound hypotension, even after a single dose, as well as potent depression of the conduction through the atrioventricular node and the bundle of His.[92] Disopyramide was recently incriminated as the cause of ventricular tachyarrhythmias in association with QT prolongation.[93,94]

3. Obstetric considerations

Disopyramide readily crosses the placenta and is also secreted in breast milk.[95,96] Fetal serum levels at birth are approximately 40% those of the mother. No teratogenic effects were observed in rats, mice, and rabbits when disopyramide in doses of 30–150 mg/kg were given orally during gestation. At the highest dose level, however, fetal body weight at term appeared to be reduced.[96,97] One detailed report of disopyramide therapy in a pregnant woman receiving 800 mg/day for 14 weeks showed no evidence of adverse effects on the course of pregnancy and on the neonate; spontaneous labor occurred at term, and the baby had a normal weight.[95] However, Leonard and coworkers[98] described a pregnant woman with cardiac arrhythmias due to mitral valve prolapse, in whom disopyramide therapy was associated with uterine contractions. The onset of contractions coincided with each successive dose of the agent and subsided after its withdrawal. The mechanism of this oxytocic-like action is unknown.

Although some European investigators[64] claim that disopyramide may be a safe alternative drug in the treatment of maternal arrhythmias, this agent has not been sufficiently evaluated to recommend its use in the obstetric patient.

F. Verapamil

Verapamil, a papaverine derivative originally developed as an antianginal agent, is a highly effective drug in the management of supraventricular arrhythmias.[99,100] Although it has not yet been released for clinical use in the United States, many studies have established its efficacy in the management of paroxysmal supraventricular tachycardia (over 80% successful reversion). In patients with atrial fibrillation and atrial flutter, reversion to sinus rhythm is less common; however, verapamil usually slows the ventricular response. The usefulness of the drug in treating patients with ventricular arrhythmias is limited, but occasionally it may successfully terminate recurrent episodes of sustained ventricular tachycardia.[101] Verapamil has also shown a beneficial effect in the treatment of angina pectoris, coronary artery spasm, systemic arterial hypertension, and idiopathic hypertrophic subaortic stenosis.

1. Electrophysiological properties

The mechanism of verapamil is to selectively block the transmembrane influx of calcium, thereby depressing activity in the sinoatrial and atrioventricular nodes, which depends, in large part, on inward calcium current for phase 0 depolarization.[102] Inhibition of calcium transport in vascular smooth muscle cells accounts for its peripheral and coronary vasodilatory effect. Verapamil slows the conduction in the sinoatrial and atrioventricular nodes and increases the duration of the effective refractory period of the atrioventricular node. Verapamil exerts a negative inotropic effect that results from its calcium antagonist effect.

2. Pharmacokinetics

Verapamil is rapidly absorbed after oral administration, but its bioavailability is very low because of the extensive first-pass hepatic effect. It is eliminated by hepatic metabolism, and only a small portion of the administered dose is excreted unchanged in the urine. It is about 90% bound to plasma proteins, and its half-life is three to seven hours.[103] The usual dosage for conversion of arrhythmias ranges from 5 to 10 mg administered intravenously at a rate of 1 mg/min under blood pressure and electrocardiographic monitoring. Long-term therapy for prophylaxis of arrhythmias or slowing of ventricular rate requires oral doses of 80–120 mg three or four times daily.

3. Adverse effects

Verapamil is usually well tolerated, but cardiovascular side effects may occur, including hypotension, bradycardia, cardiac failure, and asystole in association with the sick sinus syndrome. Occasionally it causes nausea, constipation, headache, and dizziness.[104–106]

4. Obstetric considerations

Experience with verapamil in the treatment of maternal arrhythmias is limited. However, European investigators[64] concluded that its use in the pregnant patient encounters no teratogenic hazards or adverse effects on the course of pregnancy or the neonate. One report in the literature[107] describes the beneficial effect of verapamil in combination with digoxin in the management of fetal supraventricular tachycardia in utero. The mother received oral verapamil, 240 mg/day, for six weeks, and the fetal blood level of the drug at delivery was approximately 40% that of the mother, indicating placental transfer of the drug. Additional information in pregnant patients derives from the sporadic use of verapamil in the management of premature labor[108,109] and severe eclampsia/preeclampsia.[110,111] Both the tocolytic and antihypertensive effects were attributed to the calcium antagonist properties of the drug. In neither report was the use of verapamil associated with deleterious effects. Despite these promising reports, further studies will have to substantiate the innocence of this drug when used acutely during the critical period of organogenesis as well as chronically throughout pregnancy.

G. Digitalis Glycosides

Although traditionally described as an inotropic agent, digitalis is in fact one of the most widely used antiarrhythmic agents. It is a preferred therapy in the acute management and prophylaxis of paroxysmal supraventricular tachyarrhythmias, as well as in rate control in atrial fibrillation and flutter. Its major actions are exerted by way of its vagotonic effect on sinus and atrioventricular nodes.

Extensive experience has been accumulated with the use of dogoxin during pregnancy,[112–114] making it the drug of

TABLE M.XX.1. Guide to the Use of Antiarrhythmic Drugs in Pregnancy

Drug	Route of administration	Clinical application	Therapeutic concentration	Placental transfer UV/MV ratio[a]	Secreted in breast milk	Use in pregnancy	Comment
Lidocaine	Parenteral	"Choice" in ventricular tachyarrhythmias; digitalis toxicity	2–4 μg/ml	0.5–0.7	Yes	Safe	Toxic doses and fetal acidosis may cause CNS and cardiovascular depression in the neonate.
Quinidine	Oral	Paroxysmal atrial tachyarrhythmias[b]; prophylaxis in atrial and ventricular tachyarrhythmias	2–5 μg/ml	~1.0	Yes	Relatively safe	Excessive doses may lead to premature labor, very occasionally neonatal thrombocytopenia.
Procainamide	Oral Parenteral	Termination and prophylaxis in atrial and ventricular tachyarrhythmias	4–8 μg/ml (+NAPA[c] 8–16 μg/ml)	?	?	Relatively safe	High incidence of maternal antinuclear antibodies and lupus-like syndrome with chronic use.
Phenytoin	Oral Parenteral	Digitalis toxicity; refractory ventricular tachyarrhythmias	10–18 μg/ml	0.8–1.0	Yes, at low concen- tration	Not recom- mended for chronic use[d]	High risk of malformations ("fetal hydantoin syndrome"); bleeding disorder.

Disopyramide	Oral Parenteral	Atrial and ventricular tachyarrhythmias	3–7 μg/ml	~0.4	Yes	Probably safe[e]	One report documents uterine contractions in association with the drug.
Verapamil	Oral Parenteral	Paroxysmal supraventricular tachycardia; rate control in chronic atrial fibrillation	15–30 ng/ml[f]	~0.4	?	Probably safe[e]	Rapid IV injection may occasionally cause maternal hypotension and fetal distress.
Digoxin	Oral Parenteral	Paroxysmal supraventricular tachyarrhythmias; rate control in chronic atrial fibrillation	1–2 μg/ml	~1.0	Yes, at equal to maternal serum concentration	Safe	Adjust dosage when quinidine is given concomitantly.
Propranolol	Oral Parenteral	Termination and prophylaxis in atrial and ventricular tachyarrhythmias; rate control in chronic fibrillation	75–100 ng/ml[f]	~1.0	Yes	Relatively safe	Chronic administration may be associated with intrauterine growth retardation, premature labor, neonatal hypoglycemia, bradycardia, and respiratory depression.

[a]Umbilical venous/maternal venous concentration ratio.
[b]Prior digitalization recommended.
[c]N-acetylprocainamide.
[d]Probably safe as acute therapy of digitalis-induced arrhythmia.
[e]These drugs have not been studied extensively enough in pregnant patients to establish absolute safety, but no serious adverse effects to the fetus have been reported.
[f]Large interindividual variation.

choice in the therapy of the above-mentioned rhythm disturbances. At therapeutic levels it is considered absolutely safe in the obstetric population. Whenever a patient receives diuretics or quinidine in combination with digitalis therapy, serum electrolytes and drug levels should be followed on a regular basis in order to anticipate digitalis intoxication. The pharmacokinetics of digitalis compounds and their use in pregnant patients are discussed elsewhere (Chapter M. XXIV).

H. Propranolol (Inderal)

Propranolol is a beta-adrenergic antagonist that has antiarrhythmic properties shared by lidocaine and phenytoin. Its mechanism is considered to be the combined result of inhibition of adrenergic stimulation of the heart and direct membrane mediated action on the myocardium. It is useful in the management of atrial and ventricular premature beats and in ectopic and reentrant supraventricular and ventricular tachycardia. In atrial flutter and fibrillation, propranolol acts on the atrioventricular node to reduce the rate of the ventricular response. A detailed discussion is presented in Chapter M. XIX.

IV. PRINCIPLES OF ANTIARRHYTHMIC MEDICATION IN PREGNANCY

A variety of rhythm disturbances may occur in pregnancy, and these are a source of concern to the patient and her obstetrician. The first approach to any rhythm disorder is a careful assessment of its severity and the possible underlying cardiac or metabolic defects. Most dysrhythmias that occur during pregnancy can usually be managed by reassurance and avoidance of precipitating factors, but some are distressing to the point of requiring medication. The overriding principle in medication is that, with few exceptions, all drugs given to the mother pass to the fetus and may affect it either in utero or after birth. Therefore, medication in pregnancy must always be given with great caution (see Table M.XX.1).[115]

As a general rule, the conversion of acute symptomatic arrhythmias to sinus rhythm is always indicated, but prophylactic antiarrhythmic therapy throughout pregnancy is justified only in the few cases with documented recurrent and sustained tachyarrhythmias. The development of simple long-term electrocardiographic monitoring methods has led to the recognition of considerable spontaneous variation in the frequency of arrhythmias. Thus, if a patient is taking antiarrhythmic drugs prior to conception, withdrawal of the medication may be attempted under Holter monitoring. It may become evident that some patients can be satisfactorily managed without specific therapy. Where medication is needed for continuing rhythm problems, repeated assessment of required drug dosage is necessary throughout pregnancy.

Most patients with tachyarrhythmias of supraventricular origin can be managed acutely and prophylactically by digoxin therapy, the safety of which during pregnancy has been established. Failure of this regimen will require the addition of either quinidine or propranolol, both at the lowest therapeutic doses. In paroxysmal supraventricular tachycardia, slow intravenous injection of verapamil may become the therapy of choice in the future.[116]

As an initial parenteral drug in ventricular tachyarrhythmias, lidocaine is the first choice. When given in therapeutic doses, it has no negative effect on the fetus. A history of recurrent sustained attacks of ventricular tachycardia will dictate the prophylactic use of quinidine, or if this is not tolerated or proves ineffective, procainamide. Both agents are considered relatively safe during gestation. Synchronized electrical cardioversion may become necessary in refractory atrial or ventricular dysrhythmias, especially when signs of cardiac decompensation or hypotension appear. This procedure has been performed with safety during all three stages of pregnancy.[117–121] On rare occasions, atrial overdrive pacing will be required for the termination of refractory tachyarrhythmias. This approach is of particular value in patients with digitalis intoxication and drug-induced "torsade de pointes."

Any pregnant patient, with or without organic heart disease, treated for significant rhythm disorders requires close medical surveillance during pregnancy and delivery, and should be afforded all the benefits of modern obstetric and cardiologic management.

V. ELECTRICAL CARDIOVERSION

The use of electrical energy has become standard practice for terminating various cardiac rhythm disturbances. The use of synchronized direct current countershock may significantly decrease disability and morbidity in symptomatic patients refractory to conventional pharmacologic therapy and, when properly employed, is associated with only a low risk. Though experience with transthoracic electric discharge during pregnancy is limited, both elective and emergency cardioversion have been performed safely for both mother and fetus during all three stages of pregnancy (Table M.XX.2).

Schroeder and Harrison[118] reported several episodes of successful cardioversion for paroxysmal atrial tachycardia using 100 Wsec in one patient during various stages of pregnancy. Grand and Bernard[119] used 300 Wsec to revert atrial fibrillation successfully in one pregnant patient without an apparent effect on fetal heart rhythm. Though suspected fetal distress necessitated cesarean section for delivery in this patient, cardioversion did not induce premature labor in other reports.[117,118,120,122,123] Curry and Quintana[124] described the successful termination of ventricular fibrillation during actue myocardial infarction with a single 300 Wsec shock. The fetal ECG was unaffected by the electrical discharge; the mother, however, died three months later, presumably as a result of recurrent ventricular arrhythmia.

Although the indication for and the technique of this procedure in pregnant patients are, in principle, similar to those in the nonpregnant patient, the question of potential fetal complications requires special consideration. One possible risk is the provocation of fetal ventricular fibrillation. Though the current discharge of the cardioverter is synchronized with the R wave of the ECG of the mother, if the electrical discharge coincides with the ventricular vulnerable period of the fetus, ventricular fibrillation could result. This complication is remote, however, since not only is the energy reaching the fetal heart miniscule,[121] but also young mammal hearts appear to have a high fibrillatory threshold (M. Manoach, personal communication); the latter is so presumably because a critical myocardial mass is necessary to sustain ventricular fibrilla-

TABLE M.XX.2. Electrical Cardioversion in Pregnancy—Published Reports

Arrhythmias	Trimester	DC shock (Wsec)	Outcome	Authors
Supraventricular tachycardia	1°, 2°, 3°	100 (7 episodes)	Three normal deliveries	Schroeder et al [118]
Supraventricular tachycardia	2°	?	Arrhythmia sustained until delivery	Robards et al [120]
Atrial fibrillation	2°	100	Normal delivery	Vogel et al [117]
Atrial fibrillation	3°	300	Cesarean-section for fetal distress	Grand et al [119]
Atrial flutter	1°	100	Normal delivery	Sussman et al [123]
Atrial flutter	1°	100	Normal delivery	Meitus [122]
Ventricular fibrillation	2°	300	Normal fetal ECG	Curry et al [124]

The therapy of hypertension during pregnancy consisted for many years of a low-salt diet only. However, a better understanding of the pathophysiology of gestational hypertension no longer supports the benefit of dietary or drug-induced sodium depletion. Recently, antihypertensive agents other than diuretics have become the first choice in the treatment of gestational hypertension.

It is believed that adequate control of blood pressure reduces the incidence of cardiovascular morbidity and mortality of mother and fetus. But at the same time, a decrease in blood pressure may reduce perfusion of blood through the uteroplacental unit. The possible changes in organ perfusion and the infeasibility of close observation of the developing fetus for possible side effects clearly limit the use of many antihypertensive agents. The decrease in uteroplacental perfusion is not necessarily drug related, but it correlates with the magnitude of the fall in blood pressure. The use of high doses of the many new and potent antihypertensive agents will cause significant decreases in blood pressure and organ perfusion. Moreover, the decrease in blood pressure frequently is induced over a short period, especially after intravenous application of the drug, or by giving high doses of one or more drugs orally. The cardiovascular system will not always be able to maintain perfusion. Indeed, infusions of drugs like hydralazine, nitroprusside, or diazoxide are known to cause marked decreases in organ perfusion. It seems reasonable, in view of the high metabolic demand of the uteroplacental unit, to decrease blood pressure gradually by using the lowest possible doses of one or more antihypertensive agents. A gradual decrease in blood pressure also has been observed during the restriction of activities and with bed rest, often prescribed as the first step in the treatment of gestational hypertension. This therapeutic modality has been shown to be expensive but efficacious. Therefore, from a hemodynamic point of view, gradual decreases in blood pressure, induced by bed rest or by the careful use of low doses of antihypertensive agents, does not necessarily impair blood supply to the developing fetus.

It is obvious that drugs that are shown to cause toxic side effects in the fetus or neonate should not be used during pregnancy. Moreover, drug-related complications observed in the neonate reveal that certain agents should not be used during the last days prior to delivery.

The use of oral antihypertensive medication in the treatment of gestational hypertension is discussed in the first part of this chapter. The last part of this chapter details the use of drugs needed in the treatment of hypertensive emergencies during pregnancy.

II. DIURETICS

Oral diuretics decrease blood pressure in a large proportion of hypertensive patients. Indeed, single agents control blood pressure adequately in approximately 50% of patients with mild or moderate hypertension. It has been shown that certain subgroups of hypertensive patients respond particularly well to diuretic agents. Older patients and black patients respond better to diuretics than to such other antihypertensive agents as beta-adrenergic blocking drugs. Diuretics also are the first choice of treatment in patients with a low or suppressed activity of the renin-angiotensin system.[1,2]

Many of the commonly used nondiuretic antihypertensive agents cause some degree of volume retention, and the addition of a diuretic will enhance their antihypertensive effectiveness. Moreover, the addition of the diuretic allows the use of lower doses of the other drugs, thereby reducing the incidence of side effects.

A. Antihypertensive Actions of Diuretics

The antihypertensive actions of diuretics (Table M.XXI.1) are dependent upon the depletion of sodium and water that

TABLE M.XXI.1. Depressor and Counterbalancing Pressor Actions Induced by Diuretics

Depressor actions of diuretics
Decrease in extracellular volume
Decrease in plasma volume
Decrease in sodium and water content of arteriolar walls
Decrease in vascular reactivity to pressor stimuli
Direct vasodilatory action (thiazide diuretics)
Inhibition of aldosterone synthesis
Decrease in total peripheral resistance
Counterbalancing pressor actions of diuretics
Increase in renin activity
Increase in aldosterone secretion
Increase in catecholamine secretion
Decrease in renal function
Increase in blood viscosity

they produce. Maximal volume depletion occurs during the first three to five days of treatment and is accompanied by a decrease in cardiac output.[3] Thereafter, extracellular fluid volume and plasma volume slightly increase again but do not reach pretreatment levels.[4–7] Chronic diuretic therapy is always accompanied by some degree of volume depletion, and discontinuation of the drug can lead to symptomatic volume retention.[8] Addition of large amounts of sodium chloride to the diet (> 15 gm/day) abolishes the volume-depleting effect of diuretics and causes blood pressure to return to pretreatment levels.

Diuretic-induced volume depletion does not always result in a decrease in blood pressure. It is well established that volume depletion causes marked increases in renin secretion. In turn, renin secretion by the kidney stimulates the formation of angiotensin II, a hormone that is not only a most potent vasoconstrictor but also stimulates aldosterone secretion by the adrenal cortex. Aldosterone causes sodium retention in the kidney and a direct pressor action at the level of the blood vessel wall. Patients who do not respond to treatment with diuretics often show significant increases in renin activity and aldosterone secretion during chronic therapy. The diuretic-induced increases in angiotensin II and aldosterone counterbalance the hypotensive effect of these agents.[2,9,10]

Another mechanism related to the blood pressure lowering effect of diuretics is that they mobilize some of the excess sodium that has been demonstrated to be present in the arteriolar walls of hypertensive patients. This leads directly to widening of the vascular lumen and might also lead to a decrease in the reactivity of the vessel wall to various pressor stimuli[11–13]

Other beneficial effects of diuretics include direct vasodilatory effects. Thiazide diuretics exhibit some relaxing effect on the smooth muscle cells of the resistance vessels. Loop diuretics produce an increase in venous capacitance and a decrease in limb vascular resistance.[14–16] The role of prostaglandins in the blood pressure lowering effect of diuretics has not been established. However, treatment with the inhibitor of prostaglandin synthesis, indomethacin, reverses diuretic-induced sodium depletion and attenuates the antihypertensive effects of the diuretics.[17] Finally, the inhibitory effect of the potassium-retaining diuretic spironolactone on aldosterone synthesis appears to be of additional benefit in its hypotensive effect.[18]

B. Hemodynamic Effects of Diuretics

Although diuretics decrease cardiac output acutely and their chronic antihypertensive effects are related to a fall in total peripheral resistance, cardiac output returns to pretreatment levels.[5,6,19]

Generally, a decrease in total peripheral resistance will lead to an increase in organ perfusion. However, the increase in perfusion is offset, at least in part, by the fall in blood pressure. A reduction in perfusion can be expected to occur when blood pressure decreases markedly and suddenly or when the demand for perfusion of organs is increased. The reduction in perfusion will be worse when plasma volume is decreased prior to the start of the diuretic. The increase in viscosity and the vasoconstrictor effect of angiotensin II and catecholamines, released as a consequence of diuretic therapy, might add to a possible decrease in organ perfusion.

Dietary salt restriction enhances the effect of diuretics. Its combination can result in further decreases in blood pressure and plasma and extracellular fluid volume. However, severe electrolyte imbalance might accrue and organ perfusion might deteriorate, especially when the metabolic need is increased or the arteries supplying the organ are narrowed. Decreases in renal function have been reported to occur during diuretic therapy.[20]

C. Thiazide Diuretics

Thiazide diuretics are the most commonly used agents for the treatment of hypertension. They inhibit active reabsorption of chloride in the cortical portion of the ascending limb of the loop of Henle, with a corresponding decrease in the transport of sodium. As a result, thiazides greatly increase the amount of sodium delivered to the aldosterone-governed ion-exchange site of the distal part of the distal tubule, and more sodium–potassium exchange occurs, increasing potassium depletion.

The limited effect of thiazide diuretics on sodium transport in the proximal tubule is of less importance in increasing sodium excretion, as is their possible effect on the active transport of chloride in the medullary portion of the ascending limb of the loop of Henle. Some of the specific thiazide diuretics are listed in Table M.XXI.2. They vary according to their duration of action and their relative potency.

D. Loop Diuretics

Loop diuretics have a short duration of action and are less often used than thiazide diuretics in the treatment of hypertension. They are rapidly acting, potent diuretics. The sodium excretion is accomplished through blockade of active chloride transport at the medullary portion of the ascending limb of the loop of Henle.

Furosemide (Lasix) is the most commonly used of this group. It has a duration of action between four and six hours; it is usually prescribed in dosages ranging between 40 and 120 mg/day, usually divided into at least two separate doses. Higher dosages might be needed in patients with renal failure. Marked volume depletion can be achieved by a combination of thiazide diuretics and loop diuretics; however, the risk of serious side effects increases significantly when this combination is used.

E. Potassium-Sparing Diuretics

The primary site of action of potassium-sparing diuretics are the distal and collecting tubules of the kidney. Spironolactone (Aldactone®) binds to intracellular aldosterone receptors. It blocks the aldo-

TABLE M.XXI.2. Examples of Thiazide Diuretics

Name	Dosage (mg/day)	Duration of action (hr)
Chlorothiazide (Diuril®)	250–1,000	6–12
Hydrochlorothiazide (Hydrodiuril®, Esidrex®)	25–150	12–18
Hydroflumethiazide (Saluron®)	25–50	18–24
Bendroflumethiazide (Naturetin®)	5–20	18–36
Trichlormethiazide (Naqua®, Methahydrin®)	2–4	24–48
Polythiazide (Renese®)	1–4	24–48
Metolazone (Zaraloxin®)	1–5	12–14
Chlorthalidone (Hygroton®)	25–100	24–72

sterone-induced stimulation of Na-K ATPase, which is linked with the interstitial Na-K exchange pump. Moreover, spironolactone interferes with the biosynthesis of aldosterone. Triamterene (Dyrenium®) and amiloride (Midamor®) block the Na-K carrier in the luminal membrane of the tubular cells. The net result of treatment with either of the potassium-sparing agents is weak to moderate sodium depletion and sometimes marked potassium and hydrogen retention. Potassium-retaining diuretics often are prescribed in conjunction with thiazide or loop diuretics to minimize potassium depletion. Spironolactone is usually used in doses of 25–200 mg/day. Its duration of action is 8–12 hours. Triamterene has a duration of action of approximately 12 hours, and doses of 100–300 mg are prescribed. Amiloride has a duration of action of 16 to 20 hours, and lower doses are needed to achieve a significant effect (5–20 mg/day).

TABLE M.XXI.3. Maternal and Fetal Side Effects of Diuretics

Maternal side effects
Hyperuricemia
Hyperglycemia
Hypercalcemia
Hyponatremia
Hypokalemia
Hyperreninemia
Deterioration of kidney function
Reduction in plasma volume
Reduction in placental perfusion
Ventricular ectopic activity
Hemorrhagic pancreatitis
Thrombocytopenia
Hypersensitivity
Fetal side effects
Hyponatremia
Hypokalemia
Ventricular ectopic activity
Thrombocytopenia

F. Diuretics and Pregnancy

Edema is a common event during pregnancy: it may occur in up to 80% of pregnancies. Preeclampsia and eclampsia are usually accompanied by frank edema. Therefore, pregnant patients have been regarded as sodium retainers in whom dietary salt restriction or diuretics should be used prophylactically.[21–23] However, older data suggest that salt might be of benefit during pregnancy.[24] Recent reviews on this subject reveal that the benefits of salt restriction or diuretic therapy in mild to moderate hypertension have not been clearly shown.[25,26] In fact, hypertensive pregnant patients tended to excrete salt loads more easily than women who were normotensive during pregnancy.[27]

The side effects observed during diuretic therapy, with or without dietary sodium restriction, are listed in Table M.XXI.3.

Hypertension during pregnancy often develops in the second or third trimester, when the metabolic needs of the uteroplacental unit are markedly increased. Moreover, hypertensive pregnancy, as well as preeclampsia and eclampsia, are characterized by a diminished plasma volume and subnormal circulatory support. Therefore, further imbalance between blood flow and demand occurs in patients with severe hypertension and preeclampsia/eclampsia, possibly resulting in a poor outcome of pregnancy.[28-33] Changes in blood pressure or plasma volume, induced by diuretics or salt restriction, will worsen the clinical situation. Reductions in uterine blood flow and placental metabolic competence have been reported during diuretic therapy.[34,35] Vigorous sodium depletion can also lead to impairment of kidney function mimicking the development of preeclampsia/eclampsia.[36,37] Indeed, the hemodynamic consequences of the disease are exaggerated by the induction of volume depletion.

Hyperuricemia, and a possible decrease in kidney function, may mask the symptoms of preeclampsia/eclampsia. Diuretic-induced hyperglycemia can interfere with the proper assessment of glucose tolerance in diabetic patients. Ventricular ectopic activity have been reported in the presence of mild as well as marked hypokalemia.

The lack of proof of benefit, the severity

of possible side effects, and a better insight into the pathophysiologic characteristics of hypertension-associated pregnancies, and preeclampsia/eclampsia are arguments against the use of diuretics or severely restricted salt intake during pregnancy.

The use of diuretic therapy during pregnancy should be limited to the following cases: 1) pregnancy in a patient with renal insufficiency; 2) pregnancy in a patient with congestive heart failure; 3) oliguria and renal insufficiency during preeclampsia/eclampsia; and 4) as an adjunct to treatment with hypotensive agents that cause volume retention, such as methyldopa, hydralazine, and diazoxide. In such cases, thiazide diuretics are most commonly prescribed. If the use of a more potent diuretic is needed, furosemide can be added to, or substituted for, thiazide diuretics. Potassium-sparing diuretics have not been sufficiently tested during pregnancy. Therefore, potassium supplements probably are the best choice for the repletion of total body potassium. The limitation of indications for thiazide or loop diuretics during pregnancy further reduces the need for potassium-retaining diuretics.

III. BETA-ADRENERGIC BLOCKING DRUGS

Beta-adrenergic blocking agents are widely used as first or second choice agents in the treatment of hypertension. By themselves they lower blood pressure effectively in approximately 50% of patients with mild to moderate hypertension.[38,39] Moreover, they are useful when a diuretic alone does not lower blood pressure adequately.[40]

Many beta-blocking drugs are available. They can be sudivided according to their cardioselectivity and duration of action.[41] Cardioselective beta-adrenergic blocking drugs block the beta-1 receptors in the myocardium in a competitive fashion. Noncardioselective drugs block the beta-1 receptors in the heart and also the adrenergic beta-2 receptors in smooth muscle cells of blood vessel walls and bronchi. The difference between nonselective and selective beta blockers is relative; most cardioselective beta blockers will have beta-2-adrenergic antagonistic effects when given in high doses.

Other differences between beta-adrenergic blocking drugs include the presence or absence of membrane-stabilizing or local anesthetic-like activity, and the presence or absence of intrinsic sympathomimetic or partial agonist activity. The absence or presence of membrane-stabilizing effect does not appear to be of clinical relevance. However, drugs with partial agonist activity such as pindolol, oxprenolol, and alprenolol might cause less bradycardia and less bronchospasm than those without agonist activity.

The suppression of renin produced by most beta-blockers might be a beta-1 or beta-2 effect or both.[42]

Metabolic effects of beta-adrenergic blockers include inhibition of skeletal muscle glycolysis and lipolysis. The consequences of these effects include a possible prolongation of, or delayed recovery from, insulin-induced hypoglycemia and a reduction in plasma free fatty acid levels. Beta-blocking drugs can induce an increase in uterine tone. Moreover, they might interfere with blood flow in the myometrium because of their blockade of beta-2 vascular receptors.

A. Antihypertensive Actions of Beta-Adrenergic Blocking Drugs

Different mechanisms are believed to explain the antihypertensive effect of beta-adrenergic blocking drugs (Table M.XXI.4.). They include a decrease in cardiac output, suppression of renin secretion, central nervous system effects, and blockade of peripheral presynaptic facilitatory β-adrenoceptors.[38,39,43,45] Acute administration of beta-adrenergic blocking agents decreases cardiac output, but the antihypertensive action of the drugs is apparent only after one or two days of

TABLE M.XXI.4. Depressor and Counterbalancing Pressor Actions Induced by Beta-Adrenergic Blocking Drugs

Depressor actions of beta-adrenergic blocking drugs
Decrease in renin secretion
Decrease in aldosterone secretion
Unspecified action in the central nervous system
Blockade of peripheral presynaptic facilitatory beta-receptors
Decrease in cardiac output
Decrease in total peripheral resistance
Counterbalancing pressor actions of beta-adrenergic blocking drugs
Presence of intrinsic agonist activity
Increase in alpha-adrenergic-mediated vasoconstriction
Sodium retention (rare)
Decrease in kidney function

therapy.[46] When blood pressure is significantly decreased, cardiac output usually is only slightly lower than pretreatment levels while peripheral resistance is decreased. In patients who show an increase in blood pressure during therapy with a beta-blocker, peripheral resistance is believed to be increased.[39,47] The main hemodynamic correlate to the decrease in blood pressure induced by chronic treatment with beta-blockers is the fall in total peripheral resistance, enhanced by possible decreases in cardiac output.[46] The beta-blocker-induced decrease in cardiac output might be the main mechanism of its antihypertensive action in patients with a high pretreatment cardiac output.

Most beta-blockers reduce renin secretion. The antihypertensive effect of the agents seems related, at least in part, to this ability. Patients with higher pretreatment renin values respond better to beta-blockers than patients with lower renin values. The changes in aldosterone secretion determine, in addition to the effects on renin secretion, the ultimate outcome of therapy.[48]

Central nervous system effects might also be involved in the antihypertensive effect of these drugs. Although many nonselective beta blockers cause side effects such as sedation, vivid dreams, and depression, the role of the central nervous system in their blood pressure lowering action remains to be elucidated.

Finally, blockade of epinephrine-induced stimulation of presynaptic facilitatory β-adrenoceptors might contribute to the antihypertensive effects of these drugs.[44]

As a general rule, beta-blockers do not interfere with renal function and do not cause volume retention. However, reversible decreases in creatinine clearance have been observed in some patients, and significant volume retention may rarely occur.[39,42] These effects may counterbalance the antihypertensive effect of beta-blockers.

As mentioned earlier, blood pressure increases in some patients during treatment with beta-blockers. The rise in blood pressure in these patients is related to increased alpha-adrenergic activity during beta-blockade present when alpha-receptors are unopposed by beta-2-mediated vasodilation. Obviously, this increase in alpha-adrenergic activity reduces the antihypertensive efficacy of beta-blockers, particularly that of noncardioselective agents. Black patients and older patients do not respond as well to therapy with beta-blockade as do white or younger patients.[2,49] Differences in sodium intake and in resting beta-adrenergic activity might explain these findings.

A list of commonly used beta-adrenergic blocking drugs is given in Table M.XXI.5. Propranolol (Inderal®), timolol (Blocadren®), nadolol (Corgard®), metoprolol (Lopressor®), and atenolol (Tenormin®) are currently available in the United States; the other agents listed probably will be released in the near future. Dosages most frequently used are 40–160 mg bid for propranolol, 10–20 mg bid for timolol, 40–120 mg/day as a single dose for nadolol, 50–200 mg bid for metoprolol, and 50–100 mg per day for atenolol.

Labetalol is a beta-adrenergic blocking drug also possessing alpha-adrenergic antagonist properties. It blocks the increase in alpha-adrenergic activity accompanying peripheral beta-blockade. Therefore, when comparable degrees of beta-block-methyl-norepinephrine, whereas clonidine acts as an alpha-adrenergic agonist without first requiring metabolic conversion. A consequence of this difference is that clonidine exhibits alpha-agonistic properties when exposed to the alpha-adrenergic receptors of the peripheral sympathetic nervous system. Indeed, clonidine has been shown to induce pressor responses shortly after its intravenous or oral administration.[7] However, the peripheral agonist activity of the drug is overwhelmed by its central action during chronic therapy using low doses of the drug and does not interfere with its antihypertensive effect.[72]

Clonidine and methyldopa have a suppressive effect on renin secretion that might enhance their blood pressure lowering action in certain patients.[73,74] Clonidine's decelerating effect on heart rate is a consequence of its enhancement of vagal mechanisms and cardiac alpha receptors.

A third drug that interferes with the function of the alpha-adrenergic system is prazosin. The action of this drug is quite different from that of alpha-methyldopa and clonidine. Prazosin blocks the postsynaptic alpha-1-receptor in the periphery. It does not possess a central action. The antihypertensive effect of the drug may be less than that of clonidine.[72]

B. Hemodynamic Effects of Drugs Interfering With the Alpha-Adrenergic System

Ultimately the decrease in blood pressure induced by alpha-adrenergic drugs is related to a fall in total peripheral resistance. Moreover, clonidine and alpha-methyldopa cause some decrease in cardiac output, which might add to the antihypertensive potency of these drugs. Alpha-methyldopa and prazosin can cause symptomatic orthostatic changes in the blood pressure.

Clonidine (Catapres) is usually prescribed in doses ranging from 0.1 to 1.2 mg per day in a bid regimen. Its duration of action is 8–12 hours. Higher doses, or its combination with drugs such as propranolol, might rarely induce symptomatic rebound or overshoot hypertension.[75] Alpha-methyldopa (Aldomet®) also may produce rebound hypertension after abrupt discontinuation of the drug. It is usually prescribed in doses ranging from 125 to 1,500 mg per day, in a bid fashion. Its duration of action is 12–16 hours. Rebound hypertension or overshoot hypertension can be prevented by stepwise decreases in the daily doses of the drugs.

Prazosin (Minipress, 4–30 mg/day, in a bid or tid fashion) might cause symptomatic orthostatic hypotension, especially after the first dose of the drug. Its duration of action is approximately six hours. It has been suggested to give the very first dose of the drug at night. Rebound hypertension has not been reported after discontinuation of prazosin.

C. Drugs Interfering With the Alpha-Adrenergic Nervous System During Pregnancy (Table M.XXI.8)

As discussed earlier, a decrease in both peripheral resistance and cardiac output might interfere with organ perfusion and function. The decrease in organ function might be worse when orthostatic hypotension occurs. Orthostatic hypotension can be induced by both alpha-methyldopa and prazosin and usually is worse when high doses of the drugs are prescribed or when the drugs are given during volume depletion.

A decrease in plasma volume often is present in patients with gestational hy-

TABLE M.XXI.8. Maternal and Fetal Side Effects of Drugs Interfering With the Alpha-Adrenergic Sympathetic System

Maternal side effects
Orthostatic hypotension (prazosin, alpha-methyldopa)
Central nervous system effects (clonidine, alpha-methyldopa)
Fetal side effects
Possible effect on fetal growth (alpha-methyldopa)

pertension. Moreover, especially during the last trimester of pregnancy, orthostatic symptoms can be present in the absence of drug treatment. Orthostatic symptoms and thus possible decreases in uteroplacental perfusion might also be more pronounced when these drugs are added to patients who are being treated with a diuretic.

Alpha-methyldopa has been widely used as an antihypertensive agent during pregnancy. It has been shown to be safe for mother and fetus. One study claims that fetal growth was greater in patients treated with the beta-adrenergic blocking drug oxprenolol than in those treated with alpha-methyldopa.[76] Alpha-methyldopa crosses the placenta,[77] and some authors claim that the use of drugs interfering with the action of the central nervous system might interfere with the normal development of the brain.[68] Others claim that treatment with methyldopa might improve future child development. Infants whose mothers had received methyldopa between the 16th and 20th weeks of gestation had smaller heads at birth than did those whose mothers had no specific treatment.[78]

Clonidine has been used in a fairly small number of patients with gestational hypertension without measurable drug-related side effects in mother or fetus. The drug has been insufficiently tested to warrant its unrestricted use throughout pregnancy.

Prazosin has not been used as an antihypertensive agent in pregnant women.

V. VASODILATORS

A. Antihypertensive Action of Vasodilators in Combination Therapy

Vasodilators are being used in the treatment of hypertensive patients when a combination of a diuretic and a beta-adrenergic blocking drug or a drug that interferes with the alpha-adrenergic system does not decrease blood pressure adequately. It is not surprising that vasodilators are not being used as single agents in the treatment of hypertensive patients (Table M.XXI.9). Since vasodilators reduce peripheral resistance through nonspecific mechanisms, they evoke responses such as increases in renin activity, aldosterone secretion, and cardiac output. Their blood pressure lowering effect results in marked sodium retention. The increase in aldosterone secretion might add to that effect and cause further sodium retention.

TABLE M.XXI.9. Depressor and Counterbalancing Pressor Actions of Vasodilator Drugs

Depressor actions of vasodilators
Decrease in peripheral resistance
Counterbalancing pressor actions of vasodilators
Sodium retention
Increase in renin activity
Increase in aldosterone
Increase in cardiac output

Hydralazine is the vasodilator most frequently used in the long-range treatment of hypertensive patients. Vasodilators interfere with movements of calcium in the vascular smooth muscle cells. Because of their action, intracellular calcium concentration falls, resulting in a decrease in the vascular force of contraction.[79–81]

B. The Use of Vasodilators During Pregnancy (Table M.XXI.10)

Hydralazine has been used for the treatment of hypertensive pregnant women as

TABLE M.XXI.10. Maternal and Fetal Side Effects of Vasodilators

Maternal side effects
Sodium and water retention
Tachycardia
Headaches, flushing
Angina pectoris
Orthostatic hypotension
Symptomatic hypotension
Fetal side effects
Bradycardia in the presence of maternal hypotension after IV application

mortality and the prematurity rate. The value of prophylactic thiazides in juveniles. JAMA 1966; 195:429–432.
23. Lindheimer MD, Katz AI. The kidney in pregnancy. N Engl J Med. 1970; 283:1095–1097.
24. Robinson M. Salt in pregnancy. Lancet. 1958; 1:178–181.
25. Lindheimer MD, Katz AI. Sodium and diuretics in pregnancy. N Engl J Med. 1973; 288:891–894.
26. Lindberg BS. Salt, diuretics and pregnancy. Gynecol Obstet Invest. 1979; 10:145–156.
27. Sarles HE, Hill SS, LeBlanc AL, Smith GH, Canales CO, Remmers AG. Sodium excretion patterns during and following intravenous sodium chloride loads in normal and hypertensive pregnancies. Am J Obstet Gynecol. 1968; 102:1–7.
28. Gant NG, Madden JD, Chand S, Worky RJ, Strong JD, MacDonald DC. Metabolic clearance rate of dehydroisoandrosterone. Obstet Gynecol. 1976; 47:319–326.
29. Worley RJ, Everett RB, MacDonald PC, Gant FN. Placental clearnace of dehydroisoandrosterone sulfate and pregnancy outcome in three categories of hospitalized patients with pregnancy induced hypertension. Gynecol Invest. 1975; 6:28–29.
30. Bletka M, Hlavaty V, Trukova M, Bendl J, Bendova L, Chytil M. Volume of whole blood and absolute amount of serum proteins in the early stage of late toxemia of pregnancy. Am J Obstet Gynecol. 1970; 106:10–13.
31. Gallery EDM, Hunyor SN, Gyorky AZ. Plasma volume contraction: A significant factor in both pregnancy-associated hypertension (preeclampsia) and chronic hypertension in pregnancy. Q J Med. 1979; 48:593–602.
32. Soffronoff EC, Kaufmann BM, Connaughton JF. Intravascular volume determinations and fetal outcome in hypertensive disease of pregnancy. Am J Obstet Gynecol. 1977; 127:4–9.
33. Arias F, Zamora J. Antihypertensive treatment and pregnancy outcome in patients with mild chronic hypertension. Obstet Gynecol. 1979; 53:489–494.
34. Gant NF, Madden JD, Sitteri PK, MacDonald PC. The metabolic clearance rate of dehydroisoandrosterone sulfate III. The effect of thiazide diuretics in normal and future pre-eclamptic pregnancies. Am J Obstet Gynecol. 1975; 123:159–163.
35. Gant NF, Madden JD, Sitteri PK, MacDonald PC. The metabolic clearance rate of dehydroisoandrosterone sulfate IV. Acute effects of induced hypertension hypotension and natiuresis in normal and hypertensive pregnancies. Am J Obstet Gynecol. 1976; 124:143–148.
36. Palomaki JF, Lindheimer MD. Sodium depletion simulating deterioration in a toxcemic pregnancy. N Engl J Med. 1970; 282:88–89.
37. Macleon AB, Doig JR, Aickin DR. Hypovolemia, preeclampsia and diuretics. Br J Obstet Gynecol. 1978; 85:597–603.
38. Buhler FR, Laragh JH, Baer L, Vaitghan O, Brunner HR. Propranolol inhibition of renin secretion: A specific approach to diagnosis and treatment of renin-dependent hypertensive diseases. N Engl J Med. 1972; 287:1209–1214.
39. Drayer JIM, Weber MA, Longworth DL, Laragh JH. The possible importance of aldosterone as well as renin in the long-term antihypertensive action of propranolol. Am J Med. 1978; 64:187–193.
40. Weber MA, Lopez-Ovejero JA, Drayer JIM, Case DB, Laragh JH. Renin reactivity as a determinant of the response to combined treatment with a beta-adrenergic blocking agent and a diuretic in hypertensive patients. Arch Intern Med. 1977; 137:284–289.
41. Frishman W. Clinical pharmacology of the new beta-adrenergic blocking drugs. Part 1. Pharmacodynamic and pharmacokinetic properties. Am Heart J. 1979; 97:797–807.
42. Weber MA, Drayer JIM. Renal effects of beta-adrenoceptor blockade. Kidney Int. 1980; 18:686–699.
43. Frishman W, Silverman R. Clinical pharmacology of the new beta-adrenergic blocking drugs. Part 2. Physiologic and metabolic effects. Am Heart J. 1979; 97:797–807.
44. Langer FZ, Cavero I, Massingham R. Recent developments in noradrenergic neurotransmission and its relevance to the mechanism of action of certain antihypertensive agents. Hypertension. 1980; 2:372–382.
45. Vlachakis ND. Hemodynamic effects of propranolol therapy in relationship to renin status and plasma catecholamines in primary hypertension. J Clin Pharmacol. 1980; 20:20–29.
46. Simon G, Franciosa JA, Gimenez HJ, Cohn JN. Short-term systemic hemodynamic adaptation to beta-adrenergic inhibition with atenolol in hypertensive patients. Hypertension. 1981; 3:262–268.
47. Tarazi RC, Dustan HP. Beta-adrenergic blockade in hypertension. Am J Cardiol 1972; 29:633–640.
48. Drayer JIM, Keim HJ, Weber MA, Case DB, Laragh JH. Unexpected pressor responses to propranolol in essential hypertension. Am. J. Med. 1976; 60:897–903.
49. Buhler FR, Burkart F, Lutold BE, Kunk K, Marbet G, Pfisterer M. Antihypertensive beta blocking action as related to renin and age. Am J Cardiol. 1975; 36:653–669.
50. Wilson M, Morganti AA, Zervoudakis I, Letcher RL, Romney BM, VonOeyon P, Papera S, Sealey JE, Laragh JH. Blood pressure, the renin-aldosterone system and sex steroids throughout normal pregnancy. Am J Med. 1980; 68:97–104.
51. Bay WH, Ferris TF. Factors controlling plasma renin and aldosterone during pregnancy. Hypertension. 1979; 1:410–415.
52. Worley RJ, Gant Jr. NF, Everett RB, MacDonald PC. Vascular responsiveness to pressor agents during human pregnancy. J Reprod Med. 1979; 23:115–128.
53. Eliahou HE, Silverberg DS, Reisin E, Romeru

I, Mashiach S, Serr DM. Propranolol for the treatment of hypertension in pregnancy. Br J Obstet Gynecol. 1978; 85:431–436.
54. Pruyn SC, Phelan JP, Buchanan GC. Long-term propranolol therapy in pregnancy: Maternal and fetal outcome. Am J Obstet Gynecol. 1979; 135:485–489.
55. Bott-Kanner G, Schweitzer A, Reisner SH, Joel-Cohen SJ, Rosenfeld JB. Propranolol and hydralazine in the management of essential hypertension in pregnancy. Br J Obstet Gynecol. 1980; 87:110–114.
56. Cotteel M, Dequiedt PH, Potier A, Puech F, LeLievre G, Leroy JL, Tacquet A, Delecour M. Influence des therapeutiques actuelles et notamment des beta-bloquants sur le prognostic foetal et maternel des syndromes hypertensifs de la grossesse. J Gynecol Obstet Biol Reprod. 1979; 8:253–259.
57. Redman CWG. Treatment of hypertension in pregnancy. Kidney Int. 1980; 18:267–278.
58. Sandstrom B. Antihypertensive treatment with the adrenergic beta-receptor blocker metoprolol during pregnancy. Gynecol Obstet Invest. 1978; 9:195–204.
59. O'Hare MF, Russell CJ, Leahey WJ, Varma MPS, Murnaghan GA, McDevitt DG. Sotalol in the management of hypertension complicating pregnancy. Br J Clin Pharmacol. 1979; 8:390P–391P.
60. Pritchard BNC, Richards DA. Labetalol, an α- and β-adrenoceptor-blocking agent: Its use in therapeutics. Br J Clin Pharmacol. 1979; 8:239S–244S.
61. Michael CA. Use of labetalol in the treatment of severe hypertension during pregnancy. Br J Clin Pharmacol. 1979; 8:211S–215S.
62. Lamming GD, Symonds EM. Use of labetalol and methyldopa in pregnancy-induced hypertension. Br J Clin Pharmacol. 1979; 8:217S–222S.
63. Tcherdakoff Ph, Colliard M, Berrard E, Kreft C, Dupay A, Bernaille JM. Propranolol in hypertension during pregnancy. Br Med J. 1978; 2:670.
64. Cottrill CM, McAllister Jr. RG, Gettes L, Noonan JA. Propranolol therapy during pregnancy, labor, and delivery: Evidence for transplacental drug transfer and impaired neonatal drug disposition. J Pediatr. 1977; 91:812–814.
65. Habib A, McCarthy JS. Effects on the neonate of propranolol administered during pregnancy. J Pediatr. 1977; 95:808–811.
66. Redmond GP. Effect of drugs on intrauterine growth. Clin Perinatol. 1979; 6:5–19.
67. Lieberman BA, Stirrat GM, Cohen SL, Beard RW, Pinker GD, Belsey E. The possible adverse effects of propranolol on the fetus in pregnancies complicated by severe hypertension. Br J Obstet Gynecol. 1978; 85:678–683.
68. Lewis PD. Do drugs acting on the nervous system affect cell proliferation in the developing brain. Lancet. 1977; 1:399–401.
69. Van Zwieten PA. Pharmacology of centrally acting hypotensive drugs. Br J Clin Pharmacol. 1980; 10:13S–20S.
70. Weber MA, Drayer JIM. The sympathetic nervous system in primary hypertension. Mineral Electrolyte Metab. (in press).
71. Drayer JIM, Weber MA, Lipson JL. Captopril-based multiple drug therapy improves blood pressure control and decreases the incidence of hypokalemia in patients with severe hypertension. Proceedings of the 8th International Meeting on Hypertension. Milan, Italy, 1981 (abstr).
72. Hubbell FA, Weber MA, Drayer JIM, Rose DE. Manuscript in preparation.
73. Weber MA, Drayer JIM, Laragh JH. The effects of clonidine and propranolol, separately and in combination, on blood pressure and plasma renin activity in essential hypertension. J Clin Pharmacol. 1979; 18:233–240.
74. Weber MA, Case DB, Baer L, Sealey JE, Drayer JIM, Lopez-Ovejero JA, Laragh JH. Renin and aldosterone suppression in the antihypertensive action of clonidine. Am J Cardiol. 1976; 38:825–830.
75. Garbus SB, Weber MA, Priest RT, Brewer DD, Hubbell FA: The abrupt discontinuation of antihypertensive treatment. J Clin Pharmacol. 1979; 19:207–217.
76. Gallery EDM, Saunders DM, Hunyor SN, Gyorky AZ. Ramdomized comparison of methyldopa and oxprenolol for treatment of hypertension in pregnancy. Br Med J. 1919; 1:1591–1594.
77. Ounsted MK, Moak VA, Good EJ, Redman CWG. Hypertension during pregnancy with and without specific treatment: The development of the children at the age of four years. Br J Obstet Gynecol. 1980; 87:19–24.
78. Jones HMR, Cummings AJ, Setchell KDR, Lawson AM. A study of the disposition of α-methyldopa in newborn infants following its administration to the mother for the treatment of hypertension during pregnancy. Br J Clin Pharmacol. 1979; 8:433–440.
79. Limas CJ, Cohn JN. Stimulation of vascular smooth muscle sodium potassium-adenosinetriphosphatase by vasodilators. Circ Res. 1974; 35:601–607.
80. Koch-Weser J. Vasodilator drugs in the treatment of hypertension. Arch Intern Med. 1974; 133:1017–1027.
81. Zacest R, Gilmore E, Koch-Weser J. Treatment of essential hypertension with combined vasodilation and beta-adrenergic blockage. N Engl J Med. 1972; 286:617–622.
82. Lammintausta R. The renin-aldosterone system in dihydralazine therapy during hypertensive pregnancy. Int J Clin Pharmacol. 1978; 16:581–584.
83. Curet LB, Olson RW. Evaluation of a program of bed rest in the treatment of chronic hypertension in pregnancy. Obstet Gynecol. 1979; 53:336–340.
84. Vink GJ, Moodley J, Philpott RH. Effect of dihydralazine on the fetus in the treatment of ma-

ternal hypertension. Obstet Gynecol. 1980; 55:519–522.
85. Berkowitz RC. Antihypertensive drugs in the pregnant patient. Obstet Gynecol Surv. 1980; 35:191–204.
86. Case DBC, Wallace JM, Keim HJ, Weber MA, Sealey JE, Laragh JH. Possible role of renin in hypertension as suggested by renin-sodium profiling and inhibition of converting enzyme. N Engl J Med. 1977; 296:641–646.
87. Drayer JIM, Boers GHJ, Kloppenborg PWC, Stevens JVC. Renin blockade in the treatment of hypertension, a role for the oral converting enzyme inhibitor captopril. In: Weber MA, ed. Treatment Strategies in Hypertension. Miami: Symposia Specialists, 1981:151–166.
88. Broughton Pipkin F, Turner SR, Symonds EM. Possible risk with captopril in pregnancy: Some animal data. Lancet. 1980; 1:1256.
89. Perkins RP. Diazoxide in treatment of severe preeclampsia and hypertensive encephalopathy. Am J Obstet Gynecol. 1976; 126:296–297.
90. Perkins RP. Treatment of toxemia of pregnancy. JAMA. 1977; 238:2143–2144.
91. Thien Th. Treatment of hypertension with diazoxide. Thesis, University of Nijmegen, The Netherlands, 1980.
92. Kumar GK, Dastoor FC, Rabayo JR, Razzague MA. Side effects of diazoxide. JAMA. 1976; 235:275–276.
93. Morris JA, Arce JJ, Hamilton CJ, Davidson EC, Maidman JE, Clark JH, Bloom RS. The management of severe preeclampsia and eclampsia with intravenous diazoxide. Obstet Gynecol. 1977; 49:675–680.
94. Pritchard JA. Management of preeclampsia and eclampsia. Kidney Int. 1980; 18:259–266.
95. Thien ThA, Huysmans FTM, Gerlag PGG, Koene RAP, Wijdeveld PGAB. Diazoxide infusion in severe hypertension and hypertensive crisis. Clin Pharmacol Ther. 1979; 25:795–799.
96. Milsap RL, Auld PAM. Neonatal hyperglycemia following maternal diazoxide administration. JAMA. 1980, 243:144–145.
97. Johnson RA. Adverse neonatal reaction to maternal administration of intravenous chlormethiazole and diazoxide. Br Med J. 1976; 1:943.
98. Fidler J, Bennett MJ, DeSwiet M, Ellis C, Lewis PJ. Treatment of pregnancy hypertension with prostacyclin. Lancet. 1980; 2:31–32.

M.XXII

Anticoagulation in Pregnancy

Lee B. Berman, MD, and Louis Aledort, MD

I. INTRODUCTION

The indications for anticoagulation include recurrent deep vein thrombosis, pulmonary emboli, recurrent emboli due to valvular disease, and prevention of thrombosis and/or emboli in patients with arrhythmia, prosthetic heart valve, and/or congestive heart failure. These are also the indications for anticoagulation in pregnancy.

Pregnancy causes changes in concentrations of several clotting factors, with factors II, VII, VIII, IX, and X being increased. Platelet counts are unchanged in pregnancy. Fibrinogen (factor I) is also increased during pregnancy, with increased synthesis and catabolism of the molecule. Soluble fibrin monomer complexes (SFMC) increase progressively during pregnancy, and there are further increases in the immediate postpartum

Cardiac Problems in Pregnancy, pages 261–272

period; this results in eventual doubling of the normal level of SFMC, which is approximately 2.6% the total fibrogen content.[1]

Other changes in pregnancy have been thought to predispose to thrombosis. These include decreased blood flow in the legs, increased blood viscosity, and decreased deformability of erythrocytes.[2] The clinical significance of the alterations in the clotting factor levels is probably not great during the prepartum period. The incidence of thrombophlebitis in a general office practice has been reported to be 1.3 cases per 1,000 women examined per year, with one-fourth of these being deep vein phlebitis.[2] In another series, Drill calculated the incidence of thrombophlebitis to be 2.2 per 1,000 nonpregnant women per year.[3] Aaro found superficial phlebitis in 1.7 per 1,000 pregnancies and deep vein phlebitis in 0.36 per 1,000 during the antepartum period.[4] This is not much different from the incidence in the general nonpregnant population. The reported incidence of thrombophlebitis complicating pregnancy has varied from 0.018% to 0.29%, with an average of 0.1%.[5] Therefore, pregnancy does not appear to be a strong predisposing factor to thrombophlebitis.

There is, however, an increased risk of thromboembolic disease in the first four weeks of the postpartum period. During this period incidences of 12 per 1,000 and 1.5 per 1,000 cases of superficial and deep vein phlebitis have been reported, respectively. This is 49 times the risk of the general population.[2] Aaro found most cases of superficial phlebitis (87%) occur in the first 72 hours after delivery. However, the risk for deep vein phlebitis and pulmonary embolism remains high for three weeks.[4] In this series ten of 13 pulmonary emboli complicating pregnancy appeared in the first three weeks postpartum. Only three pulmonary emboli were seen in the antepartum period. Most instances of postpartum pulmonary embolism are seen in patients with obstetrical complications such as pelvic hematoma, ruptured tubal pregnancy, septic abortion, placenta previa, and difficult forceps delivery.[4] Cesarean section is complicated by fatal pulmonary embolism nine times as often as vaginal delivery.

Pulmonary embolism is the most common cause of maternal death resulting in 30 deaths per 10^6 deliveries. Untreated pulmonary embolism complicating pregnancy will result in a 13% mortality.[4] Treated, this can be reduced to a 1% mortality rate. Nonpregnant patients have been reported to have 28% mortality from untreated pulmonary emboli.[2] Twenty percent of patients with deep vein phlebitis will have pulmonary emboli.[2,4] Therefore, all pregnant patients with pulmonary emboli or deep vein phlebitis must be anticoagulated.

Recognition of diffuse intravascular coagulation (DIC) requires consideration of heparin therapy. The presence of overt thrombosis is usually considered to be an indication for heparinization. Hemorrhage as a manifestation of DIC is another matter. No firm conclusions can be drawn from this controversy. Some clinicians do not treat, others heparinize, and still others administer heparin followed by replacement of coagulation factors. It is essential that each case be carefully evaluated before making any decision regarding therapy. This is unfortunately also true for amniotic fluid embolism, a condition in which DIC may result from thromboplastic material entering the circulation during parturition. Some clinicians have advocated early use of heparin[6], but this is not generally agreed upon.

Diagnostic tests for thrombotic and embolic events have limitations in nonpregnant patients. Clinical diagnosis is nonspecific and frequently is insensitive. Diagnosis of thromboembolic disease in pregnancy is complicated by the risk to the fetus of radiation from diagnostic procedures. Lung scans, radioiodine fibrinogen scans, and venograms are contraindicated[7]; pulmonary angiography can be done with shielding of the abdomen. Venous plethysmography and ultrasound may have a false-positive result due to compression of the pelvic veins from the gravid uterus. A negative venous plethysmograph is always of limited clinical usefulness, because this technique, while sensitive to popliteal and proximal vein thrombosis, is insensitive to calf vein thrombosis.

The choice of anticoagulant in the pregnant patient must be made with consideration of the toxicity to the fetus and the mother. Toxicity to both fetus and mother have been reported for both heparin and warfarin (Coumadin).[8] Coumadin is not approved by the manufacturer for use in pregnant patients.[9] It is probably more toxic than heparin and should not be used in pregnancy. The drug of choice for anticoagulation in pregnancy is heparin. Coumadin may be used in the postpartum period.

II. HEPARIN

A. History

Heparin, recognized as an anticoagulant in the early 1900s, is a naturally occurring mucopolysaccharide found in mast cells. Purified heparin is still not available, and there is continued investigation into identification and isolation of the active material. Heparin preparations, noted as units, are now based on a crude standardization: the prolongation of the clotting time of sheep plasma. Commercial products are noted in units per milligram. Since the number of units per milligram varies among products, it is important to order heparin in units rather than in milligrams. It is also important to note the source of the heparin (ie, lung or intestinal mucosa), since neutralization of these preparations also varies.

B. Mechanics of Action of Heparin

Heparin is a potent anticoagulant both in vivo and in vitro. Its major effect is to inhibit factors in the intrinsic pathway of coagulation. In addition, it can affect the fibrinolytic pathway. A recent important finding—that antithrombin III activity and heparin cofactor activity are properties of a single molecular species—has helped shed light on the mechanism of action of the heparins.

The inhibitor is responsible for most thrombin-neutralizing and heparin cofactor activity in normal blood. The neutralization of thrombin occurs at a 1:1 stoichiometric ratio of enzyme to inhibitor. Heparin addition does little to alter this, but it dramatically accelerates the rate of reaction.[10]

The coagulation cascade is composed of a series of interrelated reactions (Fig. M.XXII.1). A precursor zymogen is changed into a related serine protease. This serine protease catalyzes the subsequent zymogen, leading in turn to its related serine protease. In the presence of antithrombin III, the serine protease of factors XII (XIIa), XI (XIa), X (Xa), and IX (IXa) can each be slowly neutralized by antithrombin without heparin. In the presence of heparin, the factors are rapidly inhibited by antithrombin.[10]

It is postulated that the arginine of antithrombin III and the serine of the serine proteases associate to produce neutralization. Heparin may accelerate this association by altering the lysines of the antithrombin molecule. In addition to neutralizing the effect of the serine proteases of the clotting cascade, antithrombin can neutralize plasmin, which is critical for fibrinolysis. The neutralization is accelerated by heparin.[10]

Antithrombin III is probably critical for maintaining the nonthrombogenic state. Major clotting factor deficiencies must be present before spontaneous bleeding occurs. In contrast, a minor congenital deficiency of antithrombin III leads to profound thrombosis, and then heparin is not as effective for therapy of the thrombosis.[10]

C. Heparin-Associated Thrombocytopenia

For more than 30 years, heparin has been associated with thrombocytopenia. This has been observed both in humans and in animal models. It can be of sufficient magnitude to produce clinical hem-

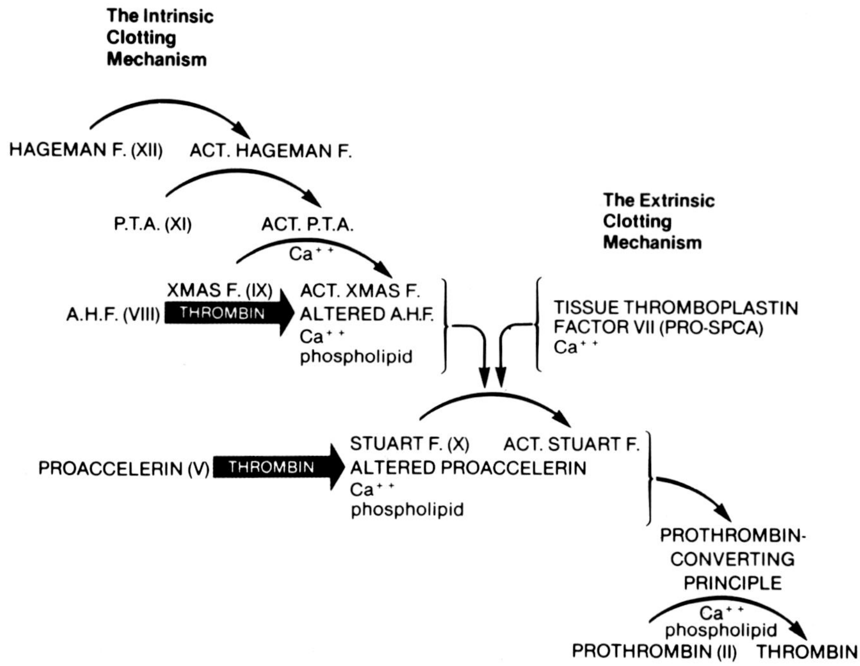

Fig. M.XXII.1. The mechanism of normal coagulation. (Reproduced with permission from Aledort LM. Anticoagulation with coumarin drugs. Primary Cardiol. 1977; 3:34–47.)

orrhage and death. The mechanism is not completely understood. The possibility that it will occur must be acknowledged, and the patient must be monitored.

In a recent prospective double-blind study, a bovine lung and two different intestinal mucosa-derived heparin preparations were evaluated. Of 149 patients studied, a platelet count of less than 100 $\times$ 10^9/liter was noted in 21 patients. Of these there were 13 of the 50 receiving bovine lung heparin, four of the 45 receiving intestinal mucosa A-heparin (Pan-heparin-Abbott Labs), and four of the 50 receiving intestinal mucosa O-heparin (Liquaemin, Sodium, Organon Labs). There was a significantly increased incidence of thrombocytopenia in the bovine lung group. Thrombocytopenia appeared as early as the third day and disappeared in all groups three to eight days after discontinuation of heparin.[11]

D. Acute Therapy

When given intravenously, heparin is rapidly cleared. Drug disappearance approximates a linear relationship. By increasing the dose, the half-life is increased, thus maintaining more heparin in the body longer. This pattern is characteristic for normal recipients. There are, however, some interesting data relating to the differences in effects and duration of activity of heparin in patients with phlebitis and pulmonary embolism.[10]

When plasma heparin levels were measured following intravenous bolus doses in patients with pulmonary embolism, the heparin half-life was 52 minutes, in contrast to 93 minutes in those who had thrombophlebitis. These data were obtained using activated partial thromboplastin time as a measure of heparin activity. When more sensitive assays of heparin activity were used, the respective half-lives appeared to be even shorter.[10]

These findings were corroborated in other excellent experiments, in which the inhibition of factor Xa was used to explore the relationship of dose to clearance in patients with phlebitis and emboli. In disease states the disappearance patterns changed and more closely approximated a first-order function. In patients with pulmonary embolism, half the heparin dose was cleared within 80 minutes; in those with phlebitis, half the heparin was cleared within 106 minutes. Evaluation of the postinfusion plasma level as a function of heparin dose in disease states revealed that more heparin was needed to reach a given level in patients with emboli than in those with phlebitis. In pregnant patients who have physiologic increases in their clotting factors, the required heparin dosage has been observed to increase at about the 28th gestational week.[12]

E. Prophylaxis

It has long been recognized that there is a group of "high-risk" patients in whom safe and effective prevention of thrombosis and embolism is highly desirable. This group includes patients undergoing general abdominothoracic surgery, elective surgery, or emergency hip surgery. Medical patients with myocardial infarction and congestive heart failure are also at risk. Multiple heparin regimens have been tried in an attempt to provide these patients with a prophylactic plan that would work.

Well-controlled clinical trials have been carried out using low dose heparin. Although endpoints for measuring thrombosis were difficult to attain, this has been successfully accomplished. The most important endpoint is fatal pulmonary embolism, but others include major pulmonary emboli and/or acute deep vein thrombosis.[13]

Prophylaxis has been advocated for pregnant patients with a history of deep vein thrombophlebitis.[14] For these patients the risk of recurrent thromboembolism during pregnancy is 9–12%.[14,15] If deep vein phlebitis is associated with use of birth control pills, the risk of recurrent phlebitis may be less than in those in whom deep vein phlebitis is due to intrinsic venous disease.[15] Heparin, in a dose of 5,000 units every eight hours, has been reported to be safe and effective in preventing recurrent thrombophlebitis complicating pregnancy. However, the number of patients at risk in this series (n = 7) was insufficient to draw any firm conclusion.[11]

F. Route of Administration

No oral heparin preparation exists at present. Intramuscular administration is painful, may produce hemorrhage, is absorbed capriciously, and is rarely used. Intravenous or subcutaneous injection are the preferred routes. Long-term self-administered subcutaneous heparin has been used successfully in pregnant outpatients after initial intravenous heparin therapy.[12]

When heparin is given to a patient with acute thrombosis, one must administer enough to arrest the process. In the present state of the art, we can only measure the ability of heparin to inhibit either whole blood clotting time or partial thromboplastin time. We cannot easily assess whether the heparin has aided inactivation of the serine proteases or stopped the generation of thrombin, thus inhibiting the conversion of fibrinogen to fibrin. More sophisticated methods will have to be more easily applied in routine laboratory procedures if we are to feel confident about the accuracy and effectiveness of our heparin dose.

For acute thrombosis, it may be necessary to give anywhere from 2,500 to 10,000 units every four hours, or 4,000–15,000 units every six hours, to achieve a prolongation of whole blood clotting time to 2–$2^1/_2$ times normal, or partial thromboplastin time to $1^1/_2$–$2^1/_2$ times normal. Continuous infusion of heparin requires more care, but produces fewer bleeding complications and can be achieved with an initial loading dose of approximately 10,000 units, followed by 1,500 units/hr.

For diffuse intravascular coagulation, lower doses can be utilized without a loading dose, and only 500 units are required per hour by continuous infusion. Evidence of reversal of this process in 24–48 hours indicates a correct dose. If the dose is too low, it can be increased.

The question of what constitutes an ideal method of monitoring heparin remains controversial. It is clear, however, that whether one uses clotting time or partial thromboplastin time, a baseline value should be obtained, and within the first day of therapy, in vivo prolongation should be evaluated and the dose altered appropriately. Once the dosage is established, it is safest to measure effectiveness daily. More frequent evaluation is not necessary. Low-dose constant infusion of heparin for DIC may not alter the clotting time or partial thromboplastin time.

Heparin therapy for acute thrombosis should be continued for a period of seven to ten days to ensure fixation of the vessel wall. Oral anticoagulants should be started before heparin is discontinued. Baseline prothrombin times and follow-up levels should be measured at a time when the effects of heparin are minimal—ie, just before the next dose, when treatment is bolus and intermittent.

The optimal time for initiating treatment and the ideal regimen for prophylaxis in high-risk patients are not absolute, but at present, it appears that 5,000 units given subcutaneously two hours before surgery and 5,000 units either every eight or every 12 hours provides safe and effective treatment. Therapy with that regimen is usually continued until the high-risk period is over. In the case of the pregnant patient anticoagulation should generally be continued for four weeks after delivery.

G. Reversal of Heparin Effect

If heparin use is complicated by hemorrhage, heparin can be neutralized by protamine sulfate. One milligram of protamine sulfate by intravenous infusion will neutralize 100 USP units of heparin.[9]

H. Fetal Toxicity of Heparin

The sequels of anticoagulation in pregnancy have recently been reviewed by Hall.[8] She was able to find 135 published cases of heparin used in pregnancy without Coumadin. One-eighth of the infants were stillborn; one-fifth, premature (a third of whom died); and only two-thirds were normal. Maternal hemorrhage complicated heparin administration in 14 patients (10%) with three deaths (2%). The methodology of this study would be expected to overestimate the toxicity of heparin, since uncomplicated uses of this drug would not necessarily be reported. Heparin is a relatively large molecule (mol wt $\simeq$ 16,000) and does not cross the placenta.[16] It is a physiologic anticoagulant that is found in all normal subjects. Intuitively, therefore, one would not anticipate significant fetal toxicity from this drug. Without a prospective study to include all uncomplicated uses of heparin in the denominator, we will be unable to determine the percentage of fetuses adversely affected by this drug.

III. COUMADIN

The major types of anticoagulants used today are the heparins, which directly prevent the clotting of blood, the antiplatelet agents, which impair the role platelets may play in thrombosis, and the coumarin-like drugs, which lower the plasma levels of proteins involved in the coagulation mechanism.

The coumarin-like drugs were first recognized in the early 1900s. A veterinarian noted a coagulation disorder produced in animals when improperly cured hay made with common varieties of sweet clover was included in the feed. This disorder, known as "sweet clover disease," developed over a two-week period as a result of a slow inhibition of the coagulation process. In 1934 the anticoagulant bishydroxy-coumarin was purified and isolated. The coumarin anticoagulants also include the numerous coumarin derivatives and the indandiones, a group of drugs shown to have similar action in almost all respects and to be qualitatively indistinct from the coumarins.

A. Mechanism of Action

The coumarin-like drugs function as anticoagulants by decreasing the amount of four coagulation factors: II, VII, IX, and X. These factors are synthesized in the liver and are vitamin K dependent. It appears that the only physiologic function of vitamin K is the activation of these four factors. Its role in the coagulation mechanism was first noted when it was discovered that the hemorrhage associated with obstructive jaundice could be prevented or stopped by the administration of this fat-soluble vitamin. Whereas natural forms of the vitamin are fat soluble, some synthetic products are water soluble.

The vitamin in food is absorbed in the upper part of the small intestine and rapidly appears in chylomicrons in serum. Some vitamin K is synthesized by intestinal microorganisms and is also absorbed and utilized. The vitamin is rapidly concentrated in the liver, but it disappears within 24 hours. The capacity to store vitamin K is thus limited. Dietary deficiency of vitamin K is rare; however, older patients maintained on deficient diets become depleted in 30 to 32 days. If oral antibiotics are added, depletion occurs in 21 to 28 days.

The coumarin-like drugs function by being vitamin K antagonists; thus they work at a stage subsequent to peptide synthesis. Following administration of the drug, an abnormal prothrombin is produced. This protein does not complex with calcium or absorb to barium, and it lacks coagulant activity. Vitamin K is needed to convert the precursors into active form.

The coumarins are rapidly absorbed, bind tightly to albumin, and are transported to the liver. They function in the liver and are detoxified in hepatic microsomes. Their effect on coagulation factors is a function of the relative rates of synthesis and turnover of the four coagulation factors. Based on this, the factors are inhibited in the following order: factor VII, IX, X, II.

The schematic shown in Figure M.XXII.1 demonstrates the intrinsic and extrinsic coagulation mechanism. Factor IX is in the intrinsic mechanism, factor VII is part of the extrinsic mechanism, and factor X is in both. As a result, these anticoagulants will prolong both the one-stage prothrombin time (PT), which measures the tissue thromboplastin-activated extrinsic system, and the partial thromboplastin time (PTT), which assays the intrinsic system. Throughout the world, patients on these anticoagulants are monitored by measuring the prothrombin time.

B. Therapy

These drugs require about 24 hours or more to produce their maximal effect. They differ in dose and in rapidity and duration of action.

If patients on heparin therapy are to be changed to coumarin-like drugs, it is important to follow some general principles (Table M.XXII.1). The baseline PT should be drawn at a time when heparin is not affecting this measurement. On bolus therapy, the effect is usually dissipated between four and six hours after intravenous heparin administration. Daily follow-up examinations of PT should be carried out under the same circumstances.

TABLE M.XXII.1. General Rules for Changing From Heparin to Coumarin

Baseline prothrombin time (PT) should be drawn when heparin is not affecting the measurement (on bolus therapy)—between four and six hours after intravenous heparin injection).
Daily follow-up measurements of PT should be done under similar conditions.
Careful monitoring is necessary initially to determine appropriate dosage.
When patient leaves hospital, weekly or biweekly PT measurement may be necessary to assure coagulation of a 2- to 2½-fold prolongation of baseline PT levels.
Once dosage is established, and if patient is reliable, PT may be monitored as infrequently as once a month.
Clinician must be constantly aware of factors influencing activity of the drugs.
Do not change to Coumadin until nursing is terminated.

Because the effect of these oral anticoagulants depends upon synthesis and turnover of the clotting factors, time must be allowed for them to act.[17]

Although there is controversy over larger initial doses versus smaller doses over time, each clinician chooses that regimen with which he is comfortable and familiar. However, first it is important to monitor each patient carefully to determine the appropriate dosage. Weekly or biweekly PTs may be necessary when the patient leaves the hospital to assure anticoagulation by a 2- to 2-1/2 fold prolongation of baseline PT levels.[17]

Adequate anticoagulation is critical in that thrombosis may not be prevented if the inhibition of coagulation factors is insufficient. On the other hand, over-anticoagulation may lead to serious if not life-threatening hemorrhage.[17]

In general, most patients, once in therapeutic range, need little alteration of the dosage of anticoagulant. Therefore, if the patient is reliable and there has not been any change in the clinical picture or lifestyle, the PT may be monitored as infrequently as once a month. However, it is becoming increasingly clear that the clinician must be constantly aware of the factors that influence the activity of these anticoagulant drugs.[17]

C. Potentiating Agents

An increasing number of agents are capable of intensifying the activity of coumarin-like drugs. Potentiation may occur by a) displacement of anticoagulant from albumin binding, b) inhibition of vitamin K production by gastrointestinal bacteria, c) inhibition of hepatic microsomal enzymes that degrade coumarin; and d) competition for vitamin K, or some unknown mechanism (Table M.XXII.2).[17]

TABLE M.XXII.2. Drugs Reported to Potentiate Effects of Oral Coumarin Anticoagulants

Drug	Mechanism of action
Tolbutamide Ethacrynic acid Nalidixic acid Diazoxide Sulfasoxazole Diphenylhydantoin Phenylbutazone Oxyphenbutazone Salicylates Indomethacin Chloral hydrate (Cl_3C-COOH)	Displacement of the anticoagulant from the protein-binding sites in plasma. Increase in the peak plasma concentration of free coumarin
Chloramphenicol Neomycin Sulfasoxazole Tetracycline	Interference with vitamin K production by gut bacteria?
Chloramphenicol? Disulfiram Methylphenidate Phenyramidol Allopurinol Nortiptyline	Inhibition of hepatic microsomal enzymes that metabolize coumarin anticoagulants and thereby raise levels in plasma
Acetaminophen Methylthiouracil Propylthiouracil Quinidine Quinine Anabolic steroids D-thyroxine Glucagon Clofibrate	Unknown
Salicylates	Competition with vitamin K site

Magnesium hydroxide, not aluminum hydroxide, can increase absorption of Dicumarol but not Coumadin. D-thyroxine and clofibrate and norethandrolone increase the sensitivity of the patient to the oral anticoagulant without affecting metabolism.[17]

D. Drugs That Reduce Activity

The major mechanism is a) increased metabolism of anticoagulant, or b) decreased absorption (Table M.XXII.3).

The drug phenylbutazone has an unusual mechanism of action; first it potentiates coumarin-like drugs by displacing albumin, but then it inhibits their action by increasing their metabolism.[17]

E. Resistance

Occasionally there is a genetic predisposition that makes patients resistant to the coumarin drugs. One type is an autosomal dominant trait that renders the patient sensitive to vitamin K. Another type is due to enhanced metabolism.[17]

TABLE M.XXII.3. Drugs Reported to Reduce Effects of Oral Coumarin Anticoagulants

Drug	Mechanism of action
Diphenylhydantoin Heptabarbital Amobarbital Secobarbital Phenobarbital Phenylbutazone Ethchlorvynol Glutethimide Griseofulvin Haloperidol Meprobamate Tolbutamide	Increases the rate of metabolism of coumarin anticoagulants by stimulating the hepatic microsomal enzymes responsible for their metabolism
Oral contraceptives	Decrease the hypoprothrombinemic response to the coumarin anticoagulants by increasing factor production
Cholestyramine Heptabarbital	Decrease absorption

F. Toxicity

The major hazard to over-anticoagulation is bleeding. Renal and gastrointestinal bleeding are easily noted, but less commonly retroperitoneal hemorrhage may occur. Mild to moderate increments in the PT, without bleeding, can be controlled by withholding anticoagulants. More severe increases in the PT, without bleeding, can be reversed by the administration of oral or subcutaneous vitamin K in low doses (1–10 mg may be sufficient).[17]

Patients with hemorrhage present another problem. Because vitamin K takes an average of six hours to produce an effect, one may be faced with an acute medical emergency. In addition to dealing with the hemorrhage, one may not desire full or rapid reversal of the "anticoagulated" state for fear of potentiating thrombosis. Therefore, it is frequently necessary to treat the patient by replacing depressed factors through transfusion of fresh frozen plasma. Such plasma retains all the essential factors; rarely, if large quantities of factors are required, volume overload may be a problem, and it may be necessary to administer factor concentrates. Two concentrates containing factors II, VII, IX, and X are commercially available (Konyne-Cutter and Proplex-Hyland). A major complication of the use of prothrombin complexes, however, is the very high incidence of hepatitis. In addition, a recently recognized complication of these materials is thrombosis.[17]

G. Fetal Toxicity of Coumadin

Coumadin is toxic to the fetus. Hall found 418 reported cases of Coumadin abuse in pregnant patients. One-sixth of these cases resulted in abnormal live-born infants, and one-sixth resulted in abortion or stillbirth, with only two-thirds apparently normal infants.[8] The design of this study, in which the literature (often consisting of single case reports) was reviewed, does not allow an assessment of the true toxicity of coumarins, which undoubtedly is over-estimated. Nonetheless, there is compelling evidence that coumarins are teratogenic. There is a distinctive syndrome of warfarin embryopathy with 29 reported cases.[8,18,19,20] Also called chondrodysplasia punctata, warfarin embryopathy is characterized by nasal hypoplasia and stippled epiphyses (Fig. M.XXII.2). All patients with warfarin embryopathy have been exposed to warfarin between the sixth and ninth weeks of gestation. Because of this fact, some have felt that Coumadin can be safely administered in the second and third trimester. This is probably not a justifiable conclusion, since Coumadin seems to have neurological toxicity that is not confined to the first trimester.[8]

Should a patient taking Coumadin become pregnant, the manufacturer advises that the patient be informed of the risks and that the possibility of termination of pregnancy be discussed with the patient.[9]

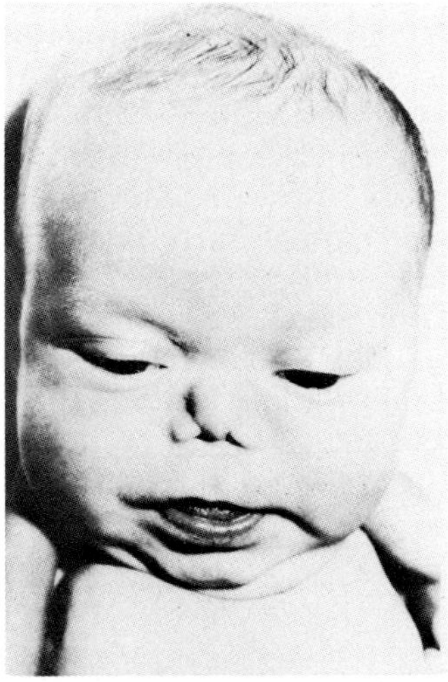

Fig. M.XXII.2. Typical facies of infant with warfarin embryopathy. Note the hypoplastic nose. (Reproduced with permission from Pettifor JM, Benson R. Congenital malformations associated with the administration of oral anticoagulants during pregnancy. J Pediatr. 1975; 86:459–462.)

Coumarins may pass into the milk of mothers and therefore should not be administered to nursing mothers.[9]

IV. DEXTRAN

In addition to heparin and coumarins, other anticoagulants have been used in pregnancy. Dextrans are high molecular weight polysaccharides that would not be expected to cross the placenta. The mechanism of antithrombotic action of dextran is unknown, but it has been postulated to be coating of the vascular endothelium and coating of the formed blood elements, including platelets, thus inhibiting the release of platelet factor III.

Dextran has been reported by Wallach to be an effective treatment for thrombophlebitis in pregnancy.[21] In that series, however, 10% of dextran-treated patients had suspected pulmonary embolism while receiving dextran and had to be treated with heparin. Other investigators have found dextran to be an ineffective treatment for thrombophlebitis in pregnancy.[22] There is insufficient experience with this therapy to recommend it.

V. THROMBOLYTIC THERAPY

Kinases catalyze the conversion of plasminogen to plasmin. Streptokinase and urokinase, which has been advocated as a treatment for massive pulmonary embolism with shock,[23] is now approved for use in the United States. Although the manufacturer considers pregnancy a contraindication, thrombolytic therapy has been used successfully in pregnancy, including the prepartum period.[24] It has been suggested that aminocaproic acid, which usually is used to reverse kinase-induced fibrinolysis, should not be used in the prepartum period because it crosses the placenta. Trasylol, a serine protease inhibitor, has a high molecular weight, does not cross the placenta, and has been recommended for prepartum reversal of fibrinolysis. Relative uterine atonia requiring pitressin at the time of delivery has been reported as an effect of thrombolytic therapy.[24]

VI. ADDITIONAL MEASURES

In cases of massive pulmonary embolism complicating pregnancy, both pulmonary embolectomy[25] and vena cava ligation[26] have been successfully performed. Although we are unaware of any case reports, placement of an "umbrella" in the inferior vena cava can no doubt also be done in a pregnant patient. Umbrella placement is usually done under fluoroscopic control, but it could probably be accomplished without fluoroscopy or with sonographic control. Placed below the renal arteries, an umbrella would still allow embolization from the left ovarian vein, which drains to the left renal vein.

During the acute attack of thrombophlebitis the patient should be kept in bed. The Trendelenberg position is better than simple elevation of the legs, which may compress the vena cava. Ambulation should begin a few days after haparin has been started, but the patient must wear elastic hose.

VII. CONTRAINDICATIONS TO ANTICOAGULATION

Bleeding is always a relative contraindication to anticoagulation. One must use clinical judgment in assessing the risk:benefit ratio in a patient with pulmonary emboli and a small gastrointestinal, pulmonary, urogenital, or wound hemorrhage. Bleeding into the cranium is an absolute contraindication to anticoagulation. Bacterial endocarditis and pericarditis greatly increase the risk of anticoagulation.

Placenta previa, threatened abortion, preeclampsia/eclampsia, and delivery are obstetrical contraindications to anticoagulation. Delivery, like abdominal and thoracic surgery, can be done in patients receiving full-dose heparin, if absolutely necessary. However, we recommend that heparin be discontinued several hours before delivery and be restarted several hours after delivery.

VIII. ACKNOWLEDGMENTS

This work was supported in part by Health Services Administration grant MCB-360001-04-01, Regional Comprehensive Hemophilia Diagnostic and Treatment Center, and NHLBI Contract N01-HD-53020; the Margie Boas Fund, the Polly Annenberg Levy Hematology Center, Department of Medicine, Mt. Sinai School of Medicine of the City University of New York.

IX. REFERENCES

1. Graeff H, Kuhn W, eds. Coagulation Disorders in Obstetrics. Philadelphia: W.B. Saunders, 1980:7–9.
2. Handin RI. Thromboembolic complications of pregnancy and oral contraceptives. Prog Cardiovasc Dis. 1974; 16:395–405.
3. Drill VA. Oral contraceptives and thromboembolic disease. JAMA. 1968; 206:77–84.
4. Aaro LA, Juergens JL. Thrombophlebitis associated with pregnancy. Am J Obstet Gynecol. 1971; 109:1128–1136.
5. VillaSanta V. Thromboembolic disease in pregnancy. Am J Obstet Gynecol. 1965; 93:142–160.
6. Chuang AF, Merkatz IR. Survival following amniotic fluid embolism with early heparinization. Obstet Gynecol. 1973; 42:809–814.
7. Editorial. Venous thromboembolism and anticoagulation in pregnancy. Br Med J. 1975; 4:421–422.
8. Hall JG, Paull RM, Wilson KM. Maternal and fetal sequelae of anticoagulation during pregnancy. Am J Med. 1980; 68:122–140.
9. Physicians' Desk Reference. Oradell, N.J.: Medical Economics Co, 1980:869–871, 1043–1044.
10. Aledort LM. Heparin dosage is it disease specific. Primary Cardiol. 1979; 5:8–10.
11. Bell WR, Royall RM. Heparin-associated thrombocytopenia: A comparison of three heparin preparations. N Engl J Med. 1980; 303:902–907.
12. Spearing G, Fraser I, Turner G, Dixon G. Long-term self-administered subcutaneous heparin in pregnancy. Br Med J. 1978; 1:1457–1458.
13. Prevention of fatal postoperative pulmonary embolism by low dose heparin: An international multicentre trial. Lancet, 1975; 2:45–51.

14. Baskin HF, Murray JM, Harris RE. Low-dose heparin for prevention of thromboembolic disease in pregnancy. Am J Obstet Gynecol. 1977; 129:590–591.
15. Badaracco MA, Vesseg MP. Recurrence of venous thromboembolic disease and use of oral contraceptives. Br Med J. 1974; 1:215–217.
16. Flessa HC, Kapstrom AB, Glueck HI, Will JS. Placental transport of heparin. Am J Obstet Gynecol. 1956; 93:570–573.
17. Aledort LM. Anticoagulation with coumarin drugs. Primary Cardiol. 1977; 3:34–37.
18. Becker MH, Genieser NB, Finegold M, Miranda D, Sparkman T. Chondrodysplasia punctata: Is maternal warfarin therapy a factor? Am J Dis Child. 1975; 129:356–359.
19. Shaul WL, Emery H, Hall JG, Chondrodysplasia punctata and maternal warfarin use during pregnancy. Am J Dis Child. 1975; 129:360–362.
20. Pettifor JM, Benson R. Congenital malformation associated with the administration of oral anticoagulants during pregnancy. J Pediatr. 1975; 86:459–462.
21. Wallach RC. Dextran therapy for pregnancy-associated deep thrombophlebitis. Am J Obstet Gynecol. 1972; 112:613–618.
22. Mueller MJ Sr, Lebherz TB. Antepartum thrombophlebitis, morbidity with long-term heparin and a proposed regimen of therapy. Obstet Gynecol. 1969; 34:874–880.
23. Sharma GURK, Sasahara AA. Diagnosis and treatment of pulmonary embolism. Med Clin North Am. 1979; 63:239–250.
24. Hall, RJC, Young C, Sutton GC, Campbell S. Treatment of acute massive pulmonary embolism by streptokinase during labor and delivery. Br Med J. 1972; 4:647–649.
25. Cohn LH, Shumway NE. Pulmonary embolectomy during pregnancy. Arch Surg. 1973; 106:214–215.
26. Sauter RD, Fletcher FW, Lewis RF, Wentzel FJ. Inferior vena caval and ovarian vein ligation for antepartum pulmonary thromboembolization. JAMA. 1966; 196:290–292.

M.XXIII

Tocolytic Drugs and the Cardiac Patient

Niels H. Lauersen, MD

I. INTRODUCTION

Recent physiologic understanding combined with pharmacologic advances has provided physicians with a new clinical capability, the ability to control the forces of labor. Drugs that inhibit the activity of the uterus are termed tocolytic drugs. Because of their effect on the cardiovascular system of mother and fetus, their discussion within the present framework seems indicated.

Prematurity remains a major health problem, accounting for 8% of births but 75% of perinatal deaths.[1] A major contemplated indication for tocolytic agents is the prevention of premature delivery.[2] Situations can arise, however, in which prevention of delivery until term is either not feasible or not clinically desirable. In these instances, when amniocentesis indicates that the fetal lungs are not mature, a tocolytic agent may be administered in conjunction with corticosteroids. The goal of this therapy is for the tocolytic drug to prevent delivery for a limited period of time (24 to 48 hours) so that the corticosteroids can act to enhance fetal lung maturation.[3]

The tocolytic drugs have clinical usefulness beyond the delay of parturition; they may be employed when temporary uterine relaxation is desired. The occurrence of very frequent uterine contractions with hypertonicity can result in fetal distress. The administration of tocolytic agents can inhibit this hyperactivity and result in an improved fetal environment.[4,5] Tocolytic drugs can provide the obstetrician with the time necessary for accurate evaluation of the situation and preparation for a safe delivery. Transient uterine relaxation can also be useful for certain obstetrical manipulations. Tocolytic drugs have been administered for this purpose to allow external cephalic version of breech presentations.[6] This maneuver can help avoid operative delivery.

The decision to interfere with the forces of labor through the administration of a tocolytic drug always requires a careful consideration of the potential benefit to be achieved versus the potential hazard of the therapy. If the patient who is a candidate for labor inhibition has cardiovascular problems, the assessment of the risk–benefit ratio must be particularly precise. The usefulness of tocolytic agents

Cardiac Problems in Pregnancy, pages 273–280

to the cardiac patient in labor directly depends on the knowledge of the physician concerning the nature, effectiveness, and side effects of these drugs.

II. TOCOLYTIC AGENTS: UTERINE AND CARDIOVASCULAR EFFECTS

Tocolytic agents can inhibit uterine activity either by direct action at the level of the myometrium or by central inhibition of substances that stimulate the uterus or, at times, by a combination of both effects. Beta mimetics, diazoxide, and magnesium sulfate are direct inhibitors; the prostaglandin synthesis inhibitors work centrally; and alcohol has both a central effect and some residual direct inhibitory effect.

The smooth muscle of the uterus contains both alpha- and beta-adrenergic receptors.[7] Stimulation of the uterine beta-receptors by beta-mimetic drugs results in muscle relaxation. The smooth muscle of the heart also has beta-receptors, but stimulation of the heart beta-receptors results in positive inotropic as well as chronotropic effects. In addition to these effects, activation of extracardiac beta-receptors causes dilation of vascular and bronchial smooth muscle. The characteristic cardiocirculatory response to beta-mimetics is therefore tachycardia, increase in cardiac output, a rise in systolic blood pressure, a fall in diastolic pressure, and a decrease in systemic vascular resistance.[8] These cardiovascular effects limited the clinical application in obstetrics of early beta-mimetics such as isoxsuprine*[9,10] and initiated the search for more uterine-specific drugs. Lands et al[11] theorized that there were two types of beta-receptors defined as beta-1- and beta-2-receptors. Beta-2-receptors are predominant in the uterus and relax on stimulation. Most of the newer beta-mimetics used as tocolytic agents such as ritodrine,† terbutaline,‡ fenertol, and salbutamol are chiefly beta-2-receptor stimulators, but they also retain certain beta-1 characteristics and evoke some degree of cardiovascular response.[12]

Diazoxide§ is a potent inhibitor of uterine activity in both humans[13,14] and nonhuman primates.[15] The drug, a benzothiadiazine, also relaxes vascular smooth muscle and is an antihypertensive agent. Research demonstrated that this drug could effectively inhibit labor at term, but it also appeared to have unpredictable antihypertensive effects in normotensive patients.[14] Administration of diazoxide also produces some degree of tachycardia.

Magnesium sulfate directly and immediately inhibits uterine activity,[16,17] probably through calcium displacement as the two ions compete for the same receptor site.[18] The cardiovascular effects of magnesium can be profound, with tachycardia, a decrease in peripheral vascular resistance, and an increase in stroke volume. The cardiovascular effects of magnesium sulfate may be comparable to those of the beta-mimetics.[19]

The precise role of the prostaglandins in the initiation and maintenance of labor remains to be clarified.[1] Agents that inhibit prostaglandin synthesis can prolong parturition[20,21] and control premature labor.[22,23] The list of prostaglandin inhibitors is expanding with recent pharmacologic developments and now includes aspirin, indomethacin,** ibuprofen,†† and naproxen.‡‡ The cardiovascular effects of the prostaglandin inhibitors in the pregnant patient have not been documented. Primary pulmonary hypertension of the newborn, however, has been reported in association with indomethacin therapy.[24] In nonpregnant patients cardiovascular effects associated with prostaglandin inhibitor administration appear to be rare, but, in a very small number of cases, less than 1% of hypertension tachycardia and chest pain have been reported.

*Vasodilan®, Mead Johnson Pharmaceutical, Evansville, IN.

†Yutopar®, Merrell-National Laboratories, Division of Richardson-Merrell Inc., Cincinnati, OH.

‡Brethine®, Geigy Pharmaceuticals, Ardsley, NY; Bricanyl®, Astra Pharmaceutical Products, Worcester, MA.

§Hyperstat®, Schering Corp., Kennilworth, NJ.

**Indocin®, Merck Sharp & Dohme, West Point, PA.

††Motrin®, The Upjohn Company, Kalamazoo, MI.

‡‡Naprosyn®, Syntex Puerto Rico, Inc., Humacao, PR.

Ethyl alcohol administration can arrest labor and postpone premature delivery.[25] Its effectiveness may be due in part to the ability of ethanol to suppress the release of oxytocin from the posterior pituitary.[26] Some direct relaxant effect on the myometrium, however, cannot be ruled out. Bueno-Montano and co-workers[27] and Wilson et al,[28] have demonstrated that ethyl alcohol inhibits the activity of isolated human myometrium. Furthermore, in a series of in vivo experiments, Mantell and Liggins[29] and Lauersen et al[30] reported that ethanol administration reduced the uterine responsiveness to a concomitant exogenous oxytocin infusion. The cardiovascular effects of acute ethanol administration are usually mild, with an increase in heart rate and cardiac output and a decrease in total peripheral vascular resistance.[31,32] At high doses of alcohol, there can be a depression in ventricular contractility.

III. TOCOLYTIC AGENTS AND CARDIOVASCULAR DISEASE IN PREGNANCY

At present the prevention of premature delivery must be considered the primary target for the use of tocolytic agents in pregnancy. The decision to arrest the progress of labor through the administration of a tocolytic agent must always be based on the careful assessment of a number of factors. These factors include the presence of fetal abnormality, evidence of a compromised fetal environment, and the possibility of infection such as amnionitis. The goal of this assessment is to determine whether the fetus could be and should be provided a superior chance for survival in or outside the womb. When the patient in premature labor is a cardiac patient, another dimension of complexity is added to the problem. It then must be determined whether postponement of delivery will threaten the health of the mother or be in her best interest. If it is determined that both fetus and mother will benefit or, at minimum, will not be harmed if delivery is delayed, then the appropriate pharmacologic tool must be chosen. The choice is determined by the condition of the pregnancy and the cardiac problem of the mother.

The cardiac patient can run a higher risk of premature labor. She should be informed of this risk early in pregnancy and advised to avoid situations that might precipitate labor such as unnecessary stress. She should be alerted to the early signs of premature labor, for the earlier labor is detected, the more effective the treatment, and with less medication. The physician of the known cardiac pregnant patient should determine whether this patient would be a candidate for a tocolytic drug and, if so, which drug. If a patient is in premature labor and a cardiac condition is suspected, that condition must be fully evaluated prior to the choice or administration of a tocolytic agent.

Cardiac patients have been classified according to functional capacity by the Criteria Committee of the New York Heart Association, Inc.[33]:

Class I—Patients who are not limited by cardiac disease in their physical activity. Ordinary physical activity does not precipitate the occurrence of symptoms such as fatigue, palpitation, dyspnea or anginal pain.

Class II—Patients in whom the cardiac disease causes a slight limitation in physical activity. These patients are comfortable at rest, but ordinary physical activity will precipitate symptoms.

Class III—Patients in whom the cardiac disease results in a marked limitation of physical activity. They are comfortable at rest, but less than ordinary physical activity will precipitate symptoms.

Class IV—Patients in whom the cardiac disease results in the inability to carry on physical activity without discomfort. Symptoms may be present even at rest, and discomfort is increased by any physical activity.

In general, prevention of premature delivery by any tocolytic agent, even one with minimal cardiovascular effects, would be contraindicated in those patients for whom pregnancy itself was contraindicated; this would include class IV and most class III cardiac patients. If, however, a cardiac patient, even a class III patient, had been adequately compensated and had tolerated the pregnancy well, then postponement of premature delivery by a tocolytic agent might be considered.

The use of a beta-mimetic in premature labor in a cardiac patient is not advised. At present the only beta-mimetic approved by the U.S. Food and Drug Administration (FDA) for the control of premature labor is ritodrine (Yutopar). Extensive clinical testing has demonstrated ritodrine's ability to delay delivery but also revealed the frequent cardiovascular effects of the drug.[34,35] Administration of ritodrine for premature labor increased maternal heart rate by a mean of 38 beats per minute[35]; the tachycardia thus induced would place impermissible strain on the system of a cardiac patient. A second hazard is that the drug-induced tachycardia could mask an idiopathic tachycardia that is one of the most important symptoms of imminent cardiac failure.[36] The effects of magnesium sulfate and diazoxide can be similar to those of the beta-mimetics, so these drugs would be similarly contraindicated for the prevention of premature delivery in the cardiac patient.

The use of tocolytic agents during pregnancy may adversely affect both mother and infant. The FDA has received reports of several cases of maternal pulmonary edema and serious cardiovascular side effects (adult respiratory distress syndrome, hypokalemia, angina pectoris, etc), occasionally resulting in the death of mother or child. In addition, adverse effects such as hypoglycemia, ileus, and hypocalcemia have been reported in the offspring of pregnant women treated with these drugs.[38]

Intravenous administration of ethyl alcohol may be the therapy of choice for premature labor for selected cardiac patients. Although alcohol has some cardiovascular effects, they usually are minor. Prior to the administration of the drug the patient's vital signs are evaluated and she should be placed on a continuous ECG monitor if possible. A 10% alcohol solution is administered at a rate of 7.5 ml/kg body weight/hr for two hours, followed by a maintenance dose of 1.5 ml/kg body weight/hr for ten hours. The patient may receive up to 1,800 ml of fluid over a 12-hour period, 900 ml in the first two hours. This amount of fluid alone may be cause for concern in the cardiac patient, and the patient's liquid intake and output must be carefully monitored. It would be advisable to administer the alcohol in 5% dextrose in water to prevent salt retention. The patient's vital signs should be monitored throughout the infusion, and administration should be terminated at any indication of cardiac decompensation.

Prostaglandin inhibitors might be considered as therapy for the cardiac patient in premature labor. The major problem with these drugs appears to be their effects on the fetal cardiovascular system. Premature closure of the ductus arteriosus has been reported with administration of indomethacin for premature labor.[37] Although the study of Niebyl and co-workers[23] failed to reveal any evidence of premature closure in 16 infants of indomethacin-treated mothers, these authors, however, point up another potential problem area with antiprostaglandin administration for both mother and fetus; indomethacin and aspirin cause platelet dysfunction in vitro.

If it were determined that the risk from delivery significantly outweighed the risk from the administration of the prostaglandin blocker, then an administration schedule for indomethacin as outlined by Niebyl and co-workers[23] could be followed.

The patient receives an initial 50 mg dose of indomethacin orally, followed by 25 mg every four hours for 24 hours. As with ethanol, administration of this drug to a cardiac patient must be accompanied by careful monitoring of the mother's vital signs and ECG.

When the clinical picture indicates that delivery cannot be postponed until term or if it is determined that prolonging the pregnancy for a number of weeks would not be in the best interest of either mother or fetus, the tocolytic agents can be used to delay delivery for 24 to 48 hours to permit administration of a corticosteroid to hasten fetal lung maturity.[3] In such a case ultrasonography should be done to determine fetal size and condition, and amniocentesis should be performed to assess fetal lung maturity by L/S ratio or fluorescence polarization and to rule out infection.

The administration of corticosteroids to a cardiac patient can be cause for concern. These drugs can lead to water retention and result in pulmonary edema. If a cardiac patient is not well compensated or has mitral stenosis and is prone to pulmonary edema, administration of the steroid alone would be contraindicated. Furthermore, the steroids are only significantly effective within a range, between 28 and 32 gestational weeks.[3] Administration before or after that time could expose both mother and fetus to the risks of drug administration without a concomitant potential benefit.

Once it has been determined that a cardiac patient is a candidate for steroid administration, the appropriate tocolytic agent for suppression of labor must be chosen.

Beta-mimetics might be considered in this case, because only a short-term administration of the drug is required. It would appear that the cardiovascular stress they induce might be offset by their potent uterine relaxant effects. Maternal pulmonary edema has been reported, however, after concurrent administration of corticosteroids and the beta-mimetics ritodrine[39,40] and terbutaline.[40–42] Beta-mimetics would not be the drugs of choice in association with corticosteroid administration in patients with moderate to severe cardiac disease, particularly patients with aortic stenosis, idiopathic hypertrophic subaortic stenosis, pulmonic stenosis, or mitral stenosis.[42] The occurrence of pulmonary edema is quite rare, but reasons for its occurrence have been offered. Ritodrine and terbutaline are specific beta-2-stimulators, but they still possess cardiovascular side effects and result in increased pulse rate and peripheral vasodilatation. These drugs also increase cardiac output and could result in sodium and water retention, and might produce paradoxic pulmonary venoconstriction. These effects could become exaggerated and lead to cardiac failure and pulmonary edema. In addition, the glucosteroids, which also have a sodium retention effect, can also cause water retention, which would lead to increased fluid conservation in the pregnant patient. The combination of beta-mimetics and glucocorticoids might thus cause heart failure and pulmonary edema.

In well-compensated class I or II cardiac patients, administration of a beta-mimetic to delay delivery for corticosteroid administration might be attempted. Prior to the administration of the drugs, the patient's vital signs should be carefully ascertained and her ECG should be continuously monitored during administration. If ritodrine is to be administered, the starting dose should be 50 mcg/min administered intravenously in 5% dextrose in water by a constant rate infusion pump. The maternal pulse rate and blood pressure should be checked every five minutes. The infusion rate of ritodrine would be increased to 50 mcg/min every ten to 20 minutes until labor stops or maternal pulse rate reaches 120 beats per minute. The maximum infusion rate should be no more than 300 mcg/min. If the maternal pulse rate rises above 120 beats per minute, then the infusion rate should be cut back or discontinued until the pulse rate is acceptable. When a steady infusion rate has been achieved, the maternal pulse and blood pressure should be assessed every 15 minutes. Once the patient's tolerance to the drug and the uterine relaxant effectiveness of the beta-mimetic have been established, the corticosteroid may be administered. A suggested treatment dose is 12 mg of betamethasone intramuscularly, followed by another 12 mg in 12 hours. The ritodrine infusion should be terminated after 12 hours. If the patient develops any respiratory changes indicative of the development of pulmonary edema, the beta-mimetic administration should be immediately discontinued and the second injection of steroid should not be administered. The serum electrolytes should be immediately checked, because beta-mimetics can decrease potassium stores. If the potassium levels are within the normal range diuretics should be given.[42] Even if there is no sign of pulmonary edema, the patient's electrolytes should be checked at 12 hours, the end of the beta-mimetic infusion, and prior to the administration of the second dose of steroid. After the second dose of steroid, the patient should be carefully observed for the next 12 hours, and vital signs should be checked every 30 to 60 minutes.

The effectiveness of diazoxide for this indication has not been reported, and the drug cannot be recommended. Magnesium sulfate has been administered with corticosteroids, and development of pulmonary edema associated with this therapy has been reported.[19] As previously described, the cardiovascular effects of magnesium sulfate approximate those of the beta-mimetics, and no advantage appears to be gained by the administration of this agent in place of the beta-mimetics.

If a cardiac patient should not receive or cannot tolerate a beta-mimetic for even a single administration, alcohol would be the therapy of choice. The alcohol would be administered in the same manner as for long-term prevention of premature delivery. If, however, the cardiac patient is in very active labor, with cervical dilation beyond 4 cm, administration of alcohol must be carefully weighed. If the alcohol does not inhibit the labor (and the drug is less effective in the more advanced labor) delivery can occur. The fetus will be under the influence of the alcohol and can be depressed upon delivery.[43]

The use of prostaglandin blockers to inhibit labor for the administration of corticosteroids has not been reported. The short-term cardiovascular effects of these drugs appear to be minimal. It is possible that the potential fetal cardiovascular problems encountered when the drugs are given over an extended time for the prevention of premature delivery could be avoided by giving a single, short-term administration.

Tocolytic agents have been employed in the management of acute labor problems, including external cephalic version[6,44] and fetal distress.[4,5] In these cases, a rapid and profound uterine relaxation is required. The centrally acting drugs, prostaglandin blockers and alcohol, would not be effective; the onset of their inhibitory activity is too gradual to be clinically efficacious in the acute situation. Also, as already mentioned, administration of alcohol at a time proximal to birth could result in the delivery of a depressed fetus.[43] Acute situations require the potent, direct-acting myometrial inhibitors. In this situation, the choice of the agent required to produce uterine relaxation is not difficult, but the decision to administer such an agent to a cardiac patient is complex. This decision must be made on a case-by-case basis by thorough and sensitive assessment of the possible benefits to mother and infant and potential harm to the mother. None of the direct myometrial inhibitors is free of cardiovascular effects, even in short-term administration. It is these cardiovascular effects that must be weighed against the benefit of a brief, profound uterine relaxation.

The clinician may encounter a cardiac patient with a breech presentation who would require delivery by cesarean section. In this case, the physician is faced with the dilemma of whether the operative delivery would be more stressful to the patient than external cephalic version achieved with the administration of a tocolytic agent. If the clinical factors balance in favor of version, the directly acting tocolytic drug should be administered with great caution. The patient must be monitored as previously described. Uterine relaxation could be achieved by intravenous administration of a beta-mimetic, such as ritodrine, starting at a low dose and increasing the rate until a sufficient degree of relaxation is achieved. The infusion is then continued throughout the version maneuver, which should be performed under the guidance of ultrasonography.[6,44,45] The version is performed by lifting the breech and gently rotating the fetus forward as described by Fall and Nilsson.[6] When the version is complete and the fetal status established by sonography, the infusion may be discontinued. The entire procedure should take no more than 30 minutes, and this brief time would not impose extreme stress on a well-compensated cardiac patient.

The occurrence of fetal distress in labor caused by uterine hypertonicity is another indication for the acute administration of a directly acting tocolytic agent.[4,5] The risk–benefit ratio in this instance involves balancing the potential benefit to the fetus from relief of the hypertonicity versus the possible stress to the mother from the drug administration. If it is determined that the clinical factors favor intervention with a tocolytic agent, the administration would be similar to that for version. In this case, both the maternal and fetal hearts must be continuously monitored to determine the drug effects. Cesarean section may not be avoided in these cases, but the uterine relaxation might provide valuable time for intrauterine resuscitation[46] and adequate preparation for operative delivery.

The control of uterine activity provided by tocolytic agents is a potent clinical tool for the practicing obstetrician. The benefits that can accrue from the use of tocolytics should not be denied cardiac patients. The use of these drugs with a cardiac patient, however, is a complex problem. The physician must be well acquainted not only with the cardiac condition of the patient but also with the cardiac effects of the various drugs. The risk–benefit ratio must be assessed with particular skill whenever a tocolytic agent is to be administered to a cardiac patient.

IV. REFERENCES

1. Fuchs F. Prevention of prematurity. Am J Obstet Gynecol. 1976; 126:809–820.
2. Niebyl JR, Blake DA, Johnson JWC, King TM. The pharmacologic inhibition of premature labor. Obstet Gynecol Surv. 1978; 33:507–515.
3. Liggins GC, Howie RN. A controlled trial antepartum glucocorticoid treatment for the prevention of respiratory distress syndrome in premature infants. Pediatrics. 1972; 50:515–525.
4. Caldeyro-Barcia R, Magana JM, Castillo JB, Poseiro JJ, Mendez-Bauer C, Pose SV, Escarcena L, Casacuberta C, Bustos JR, Giussi G. Nuevo enfoque para el tratamiento del sufrimiento fetal agudo intraparto. Arch Gynecol Obstet. 1969; 24:15–24.
5. Lipshitz J. The use of a β_2-sympathomimetic drug as a temporizing measure in the treatment of acute fetal distress. Am J Obstet Gynecol. 1977; 129:31–36.
6. Fall O, Nilsson BA. External cephalic version in breech presentation under tocolysis. Obstet Gynecol. 1979; 53:712–715.
7. Ahlquist RP. A study of the adrenotropic receptors. Am J Physiol. 1948; 153:586–600.
8. Sackner MA. Changes in blood oxygen and in cardiac function following $beta_2$ and other bronchodilator drugs. Chest. 1978; 73:985.
9. Bishop EH, Woutersz TB. Isoxsuprine, a myometrial relaxant. A preliminary report. Obstet Gynecol. 1961; 17:442–446.
10. Hendricks CH, Cibils LA, Pose SV, Eskes T. The pharmacologic control of excessive uterine activity with isoxsuprine. Am J Obstet Gynecol. 1961; 82:1064–1075.
11. Lands AM, Luduena FP, Buzzo HJ. Differentiation of receptors responsive to isoproterenol. Life Sci. 1967; 6:2241–2249.
12. Bieniarz J, Ivankovich A, Scommegna A. Cardiac output during ritodrine treatment in premature labor. Am J Obstet Gynecol. 1974; 118:910–920.
13. Landesman R, Coutinho EM, Wilson KH, Lopes ACV. The relaxant effect of diazoxide on nongravid human myometrium in vivo. Am J Obstet Gynecol. 1968; 102:1080–1084.
14. Landesman R, de Souz JA, Coutinho EM, Wilson KH, de Sousa MB. The inhibitory effect of diazoxide in normal term labor. Am J Obstet Gynecol. 1969; 103:430–433.
15. Wilson KH, Lauersen NH, Raghavan KS, Fuchs F, Niemann WH. Effects of diazoxide and beta adrenergic drugs on spontaneous and induced

uterine acitvity in the pregnant baboon. Am J Obstet Gynecol. 1974; 118:499–509.

16. Hutchinson HT, Nichols MM, Kuhn CR, Vasicka A. Effects of magnesium sulfate on uterine contractility, intrauterine fetus and infant. Am J Obstet Gynecol. 1964; 88:747–758.
17. Steer CM, Petrie RH. A comparison of magnesium sulfate and alcohol for the prevention of premature labor. Am J Obstet Gynecol. 1977; 129:1–4.
18. Coutinho EM. Calcium, magnesium, and local anesthesia. J Gen Physiol. 1966; 49:845–846.
19. Elliott JP, O'Keeffe DF, Greenberg P, Freeman RK: Pulmonary edema associated with magnesium sulfate and betamethasone administration. Am J Obstet Gynecol. 1979; 134:717–719.
20. Waltham R, Tricomi V, Palav A. Mid-trimester hypertonic saline-induced abortion: Effect of indomethacin on induction/abortion time. Am J Obstet Gynecol. 1972; 114:829–831.
21. Lewis RB, Schulman JD. Influence of acetylsalicylic acid, an inhibitor of prostaglandin synthesis, on the duration of human gestation and labor. Lancet. 1973; 2:1159–1161.
22. Zuckerman H, Reiss U, Rubinstein I. Inhibition of human premature labor by indomethacin. Obstet Gynecol. 1974; 44:787–792.
23. Niebyl JR, Blake DA, White RD, Kumor KM, Dubin NH, Robinson JC, Egner PG. The inhibition of premature labor with indomethacin. Am J Obstet Gynecol. 1980; 136:1014–1019.
24. Manchester D, Margolis HS, Sheldon RE. Possible association between maternal indomethacin therapy and primary pulmonary hypertension of the newborn. Am J Obstet Gynecol. 1976; 126:467–469.
25. Zlatnik F, Fuchs F. A controlled study of ethanol in threatened premature labor. Am J Obstet Gynecol. 1972; 112:610–612.
26. Wagner G, Fuchs A-R. Effect of ethanol on uterine activity during suckling in post-partum women. Acta Endocrinol. 1968; 58:133–141.
27. Bueno-Montano M, McGaughey HS Jr, Harbert GM, Thornton WN Jr. Drug preservatives and uterine contractility. Am J Obstet Gynecol. 1966; 94:1–5.
28. Wilson KH, Landesman R, Fuchs A-R, Fuchs F. The effect of ethyl alcohol on isolated human myometrium. Am J Obstet Gynecol. 1969; 104:436–439.
29. Mantell CD, Liggins GC. The effect of ethanol on the myometrial response to oxytocin in women at term. J Obstet Gynaecol Br Commonw. 1970; 77:976–981.
30. Lauersen NH, Wilson KH, Fuchs F. The inhibitory effect of ethanol on oxytocin induced labor at term. J Reprod Med. 1981; 26:547–550.
31. Becker CE, Roe RL, Scott RA (eds). Alcohol as a Drug: A Curriculum on Pharmacology, Neurology and Toxicology. New York: Medcom Press, 1974:70.
32. Silber EN, Katz LN eds. Heart Disease. New York: Macmillan Publishing Co., Inc., 1975:1035.
33. New York Heart Association. Nomenclature and Criteria for Diagnosis of Diseases of the Heart and Blood Vessels, Ed. 5, New York: Peter F. Mallen, Inc., 1953.
34. Bieniarz J, Motew M, Scommegna A. Uterine and cardiovascular effects of ritodrine in premature labor. Obstet Gynecol. 1972; 40:65–73.
35. Lauersen NH, Merkatz IR, Tejani N, Wilson KH, Roberson A, Mann LI, Fuchs F. Inhibition of premature labor: A multicenter comparison of ritodrine and ethanol. Am J Obstet Gynecol. 1977; 127:837–845.
36. Mendelson CL, Pardee HEB. The pulse and respiratory rates during labor as a guide to the onset of cardiac failure in women with rheumatic heart disease. Am J Obstet Gynecol. 1942; 44:370–383.
37. Sharpe GL, Thalme B, Larsson KS. Studies on closure of the ductus arteriosus. XI Ductal closure in utero by a prostaglandin synthetase inhibitor. Prostaglandins. 1974; 8:363–368.
38. F.D.A. Drug Bulletin, Vol 11 (2), July 1981.
39. Elliot HR, Abdulla U. Pulmonary edema associated with ritodrine infusion and betamethasone administration in premature labor. Br Med J. 1978; 2:799–800.
40. Tinga DJ, Aarnoudse JG, Rogge P, Young S, Goodin R. Postpartum pulmonary edema associated with preventative therapy for premature labor. Lancet. 1979; 1:1026–1027.
41. Stubblefield PG. Pulmonary edema occurring after therapy with dexamethasone and terbutaline for premature labor: A case report. Am J Obstet Gynecol. 1978; 132:341–342.
42. Jacobs MM, Knight AB, Arias F. Maternal pulmonary edema resulting from betamimetic and glucocorticoid therapy. Obstet Gynecol. 1980; 56:56–59.
43. Zervoudakis IA, Krauss A, Fuchs F, Wilson KH. Infants of mothers treated with ethanol for premature labor. Am J Obstet Gynecol. 1980; 137:713–718.
44. Saling E, Müller-Holve W. External cephalic version under tocolysis. J Perinatal Med. 1975; 3:115–119.
45. Hartikainen-Sorri A, Ylikorkala O. Value of external version in fetal malpresentation in combination with use of ultrasound. Acta Obstet Gynecol Scand. 1977; 56:63–67.
46. Lauersen NH. Clinical methods and use of fetal acid-base measurements. In: Lauersen NH, Hochberg HM (eds). Clinical Perinatal Biochemical Monitoring. Baltimore: Williams & Wilkins, 1981:36–37.

M. XXIV

Cardiac Glycosides and Pregnancy

Warren D. Johnston, MD, and Uri Elkayam, MD

Digitalis has been a mainstay in the treatment of congestive heart failure for almost two centuries. It remains today as one of the more commonly used drugs in clinical practice. It is currently the only oral drug approved in the United States for use as a positive inotropic agent in the treatment of ventricular failure, although newly developed oral catecholamines also appear to hold promise in this regard.[1] The efficacy of digitalis in the management of chronic heart failure is considered time honored but is not altogether unchallenged.[2] However, recent hemodynamic studies have reiterated the value of long-term digitalis therapy in congestive heart failure.[3] Digitalis preparations are also widely used for the treatment of certain cardiac arrhythmias.

Throughout the years large numbers of women taking digitalis preparations have undergone pregnancy. Relatively recent advances in medicine, such as surgical modification or correction of congenital defects, development of prosthetic heart valves, implantation of pacemakers, improved pharmacotherapy of congestive heart failure, and improvements in the management of high risk obstetrical patients, have undoubtedly increased the percentages of pregnant women who are maintained on digitalis. Thus, a thorough knowledge of the cardiac glycosides and their usage in pregnancy has become increasingly pertinent. Before turning to the specifics of digitalis in pregnancy, a brief general review of the cardiac glycosides is presented.

Cardiac Problems in Pregnancy, pages 281–288

I. CARDIAC GLYCOSIDES

Digitalis glycosides are steroid or steroid-glycoside compounds that possess positive inotropic activity and exert specific electrophysiologic effects on the heart. Digitalis preparations increase the force and velocity of myocardial contractions. The mechanism for this positive inotropic effect is incompletely elucidated. Current evidence supports the concept that cardiac glycosides increase the availability of calcium to the contractile element during excitation-contraction coupling. Further, this action may be related in some fashion to digitalis-induced Na^+-K^+-activated ATPase inhibition.[4] The clinically important antiarrhythmic properties of digitalis preparations result from electrophysiologic effects primarily on the atria and atrioventricular node. Specifically, digitalis slows AV node conduction and prolongs its effective refractory period. Digitalis may also suppress ectopic atrial pacemakers and alter propagation through reentrant pathways in the atrium.[5] The mechanism of these events probably involves inhibition of Na^+ and K^+ transport, as well as autonomic nervous system influences.[6]

There are over 300 cardiac glycoside compounds known to exist. However, only five of these preparations have enjoyed widespread clinical use; namely, digitalis leaf, digitoxin, digoxin, ouabain, and deslanoside. The choice of the chemical formulation used in specific circumstances is usually dictated by the pharmocokinetics of the individual preparations. Thus, differences in routes of administration, speed of onset of action, peak effects, and duration of action often determine which preparation is used. (See Table M.XXIV.1)

A. Digoxin

Digoxin is the most commonly used preparation in clinical practice and therefore is discussed here in some detail. Its popularity is due primarily to its intermediate duration of action and the availability of oral and parenteral administration. The clinical pharmocokinetics of digoxin has recently been reviewed by Lisalo[7] and Aronson.[8] Absorption of the orally administered compound occurs primarily from the proximal small intestine. In patients with normal gastrointestinal function, approximately 67% of the drug is absorbed when administered in tablet form, 80% from elixir, and almost 100% from encapsulated elixir.[7] The absorption of the drug can be impaired by concomitant administration of cholestyramine or nonabsorbable antacids, and it is both diminished and erratic in patients with malabsorption syndrome. Approximately 20–30% of digoxin is protein bound, but due to its apparent high volume of distribution, this protein binding is clinically unimportant.[7] The onset of action occurs

TABLE M.XXIV.1. Properties of the Commonly Used Cardiac Glycosides

Drug	Route of administration	Onset of effect	Peak effect	Route of metabolism
Ouabain	Intravenous	5–10 minutes	0.5–2 hours	Predominantly renal; some gastrointestinal
Deslanoside	Intravenous	10–30 minutes	1–2 hours	Renal
Digoxin	Intravenous	15–30 minutes	1–5 hours	Predominantly renal; some gastrointestinal
	Oral	1–2 hours	1.5–5 hours	
Digitoxin	Intravenous	25–125 minutes	6 hours	Predominantly hepatic with renal excretion of metabolites
	Oral	2–4 hours	8–12 hours	

within 15–30 minutes after intravenous dosage and reaches peak effect within one to five hours. Given orally, the onset of action is between one to two hours, with a maximum effect reached at between one and one-half to five hours. The average time of elimination is 40 hours in patients with normal renal function.[7] Excretion is primarily via the kidneys and is dependent upon glomerular filtration rate. Approximately one-third of body stores are lost daily in patients with normal renal function.[6] The average digitalizing dose is 0.75–1.00 mg intravenously or 1.25–1.50 mg orally. Maintenance dosage averages 0.25–0.50 mg daily. If no loading dose is used, steady-state equilibrium on maintenance dosage will be reached in approximately five to seven days in patients with normal kidneys.[9] Maintenance dosages need to be adjusted for diminished renal function. Quinidine administration to a patient on maintenance digoxin therapy can lead to a significant increase in plasma digoxin levels.

B. Digitoxin

Digitoxin is the principal active agent in digitalis leaf and therefore shares comparable pharmacokinetics. Digitalis leaf has largely been replaced by pure glycoside preparations, allowing for more accurate standardization of the active drug contents.[6] Digitoxin is characterized principally by its long half-life of four to six days. Its principal excretory pathway is via the liver and, thus, its half-life varies little with changing renal function. This may be considered an advantage since half-lives are relatively constant and dosing schedules may be formulated with greater ease and accuracy.[10] The absorption of orally administered digitoxin is 90–100% complete. Approximately 97% of digitoxin in plasma is bound to albumin.[11] The onset of action is 25–125 minutes for intravenous dosage, with the peak effect being reached in six hours. When given orally, the onset of action is within two to four hours, and the maximum effect is reached in eight to 12 hours. The average digitalizing dose is 0.70–1.20 mg in divided oral doses and 1 mg intravenously in incremental doses. The usual maintenance dose is 0.10 mg, and steady state is reached with this dosage in approximately three to four weeks if no loading dose is administered.

C. Ouabain and Deslanoside

Ouabain and deslanoside are both poorly absorbed from the gastrointestinal tract and are available only for intravenous use. Ouabain has an onset of action of approximately five to ten minutes. This fast action can be clinically useful in situations where a rapid effect is required. Its half-life averages 21 hours. Excretion is via the

	Loading dose		
Half-life	Oral	IV	Maintenance dose
21 hours	—	0.3–0.5 mg	0.1 mg q 4 h
33 hours	—	0.8 mg	—
36–48 hours	1.25–1.5 mg	0.75–1.0 mg	0.25–0.5 mg/day
4–6 days	0.7–1.2 mg	1.0 mg	0.1–0.2 mg/day

kidneys, but gastrointestinal excretion can also be substantial.[12] Deslanoside is structurally very similar to digoxin. Its onset of action is somewhat more rapid than digoxin, but the half-lifes of the drugs are essentially identical. Thus it enjoys no substantial advantages over parenteral use of digoxin. If rapidity of action is essential, ouabain is preferable to deslanoside.

D. Toxicity

Unfortunately, toxicity due to digitalis administration remains a major clinical problem. Beller et al, using electrocardiographic criteria, found in a prospective study, 22% of a digitalized hospital population to be definitely digitalis toxic and 6% to be possibly toxic.[13] It was hoped that the availability of serum digitalis levels would substantially mitigate this problem. However, it is now clear that individual differences in response sensitivity to cardiac glycosides gives rise to significant overlap between toxic and nontoxic serum levels.[6] Predisposing factors to toxicity include hypoxia, pulmonary disease, acid base disorders, renal insufficiency, type and severity of heart disease, concomitant drug administration (such as diuretics, anesthetics, and quinidine), and serum electrolyte disorders (such as hypokalemia, hyperkalemia, hypomagnesemia, hypercalcemia, and hyponatremia). Manifestations of digitalis toxicity are both cardiac and extracardiac. Unfortunately, cardiotoxic rhythm disturbances precede the development of extracardiac signs and symptoms in approximately 50% of cases.[6] The extra-cardiac findings include anorexia, nausea and vomiting, headache, fatigue, malaise, and visual symptoms such as scotomas, haloes, changes in color perception, and flashing vision. Other neurologic symptoms include confusion, delirium, disorientation, and convulsions. Cardiac toxicity includes virtually every known rhythm disturbance. Some common arrhythmias seen with toxicity include premature ventricular captures, ventricular tachycardia, atrial tachycardia with atrioventricular (AV) nodal block, AV junctional tachycardia, sinus arrest, Mobitz type I second-degree AV nodal block, and third-degree AV nodal block. Treatment of toxicity includes, most importantly, recognition of the problem and withdrawal of the digitalis preparation. Potassium should be given in cases with hypokalemia, but caution should be observed if conduction disturbances are present, as elevation of serum potassium may further impair atrioventricular nodal conduction. Phenytoin, lidocaine, and propranolol are often recommended to treat ectopic tachyarrhythmias due to digitalis toxicity. The use of these drugs in pregnancy is discussed in detail in Chapters M.XIV and M.XX. Occasionally electrical cardioversion[14] or pacemaker insertion may be required. Steroid binding resins may be tried to decrease gastrointestinal absorption. Specific antibodies to cardiac glycosides are potentially useful and may hold promise for the future.[15]

II. DIGITALIS AND PREGNANCY

Given the number of years digitalis preparations have been used therapeutically, and the large number of women who have been exposed to the drug during pregnancy, it is surprising that the available data on the effects of digitalis on the mother and fetus is relatively recent and still incomplete. This is probably because the overwhelming clinical impression and experience accumulated throughout the years suggested that digitalis preparations had been quite safe for use in pregnancy. This conclusion has, in fact, essentially withstood more recent experimental inquiry.

A. Pharmocokinetics

Although pregnancy is associated with marked hemodynamic changes in the maternal circulation, it does not appear to have a significant effect on the pharmacokinetics of digitalis preparations. It has therefore been suggested by some authors that digitalis requirements should remain the same and standard doses should be given during pregnancy.[16] Rogers et al, however, noted relatively low serum digoxin levels in pregnant women at term and found that these levels nearly doubled in the month after delivery without changes in digoxin dosages.[17] It was felt that increases in maternal blood volume and glomerular filtration during pregnancy were not of significant enough magnitude to fully explain these low levels at term. The authors postulated that delayed gastric emptying during labor may have impaired immediate absorption of the drug leading to the lower serum levels. However, a participation of the fetus in the metabolic process of the drug could not be excluded.

B. Animal Studies

Before the availability of radioactive digitalis and the radioimmunoassay for measurement of serum and tissue digoxin levels a placental barrier to the passage of digitalis to the fetus was though to exist. Okita et al in 1952 demonstrated clearly that digitoxin crossed the placenta of pregnant guinea pigs, with 23% of the dose appearing in the fetus in one hour.[18] They also found that in rats given digitoxin only 0.7% of the dose appeared in the fetuses at one hour, thus demonstrating that there are marked species difference in the placental passage of digitoxin. Tissue binding of digitoxin and its metabolites were found in the fetal heart of the guinea pig. On a tissue-weight basis, higher levels of digitoxin were found in the fetal heart than in the maternal heart. Fouron[19] studied dogs whose metabolism of digoxin is known to be similar to humans[20] and found that transplacental passage of digoxin occurred almost immediately but that fetal levels were lower than maternal levels until after four days, when equilibrium was reached. A significant level of digoxin was also found by this investigator in the amniotic fluid. The level was equal to or higher than levels found in maternal blood after one week of digoxin administration. Hernandez et al[21,22] and Singh et al[23] have demonstrated rapid placental passage of digoxin in pregnant ewes. Hernandez et al found a longer half-life of digoxin in the fetal serum when compared to the mother following a single bolus dose of tritiated digoxin. Although it could be demonstrated by these investigators that after chronic dosing the feto-maternal levels were essentially equal, the tissue binding of digoxin in all fetal tissues was significantly less than that which occurred in maternal tissue. The feto-maternal tissue level ratio of digoxin was found to be 0.25. The level of digoxin in the amniotic fluid of the mother was almost equal to the levels in the fetal and maternal blood.

C. Human Studies

Placental transport of digitalis has been clearly demonstrated to occur in humans. Okita et al[24] studied digitoxin levels in 11–12-week-old human fetuses three to five hours following an intravenous injection to the mother. Transplacental passage of digitoxin to the fetus was observed, but in very low concentrations. Soyka[25] subsequently pointed out that the low concentration of digitoxin observed in the fetus does not suggest a placental barrier to the passage of the drug but rather reflects the extensive serum binding and long half-life of digitoxin.

Digoxin has been shown by numerous workers to cross the placenta. Rogers et al[17] demonstrated nearly equal fetal and maternal serum levels at term five to six hours after the last maternal oral dosage of maintenance digoxin. Passive diffusion of digoxin across the placenta was postulated. Saarikoski[26] injected pregnant women with radioactive digoxin five minutes to two hours prior to legal abortion and found rapid transplacental passage, with equilibrium between fetal and maternal blood in about 30 minutes. Low uptake of digoxin by fetal tissue was noted, the highest tissue level was seen in the fetal heart with a concentration approximately equal to but not higher than the plasma level. It has therefore been concluded that the capacity of the human fetal heart to bind and accumulate digoxin during the first half of gestation is limited. Digoxin was also found in the amniotic fluid but in lower levels than noted in fetal or maternal plasma. Allonen et al[27] administered two doses of 0.5 mg oral digoxin to pregnant females at about 24 hours and two to six hours prior to abortion of 12–16-week fetuses. The detection of digoxin in the fetal serum demonstrated transplacental passage of the drug. The fetal-to-maternal serum ratio was 0.6. No detectable digoxin level could be found in fetal heart tissue. Allonen et al concluded that the major limiting factor in digoxin passage is probably poor lipid solubility of the drug, which may limit its diffusion through biological membranes. Padeletti et al[28] have also found rapid placental passage of intravenously administered digoxin in pregnant humans with fetal-maternal equilibrium reached at about 75 minutes. They postulated that tissue and protein-binding of digoxin in both the mother and fetus accounts for the delay in the equilibrium between the two circulations. Digoxin was also found in significant amounts in the amniotic fluid in three out of five of their cases.

Saarikoski[29] showed rapid transplacental passage of ouabain in pregnant women during the second trimester of pregnancy. Equilibrium time of over two hours between maternal and fetal circulations was observed. Tissue binding and possible placental uptake of ouabain were implicated in this lag phase. The concentration of ouabain in the fetal heart was found to be three to ten times that of fetal plasma. Thus, an uptake mechanism for ouabain apparently exists in the fetal heart by the second trimester of pregnancy. Ouabain was also found in low concentration in the amniotic fluid.

In summary, digitalis preparations have been found to pass into the fetal circulation in both animals and man. The rapidity of passage and equilibrium and the degree of tissue binding of the cardiac glycosides differ markedly between species and between different digitalis preparations. Digitalis is also present in the amniotic fluid and may serve as a potential reservior both for maternal reabsorption or fetal exposure.

D. Adverse Effects in Pregnancy

Despite the transplacental passage of digitalis, remarkably few adverse effects on the fetus have been demonstrated. Fouron[19] found digitalis effects on fetal electrocardiograms three hours after toxic dosages were administered to pregnant dogs. Potondi[30] reported a case of digitalis overdosage in a pregnant women whose subsequent miscarriage was attributed to digitalis poisoning. Sherman and Locke[31] also reported a case of maternal digitalis toxicity associated with electrocardiographic changes in the newborn and subsequent death of the infant, presumably secondary to the effects of intrauterine anoxia.

Concern has been raised that digitalis may play a role in low birth weights observed occasionally in infants of mothers with heart disease. It is postulated that digitalis, by binding in the placenta, might alter the placental transport of amino acids to the fetus.[32] Another possible explanation for low birth weight may be related to the observation of Weaver and Pearson,[33] who showed that women on digitalis had earlier onset of spontaneous labor. They noted lower birth weights of infants of these mothers. After adjusting for gestational age, they concluded that the weight differences were due to relative prematurity and not to growth retardation. They attributed the early onset and shorter labors in digitalized patients to a direct effect of digitalis on the myometrium.

Digoxin has also been noted to be secreted into human breast milk.[34–36] However, the amount of exposure to the infant is calculated to be in the range of 1–2 μg/day.[34] This amount is probably insufficient to adversely affect the child.

Despite these isolated reports, in large series of pregnant patients, no demonstrable clinical or electrocardiographic adverse effects have been demonstrated in the fetuses of mothers who consumed digitalis during pregnancy.[37,38] This may be in part due to the relatively low binding of digitalis in fetal tissues and a relative resistance of the fetal heart to digitalis effects.[23,24,39]

III. FETAL TREATMENT WITH DIGITALIS

The passage of digitalis from the maternal to the fetal circulation and the apparent lack of adverse effects upon the fetus suggests the possibility of treatment of fetal tachycardia and congestive heart failure by maternal administration of the drug. Kerenyi et al[40] reported the first successful transplacental pharmacocardioversion with digitalis. A year later Harrigan et al[41] reported the successful termination of a fetal tachyarrhythmia by maternal treatment with digoxin. A fetus of 26 weeks gestation was noted to develop a tachycardia of 260 beats per minute (bpm) complicated by congestive heart failure. Treatment of the mother with 1.5 mg of digoxin orally over 14 hours was associated with abrupt conversion of the heart rate to 125–130 bpm. A normal infant was subsequently delivered at term. Other attempts at pharmocologic conversion of fetal tachycardias with digitalis that have been reported in the literature were less successful.[41,42] However, given the relative safety of fetal exposure to digitalis and the possible threat of fetal death or forced early delivery posed by fetal tachycardia, a trial of maternal digitalis therapy is indicated in an in utero attempt to convert these arrhythmias. (For further details, see chapters F.XIII and F.XIV.)

IV. SUMMARY

Digitalis preparations have enjoyed widespread usage in both the pregnant and the nonpregnant state. Pregnancy does not markedly alter the mechanisms of action, pharmacokinetics, or toxic effects of the drug. The cardiac glycosides traverse the placenta and appear in the fetal circulation. They are also excreted into breast milk and amniotic fluid. Despite these sources of fetal exposure, few adverse effects have been reported, and thus the digitalis preparations are considered safe for usage in pregnancy. The presence of digitalis in the fetal circulation may occasionally be used for therapeutic advantage in the treatment of fetal arrhythmias.

V. ACKNOWLEDGMENTS

We gratefully acknowledge the expert secretarial assistance of Ellen Mansour in the preparation of this manuscript.

VI. REFERENCES

1. Awan NA, Needham KE, Evenson MK, Mason DT. Comparison of hemodyamic actions of pirbuterol and dobutamine on cardiac function in severe congestive heart failure. Am J Cardiol. 1981; 47:665–669.
2. Fleg JL, Gottlieb SH, Lakatta EG. Is digitalis really useful in therapy of chronic congestive heart failure? Circulation. 1979; 59, 60 (Suppl II):178.
3. Arnold SB, Byrd RC, Meister W, Melmon K, Cheitlin MD, Bristow JD, Parmley WW, Chatterjee MB. Long term digitalis therapy improves left ventricular function in heart failure. N Engl J Med. 1980; 303:1443–1448.
4. Lee KS, Klaus W. The subcellular basis for the mechanism of inotropic action of cardiac glycosides. Pharmacol Rev. 1971; 23:193–244.
5. Rosen MR, Wit AL, Hoffman BF. Electrophysiology and pharmacology of cardiac arrhythmias. IV. Cardiac antiarrhythmias and toxic effects of digitalis. Am Heart J. 1975; 89:391–399.
6. Smith TW. Digitalis glycosides. N Engl J Med. 1973; 288:719–722, 942–946.
7. Lisalo E. Clinical pharmacokinetics of digoxin. Clin Pharmacokinet. 1977; 2:1–16.
8. Aronson, JK. Clinical pharmacokinetics of digoxin. Clin Pharmacokinet. 1980; 5:137–149.
9. Marcus FL, Burkhalter CL, Pavlovich J, Kapadia GG. Administration of tritiated digoxin with and without a loading dose: A metabolic study. Circulation. 1966; 34:865.
10. Lukas DS. Of toads and flowers. Circulation. 1972; 46:1–4.
11. Lukas DS, DeMartino AG. Binding of digitoxin and some related cardenolides to human plasma

proteins. J Clin Invest. 1969; 48:1041–1053.
12. Selden R, Margolies MN, Smith TW. Renal and gastrointestinal excretion of ouabain in dog and man. J Pharmacol Exp Ther. 1974; 188:615–623.
13. Beller GA, Smith TW, Abelman WH, Haber E, Hud WB. Digitalis intoxication. N Engl J Med. 1971; 284:989–997.
14. Schroeder S, Harrison DC. Repeated cardioversion during pregnancy. Am J Cardiol. 1971; 27:445–446.
15. Smith TW, Haber E. Digitalis. N Engl J Med. 1973; 289:945–952.
16. Conradsson TB: Werko L. Management of heart disease in pregnancy. Prog Cardiovasc Dis. 1974; 16:407.
17. Rogers MC, Willerson JT, Goldblatt A, Smith TW. Serum digoxin concentrations in the human fetus, neonate and infant. N Engl J Med. 1972; 287:1010–1013.
18. Okita GT, Gordon RB, Geiling EMK. Placental transfer of radioactive digitoxin in rats and guinea pigs. Proc Soc Exp Biol Med. 1952; 80:536–538.
19. Fouron JC. Dynamic of the placental transfer of digoxin in the dog. Biol Neonate. 1973; 23:116–122.
20. Doherty JE, Perkins WH. Tissue concentration and turnover of tritiated digoxin in dogs. Am J Cardiol. 1966; 17:47–52.
21. Hernandez A, Burton RM, Goldring D, Klint R. The effects of maternally administered digoxin upon the cardiovascular hemodynamics of fetal lamb. Am Heart J. 1973; 85:511–517.
22. Hernandez A, Strauss AW, Burton RM, Goldring D. The effects of long term administration of ^{3}H-digoxin to the pregnant ewe upon the cardiovascular hemodynamics of the fetal lamb. Am J Obstet Gynecol. 1975; 121:1100–1102.
23. Singh PEF, Mirkin BL. Elimination kinetics and placental transfer of digoxin in pregnant and nonpregnant ewes. Res Commun Chem Pathol Pharmacol. 1978; 20:31–42.
24. Okita GT, Plotz EJ, Davis ME. Placental transfer of radioactive digitoxin in pregnant women and its fetal distribution. Circ Res. 1956; 4:376–380.
25. Soyka LF. Digoxin: Placental transfer, effects on the fetus and therapeutic use in the newborn. Clin Perinatol. 1975; 2:23–35.
26. Saarikosh S. Placental transfer and fetal uptake of ^{3}H-digoxin in humans. Br J Obstet Gynaecol. 1976; 83:879–884.
27. Allonen H, Kanto J, Iisalo E. The foeto-maternal distribution of digoxin in early human pregnancy. Acta Pharmacol Toxicol. 1976; 39:477–480.
28. Padeletti L, Porclani MC, Scimone G. Placental transfer of digoxin (beta-methyl-digoxin) in man. Int J Clin Pharmacol Biopharmacol. 1979; 17:82–83.
29. Saarikoski S. Placental transmission and foetal distribution of ^{3}H-ouabain. Acta Pharmacol Toxicol. 1980; 46:272–282.
30. Potondi A. Congenital rhabdomyoma of the heart and intrauterine digitalis poisoning. J Forensic Sci. 11:81–88.
31. Sherman JL, Locke RU. Transplacental neonate digitalis intoxication. Am J Cardiol. 1960; 6:834–837.
32. Whitsett JA, Wallick ET. [^{3}H]ouabain binding and Na^+-K^+-ATPase activity in human placenta. Am J Physiol. 1980; 238:E38–E45.
33. Weaver JB, Pearson JF. Influence of digitalis on time of onset and duration of labour in women with cardiac disease. Br Med J. 1973; 3:519–520.
34. Levy M, Granit L, Laufer N. Excretion of drugs in human milk. N Engl J Med. 1977; 297:789.
35. Loughnan PM. Digoxin excretion in human breast milk. J Pediatr. 1978; 92:1019–1020.
36. Chan V, Tse TF, Wong V. Transfer of digoxin across the placenta and into the breast milk. Br J Obstet Gynaecol. 1978; 85:605–609.
37. Szekely P, Desmond GJ. Heart disease and pregnancy. Current Problems Cardiol. 1979; 4:1–74.
38. Mendelson CL. Cardiac disease in pregnancy. Philadelphia: Davis, 1960:68.
39. Papp J, Nemeth M, Resch B. Foetal development of responsiveness to cardiotonic drugs in human foetus, neonate and infant. N Engl J Med. 1972; 287:1010–1013.
40. Kerenyi TD, Gleicher N, Meller J, et al. Transplacental cardioversion of intrauterine supraventricular tachycardia with digitalis. Lancet. 1980; 2:393–395.
41. Harrigan JT, Kangos JJ, Sikka A, Spisso KR, Natarajan N, Rosenfeld D, Leiman S, Korn D. Successful treatment of fetal congestive heart failure secondary to tachycardia. N Engl J Med. 1981; 304:1527–1529.
42. Newburger JW, Keane JF. Intrauterine supraventricular tachycardia. J Pediatr. 1979; 95:780–786.
43. Kesson CW. Foetal paroxysmal auricular tachycardia. Br Heart J. 1958; 20:552–556.

M. XXV

Antibiotic Therapy in Pregnancy

Thomas C. Cesario, MD

I. INTRODUCTION

Antibiotics are frequently administered during pregnancy to treat acquired bacterial infections. In one study[1] 37% of pregnant women were found to have received these drugs. Many of the infections acquired during gestation, such as those involving the genital or urinary tracts, are beyond the scope of this book; however, antibiotics may be required during pregnancy either to prevent or to treat diseases of the heart. Thus the discussion that follows details the antibiotic usage required during pregnancy for the treatment and prevention of cardiac damage arising from the complications of bacterial infections. Furthermore, because a wide range of antibiotics may be required for these situations, a section on antibiotic pharmacology during pregnancy is provided.

II. PROPHYLACTIC ANTIBIOTICS

There are at least two situations arising during pregnancy that necessitate the use of prophylactic antimicrobial agents.

The first of these conditions involves individuals with a prior history of rheumatic fever. In this group prophylaxis against future attacks is warranted. Although there is not a consensus, it is recommended[2] that prophylaxis for recurrent streptococcal infections be continued for life in individuals who have had at least one attack of rheumatic fever. This of course means that certain people will be required to maintain dosage schedules for

Cardiac Problems in Pregnancy, pages 289–301

the prevention of such infections during gestation, despite the fact that rheumatic fever is rare during pregnancy.[3] The most effective regimen[4] for rheumatic fever prevention is the intramuscular administration of 1.2 million units of benzathine penicillin G every four weeks. Other suitable alternatives include oral penicillin V 250,000 units (approximately 150 mg) once or twice a day (preferably twice) or sulfadiazine, 1 gm per day. The latter drugs in the fetus are well known to compete with conjugated bilirubin[5] for sites on albumin, and hence may interfere with transport of this pigment to the liver and ultimate excretion. This in turn permits the deposition of bilirubin in body tissues, including the central nervous system, thereby predisposing to kernicterus. Although all cases of sulfonamide-related kernicterus appear to be caused by long-acting preparations,[6] there is still some concern over the use of this class of agents during the last trimester of pregnancy, and it has been suggested they not be given at all during that time.[7] It has also been suggested that sulfonamides not be given during pregnancy to women with a previous history of having a child with neonatal jaundice or blood group (either Rh or ABO) incompatibility.[7] A possible consideration in the penicillin-allergic patient who requires rheumatic fever prophylaxis would be erythromycin, although, as discussed later, the estolate salt probably should not be used during pregnancy.

The second situation that can occur during pregnancy and will require antibiotic prophylaxis is the prevention of endocarditis in the patient with underlying heart disease.

The first question to resolve when considering prevention of valvular infection relates to the forms of underlying cardiac disease that pose enough risk to require prophylaxis. The American Heart Association, in its most recent committee report,[8] takes a broad view of this question and suggests that patients with valves damaged by rheumatic or congenital processes should be given antibiotics to prevent endocarditis prior to various surgical and diagnostic procedures (see below). Individuals with prolapsing mitral valves[8] are also prone to endocarditis and should be considered for prophylaxis. Patients with prosthetic valves also are at risk of endocarditis and definitely warrant prophylactic antibiotics to prevent valvular infection.

In reviewing this topic Sipes and associates[9] point out that rheumatic heart disease accounts for 40–60% of cases of infective endocarditis, while congenital disease is responsible for only 7–16%. Conditions that are congenital in nature and that are associated with a significant risk of infective endocarditis include ventricular septal defect, patent ductus arteriosus, tetralogy of Fallot, pulmonic stenosis, coarctation of the aorta, and bicuspid aortic valve.

It appears that a basic event in the process leading to endocarditis is the transient bacteremia known to occur following many types of medical–surgical procedures or activities involved in daily living. In this regard, it is important to realize how frequently various essential procedures predispose to bacteremia. Everett and Hirschman[11] have recently reviewed this topic in detail. Table M.XXV.1 lists representative types of procedures and the risks they carry of inducing transient bacteremias.

The precise risk of endocarditis after various medical–surgical procedures is unknown and relates to a number of factors, including the type of heart disease, the number and type of organisms entering the bloodstream, and the immunologic status of the host.[9] Hook and Kaye have estimated the risk of infective endocarditis after one type of procedure, tooth extraction, and have suggested that one case of infective endocarditis will develop per 500–3,000 tooth extractions.

Patients, including gravidas, who have abnormal heart valves should be given antibiotic prophylaxis during the course of the procedures listed in Table M.XXV.1

TABLE M.XXV.1. Risk of Bacteremia After Various Medical–Surgical Procedures

Procedures	Percentage of cases with bacteremia detected	Reference
Dental extraction	60–90	Rogosa et al[12] Khairat, O.[13]
Tonsillectomy	28	Rhoads et al[14]
Upper GI endoscopy	8–12	Shull et al[15] Baltch et al[16]
Cystoscopy	17	Sullivan et al[17]
Urethral dilation	24	Sullivan et al[17]
Parturition	0–5	Ramsey et al[18] Redleaf et al[19] Baker et al[20] McCormack et al[21]

to be sure that anticipated episodes of bacteremia do not lead to endocarditis.

During manipulation of the mouth and upper respiratory tract, prophylaxis is directed toward oral streptococci and oral anaerobes, whereas during lower gastrointestinal and genitourinary manipulations enterococci are the major concern. The American Heart Association[8] recommends that prophylactic antibiotics be employed in patients susceptible to endocarditis during all manipulations of the upper GI tract, including the mouth, and during manipulation or procedures involving the urinary or gastrointestinal tract, including the biliary tree. They also recommend that antibiotics be similarly given for procedures involving manipulation of septic complications in the female genital tract; however, because the incidence of endocarditis is low after uncomplicated vaginal delivery they suggest that the use of antibiotic prophylaxis to prevent endocarditis in this circumstance is open to debate.

Individuals with prosthetic valves represent a special circumstance. Because the development of endocarditis in patients with artificial valves can be devastating, and because the incidence of endocarditis in these patients is high, it has been suggested that such individuals be considered for antibiotic prophylaxis for many procedures, including routine vaginal delivery. Although some investigators[10] favor routine antibiotic use during parturition to prevent endocarditis in patients with valvular heart disease, it must be pointed out that the institution of such therapy does not guarantee against endocarditis.[22] Opinion regarding routine institution of prophylaxis during delivery remains divided.[23] Furthermore, when the attending physician believes that special risks require prophylactic antibiotics to prevent endocarditis during the time of labor and delivery, a 48-hour maximum of antibiotic coverage should provide more than adequate protection. The use of antibiotics at any time carries the risk of producing superinfection with resistant organisms.

In summary, it is important to protect against endocarditis during the course of pregnancy in the same situations where prophylactic antibiotics would be employed in the nongravid state. During routine vaginal delivery the risk of endocarditis seems low, and routine antibiotics do not seem warranted except in patients with prosthetic valves.

Recently the American Heart Association published its recommendations for the prophylaxis of endocarditis.[8] These recommendations apply to pregnant patients as well as to others. The recommendations are outlined in the following section.

A. Dental Procedures and Upper Respiratory Tract Surgical Procedures

1. Regimen A

a. Penicillin regimens

1) Parenteral-oral combined. Aqueous crystalline penicillin G (1 million units intramuscularly), mixed with procaine penicillin G (600,000 units intramuscularly), is given 30–60 minutes prior to the procedure. The parenteral penicillin is then followed by penicillin V, 500 mg orally every six hours for eight doses.

2) Oral only. Penicillin V (2.0 gm orally) is given 30–60 minutes prior to the procedure, followed by 500 mg orally every six hours for eight doses.

b. Nonpenicillin regimens

1) Erythromycin. One gram orally of erythromycin is given 90–120 minutes before the procedure, followed by 500 mg every six hours thereafter for eight doses.

2) Vancomycin. One gram intravenously of vancomycin is given over 30–60 minutes, starting one hour before the procedure, followed by erythromycin 500 mg every six hours for eight doses.

2. Regimen B–penicillin plus streptomycin.

Penicillin, exactly as under Regimen A, plus streptomycin (1 gm IM) is given 30–60 minutes prior to the procedure. (This regimen or that using vancomycin may be particularly well suited to the patient taking daily medication to prevent rheumatic fever recurrences because oral bacteria under these circumstances may prove more resistant to antibiotics.)

B. Gastrointestinal and Genitourinary Instrumentation or Surgery

Aqueous crystalline penicillin G (2 million units intramuscularly or intravenously) OR ampicillin (1 gm intramuscularly) plus streptomycin (1 gm intramuscularly) or gentamicin (1.5 mg/kg not to exceed 80 mg intramuscularly or intravenously) is given 30 minutes to one hour prior to the procedure. The gentamicin and penicillin combinations are to be repeated for two additional doses eight hours apart, and the penicillin-streptomycin combination is to be repeated twice at 12-hour intervals. For patients allergic to penicillin, vancomycin (1 gm intravenously over 30–60 minutes) plus streptomycin (1.0 gm intramuscularly) is given 30–60 minutes before the procedure and repeated once at 12 hours.

III. ENDOCARDITIS THERAPY

Another situation involving the heart that might necessitate the administration of antibiotics during pregnancy is the development of endocarditis. Although this situation is unusual, it does happen. Nazarian[24] has estimated that one in 8,000 deliveries is complicated by bacterial endocarditis. In 1953 Pedowitz and Hellman[25] reviewed the relationship between pregnancy and subacute bacterial endocarditis. They reported on a survey received from 102 hospitals, each with 2,000 or more deliveries per year, and on a review of the English literature. These authors identified 35 cases of endocarditis occurring during pregnancy. In this group 28.5% developed cardiac failure and 14.2% died. Since the study of Pedowitz and Hellman was published, a number of reports have appeared detailing cases of endocarditis diagnosed and treated during pregnancy. In most recent reports of bacterial endocarditis occurring in pregnancy, Streptococcus viridans has been the organism implicated. Thus, Szekely and Snaith[26] described three cases due to this organism among a total of six cases they described. Likewise, Ward and Hickman[27] reported five cases of endocarditis in pregnancy, two of which were due to S viridans; culture results were not available for the other three. Crockett et al[28] also described a case involving the same organism. Staphylococci have also been found to produce endocarditis in pregnancy as noted by Holt et al.[29] Furthermore, we have recently treated a woman who was found to have infected cardiac valves due to Staphylococcus aureus and who was in her third trimester of pregnancy. The prevalence of streptococci and staphylococci as major causes of this disease entity during pregnancy is in keeping with the spectrum of endocarditis occurring on natural heart valves[30] as seen in North America.

Treatment of endocarditis during pregnancy should be conducted along currently recommended lines.[31] All patients will require parenteral antibiotics, usually for four to six weeks. Antibiotics chosen in this setting should always be bacteriocidal. Dosages should be maintained to provide a serum level, during the peak concentration, of at least ten times the amount required to kill the organism. The specific antibiotics chosen will depend upon the organism isolated and on sensitivity tests performed in the clinical laboratory.

Table M.XXV.2 lists treatment regimens for specific organisms likely to cause endocarditis in pregnancy.

Increasing evidence suggests that certain patients with infective endocarditis may benefit from cardiac surgery.[31] Patients particularly likely to benefit from operative intervention include those with endocarditis who develop congestive heart failure, especially if medical management fails to produce a prompt response. Repeated embolic phenomena likewise demand consideration for early surgery,[31] as does inability to control the infection. The timing of surgery for endocarditis during the course of pregnancy should be influenced by the clinical status of the patient and by the usual considerations for cardiac surgery during pregnancy.

Having detailed the specific situations in which antibiotics might be used during pregnancy for either the treatment or the prevention of cardiac disease, we now turn to a discussion of the pharmacology of antibiotics in the gravid state. Several ex-

TABLE M.XXV.2. Suggested Treatment Regimens for Specific Forms of Endocarditis Likely To Occur in Pregnancy

Organism	Antibiotic	Route	Dose	Frequency	Duration
Streptococcus viridans	Penicillin G	IV	1 million units	Every 2 hours	4 weeks
Alternative:	Cephalothin	IV	1 gm	Every 2 hours	4 weeks
Streptococcus fecalis (enterococci)	Penicillin plus	IV	1.5 million units	Every 2 hours	6 weeks
	streptomycin[a,c]		10 mg/kg (not to exceed 500 mg)	Every 12 hours	
Alternative:	Ampicillin plus	IV	1 gm	Every 2 hours	6 weeks
	gentamicin[a]	IM	1.5 mg/kg	Every 8 hours	
Alternative[b]:	Vancomycin[a] plus	IV	10 mg/kg (not to exceed 500 mg)	Every 6 hours	6 weeks
	streptomycin[a,c]	IM	10 mg/kg (not to exceed 500 mg)	Every 12 hours	
Staphylococcus aureus	Nafcillin	IV	1.5 gm	Every 2 hours	6 weeks
Alternative:	Keflin	IV	1.5 gm	Every 2 hours	6 weeks
Alternative:	Vancomycin[a]	IV	10 mg/kg (not to exceed 500 mg)	Every 6 hours	6 weeks

[a]Dosage must be altered if patient does not have normal renal function.
[b]This combination involves two potentially nephrotoxic agents and should be used with great caution.
[c]This drug has been found to have significant effect on fetal hearing[74] and should be avoided if possible.

cellent reviews of the subject have recently been published, and together they constitute an excellent survey of the body of available information.[32–34]

In introducing this topic several comments must be made. First we must realize that when any therapy is given to the pregnant woman, two patients are exposed to the drug—ie, mother and child. Second, much of the available knowledge of pharmacology in the gravid patient concerns the mother and not the child, because serial pharmacological studies are either not possible or not ethical on fetal samples. The limited information available on fetal pharmacology has been provided by studies of drug distribution done either at the time of abortion or at the time of delivery. Furthermore, pregnancy is a dynamic state, and drug distribution in the mother may vary at different times in the course of gestation. Finally, many studies of antibiotic pharmacology have compared data derived from pregnant women with data obtained by other authors from nonpregnant patients. Comparisons of this type are well known to be hazardous. Ideally, the best comparative studies of antibiotic pharmacology should be done in the same women during pregnancy and at later times when their physiology has returned to the nonpregnant status.

Maternal pharmacology is influenced during pregnancy by several major events. First, in pregnancy maternal circulatory volume increases so that any agent introduced into the circulation will be diluted to a greater extent. Second, during pregnancy, drugs may be sequestered in the intravascular compartment.[35] Third, the uterus and its contents provide a significant area to which most agents given the mother will be distributed. Fourth, methods of drug elimination may be enhanced during pregnancy; thus, elimination via the kidney is accelerated because of increased renal blood flow.[36] Furthermore, metabolism of drugs by certain organs may be altered[37] during pregnancy.

Any drug given to the mother during pregnancy which is absorbed into the circulation will probably encounter the placenta and then be distributed to the fetus. In the excellent review of placental transfer of antibiotics provided by Charles, he notes that it is doubtful that anything besides gases pass the placenta merely by diffusion.[33] Furthermore, most transfer mechanisms appear bidirectional, with fetal metabolic products usually being the only substances returned to the mother. Distribution of drugs to the fetus can be affected by various factors, including a number of disease states that may alter the ability of the placenta to transfer substances. Eclampsia, hypertension, and diabetes are among the more common diseases thought to affect placental transfer. Furthermore, certain properties of the therapeutic agent itself may influence passage; protein binding, for example, is thought to impede drug transfer.

Once drugs enter the fetal circulation, distribution of those drugs is significantly different from that in children or adults. The patent ductus arteriosus serves to route drugs around the fetal lung, and the ductus venosus routes them around the fetal liver. Immature kidneys probably excrete drugs at a considerably different rate than the mature kidneys, and when fetal renal excretion of the drug occurs, it probably results in deposition of the agent in the amniotic fluid. Indeed, this may be a major mechanism by which drugs enter this compartment. Drugs entering the fetus have the greatest chance of inducing teratogenesis if given in the first trimester; however, the fetal central nervous system is susceptible to damage even in the last trimester.

IV. SPECIFIC ANTIBIOTICS

A. Penicillins

1. Ampicillin

A number of studies have reported the use of ampicillin during gestation. Among the most unique and most enlightening of these studies were those of Philipson[38] who studied 26 women in the ninth to the thirty-sixth week of pregnancy. At a later date each woman had similar studies performed in the nongravid state. By this means the women served as their own controls. In this way Philipson demonstrated that, during pregnancy, serum levels of antibiotics are approximately half those found during the nonpregnant period. For example, the serum levels one hour after 500 mg of intravenous ampicillin ranged from 6 to 8 μg/ml.[38–40] Perry and LeBlanc,[41] however, found a higher concentration (15 μg/ml) during pregnancy but did not attempt to determine serum concentration after the pregnancy was completed. The half-life of ampicillin in the mother as determined during the last trimester has generally ranged from 30 to 45 minutes.[41–43]

Boreus[42] has shown that ampicillin crosses the placenta. Ninety minutes after administration of a single dose Boreus found that ampicillin was present in equal concentrations in maternal and fetal samples. Similarly, Bray et al[39] confirmed fetal transfer of ampicillin and determined that the fetal serum level one hour after administration was approximately 7 μg/ml.

No apparent contraindication for ampicillin exists in pregnancy other than allergy, although some authors have noted that this antibiotic may diminish urinary estrogen levels.[34] Ampicillin is an excellent drug for treating a number of gestational infections, including those involving the urinary tract if caused by susceptible organisms.

2. Other penicillins

The pharmacology of methicillin and oxacillin has been studied during gestation. MacAulay et al[44] administered intravenous methicillin to 57 patients either during labor or at the time of delivery. They found serum levels to be slightly lower than anticipated in maternal serum, but detectable antibiotic was found in fetal serum. They also found that the elimination half-life was increased during pregnancy.

Bastert et al[45] determined oxacillin levels on samples taken during amniocentesis and just prior to delivery. They found the clearance of the drug at this time to be increased. Methicillin and oxacillin have their greatest application in the treatment of staphylococcal infections and should be relatively safe to use in pregnancy. Drug allergy is the major problem associated with their use.

B. Cephalosporins

1. Cephalothin

Several studies of cephalothin's gestational pharmacology have been reported. Stewart and associates[46] administered 1 gm of cephalothin intravenously and found that the peak concentration of this drug in maternal serum was 24 μg/ml immediately after administration. Concentrations fell in two to three hours to undetectable levels. The drug appeared in the amniotic fluid in 30 minutes, gradually increasing in concentration to a level of 4.7 μg/ml at two hours. Only two of 19 specimens of umbilical cord serum contained cephalothin.

MacAulay et al[47] also gave an intravenous dose of 1 gm cephalothin to 54 patients during labor. They found that the peak maternal serum concentration was 30 μg/ml and that peak fetal concentrations approximated 10μg/ml. These investigators also detected the antibiotic in the amniotic fluid.

Bastert[48] has reported that after a single 2 gm dose of cephalothin given to the mother, amniotic fluid levels of 10 μg/ml were achieved. With repeated doses, amniotic fluid levels of 25 μg/ml were found.

Philipson,[32] summarizing the data with cephalothin, concluded that, when compared to levels in nonpregnant patients, maternal cephalothin levels were generally lower during gestation.

Cephalothin appears to be a safe drug during pregnancy, with drug allergy again being the major problem with its use. Significant levels of the drug can be expected to reach the fetus within 30 minutes of administration. It is a useful drug, especially in the penicillin-allergic patient, to treat infections caused by staphylococci and streptococci, although cross-sensitization with penicillins may occur.[49]

2. Cephazolin

The pharmacokinetics of cephazolin have been studied during pregnancy by Hannay et al,[50] who gave 1 gm intramuscularly to women one to three hours prior to delivery. They found that the maternal level one hour after administration of the drug was 25 μg/ml. Peak cord levels in their study were reached at five hours and approximated 13 μg/ml. Concentrations of the antibiotic were also found in the amniotic fluid.

The maternal peak serum concentration reported appears to be below levels found in nonpregnant patients.[51]

Cephazolin is another useful drug in pregnancy, especially for the treatment of streptococcal or staphylococcal infections in patients who are allergic to penicillins. Cross-sensitization between cephazolin and penicillin may occur as it does between cephalothin and penicillins. The major advantage of cephazolin is the ability to administer the drug intramuscularly without pain.

3. Cephalexin

Cephalexin pharmakokinetics during pregnancy have been studied by Duval[52] at the time of cesarean section. Serum levels were generally lower than might have been predicted.[32]

Cephalexin has a limited usage. It is administered orally and can be used to treat urinary tract infections if the causative organism is resistant to ampicillin and known to be sensitive to cephalexin.

4. Other cephalosporins

Several other cephalosporins have been investigated during gestation. Cephaloridine has been studied, but its potential for renal toxicity would favor the use of other cephalosporins especially in pregnant women. Cephatrizine, given orally to gravidas in a dose of 1 gm achieved peak serum levels of almost 8 μg/ml at two hours,[53] and low levels of the drug were found in fetal tissues. Charles[33] also quotes a study regarding cephacetrile[54] in which a 500 mg loading dose was followed by 500 mg of drug given by intravenous infusion every hour. In that study peak cephacetrile concentrations of 8 μg/ml were found in amniotic fluid at three hours and peak cord levels of 10–25 μg/ml were found at five hours.

C. Tetracyclines

Although ample information is available to demonstrate the fact that tetracycline can be identified in fetal tissue, especially bone,[55] the potential toxicity of this drug to the fetus (mainly dental mottling and retarded bone growth), as well as the rare massive hepatic necrosis that occurs in gravid women, have largely precluded its usefulness,[56] and it is contraindicated in pregnancy. Le Blanc and Perry[57] have noted that after 100 mg of IV tetracycline peak levels of 0.53 μg/ml are attained in amniotic fluid and of 1.5 μg/ml in cord blood. These were compared to a maternal peak concentration of 2.8 μg/ml, which came at 30 minutes after the dose.

D. Erythromycin

Philipson et al[58] studied the gestational pharmacokinetics of erythromycin. Using the estolate salt of this antibiotic, they gave 500 mg of the drug orally to women in the first half of pregnancy. The maternal peak serum level was 2.5 μg/ml with a single dose and 4.9 μg/ml with multiple doses. Drug was detected in fetal liver and amniotic fluid. Fetal serum levels of the drug were found to be 0.06 μg/ml of the multiple doses. Two patients were given the free erythromycin base, and in these women no antibiotic activity was found at three and three and one-half hours in fetal tissues. Multiple doses, however, may allow detectable fetal levels. Philipson has reported that the maternal blood levels were less than anticipated in nongravidas.

McCormack et al[59] gave pregnant women 250 mg of erythromycin four times a day. They found that 9.9% of 161 women so treated developed elevated SGOT levels. This was significantly greater than a similar number among controls. It has been suggested that the estolate salt of erythromycin not be used in pregnancy because of these findings.

Erythromycin appears to be relatively safe in pregnancy and does cross the placenta. It is a particularly useful drug in treating streptococcal infections in patients who are allergic to penicillin. It is also useful in the therapy of Mycoplasma pneumoniae infections. To be useful in pregnancy, increased quantities may be required.

E. Clindamycin

Philipson et al[58] also studied clindamycin pharmacokinetics in pregnancy. They gave a single 450 mg dose to 22 women at the time of abortion (in the first half of pregnancy) and found a mean maternal serum concentration of 5.2 μg/ml. Antibiotic was detected in many fetal tissues, including liver, spleen, lung, brain, muscle, and bone. Philipson suggested that maternal serum levels in the gravid state did not differ from those in the nongravid state.

Weinstein et al[60] gave 600 mg of clindamycin intravenously 30 minutes prior to cesarean section. They found peak maternal levels of 6–9 μg/ml and a peak umbilical vein level of 3 μg/ml at 30 minutes.

These data indicate that clindamycin serum concentrations appear to be unaffected by pregnancy. Placental transfer, however, does occur.

Clindamycin has been a useful drug, particularly for anaerobic infections. Its usefulness has been limited by the development of pseudomembranous enterocolitis[61] in a number of cases. If required in pregnancy for the treatment of infections due to Bacteroides fragilis, it appears to require the same dosage necessary for nongestational states.

F. Chloramphenicol

Chloramphenicol has been restricted in its use to serious, life-threatening situations because of the occurrence of aplastic anemia. It does, however, have a broad spectrum of antimicrobial activity, and because it is lipid-soluble, it is able to achieve significant concentrations in relatively inaccessible areas. Chloramphenicol has been a useful drug on many gynecological services because of its ability to eradicate infection by both aerobic and anaerobic organisms, as might be encountered in serious pelvic infections.

Neonates exposed to chloramphenicol in the first ten days of life may develop a serious, often fatal syndrome[62] characterized by abnormal respiratory patterns, lethargy, and hypothermia. This syndrome is an apparent result of the inability of the fetal liver to metabolize the drug. The immature liver fails to glucuronidate chloramphenicol into water-soluble derivatives. Whether other factors are also operative in the "gray baby syndrome" has not yet been established. This syndrome should not, however, occur if the dosage is restricted.

Despite the potential for toxicity, there are no reports of an adverse effect of chloramphenicol on the fetus; however, because of the possibility of such effects, the use of chloramphenicol is contraindicated in the third trimester, especially near term. Charles[33] has also advised that the drug not be given in the first trimester because of its action on mitochondrial protein synthesis.

Scott and Warner[63] have studied the transplacental passage of chloramphenicol and have found that after a 2 gm oral dose fetal serum levels ranged from 3 to 36 μg/ml.

G. Aminoglycosides

1. Kanamycin

Kanamycin is a broad-spectrum antibiotic that is useful in treating aerobic gram-negative bacillary infections. It is a drug to consider when the organism is likely to be resistant to agents such as ampicillin. In the treatment of hospital-acquired infections, sensitivities must usually be determined before kanamycin can be used, because many nosocomial infections are due to organisms resistant to this antimicrobial. Pseudomonas aeruginosa is uniformly resistant to kanamycin.

Good and Johnson[64] administered 500 mg of kanamycin to 27 pregnant women. They found that the peak serum level (at one hour) was 18.6 μg/ml, a level slightly below that expected in normals.[65] Transfer to the fetus was rapid, with peak levels in the cord blood of 9.0 μg/ml at 105 minutes after administration. Amniotic fluid levels were 5.5 μg/ml six hours after dosing.

No data on possible renal sequestration in the fetus are available. It is suggested that any child whose mother receives an aminoglycoside during pregnancy should be observed for otological or renal dysfunction during childhood.

2. Gentamicin

Gentamicin is perhaps the most widely used of the aminoglycosides. It is a broad-spectrum agent effective against most gram-negative aerobic organisms, including Pseudomonas aeruginosa. Like other aminoglycosides, it is potentially nephrotoxic and vestibulotoxic, and therefore its use should be restricted to those situations which require a drug with a wide spectrum of activity against gram-negative agents. Urinary tract infections caused by organisms resistant to other antimicrobial agents or gynecological infections caused by resistant strains would be two reasonable indications.

Several groups have reported on gentamicin pharmacokinetics during pregnancy. Yoshioka et al[66] gave 40 mg of gentamicin to 37 patients. They found a peak concentration of 3.65 μg/ml at 30 minutes and an umbilical cord peak concentration of 1.25 at 60–120 minutes.

Daubenfeld et al[67] gave gentamicin by continuous intravenous infusion; after an 80 mg loading dose, they gave 40 mg/hour. Under these circumstances maternal concentrations ranged from 2.7 to 5.0 μg/ml. Amniotic fluid levels ranged from 1.5 to 2.5 μg/ml over five hours, while the highest cord blood concentration was 4.7 μg/ml. Kaufman et al[68] studied six patients in their eighteenth to twenty-third gestational week. They gave these patients a loading dose of 80 mg and an additional 18.5 mg/hour. Maternal serum concentration at 2.5 hours was 6.2 μg/ml, and the fetal serum concentration was 1.3 μg/ml at the same time.

Weinstein[60] gave 80 mg of gentamicin at the time of cesarean section and obtained levels 50% or lower than anticipated from nonparturients.

From these studies we conclude that gentamicin given to pregnant women results in maternal drug concentrations that seem to be in the range of levels for nonpregnant females, although they may be moderately lower. Furthermore, it is clear that this antibiotic crosses the placenta, although information on fetal toxicity is not yet complete. Kaufman[68] has demonstrated that the fetal kidney could excrete the drug. The same precautions applied to kanamycin should be used for all aminoglycosides, including gentamicin.

3. Tobramycin

Tobramycin is a recently introduced aminoglycoside that has a number of similarities to gentamicin. Against certain strains of Pseudomonas aeruginosa[69] it may be more effective than gentamicin, and some investigators claim that it is less toxic.[70]

Bernard[71] studied tobramycin after a single 2 mg/kg dose given to the mother in the first half of pregnancy. Maternal serum concentrations peaked at 4 μg/ml in one hour. This level is slightly lower than expected in nonpregnant individuals. Bernard reported that tobramycin was found in fetal serum, but the concentration never exceeded 0.6 μg/ml. The amniotic fluid concentration was in the same range. Levels in the fetal kidney were found as high as 7.2 μg/ml, suggesting some fetal renal concentration of the drug. Other investigators have also studied tobramycin in pregnancy. Tanaka et al,[72] for example, have verified the fetal transfer of drug.

Tobramycin is a useful drug that is very similar to gentamicin in many respects. It should be used in pregnancy according to the same criteria and restrictions noted for gentamicin.

4. Amikacin

Amikacin is the most recently introduced of the clinically available aminoglycosides. Its pharmacology is very similar to its parent compound, kanamycin. Its use is reserved essentially for organisms resistant to other aminoglycosides.

Bernard[73] gave 30 women undergoing therapeutic abortion a single intramuscular injection of 7.5 mg/kg. Bernard found a peak maternal serum concentration of 22.5 μg/ml, very similar to what might be expected in nonpregnant females. He found fetal peak serum concentrations of 3.7 μg/ml, but concentrations in fetal kidney were again higher, 22 μg/ml 12 hours after the dose, suggesting that concentration had occurred. Antibiotic was also detected in the amniotic fluid.

5. Trimethoprim–sulfamethoxazole

Because of questions concerning safety in pregnancy, it is generally felt this drug combination should not be used during pregnancy until more information becomes available. Sulfa drugs carry the potential hazard of displacing bilirubin from albumin,[5] as noted earlier, and hence predisposing to kernicterus. It is therefore suggested that sulfas be avoided, especially near term.

V. REFERENCES

1. Doering P, Stewart R. The extent and character of drug consumption during pregnancy. JAMA. 1978; 239:843–846.
2. Kaplan E, Bisno A, Derrick W, Facklam R, Gordis L, Houser H, Jackson W, Millard D, Shulman S, Taranta A, Wannamaker L. American Heart Association Committee Report: Prevention of rheumatic fever. Circulation. 1977; 55:S1–3.
3. Other specific diseases of pregnancy. In: Walker J, MacGillivery J, MacNaughton M, eds. Combined Textbook of Obstetrics and Gynecology. New York: Churchill Livingstone, 1976: 198.
4. Wood H, Feinstein A, Taranta A, Epstein J, Simpson R. Rheumatic fever in children and adolescents: A longterm epidemiologic study of subsequent prophylaxis, streptococcal infections and clinical sequelae. III Effectiveness of three prophylaxis regimens in preventing streptococcal infections and rheumatic fever recurrences. Ann Intern Med. 1964; 60(Suppl V):31–46.
5. Odell GB. The dissociation of bilirubin from albumin and its clinical implications. J Pediatr. 1959; 55:268–279.
6. Silverman W, Andersen D, Blanc W, Crozier D. A difference in mortality rate and incidence of kernicterus among premature infants allotted to two prophylactic antibacterial regimens. Pediatrics. 1956; 18:614–625.
7. McCans J, Wenger N. Problems in management of the pregnant patient with rheumatic heart disease and valve prosthesis. South Med J. 1976; 69:1007–1010.
8. Kaplan E, Anthony B, Bisno A, Durack D, Houser H, Millard HD, Sanford J, Shulman S, Stillerman M, Taranta A, Wenger N. Prevention of bacterial endocarditis. Circulation. 1977; 56:139A–143A.
9. Sipes J, Thompson R, Hook E. Prophylaxis of infective endocarditis: A reevaluation. Annu Rev Med. 1977; 28:371–391.
10. Hook E, Kaye D. Prophylaxis of endocarditis. J Chronic Dis. 1962; 15:635–646.
11. Everett ED, Hirschman JV. Transient bacteremia and endocarditis prophylaxis: A review. Medicine. 1977; 56:61–77.
12. Rogosa M, Hampp E, Nevin T, Wagner H, Driscoll E, Baer D. Blood sampling and cultural studies in the detection of post operative bacteremia. J Am Dent Assoc. 1960; 60:171–180.

13. Khairat O. The non-aerobes of post-extraction bacteremia. J Dent Res. 1966; 45:1191–1197.
14. Rhoads P, Sibley J, Billings C. Bacteremia following tonsillectomy. JAMA. 1955; 157:877–881.
15. Shull H, Greene B, Allen S, Dunn G, Schenker S. Bacteremia with upper gastrointestinal endoscopy. Ann Intern Med. 1975; 83:212–214.
16. Baltch A, Buhac I, Agrawal A, O'Connor P, Bram M, Malatino E. Bacteremia following endoscopy. Paper presented at the 15th Interscience Conference on Antimicrobial Agents and Chemotherapy, September 1957, Washington, D.C. (abstr 165).
17. Sullivan N, Sutter V, Mims M, Marsh V, Finegold S. Clinical aspects of bacteremia after manipulation of the genitourinary tract. J Infect Dis. 1973; 127:49–55.
18. Ramsey L, Swartwout J. Cited in Burwell CS, Metcalf JM (eds). Heart Disease and Pregnancy: Physiology and management. Boston: Little Brown, 1959: 277.
19. Redleaf PD, Fadell EJ. Bacteremia during parturition. JAMA. 1959; 169:1284–1285.
20. Baker TH, Hubbell R. Reappraisal of a symptomatic puerperal bacteremia. Am J Obstet Gynecol. 1967; 97:575–576.
21. McCormack W, Rosner B, Lee YH, Rankin JS, Lin JS. Isolation of genital mycoplasmas from blood obtained shortly after delivery. Lancet. 1975; 1:596–599.
22. DeSwiet M, Louvois J, Hurley R. Failure of cephalosporins to prevent bacterial endocarditis during pregnancy. Lancet. 1975; 2:186.
23. Fleming H. Antibiotic prophylaxis against infective endocarditis after delivery. Lancet. 1977; 1:144–145.
24. Nazarian M, McCullough G, Fiedler D. Bacterial endocarditis in pregnancy. Thorac Cardiovasc Surg. 1976; 71:880–883.
25. Pedowitz P, Hellman L. Pregnancy and healed subacute bacterial endocarditis. Am J Obstet Gynecol. 1953; 66:294–301.
26. Szekely P, Snaith L. Heart Disease and Pregnancy. London: Churchill Livingstone, 1974: 112.
27. Ward H, Hickman R. Bacterial endocarditis in pregnancy. Aust NZ J Obstet Gynecol. 1971; 11:189–191.
28. Crockett E, Batchelor T, Corbeil J. Pregnancy and subacute bacterial endocarditis. Obstet Gynecol. 1960; 16:93–95.
29. Holt S, Hicks D, Charles R, Coulshed N. Acute staphylococcal endocarditis in pregnancy. The Practioner. 1978; 220:619–622.
30. Garvey G, Neu H. Infective endocarditis—An evolving disease. Medicine. 1978; 57:105–127.
31. Freedman L. Endocarditis updated. Disease-a-Month. 1979; 26:1.
32. Philipson A. Pharmacokinetics of antibiotics in pregnancy and labor. Clin Pharmacokinet. 1979; 4:297–309.
33. Charles D. Placental transmission of antibiotics. Obstet Gynecol Annu 1979; 8:19–86.
34. Ledger W. Antibiotics in pregnancy. Clin Obstet Gynecol. 1977; 20:411–421.
35. Hirsch H. The use of cephalosporin antibiotics in pregnant women. Postgrad Med J. 1971; 47(Suppl):90–93.
36. Davision J, Hytten F. Glomerular filtration during and after pregnancy. J Obstet Gynecol Br Commonw. 1974; 81:588–595.
37. Feuer G, Kardish R. Hormonal regulation of drug metabolism during pregnancy. Int J Clin Pharmacol. 1975; 11:366–374.
38. Philipson A. Pharmacokinetics of ampicillin during pregnancy. J Infect Dis. 1977; 136:370–376.
39. Bray R, Boe R, Johnson W. Transfer of ampicillin into fetus and amniotic fluid from maternal plasma in late pregnancy. Am J Obstet Gynecol. 1966; 96:938–942.
40. MacAulay M, Abou-Sake M, Charles D. Placental transfer of ampicillin. Am J Obstet Gynecol. 1966; 96:943–950.
41. Perry J, Le Blanc A. Transfer of ampicillin across human placenta. Texas Rep Biol Med. 1967; 25:547–551.
42. Boreus L. Placental transfer of ampicillin in man. Acta Pharmacol Toxicol Suppl. 1971; 3:250–254.
43. Bastert G, Wallhauser K, Weinicke K, Muller W. Pharmakokinetisch untersuchungen zum ubertritt von antibiotika in das fruchtwasser am ende der schwangerschaft I. Teil: Ampicillin. Z Geburtshilfe Perinatol. 1973; 177:330–339.
44. MacAulay M, Molloy W, Charles D. Placental transfer of methicillin. Am J Obstet Gynecol. 1973; 115:58–65.
45. Bastert G, Muller W, Wallhauser K, Hebaul H. Pharmakokinetische untersuchungen zum ubertritt von antibiotika in das fruchtwasser am ende der schwangerschfat 3. Teil:Oxacillin. Z Geburtshilfe Perinatol. 1975; 179:346–355.
46. Stewart K, Shafi M, Andrews J, Williams D. Distribution of ampicillin and cephalosporins late in pregnancy. Obstet Gynecol Br Commonw. 1973; 80:902–908.
47. MacAulay M, Charles D. Placental transfer of cephalothin. Am J Obstet Gynecol. 1968; 100:940–946.
48. Bastert G, Weinicke K, Muller W, Hebaul H. Pharmakokinetische untersuchungen zum ubertritt von antibiotika in das fruchtwasser am ende der schwangerschfet 2. Teil: Cephalothin. Z Geburtshilfe Perinatol. 1974; 178:164–173.
49. Editorial: Cross-allergenicity of penicillins and cephalosporins. JAMA. 1967; 199:495.
50. Hannay W, Sharp F, Parman M, McAllister T. Cephazolin in obstetrics. Scot Med J. 1975; 20:175–177.
51. Ishiyama S, Nakayama I, Iwamoto H, Iwai S, Okin M, Matsubara T. Absorption tissue concentration and organ distribution of cefazolin. Antimicrobial Agents Chemother. 1970.
52. Duval J, More M, Charter M, Mansour N. La cephalexin. Son transfert placentaire. Nouv Presse Med. 1972; 1:1419–1420.

53. Bernard B, Thielen P, Garcia-Cazares S, Ballard C. Maternal–fetal pharmacology of cefatrizine in the first twenty weeks of pregnancy. Antimicrobial Agents Chemother 1977; 12:231–236.
54. Hirsch H, Herbst S, Lang R, Dettli L, Gablinger A. Transfer of a new cephalosporin antibiotic to the fetus and the amniotic fluid during a continuous infusion (steady state) and single repeated intravenous injections to the mother. Archiv Gynekol. 1974; 216:14.
55. Cohlan SQ, Bevelander G, Tiamsic T. Growth inhibition of prematures receiving tetracycline: A clinical and laboratory investigation of tetracycline induced bone fluorescence. Am J Dis Child. 1963; 105:453–461.
56. Tetracyclines. In: Kucers A, Bennett N, eds. The Use of Antibiotics. 3rd Ed. Philadelphia: J. B. Lippincott, 1979.
57. Le Blanc A, Perry J. Transfer of tetracycline across the human placenta. Texas Rep Biol Med. 1976; 25:541–545.
58. Philipson A, Sabath L, Charles D. Transplacental passage of erythromycin and clindamycin. N Engl J Med. 1973; 288:1219–1221.
59. McCormack W, George H, Donner A, Kodgis L, Alpert S, Lowe E, Kass E. Hepatotoxicity of erythromycin estolate during pregnancy. Antimicrobial Agents Chemother 1977; 12:630–635.
60. Weinstein A, Gibbs R, Gallagher M. Placental transfer of clindamycin and gentamicin in term pregnancy. Am J Obstet Gynecol. 1976; 124:688–691.
61. Cohen L, McNeill C, Wells R. Clindamycin-associated colitis. JAMA. 1973; 223:1379–1380.
62. Burns L, Hodgeman J, Cess A. Fetal circulatory collapse in premature infants receiving chloramphenicol. N Engl J Med. 1959; 261: 1318–1321.
63. Scott W, Warner R. Placental transfer of chloramphenicol. JAMA. 1950; 142:1331–1332.
64. Good R, Johnson G. The placental transfer of kanamycin during later pregnancy. Obstet Gynecol. 1971; 38:60–62.
65. Welch H, Wright W, Weinstein H, Ataffa A. In vitro and pharmacological studies with kanamycin. Ann NY Acad Sci 1958; 76:66.
66. Yoshioka H, Monima T, Matsuda S. Placental transfer of gentamicin. J Pediatr. 1972; 80:121–123.
67. Daubenfeld O, Modde H, Hirsch H. Transfer of gentamicin to the foetus and the amniotic fluid during a steady state in the mother. Archiv Gynakol. 1974; 217:233–240.
68. Kaufman R, Morris J, Azarnoff D. Placental transfer and fetal urinary excretion of gentamicin during constant rate maternal infusion. Pediatr Res. 1975; 9:104–107.
69. Waterworth P. The in vitro activity of tobramycin compared with that of other aminoglycosides. J Clin Pathol. 1972; 25:979–983.
70. Smith C, Lipsky J, Laskin O, Hellman D, Mellits E, Longstreth J, Lietman P. Double blind comparison of the nephrotoxicity and auditory toxicity of gentamicin and tobramycin. N Engl J Med. 1980; 302:1106–1107.
71. Bernard B, Garcia-Cazares S, Ballard C, Thrupp L, Mathies A, Wehler P. Tobramycin: Maternal fetal pharmacology. Antimicrobial Agents Chemother. 1977; 11:688–694.
72. Tanaka S, Harima M, Yamada F, Sugaw T. Placental transfer of tobramycin. Chemotherapy (Tokyo) 1975; 23:1378.
73. Bernard B, Abate M, Thielin P, Attar H, Ballard C, Wehler P. Maternal–fetal pharmacological activity of amikacin. J Infect Dis. 1977; 135:925–932.
74. Snider D, Layde P, Johnson M, Lyle M. Treatment of tuberculosis in pregnancy. Am Rev Resp Dis. 1980; 122:65–79.

Cardiac Contraindication to Pregnancy

M.XXVI

Birth Control and Abortion in the Cardiac Patient

Norbert Gleicher, MD, and Uri Elkayam, MD

I. INTRODUCTION

In the consideration of a maternal cardiac disease in pregnancy, only very limited attention has been paid in the literature to a discussion of birth control and general aspects of family planning in this patient group. A review of most standard texts in obstetrics and cardiology did, in fact, either reveal no reference to that topic or only very limited discussion. Even so, "advisability" of pregnancy is a frequently used term in most of these discussions; what the authors are generally referring to is whether a specific pregnancy should be aborted or not. It should, however, be stated that any pregnancy in a cardiac patient that has to be aborted represents something of a failure on the part of the medical community, as proper birth control should serve to prevent pregnancy in these patients.

II. COUNSELING THE PATIENT

The female patient with known cardiac disease during her reproductive years has to be properly counseled about the dangers of pregnancy in reference to her cardiac condition. Such counseling has to involve a listing of possible risks in association with pregnancy, a description of possible means to prevent pregnancy, and last but not least a detailed description of the different birth control means and their side effects, with a specific reference to the patient's condition. It would overextend the scope of this chapter to detail the various means of birth control for the individual cardiac disease groups; nevertheless, a few principles have to be noted.

Even in the normal, noncardiac patient, pregnancy has been shown to be statistically more dangerous to the mother than

Cardiac Problems in Pregnancy, pages 305–311

Such a situation is, however, the exception. In the majority of instances, any medical disease will progress with time. The maternal chance for a successful pregnancy will therefore decrease with time. Cardiac disease is no exception to the rule. As noted earlier, advanced maternal age represents an increased risk factor.[25] It is our belief that physicians frequently too quickly recommend termination of pregnancy. Such advice may frequently solve the physician's problem, but it does not necessarily solve the patient's problem.

IV. STERILIZATION

Rovinsky[25] claims that sterilization is not indicated medically in any patient in whom surgical correction of a cardiac defect seems feasible. This approach is certainly valid; nevertheless, sterilization represents a most valuable option in certain areas. As noted earlier, contraception, especially for the long term, may be difficult in the patient with cardiac disease. Sterilization often is the safest and most reliable method of birth control in these patients. There are innumerable methods for the sterilization of the female; it would exceed the scope of this chapter to describe them in detail. It should also be remembered, however, that male sterilization may represent the best method of birth control for the couple. Especially in severe cardiac disease, in which cases general anesthesia may be associated with a disproportionate risk, such an approach may be taken. Female surgical sterilization in patients with Eisenmenger syndrome should not be performed unless absolutely necessary. Maternal mortality from all kinds of surgical procedures, at least in the immediate postpartum period, seems to be very high.[4]

V. SUMMARY

Family planning and the management of pregnancy in the cardiac patient represents a formidable problem for both the obstetrician and the cardiologist. It cannot be overemphasized how important it is to reach and communicate with the cardiac patient early in her reproductive life. As mentioned throughout this chapter, a patient who conceives against her will and against medical advice represents a failure of medical care. The problem of heart disease in pregnancy has to be addressed before pregnancy occurs.

VI. REFERENCES

1. Physicians' Desk Reference (PDR), 35th ed., 1981:1639.
2. Idem, p. 1309.
3. Idem, p. 1311.
4. Gleicher N, Midwall J, Hochberger D, Jaffin H. Eisenmenger's syndrome in pregnancy. Obstet Gynecol Surv. 1979; 34:721–741.
5. Jensen J. The Heart in Pregnancy. St. Louis: The C.V. Mosby Company, 1938.
6. Berthiot A. Grossesse et maladies du coer. Thèse pour le doctorate en medicine. Paris, 1876.
7. MacDonald A. The Bearings of Chronic Disease of the Heart Upon Pregnancy, Parturition, and Childbed. London: J & A Churchill, 1878.
8. Webster JC. The conduct of pregnancy and labor in acute and chronic affections of the heart. Am J Obstet. 1913; 68:315–319.
9. Lewis T. Diseases of the Heart Described for Practioners and Students. New York: The Macmillan Company, 1933.
10. Lamab AE. Heart disease in pregnancy; preliminary report. Am J Med Sci. 1934; 187:177–184.
11. Kustner H, Schoen R. Schwangerschaft und Herzfehler. Munch Med Wochenschr. 1934; 81:739–743.
12. Flaxman N. Pregnancy and heart disease. Am J Obstet Gynecol. 1946; 39:814–817.
13. Boyer NH, Nadas AS. Ultimate effect of pregnancy on rheumatic heart disease. Ann Intern Med. 1944; 20:99–107.
14. Gorenberg H, Chesley LC. Rheumatic heart disease in pregnancy: The remote prognosis in patients with "functional severe" disease. Ann Intern Med. 1958; 49:278–304.
15. Mendelson CL. Cardiac Disease in Pregnancy: Medical Care, Cardiovascular Surgery and Obstetric Management as Related to Maternal and Fetal Welfare. Philadelphia: F.A. Davis Company, 1960.
16. Mendelson CL. Heart disease and pregnancy. Clin Obstet Gynecol. 1961; 4:603–633.
17. Metcalfe J, Ueland K. The heart and pregnancy. In Hurst JW, ed. The Heart: Arteries and Veins, 2nd ed. New York: McGraw-Hill, 1970.
18. Metcalfe J. Rheumatic heart disease in pregnancy. Clin Obstet Gynecol. 1968; 11: 1010–1025.

19. Chesley LC. The remote prognosis for pregnant women with rheumatic cardiac disease. Am J Obstet Gynecol. 1968; 100:732–743.
20. Maynard EP Jr., Grover V. The effect of childbearing on the course of rheumatic heart disease: A 25-year study. Ann Intern Med. 1960; 52:163–171.
21. Gleicher N, Knutzen VK, Elkayam U, Loew S, Kereyni TD. Rheumatic heart disease diagnosed during pregnancy: A 30-year follow-up. Int J Gynaecol Obstet. 1979; 17:51–57.
22. Nesbit REL Jr. Coincidental medical disorders complicating pregnancy Cardiovascular Diseases. In: Danforth DN, ed. Obstetrics and Gynecology, 3rd ed. New York: Harper & Row, 1977:430–437.
23. Pritchard IA, MacDonald PC. Medical and surgical illness during pregnancy and the puerperium. Diseases of the Heart. In: Pritchard and MacDonald, eds. Williams Obstetrics, 16th ed. New York: Appleton-Century-Crofts, 1980: 730–738.
24. Benson RC. Medical and surgical complications during pregnancy. Cardiovascular complications. In: Current Obstetric and Gynecologic Diagnosis and Treatment, 3rd ed. 1980:809–813.
25. Rovinsky JJ. Diseases complicating pregnancy. In: Gynecology and Obstetrics, The Health Care of Women. New York: McGraw-Hill Book Company, 1975:787–789.
26. Bunin JJ, Appel SB. A principle for determining prognosis of pregnancy in rheumatic heart disease. JAMA. 1950; 142:90–94.

FETAL SECTION

Development of the Heart

F.I

Embryology of the Heart

Robert S. Bressler, PhD

I. INTRODUCTION

Overview: The basic pattern of heart development includes the establishment of a single midline tube by fusion of bilateral endocardial elements ventral to the foregut. A series of regional expansions appear along its length. In cephalocaudal order they are the bulbus cordis, ventricle, atrium, and sinus venosus. Blood enters the sinus venosus from the placenta, yolk sac, and body of the embryo via the umbilical, vitelline, and cardinal veins, respectively. It leaves the bulbus cordis by flowing into the truncus arteriosus and its branches, the pharyngeal arch arteries. This primitive heart tube undergoes a looping, assuming an S-shaped configuration within the pericardium. Subsequently the various chambers attain the adult position and are partitioned to provide the separate left and right circuits of the adult heart and their valves.

One of the earliest of the organ systems to develop is the cardiovascular system. This is not surprising in view of the necessity for supplying the embryo with nutrients. After fertilization the embryo goes through a period of rapid mitotic divisions called cleavage. During this process it becomes a solid sphere of cells, the morula, and then a hollow sphere with an internal cluster of cells at one pole, the blastocyst. Although many cells are produced during those stages the overall size of the embryo does not increase. Nutrients and waste materials are easily handled by diffusion. This process is adequate even for a short while after growth and implantation are achieved. Eventually the size of the embryo exceeds the efficiency of diffusion. By that time the rudiments of the circulatory system are forming. This chapter does not include a detailed description of the earliest stages of embryogenesis. The reader is referred to general embryology texts such as that by Pat-

Cardiac Problems in Pregnancy, pages 317–335

ten[1] or Hamilton and Mossman[2] for in-depth accounts of cleavage, morula, blastocyst, and bilaminar germ disc stages.

The discussion that follows is based on descriptions of human heart development.[3–12] Vascular requirements in the embryo change as various organs appear, regress, are replaced by superimposition of other structures, or increase in size and activity. The complex organogenesis exhibited by the heart is a reflection of its adaptive responses to the myriad of changes in the developing embryo. When they are studied as independent events, the "logic" of the steps in heart development is not apparent. However, when examined in the context of what is happening in the entire embryo, morphogenesis of the heart can be more readily comprehended. For example, changes in the nephric system set the stage for shifts in venous drainage from the cardinal system to the inferior vena cava. This in turn produces marked changes in the heart. This discussion is confined to cardiac morphogenesis. The reviews by Netter[13], Boyd[3], and Patten[8] are particularly good beginnings for those who want detail beyond the scope of this chapter.

II. FORMATION OF THE MESODERM AND COELOM

At the end of the second week, the implanted embryo consists of trophoblast derivatives, forming an outer extra-embryonic layer, and an inner cell mass. The latter is arranged in two primary germ layers: the ectoderm and the entoderm. This is soon followed by the formation of a mound and a groove in the amnionic surface of the ectoderm. These are Hensen's node and the primitive streak. Appearance of these structures marks the migration of ectodermal cells through them to the space between the two germ layers. The migrating cells form sheets of mesodermal tissue on either side of the midline. With the addition of cells, the mesoderm spreads forward as bilateral wings whose advancing edges meet each other at the periphery of the future cephalic end of the germ disc. The mesoderm soon becomes organized into thickened paraxial portions on either side of the midline and attenuated lateral plates extending to the edge of the germ disc. Small spaces develop within the plate. They eventually become confluent to produce a single space, the coelom, dividing the lateral plate into somatic and splanchnic layers apposed to the adjacent ectoderm and entoderm, respectively. Development of the coelomic tract begins across the midline at the cephalic end of the germinal disc and proceeds caudally. As a result the intraembryonic coelom has a U-shaped distribution between the somatic and splanchnic layers of mesoderm and arching around the prochordal and neural plates. At the middle of the embryo it communicates with the extra-embryonic coelom and may expedite the transport of nutrients and wastes between the embryo and the endometrium[9] (Fig. F.I.1).

III. ESTABLISHMENT OF THE MIDLINE HEART TUBE

Overview: The first stage of cardiac development is the formation of vascular plexuses on either side of the developing head fold. These fuse in the midline to form a straight cardiac tube exhibiting a series of dilatations representing the primitive chambers. The wall of the tube consists of three layers: endocardium, cardiac jelly, and epimyocardium.

That part of the coelom forming the base of the U (ie, crossing the midline) is the pericardial cavity. The splanchnic mesoderm in this region becomes thickened. Groups of cells on its entodermal surface form anastamosing cords which, in turn, become hollowed out, establishing bilateral plexuses that communicate with each other across the midline (Figs. F.I.2A and F.I.3A and B).

In most mammals the plexuses coalesce, forming an endothelial tube or vessel on

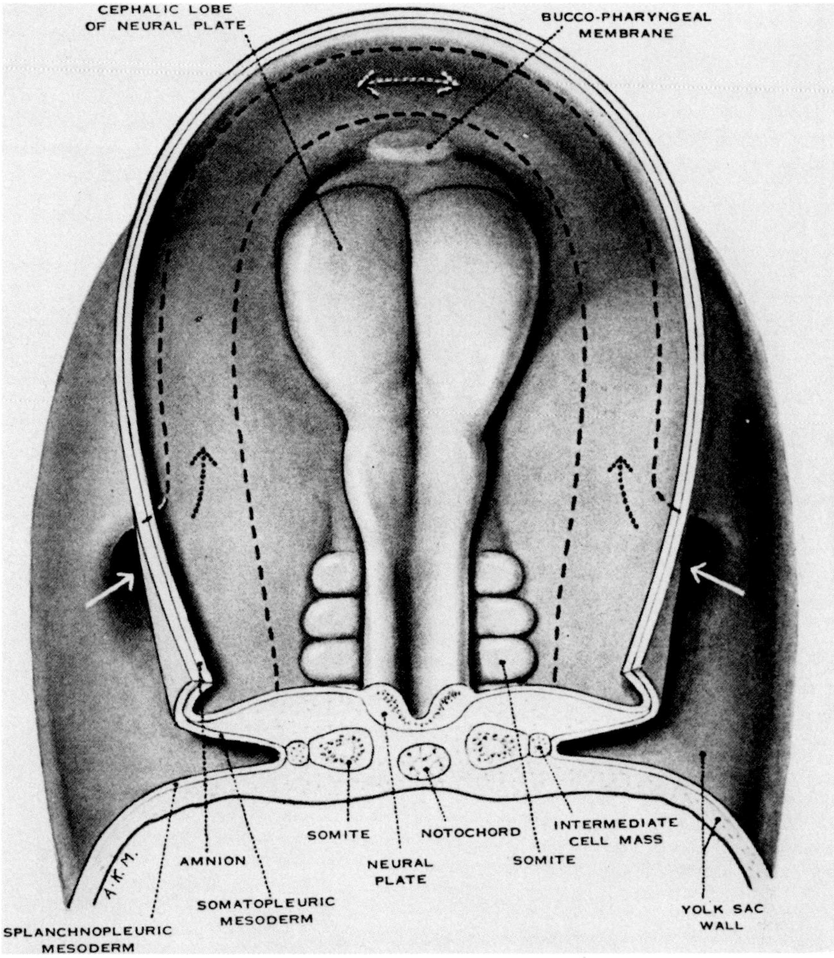

Fig. F.I.1. Schematic diagram of the cephalic portion of a neurulating embryo showing the arrangement of the intraembryonic coelom (broken lines and arrows) and its relationship to the extra-embryonic coelom at the white arrows. (Figures F.I.1, 12, 13, and 14 are from Hamilton WJ, Mossman HW. Hamilton, Boyd and Mossman's Human Embryology. ©1965 Williams & Wilkins Co., Baltimore, by permission.)

each side. In the human they may remain as plexuses until fusion of their elements in the midline produces a single heart tube[14] (Figs. F.I.2 and F.I.3). Their communication with each other by means of the midline plexus is maintained. These tubes sink into furrows within the rest of the splanchnic mesoderm. As a result, they become surrounded by a thick layer of mesoderm. The two components do not come into direct contact, but are separated by a layer of embryonic connective tissue containing few cells that is known as cardiac jelly. The outer layer will give rise to the epicardium and myocardium and therefore is called the epimyocardial mantle. The endothelial component gives rise to the endocardium of the adult (Figs. F.I.2 and F.I.3).

By this time, the head fold is forming. As it does, it rises from the germ disc and extends first directly above the cardiogenic area and then beyond it toward the periphery. Mesoderm and entoderm are incorporated into the head fold, the latter as the foregut. As a result, the area of the germ disc containing the developing heart and pericardial space is rotated 180 de-

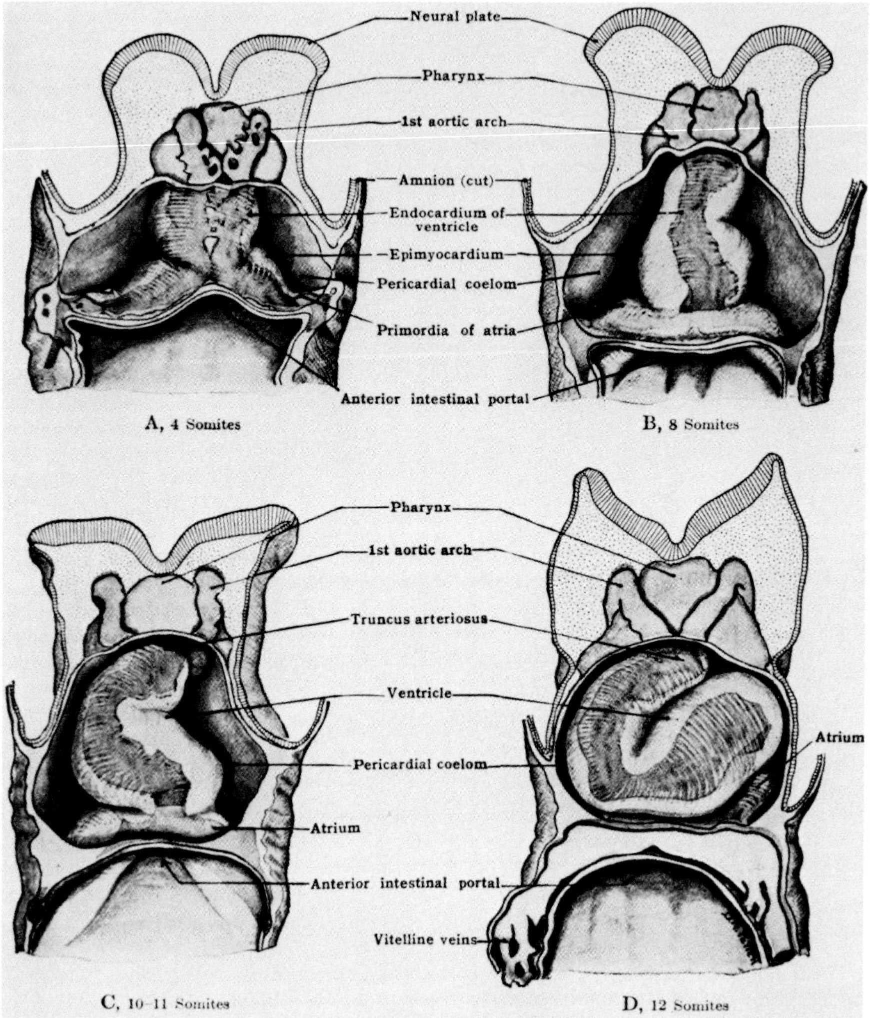

Fig. F.I.2. Ventral view of embryos of various stages illustrating fusion of the endothelial heart tubes, disposition of endocardium and epimyocardium, and early changes in the shape of the developing heart. Note the formation of the early chambers and migration of the atrium into the pericardial space from the septum transversum. Ectoderm and entoderm are cut at the reflections of the amnion and yolk sac, respectively. (From Corliss CE. Patten's Human Embryology: Elements of Clinical Development. New York: McGraw-Hill Book Company, 1976, with permission.)

grees in the sagittal plane of the embryo (Fig. F.I.4). Thus, the entoderm in the floor of the foregut now lies dorsal to the pericardial space. Mesoderm which bounded the most cephalic portion of the U-shaped coelom becomes its most caudal limit, the septum transversum.

With growth of the head fold, the bilateral rudiments of the heart are brought toward each other in the midline. They fuse, first at a region representing the bulbus cordis and then progressively in a caudal direction (Fig. F.I.2). Association of the epimyocardial mantle with the overlying entoderm is retained to form a dorsal mesocardium, which suspends the heart in the pericardial cavity (Fig. F.I.3). Between the nineteenth and twentieth days the heart bulges ventrally into the pericardial space and consists of a single midline structure composed of an endocardial tube surrounded by cardiac jelly and the epimyocardial mantle (Fig. F.I.3). Since the pericardial space was originally the base of a U-shaped cavity, it is still continuous with the rest of the coelom (the arms of the U) by means of the pleuroperitoneal canals.

Localized expansion produces four dilated regions in the developing heart tube. In cranio-caudal order, they are: bulbus cordis, ventricle, atrium, and sinus venosus. The bulbus cordis and ventricle form early since they are located at the region of initial fusion of the endocardial tubes. Their junction is marked externally by a shallow constriction. Even though the more caudal portions of the tube have not yet fused, paired atria and horns of the sinus venosus can be discerned embedded in the septum transversum (Fig. F.I.2). Branches of the paired dorsal aortae loop ventrally around the foregut as the first pharyngeal arch arteries, joining the cephalic end of the bulbus. At their caudal ends the endocardial tubes connect with vitelline, umbilical, and cardinal veins. Early in the fourth week, the dorsal mesocardium breaks down, allowing continuity between both sides of the pericardial space. This passage dorsal to the heart, between its attached arterial and venous ends, persists in the adult as the transverse sinus of the pericardium.

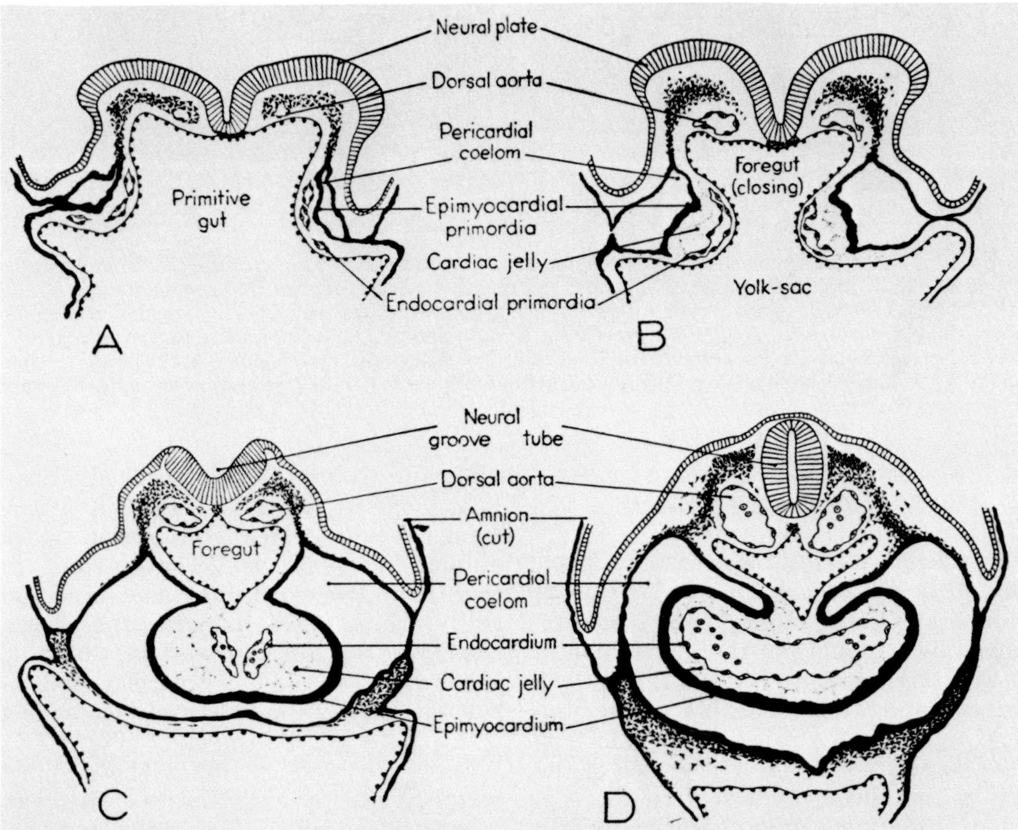

Fig. F.I.3. Cross-sections of embryos at various stages of cardiac development showing formation (**A**), approximation (**B**), and fusion (**C,D**) of endothelial heart tubes (endocardium) of each side to form the midline heart. Note the thickening of the splanchnic mesoderm to form the epimyocardial mantle, its separation from the endocardium by the cardiac jelly, and the attachment of the heart to the foregut by the forming dorsal mesocardium (unlabeled). (From Corliss CE. Patten's Human Embryology: Elements of Clinical Development. New York: McGraw-Hill Book Company, 1976, with permission.)

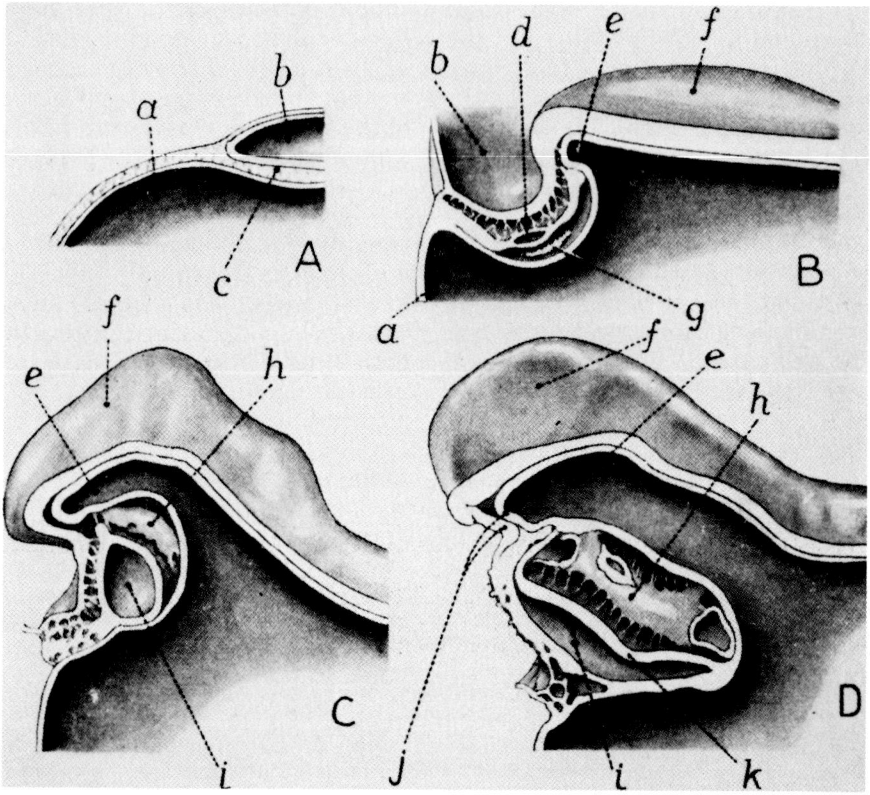

Fig. F.I.4. Diagram showing the 180 degree rotation of the cardiogenic region resulting from formation of the head fold. **A.** presomite stage; **B.** 1-somite embryo; **C.** 4-somite embryo; **D.** 7-somite embryo; a. yolk sac; b. amniotic cavity; c. intraembryonic mesoderm; d. primitive pericardial cavity; e. foregut diverticulum; f. neural fold; g. developing endothelial heart tube; h. right endothelial heart tube; i. pericardial cavity; j. buccopharyngeal membrane; k. epimyocardial mantle. (From Boyd JD. Development of the heart. In Hamilton WF, ed. Handbook of Physiology, Section 2: Circulation Volume III, 1965, by permission of the American Physiological Society.)

IV. POSITIONING OF THE CHAMBERS WITHIN THE PERICARDIUM

Overview: During this stage of development the adult orientation of the heart chambers is established. This is accomplished by a looping of the heart tube in the sagittal plane and a rotation in the frontal plane. The former places the ventricle and bulbus cordis side by side. The latter is related to the emergence of the atrium and sinus venosus from the septum transversum to assume a position dorsal to the ventricle in the pericardial space.

During its continued growth the heart tube loops in two dimensions. A loop is formed by the ventral projection of the bulbus and ventricle. Simultaneously, a counterclockwise rotation (as viewed ventrally) takes place, bringing the atrium out of the septum transversum and placing it dorsal to the left ventricle. As a result the apex of the bulboventricular loop is displaced toward the right (Fig. F.I.5).

Many authors attribute these movements to a faster growth rate of the heart tube than the pericardial space. However, explanted amphibian and chick hearts show similar looping movements when removed from their normal confines.[15,16]

These movements produce a groove between the left ventricle and the bulbus cordis that is known as the bulboventricular or conoventricular sulcus (Fig. F.I.5). A corresponding ridge in the interior of the heart tube is called the bulboventricular flange. As the atrium enters the pericardial space its connection to the ventricle, the atrioventricular junction, assumes a dorsal rather than caudal position and is shifted to the left side of the pericardium with the ventricle. By this time the caudal-most portions of the heart tube are fused to form a single middle portion of the sinus venosus. The ends of the tube diverge laterally as the left and right horns of the sinus venosus, retaining communication with the veins entering the heart.

The atrial portion now undergoes extensive dilation, but its opening to the ventricle does not. Instead, it becomes elongated to form the atrioventricular canal. With continued growth, the lateral extremities of the atrium progressively envelop the distal portion of the bulbus cordis, persisting in the adult as the right and left auricles (Fig. F.I.5). Expansion occurs in the bulbus and ventricle, too, but at their junction the lumen remains narrow, forming the primary interventricular foramen. These chambers extend caudally by growth of the epimyocardium and cavitation of its internal surface. The irregular nature of this process produces the trabeculated appearance of the future ventricles. Since this does not take place at the junction of the two chambers, a

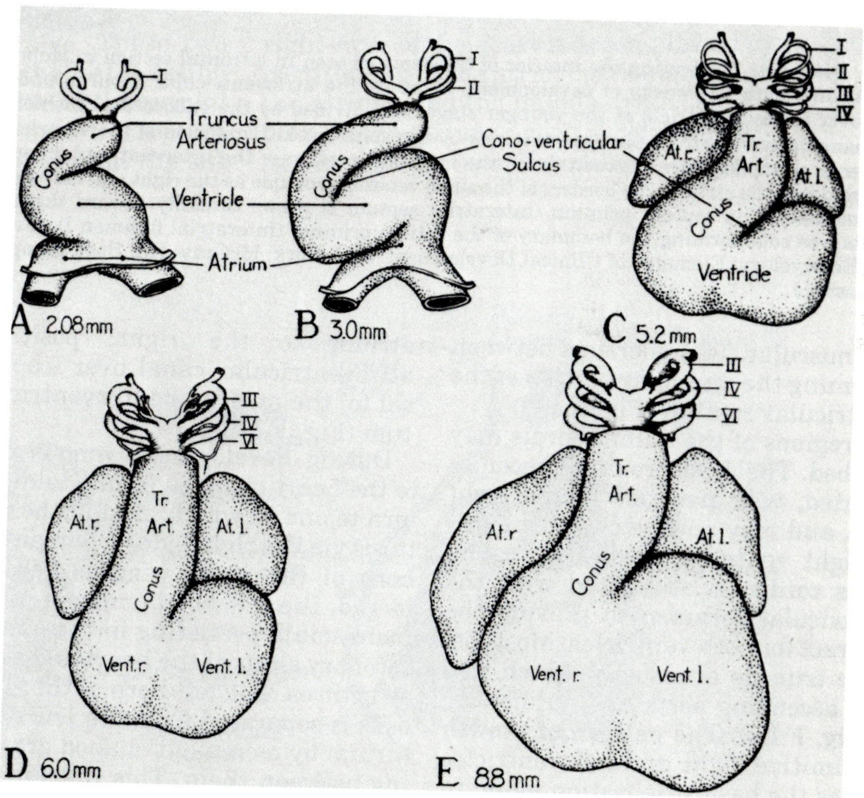

Fig. F.I.5. Ventral views of reconstructions of hearts from embryos of various stages showing the formation of the bulboventricular (conoventricular) loop and sulcus as well as the reduction in the latter and shift in position of the truncus toward the midline with age. Note the regions of the bulbus cordis: right ventricle, conus cordis, and truncus arteriosus. (From Kramer.[6])

teriosus at the level of formation of the semilunar valves; and, more proximally, in the conus. The ridges progressively protrude into the respective lumens, eventually meeting and fusing to form a septum. The most distal ridges divide the aortic sac frontally so that the sixth arch (and the pulmonary trunk arising from it) occupies a dorsal position and the fourth arch (which will form the aorta) is ventrally placed. This aorticopulmonary septum spirals as it is followed proximally to the conus. It is continuous with the truncus septum (Figs. F.I.7 and F.I.12–14).

At the level of semilunar valve formation, two minor ridges develop between the major ones. Division of the truncus results from fusion of the major ridges. Consequently, half of each major ridge and the intervening minor ridge persists as the rudiments of the semilunar valves in each vessel formed (Fig. F.I.15). The ridges forming this portion of the septum have been referred to as the distal bulbar ridges or truncus ridges. The latter name is the more commonly used. More specifically they are referred to by location as the dextro-dorsal and sinistro-ventral truncus ridges.

Similar events occur in the conus, where proximal bulbar or conus ridges produce a septum. This, too, is continuous with the more distal elements, all of them contributing to the spiral septum separating the left and right ventricles and their outlets. Considering the septum in its entirity reveals that it has rotated 180 degrees from its origin in the aortic sac to its junction with the border of the interventricular foramen. Its proximal end lies nearly in a frontal plane. It has been suggested that hemodynamic factors are responsible for the positioning of the septum. Streams of blood from each ventricle may deflect each other to form a helix when they merge at the conus cordis. This in turn may mould the cardiac jelly into a complementary configuration providing spiraling depressions and ridges along the wall of the bulbus and truncus.[5]

Formation of the endocardial cushions has been described earlier. It is important for this part of the discussion to recall that tubercles develop at the left and right

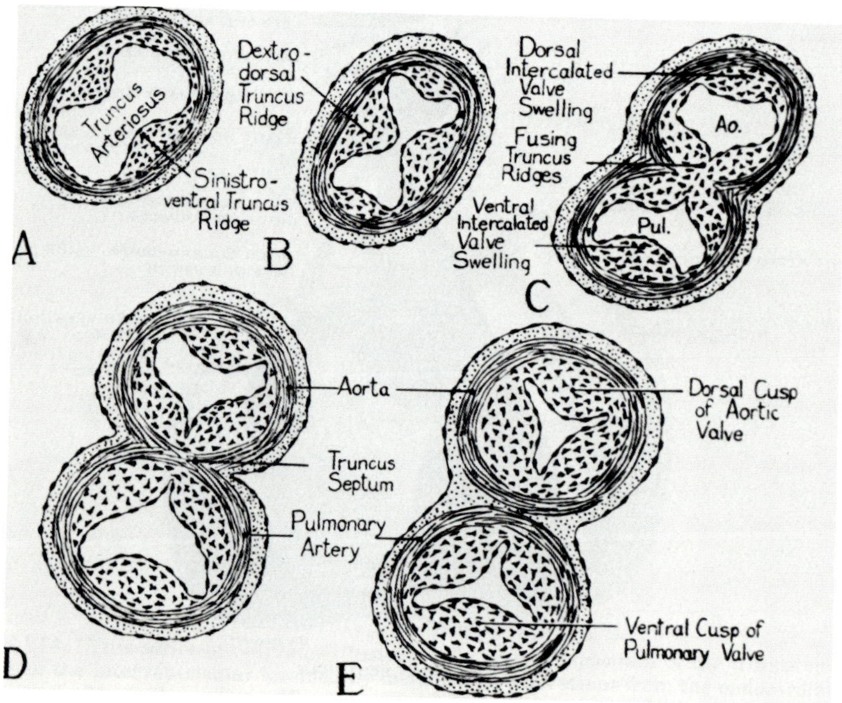

Fig. F.I.15. Schematic diagram of cross-section through the truncus arteriosus showing origin of semilunar valves from major and minor (intercalated) truncus ridges. (From Kramer.[6])

margins of each cushion. The muscular portion of the interventricular septum does not form as an upgrowth of the tissue. Rather, it is composed of the fused adjacent walls of the ventricles as they expand caudally. Hence, it never grows toward the endocardial cushions, nor does it impinge upon the interventricular foramen. The latter forms a tapering channel opening into the right ventricle just to the right of the interventricular septum. It is along the rim of the interventricular foramen that the conus ridges will fuse to separate the ventricles, converting the original interventricular foramen into the vestibule of the aorta.

The conus septum grows caudad, approaching the right border of the interventricular septum. Near its proximal edge the conus ridges diverge from each other. The sinistro-ventral conus ridge fuses with the right side of the crest of the muscular interventricular septum. The right tubercle of the ventral endocardial cushion grows toward that point. The right tubercle of the dorsal cushion expands considerably and fuses with the right side of the free edge of the dorsal extension of the muscular septum. The dextro-dorsal ridge is directed toward the right atrioventricular canal. Its lateral edge fuses with the lateral cushion of the right atrioventricular canal. The medial border merges with the right tubercle of the ventral endocardial cushion. Fusion of the conus ridges eventually extends to these divergent portions. The last vestiges of the interventricular foramen are closed by merging of three elements: the right tubercles of the endocardial cushions; mesenchyme at the apex of the muscular interventricular septum; and the conus ridges (Figs. F.I.12–14). The tissue extending between the muscular interventricular septum and the endocardial cushions becomes the interventricular portion of the membranous interventricular septum. Thus, the interventricular foramen is closed, and the left and right circuits of the heart are separated from each other.

The endocardial cushions become arched, with the concavity directed toward the muscular interventricular septum. The interatrial septum primum fuses with the convex surface at its middle. The portion of the cushions to the left of the junction gives rise to the anterior cusp of the mitral valve. The right part becomes oriented parallel to the long axis of the body and cephalic to the muscular portion of the interventricular septum. Since the conus septum attaches to the right tubercles, the interventricular septum does not meet the endocardial cushions in the midline as does the interatrial septum. Instead, it divides the right half of the cushions into medial and lateral portions. The former will give rise to the atrioventricular portion of the membranous interventricular septum, while the latter gives rise to the septal cusp of the tricuspid valve. The remaining cusps of the mitral and tricuspid valves are derived from the lateral endocardial cushions (Figs. F.I.8–10).

Associated with the thinning of the valvular cusps is the development of the connective tissue support of the valves, the annuli fibrosi. Initially the atrioventricular canal is surrounded by cardiac muscle flanked by a mesothelial-like epicardium on one side and the endocardium on the other. With the formation and fusion of the endocardial cushions, a substantial amount of connective tissue is brought to a central location between the resultant atrioventricular orifices. This is accompanied by an invagination of the epicardium in the atrioventricular sulcus. It eventually meets the endocardium, effectively separating the musculature of the atrium from that of the ventricle. Some cardiac muscle fibers remain, bridging from the floor of the right atrium to the dorsal extension of the muscular interventricular septum. There they branch, fibers continuing into each ventricle. This will become the bundle of His and its main branches. The connective tissue now surrounding the atrioventricular orifices differentiates into the annuli that make up the "cardiac skeleton" supporting the valves. Simultaneously a more differentiated connective tissue develops in the valvular projections as they become flattened out to form the definitive cusps. The cusps become elongated by an undercutting mechanism that also frees some of the trabeculae from the ventricular wall. Replacement of some of the muscle with connective tissue in the latter structures produces the chordae tendineae anchored to the still muscular papillary muscles.

VI. CORRELATION OF HEART DEVELOPMENT WITH AGE AND SIZE OF THE FETUS

The ability to correlate events of cardiac morphogenesis and growth with age and size of the embryo and fetus would be of clinical value. Unfortunately, there is much variation in the ages reported for the appearance of cardiac features, particularly during the early periods of development. This is not surprising since many studies involve a limited number of specimens. The timetable presented in Table F.I.1 is taken from Hamilton and Mossman[2] and represents a consensus for most of the events listed. However, even within that sampling there is some range in the estimated ages. Additional studies using larger numbers of specimens are needed to provide a baseline of normal heart development. Moreover, little if anything is known about the factors determining or modulating normal as well as aberrant growth of the fetal heart from the time of completion of morphogenesis until birth. By the same token, we do not know whether correlations exist between measurements of cardiac components and other parameters of fetal age. A study attempting such correlations is in progress, utilizing a large sample of autopsied midtrimester fetuses (Leslie, Shen, and Strauss, personal communication). More work of this sort is essential for the generation of accurate and clinically useful correlations.

VII. ACKNOWLEDGMENTS

I would like to thank Dr. Robert P. Goode for his helpful comments during the preparation of this manuscript and Miss Karen W. Bressler for her very capable assistance with the preparation of the figures.

TABLE F.I.1. Summary of the Development of the Heart*

Age (days)	Size	Event
18	Presomite	Angiogenetic tissue appears, reversal of cardiogenic plate
19–20	1–2 somites	Appearance of endothelial heart tubes
21	4 somites	Fusion of endothelial heart tubes
21–22	6 somites	Differentiation of atria, ventricle and bulbus cordis; first beats of heart
25	14–16 somites	Fusion of primitive atria, regression of dorsal mesocardium, formation of bulboventricular loop
26–27	20 somites to 10 mm	Circulation of blood established
32	5 mm	Septum primum appears
33	6 mm	Interventricular septum appears
35	8 mm	Foramen secundum present
36–37	9–10 mm	Atrial cushions fuse
43	15 mm	Bulbar ridges fused
46	17 mm	Interventricular foramen closed, coronary arteries formed
47	18 mm	Septum secundum appears

*Modified from Hamilton WJ, Mossman HW. Hamilton, Boyd and Mossman's Human Embryology. ©1965, Williams & Wilkins Co., Baltimore, by permission.

VIII. REFERENCES

1. Corliss CE. Patten's Human Embryology Elements of Clinical Development. New York: McGraw-Hill Book Company, 1976.
2. Hamilton WJ, Mossman HW. Hamilton, Boyd and Mossman's Human Embryology. Baltimore: Williams & Wilkins Co., 1972.
3. Boyd, JD. Development of the heart. In: Hamilton WF, ed. Handbook of Physiology. Section 2. Circulation. 1965; 3:2511–2543.
4. Davis CL. Development of the human heart from its first appearance to the stage found in embryos of twenty paired somites. Contrib Embryol Carnegie Inst Wash. 1927; 19:245–284.
5. de Vries PA, Saunders JBdeCM. Development of the ventricles and spiral outflow tract in the human heart. Contrib Embryol Carnegie Inst Wash. 1962; 37:87–114.
6. Kramer, TC. The partitioning of the truncus and conus and the formation of the membranous portion of the interventricular septum in the human heart. Am J Anat. 1942; 71:343–370.
7. Los JA. Embryology. In: Watson H, ed. Paediatric Cardiology. Saint Louis: The C.V. Mosby Co., 1968:1–28.
8. Patten BM. The development of the heart. In: Gould SE, ed. Pathology of the Heart and Blood Vessels. Springfield, Illinois: Charles C Thomas, 1968:20–90.
9. Streeter GL. Developmental horizons in human embryos. Description of age group XI, 21 to 29 somites. Contrib Embryol Carnegie Inst Wash. 1942; 30:211–245.
10. Streeter GL. Developmental horizons in human embryos. Description of age group XIII, embryos of about 4 or 5 millimeters long, and age group XIV, period of indentation of the lens vesicle. Contrib Embryol Carnegie Inst Wash. 1945; 31:27–63.
11. Streeter GL. Developmental horizons in human embryos. Description of age groups XV, XVI, XVII, XVIII, being the third issue of a survey of the Carnegie collection. Contrib Embryol Carnegie Inst Wash. 1948; 32:133–203.
12. Tandler J. The development of the heart. In: Keibel F, Mall FP, eds. Manual of Human Embryology, Vol 2. Philadelphia: J.P. Lippincott Co., 1912:534–570.
13. Netter FH. Embryology. In: The Ciba Collection of Medical Illustrations, Heart. 1969; 5:122–126.
14. Orts Llorca F, Collado JJ, Gil YDR. La fase plexiforme del desarrollo cardico en el hombre. Cited in Boyd JD. Development of the heart. In: Hamilton WF, ed. Handbook of Physiology Sect. 2, 1965; 3:2511–2543.
15. Bacon RL. Self differentiation and induction in the heart of Amblystoma. J Exp Zool. 1945; 98:87–121.
16. Butler JK. An experimental analysis of cardiac loop formation in the chick. M.A. Thesis, University of Texas.
17. Christie GA. The development of the limbus fossae ovalis in the human heart—a new septum. J Anat 1963; 97:45–54.
18. Odgers PNB. The formation of the venous valves, the foramen secundum and the septum secundum in the human heart. J Anat. 1934; 69:412–422.
19. Patten BM. Persistent interatrial foramen primum. Am J Anat. 1960; 107:271–180.
20. Patten, BM. Foundations of Embryology. 2nd Ed. McGraw-Hill Book Co. New York, 1964.

F.II

Biophysics of the Developing Heart

Page A.W. Anderson, MD, and Andrés Manring, PhD

I. INTRODUCTION

In the pages that follow we describe cardiac function in the fetus and in the neonate, emphasizing the changes that occur with development and birth. Care is taken to distinguish between fundamental changes in myocardial contractility and changes related to secondary factors such as ventricular volume. This description will serve as a basis for understanding how the heart adapts with birth.

We focus on results from the intact animal, but we also draw upon results from isolated cardiac muscle. (In the isolated preparation the force and length can be controlled precisely, whereas in the intact heart, where ventricular volume changes from one point in the cardiac cycle to another, such control is not possible.) Our focus on the intact animal is based on the concept that only by exploring the ways in which the various factors that determine cardiac function—heart rate, ventricular volume, and the inotropic state of the myocardium—interact in the intact fetal heart can we grasp how the heart functions during development and birth and in response to stress.

We consider the overall mechanical function of the heart to depend on two factors: one is muscle length or ventricular volume; the other is a broad category termed inotropy, into which fall the effects of agents such as the cardiac glycosides and β-agonists and the effects of the rate and pattern of cardiac stimulation, eg, postextrasystolic potentiation. In this context the dependence of various descriptors of fetal cardiac performance on heart rate, ventricular volume (preload), and inotropic state are described. For example, we explore the ways in which these dependencies alter cardiac output or the

Cardiac Problems in Pregnancy, pages 337–364

maximum rate of development of left ventricular pressure.

An understanding of these dependencies and their interaction is essential in explaining how the fetus deals with different forms of stress and how the fetal heart adapts with birth. The importance of this understanding is underlined by the realization that knowing what mechanisms are available to alter the function of the fetal heart will allow us to treat pathophysiologic states by using therapeutic modalities that exploit these dependencies or mechanisms. For example, a volume infusion could be used to increase end-diastolic volume, and so stroke volume, or a β-agonist could be used for its chronotropic and inotropic effects. Ultimately, when the complete characterization of the functional properties of the fetal heart has been obtained and their modulation understood, the evaluation and treatment of the stressed premature and term infant will be placed on a firm basis.

II. THE DEPENDENCIES OF THE FETAL HEART

A. The Frank-Starling Relationship

The effect of ventricular volume on the ability of the adult heart to develop pressure and eject blood was described in the late 19th and early 20th centuries by Frank[1] and Starling.[2] Frank demonstrated that when end-diastolic volume is increased, the isolated heart is able to generate a higher peak pressure and a higher maximum rate of rise of pressure ($\dot{P}_{max}$). Starling showed that an increase in stroke volume occurred with an increase in venous return. Since then, an elaborate concept has grown up around these facts.[3] Length dependence of anything—eg, peak isometric force, $\dot{P}_{max}$, cardiac output, and others—was seen as a different expression of a "Frank-Starling mechanism." Lately the experimental evidence of length-dependent activation, a mixing of the Frank-Starling mechanism and the cellular mechanisms responsible for inotropic changes in contractility, has convinced some investigators that the mechanisms are inseparable.[4,5] If they are right, the dream of finding an index of cardiac contractility is a vain one. We shall have more to say on this matter.

Although the cellular basis of the Frank-Starling mechanism is still debated, it is clear that at all stages—fetal, neonatal, and adult alike—an increase in muscle length of an isolated myocardial preparation results in an increase in tension-generating ability (Fig. F.II.1).[1,6] Even so, there is controversy about whether this relationship is of any functional importance in the intact adult animal heart[7] and about whether the relationship exists at all in the intact fetal heart.[8,9]

From in vivo studies of right ventricular output in the fetal lamb, Heymann and Rudolph[8] reported that large increases in end-diastolic pressure (from approximately 15 to 30 mm Hg, by volume infusion) produced only a small increase, at best, in cardiac output. These results generated their concept that the stroke volume of the fetal heart is somehow fixed and, by inference, that the Frank-Starling mechanism is not operative in the fetal heart. In a subsequent study[10] this group found evidence for a developmental acquisition of the heart's ability to respond to a volume infusion: left ventricular out-

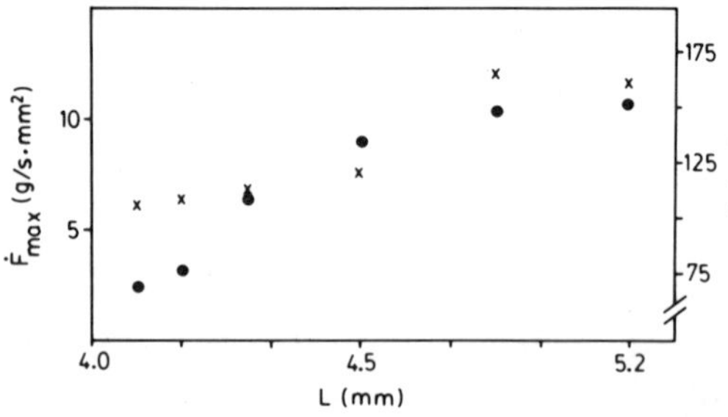

Fig. F.II.1. The maximum rate of rise of force/cross sectional area ($\dot{F}_{max}$; circles) obtained from a fetal lamb's trabeculae carneae (126 days of gestation) over a range of muscle lengths (L). The time to peak tension (T_p) for these contractions is plotted as a cross.

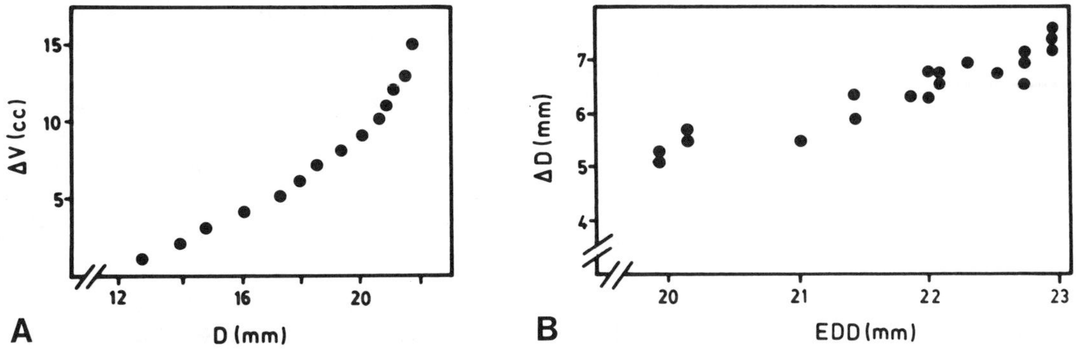

Fig. F.II.2. **A.** In vitro study of the relationship between minor axis dimension (D) and increments in ventricular volume (ΔV) in a lamb heart from a one-day-old animal (instrumented at 115 days of gestation). **B.** The in vivo relationship between end-diastolic dimension (EDD) and the amount of systolic shortening of this dimension (ΔD = EDD − end-systolic dimension) from the same lamb in A, studied the day prior to delivery at 144 days of gestation. (From the laboratory of P.A.W. Anderson).

put in the first week of life increased by a smaller percentage than in the sixth week of life. (It must be noted that the measured increase in cardiac output of the one-week-old lamb was actually *greater* than that of the older animal. The greater percent increase in the older lamb was a consequence of its control left ventricular output per kilogram being lower, perhaps because the inotropic state was different from that of the one-week-old animal.)

In contrast, Kirkpatrick et al[9] found that in the fetus an increase in end-diastolic volume is associated with a significant increase in stroke volume. The difference in the conclusions is probably the result of differences in methodology:

1) Kirkpatrick et al measured left ventricular output, whereas Heymann and Rudolph measured right ventricular output. Since fetal right ventricular output is twice that of the left ventricle,[11] the ability of the right ventricle to respond to an increase in end-diastolic volume may be nearer exhaustion than that of the left.

2) The two groups used different methods to estimate a change in ventricular volume. Heymann and Rudolph used ventricular end-diastolic pressure, whereas Kirkpatrick et al used endocardial ventricular minor axis end-diastolic dimension. The assessment of volume change with a change in end-diastolic pressure is unreliable at the high end-diastolic pressures studied by Heymann and Rudolph, since the fetal myocardium has a low compliance.[12] A large increase in end-diastolic pressure over its high range may be associated with only a small increase in end-diastolic volume. Conversely, the increase in end-diastolic volume is much greater over the low range of end-diastolic pressures (2–10 mm Hg).[12] Such an increase in end-diastolic volume is monitored accurately by an increase in left ventricular end-diastolic dimension (Fig. F.II.2).[13]

3) Different techniques were used to estimate stroke volume: electromagnetic flow probe[8] versus indicator dilution techniques or the systolic change in ventricular dimension.[9] All these techniques have their limitations. For example, systolic dimension changes will accurately reflect a change in stroke volume (Fig. 2A), but in the absence of in vitro calibration, an accurate measurement of stroke volume is difficult. In contrast, the electromagnetic flow probe can measure accurately right ventricular stroke volume, but unlike the dimension transducers, the encircling flow probe constricts the growing great vessel, produces stenosis, and increases the resistance against which the ventricle must eject. This increase in afterload may blunt or

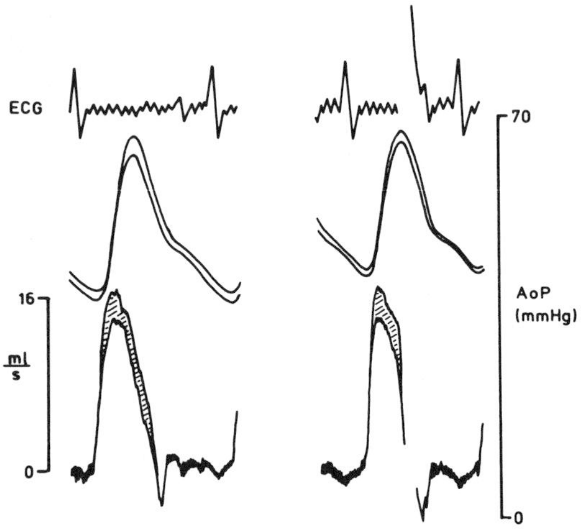

Fig. F.II.3. Volume infusions were carried out in a chronically instrumented fetal lamb during spontaneous rhythm (panel on the right) and during right atrial pacing. The stroke volume and aortic pressure both rose with 1–2 cc left atrial infusions. The cross-hatched areas demonstrated the change in stroke volume with the infusion. Left ventricular end-diastolic dimension increased by 0.6–0.8 mm with the infusion. The aortic pressure also rose. The electrocardiogram, aortic pressure, and flow waveforms are presented in that order from the top of the illustration.

obscure the effect on stroke volume of a change in a variable such as end-diastolic volume.

4) Intrinsic differences may exist between right and left ventricular myocardial contractility (although the length–tension relationships for isolated right and left ventricular fetal muscles are similar.)[6]

Whether or not the Frank-Starling mechanism is operative in the fetal animal, monitoring left ventricular volume in the chronically instrumented fetal lamb reveals large minute-to-minute changes in end-diastolic and end-systolic volume (Fig. F.II.2B).[6,9,14,15] These changes in volume sometimes occur in association with maternal movements; for example, when the ewe lies on her abdomen, precipitous decreases in fetal left ventricular end-diastolic volume may occur, followed by a return to a volume equal to or exceeding that found when the ewe was standing. Recognizing that these changes in end-diastolic and end-systolic volume occur, how

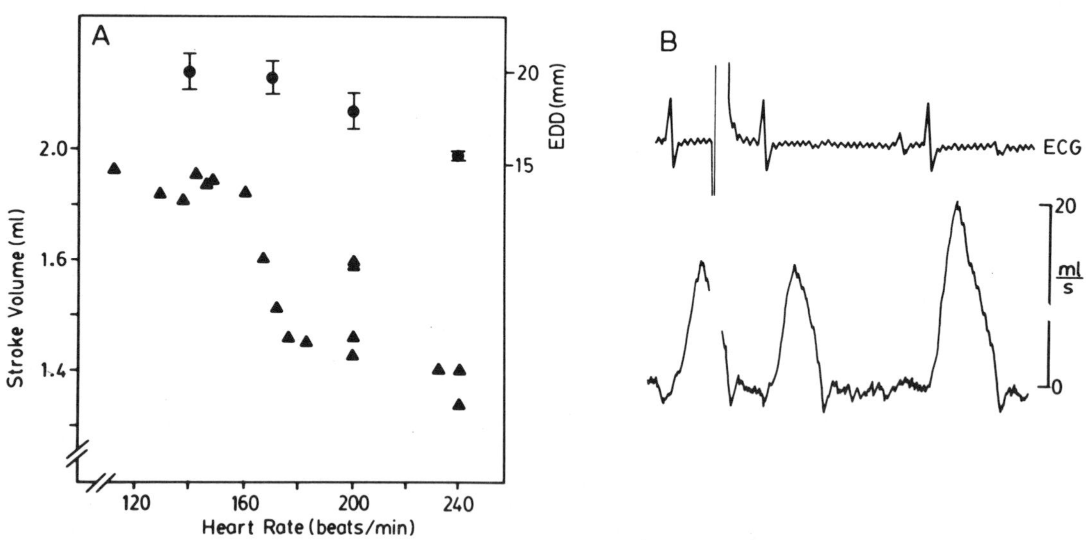

Fig. F.II.4. **A.** The left ventricular stroke volume (triangles, obtained with an electromagnetic flow probe) is presented for a fetal lamb (139 days of gestation) as a function of heart rate. The left ventricular end-diastolic dimension (EDD, circles) for that lamb at heart rates of 140, 170, 200 and 240/min demonstrates the fall in left ventricular end-diastolic volume with an increase in heart rate. **B.** The effect of introducing a pause in right atrial pacing on aortic flow (lower trace). The left ventricular end-diastolic dimension rose from 16 mm for the last paced beat to 19.5 mm after the pause. ECG, electrocardiogram.

can the fetal left ventricle have a fixed stroke volume?

When left ventricular end-diastolic volume (assessed by left ventricular dimension transducers) and stroke volume (measured by an electromagnetic flow probe) are monitored in the fetal animal, the lamb's left ventricle is shown to have a Frank-Starling mechanism (Figs. F.II.3 and F.II.4). When end-diastolic dimension is increased over a range of normal end-diastolic pressures, stroke volume is found to increase.

The Frank-Starling mechanism is clearly revealed in the chronically instrumented fetus when descriptors other than stroke volume are used to characterize left ventricular performance. For example, systolic shortening (left ventricular minor axis end-diastolic dimension − end-systolic dimension), percent fractional shortening (systolic shortening ÷ end-diastolic dimension) and $\dot{P}_{max}$ increase with an increase in left ventricular volume (Figs. F.II.5 and F.II.6).[6,14,15] These findings are consistent with an enhancement of contractility when end-diastolic volume is increased.

The presence of the Frank-Starling mechanism in the fetal left ventricle has special significance because of the large increase in left ventricular volume that occurs with birth (Fig. F.II.7).[15] The Frank-Starling mechanism must play a major role in the ability of the fetal left ventricle to increase its output with birth (eg, from 180 ml/kg/min[16] to 400–425 ml/kg/min[10,17]).

Although these findings demonstrate that the Frank-Starling relationship is operational in the fetal left ventricle, these studies do not address the following: 1) the response of the left ventricle at end-diastolic pressures of 12 mm Hg or higher, 2) the effect on right ventricular output of a change in right ventricular end-diastolic pressures over a lower range of values (consequently a larger range of right ventricular end-diastolic volumes), and 3) the effect of altering end-diastolic volume in one ventricle on the ability of the opposite ventricle to fill and to eject. Only

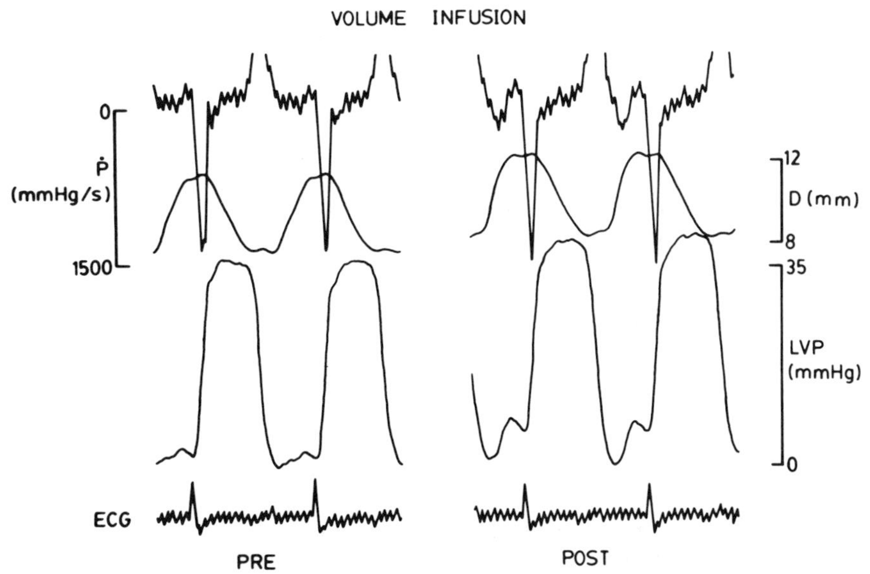

Fig. F.II.5. The response to a volume infusion in a fetal lamb (138 days' gestation). The first derivative of left ventricular pressure ($\dot{P}$), left ventricular pressure (LVP) and electrocardiogram (ECG) are presented from top of the illustration down. Pre; prior to infusion: post; following infusion.

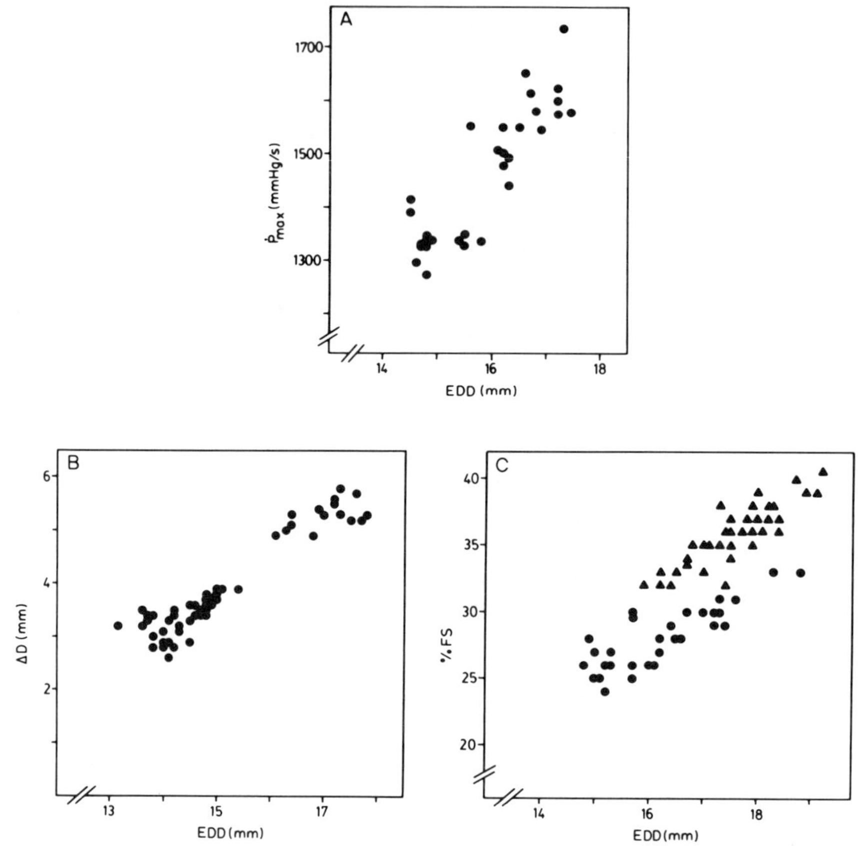

Fig. F.II.6. The effect of end-diastolic dimension (EDD) on the maximum rate of rise of left ventricular pressure (**A**; $\dot{P}_{max}$), systolic shortening (**B**; end-diastolic dimension − end-systolic dimension; ΔD) and percent fractional shortening (**C**; ΔD ÷ EDD × 100; %FS) in a fetal lamb. The heart rate was constant at a cycle interval of 300 msec. The %FS data were obtained at two infusion rates of isoproterenol: 0.006 μg/kg/min (circles) and 0.024 μg/kg/min (triangles). (Reprinted from Anderson et al[15] with permission.)

by understanding all of this potentially complex interaction will we be able to interpret how a change in ventricular volume alters the ability of the fetal heart, and so the neonatal heart, to respond to stress and to birth.

B. Heart Rate and Inotropic State (In Vivo)

An increase in heart rate has a direct inotropic effect on the chronically instrumented in vivo fetal heart.[14,15,18] When heart rate is increased, the heart shows an increase in its ability to generate pressure; eg, $\dot{P}_{max}$ increases despite a fall in left ventricular end-diastolic volume (Fig. F.II.8). When end-diastolic volume is allowed to return to its low rate value or when it does so spontaneously (Figs. F.II.6 and F.II.8), $\dot{P}_{max}$ is even further accentuated.

Similar to its effect on the ability of the heart to generate pressure, an increase in heart rate increases the ability of the ventricle to contract and so eject blood. When various ejection phase descriptors of ventricular performance are examined with end-diastolic volume being held constant, they are found to increase with an increase in heart rate. For example, the rates

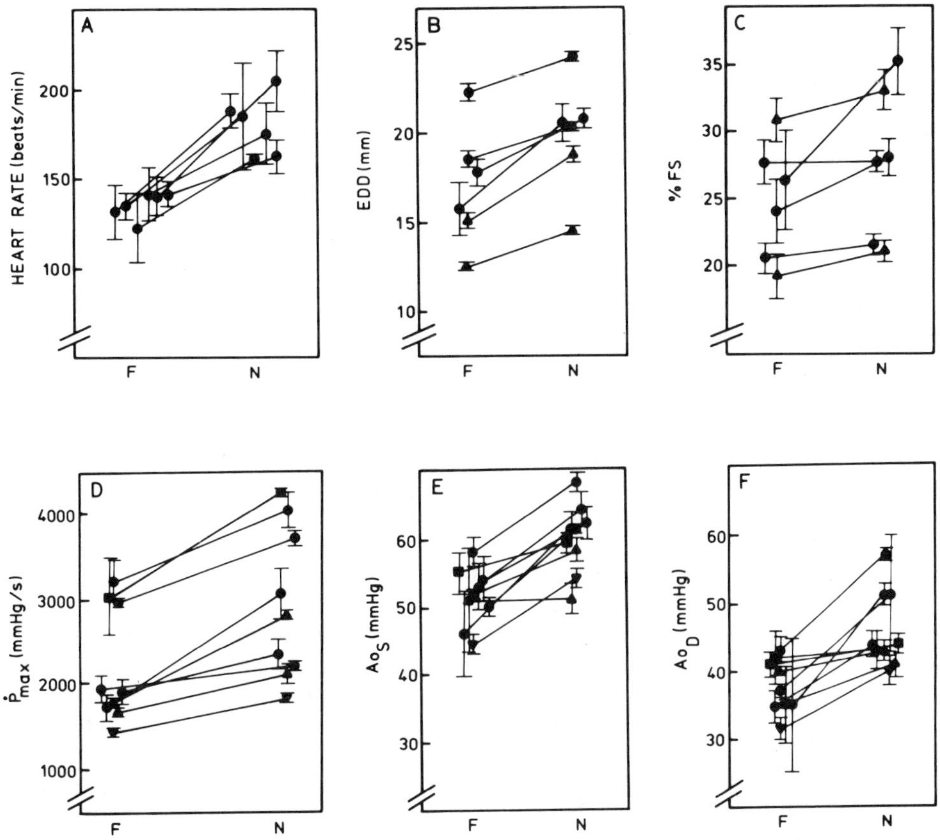

Fig. F.II.7. The change from fetal (F) to neonatal (N) life (the mean and two-standard deviations) of heart rate (**A**): ventricular end-diastolic dimension, EDD (**B**); percent fractional shortening, %FS (**C**); the maximum rate of rise of left ventricular pressure, $\dot{P}_{max}$ (**D**); aortic systolic pressure, Ao_S (**E**); and diastolic aortic pressure, Ao_D (**F**) for six lambs. The connected values in panels B, C, D, E, and F, were obtained at the same heart rates (squares, paced intervals of 250 msec; circles, 300 msec; upright triangles, 350 msec; inverted triangles, 400 msec). (Reprinted from Anderson et al[15] with permission.)

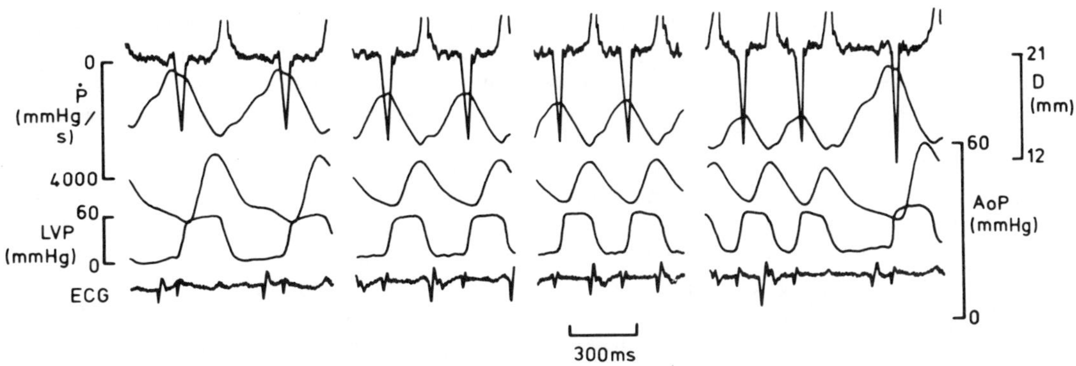

Fig. F.II.8. Data from a chronically instrumented fetal lamb (138 days of gestation) obtained at different heart rates. Traces from top: first derivative of left ventricular pressure, $\dot{P}_{max}$; left ventricular dimension, D; aortic pressure, AoP; left ventricular pressure, LVP; and electrocardiograms, ECG. The end-diastolic dimension and end-diastolic pressure fall with increasing heart rate and then, after a pause (group on far right), exceed the control values (group on far left). (Reprinted from Anderson et al[15] with permission.)

of ejection, systolic shortening, and percent fractional shortening increase as the heart rate increases (Fig. F.II.8).[14,15,18]

Thus, when end-diastolic volume is held constant, the inotropic effect of an increase in heart rate on the myocardium is revealed by the enhanced ability of the heart to generate pressure and to eject blood. However, these effects of heart rate are complicated by the decrease in diastolic filling time, and so end-diastolic volume, that accompanies an increase in heart rate. This complex interaction of diastolic filling time and enhancement of inotropic state that occurs when heart rate is increased may be the explanation for the present controversy about the effect of heart rate on cardiac output in the fetal animal.

Rudolph and Heymann[19] observed in the chronically instrumented fetus that, in general, an increase in total (biventricular) cardiac output per minute occurs when heart rate is increased over a broad range (approximately 140–250 beats per minute) and that beyond this range, output falls with a further increase in rate. These observations, coupled with their previous one that an increase in cardiac output does not occur when right ventricular end-diastolic pressure is increased (see section II.A), resulted in the following conclusion: since stroke volume is fixed in the fetus, the stressed fetus must have only one mechanism through which cardiac output can be increased—namely, an increase in heart rate.

However, the conclusion that stroke volume is fixed, and so an increase in rate results in an increase in cardiac output, is in conflict with certain of their observations. Cardiac output fell when heart rates in excess of 300 beats per minute were achieved. This fall in output could be related to the decrease in diastolic filling time, and so end-diastolic volume (Figs. F.II.4 and F.II.8), but if this explanation is correct, stroke volume must be related to end-diastolic volume. Note too that the model of Rudolph and Heymann ignores the effect of inotropy on stroke volume. Assali and his co-workers have demonstrated clearly that a positive inotropic stimulus increases fetal ventricular output.[20]

A conclusion diametrically opposite to that of Rudolph and Heymann was reached by Kirkpatrick et al[9]: an increase in heart rate does not increase ventricular output. Monitoring left ventricular volume using left ventricular dimension transducers (see section II.A; Fig. F.II.2), they found no increase in left ventricular output with an increase in heart rate. This appeared to be a consequence of a decrease in end-diastolic volume that occurred when heart rate was increased (see Fig. F.II.4). This fall in end-diastolic volume would produce a fall in stroke volume based on the Frank-Starling relationship.

In the adult animal, when an increase in heart rate is brought about by atrial pacing, end-diastolic volume falls, and cardiac output fails to increase.[21,22] Just as in the adult animal, in the fetus an increase in rate results in a fall in end-diastolic volume (see Figs. F.II.4,8,14,15, and 18). The extent to which ventricular diastolic filling time is decreased, and so end-diastolic volume and stroke volume are decreased, strongly affects whether the increase in number of beats per minute results in an increase in cardiac output. The relationship between heart rate and end-diastolic volume may not be as straightforward in the fetus as in the adult. Flow into the fetal right atrium is divided between the left and right ventricles. Consequently, a change in the site of atrial pacing, which results in alterations of right and left atrial pressure waveforms, could change flow across the foramen ovale and so alter right and left ventricular end-diastolic volumes in such a manner that the output for the right and left ventricles may change in opposite directions.[19] These considerations are consistent with the observation of Rudolph and Heymann, that increasing heart rate by right atrial pacing increases left ventricular output, and that of Kirkpatrick et al, that increasing heart rate with left atrial pacing does not increase left ventricular output.

This interaction of the effects of heart

rate on inotropic state and end-diastolic volume could be imagined easily to result in such a complicated interaction that the results of either Rudolph and Heymann or Kirkpatrick et al could be obtained (eg, see Fig. F.II.9).

These contradictory findings and opposing hypotheses need to be resolved if the control of fetal and neonatal cardiac output is to be understood. Decisions about whether a volume infusion, a diuretic, or an inotropic agent that may alter venous return should be used would be aided by understanding this interrelationship. Indeed, only through this understanding can sound therapeutic decisions be made.

When we monitored left ventricular stroke volume in the chronically instrumented fetal lamb, an increase in heart rate was shown to produce a fall in stroke volume (Fig. F.II.4). When at the higher rate, end-diastolic volume was returned to the larger low rate volume, the stroke volume of that systole could be increased by twofold or greater (Fig. F.II.4). The combined effects of rate on ventricular inotropy and end-diastolic volume were shown to result in either the results of Rudolph and Heymann or those of Kirkpatrick et al, as shown in Figure F.II.9. In that illustration the left ventricular output was essentially unchanged over a broad range of rates in one study, and in the same lamb on a subsequent date, left ventricular output increased with an increase in rate and then began to fall with a further increase in rate.

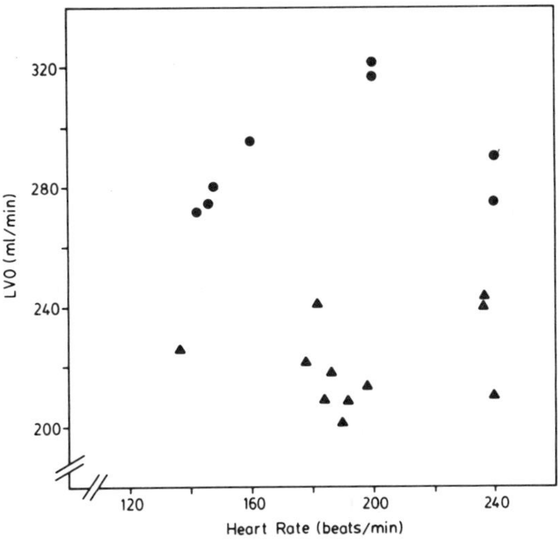

Fig. F.II.9. The fetal left ventricular stroke volume (LVO) obtained with an ascending aortic electromagnetic flow probe during a wide range of heart rates. The data were obtained from a lamb at two different gestational ages: 132 days (triangles) and 140 days (circles).

Thus, if the fall in end-diastolic volume at the faster pacing rates could be prevented, an increase in cardiac output would always occur. These results and those discussed earlier (see section II.A) demonstrate that heart rate and end-diastolic volume are both important variables in determining stroke volume, and so the cardiac output of the fetus.

C. The Force–Interval Relationship

The presence of the relationship, described above, between heart rate and ventricular performance must be considered in a more general way than simply: Does ventricular output vary with a change in heart rate? Broader questions are suggested: How does the heart, having undergone activation and contraction, return itself to a state of readiness to generate tension or eject blood by the next beat? How is its ability to contract altered by varying the pattern of stimulation? Although the underlying cellular processes are not fully understood (eg, changes in the number of cross bridges[23] or intracellular calcium availability[24]), the development of this state of preparedness following the previous activation and contraction can be followed by an experiment that measures the time course of this change in contractility from one contraction to the next (Fig. F.II.10; see also Figs. F.II.14, and F.II.25).

This general relationship between the pattern of stimulation and the ability of myocardium to contract has been termed by various authors as the force–frequency, interval–strength, or force–interval relationship.[14,25–27] Since such a relationship

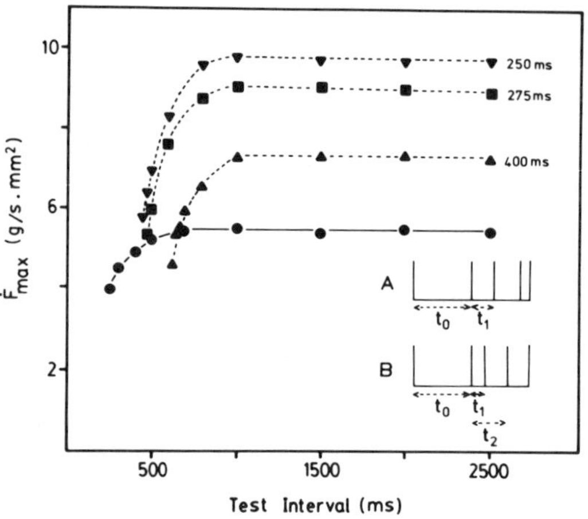

Fig. F.II.10. The force–interval curves, $\dot{F}_{max}$ (the maximum rate of rise of force) described as a function of the test interval (t_1 or t_2) from an isolated fetal trabeculae carneae cordis, 132 days' gestation, are illustrated: the basic interval, t_0 = 3,000 msec, the first-stage curve with varying t_1 (circles), and three second-stage curves with fixed t_1 and varying t_2; t_1 = 250 msec (inverted triangles), t_1 = 275 msec (squares), and t_1 = 400 msec (upright triangles). The inset is a schematic representation of the pacing sequence of the two-stage experiment. A describes the first stage; B, the second stage. (Reprinted from Anderson et al[14] with permission.)

between the rate and pattern of stimulation and the ability of muscle to contract has been shown to exist in mammalian myocardium (eg, the positive staircase that follows a change in rate or a response to paired pacing[27,28]), then the absence of such a relationship in the developing heart or the presence of one that is different from that in the adult would indicate a marked change in the manner in which contractility is modulated at different ages.

This response of the heart to a perturbation in the pattern of stimulation has been used as an index of change in myocardial performance from one stage of development to another. For example, post-extrasystolic potentiation has been shown to be less in the younger neonate than in the older infant.[29] Similarly, paired pacing produces less enhancement in contractility in isolated fetal myocardium than in that of the adult.[18] Unfortunately, since these various points in development were studied using responses to different pacing patterns, the basic characteristics of the force–interval relationship may prevent any meaningful comparison from one age to another; the more premature an extrasystole, the greater the post-extrasystolic potentiation.[14] Moreover, the sensitivity of the force–interval relationship to a change in inotropy[30] may result in quantitative differences between patient populations that reflect differences in the state of the patient's health.[31] Therefore, before we consider the presence of quantitative developmental changes in the force–interval relationship, let us 1) describe the restitution of contractility and how this restitution curve is altered by the introduction of an extrasystole, 2) examine its dependence (if any) on muscle length, and 3) examine its dependence on a change in inotropy.

Let us provide an example: if an isolated piece of cardiac muscle is stimulated every three seconds until the peak tension is constant from activation to activation, what is the peak tension of an extrasystole elicited 0.50 seconds after the previous activation? The answer depends on the species. In amphibian myocardium, the peak tension would be greater for the extrasystole than for the steady-state contraction, whereas in mammalian myocardium, the extrasystole would be the weaker one.[32] Such differences in myocardial responses from these two phyla suggest a corollary: the responses of adult and fetal mammalian myocardium may differ in a similar way; eg, the peak tension for the fetal extrasystole may be greater than the peak tension at the basic rate if ontogeny recapitulates phylogeny.

Such evaluations of the force–interval relationship can be carried out using an unlimited number of pacing patterns, as any variation in the stimulus pattern reveals to some extent the characteristics of this relationship. In other words, included in each response is a partial description of how contractility changes with time following every beat. However, this description can be obtained in a more easily interpreted manner by pacing the muscle at a constant rate (basic interval = t_0) and infrequently but regularly interpolating an extra-stimulus at various coupling intervals following the previous regular stimulus (extrasystolic interval, t_1) (Fig. F.II.10). This experiment reveals that contractility ($\dot{F}_{max}$ of the extrasystole) rises monotonically from its smallest value at the shortest t_1 to equal $\dot{F}_{max}$ of the previous contraction at the constant rate, as t_1 approaches t_0. This monotonic time course of an increase in contractility from one contraction to the next is essentially the same *throughout* the developmental period so far studied in the mammal. From mid-gestation to the adult,[14,26,30] the ability of myocardium to respond to activation is depressed immediately following a contraction. The shorter the coupling interval, the less the myocardium has recovered its ability to contract. When the coupling interval is increased, a plateau of contractility is reached finally, and the contraction has become identical to the contractions at the constant rate.

The following pacing pattern (second-stage experiment) was designed to examine how an extrasystole modifies the regeneration of contractility between contractions at the constant paced rate. Two stimuli are interpolated into the basic pacing sequence, again infrequently and regularly (Fig. F.II.10). The first of the two stimuli is introduced at a fixed t_1, and the second is applied at various intervals following the previous regular contraction (post-extrasystolic interval, or t_2).

The second-stage experimental results demonstrate that the restitution curve of contractility following an extrasystole is monotonic, like the first-stage curve, but the quantitative characteristics of the time course are altered by the presence of the extrasystole: $\dot{F}_{max}$ of the post-extrasystolic contraction again increases from its smallest value at the shortest t_2, but now rises to a plateau value that is higher than $\dot{F}_{max}$ of the regular rate. The level of the plateau and slope of the rising curve of contractility depend upon t_1: The shorter the t_1, the steeper the slope of the second-stage curve and the greater the post-extrasystolic potentiation (Fig. F.II.10). This dependence is exemplified by the different plateau values in Figure F.II.10. When the extrasystolic interval, t_1, is held constant, post-extrasystolic potentiation increases when the basic interval, t_0, is increased; and when t_0 is held constant, post-extrasystolic potentiation increases when t_1 is decreased. (However, since these contractions are interpolated into an interval that is kept constant, post-extrasystolic potentiation disappears when t_1 is so long that it approaches t_0). These characteristic features of the force–interval relationship are found in all mammalian myocardium, whether adult or fetal.[14,26,30]

Post-extrasystolic potentiation can be described by the $\dot{F}_{max}$-interval ratio; $\dot{F}_{max}$ of the second-stage curve plateau/ $\dot{F}_{max}$ of the first-stage curve plateau (ie, $\dot{F}_{max}$ of the previous regular contraction). This ratio has been used to reveal changes in inotropic state—eg, the effect of inotropic agents, disease states, and development.[30,31,33] To make such comparisons, the same rate and pattern of stimulation (ie, pacing patterns) must be used because of the dependence of the force–interval relationship, and so the $\dot{F}_{max}$-interval ratio, on t_1 and t_2.

At no stage of development studied from mid-gestation onward is the kind of behavior that characterizes amphibian myocardium observed. In amphibian myocardium contractility decreases with time following the previous contraction and post-extrasystolic potentiation is absent at all intervals of t_1. Thus, if developmental changes in the force–interval relationship recapitulate phylogenetic ones, the change must take place earlier than mid-gestation in the sheep.[14]

The possibility does exist that in other species (perhaps in those that as newborns are not able to walk or to run) such developmental changes might be found at gestational ages comparable to those studied in the sheep. To test this, the puppy was studied, and no such developmental changes were found at birth.[34] This lack of a qualitative change in the force–interval relationship demands that a quantitative change (eg, an increase or decrease in the $\dot{F}_{max}$-interval ratio) must be sought if developmental changes in contractility are to be revealed with the use of the force–interval relationship.

Examining the first derivative of left ventricular systolic pressure (say, $\dot{P}_{max}$, the maximum rate of rise of left ventricular pressure) of the extra- and post-extrasystoles in the intact animal (fetus, neonate, and adult) reveals that the general characteristics found in isolated muscle preparations are present in the intact chronically instrumented lamb beginning from 116 days of gestation to four months of life[14,33] and in the adult dog.[35]

For several reasons, the force–interval experiment had to be modified before such a comparison could be made between the relationship of the isolated preparation and that of the intact animal's heart. The new design (Fig. F.II.11) takes into consideration the fast intrinsic heart rate of the intact animal, the properties of the atrioventricular conduction system, and the variations in ventricular end-diastolic volume produced by the extrasystole:

1) The basic pacing rate (t_0) must be faster than that used in the isolated muscle experiments because of the faster intrinsic heart rate of the intact animal. The same pacing rate cannot be used throughout gestation and neonatal life because of variations in the resting heart rate. For example, the increase in heart rate that follows birth prevents the use of the same pacing rate that easily controlled the fetal heart rate one day prior to birth.[15]

2) The refractory periods and conduction times of the atrioventricular conduction system vary from one point in development to another so that it is not possible to use the same extrasystolic intervals (t_1) at the same pacing rates, t_0, at all stages of development. In general, the later in gestation or the older the lamb, the longer the refractory period and the slower the conduction velocity of the atrioventricular conduction system.[14,33] For example, an extrasystole with a t_1 of 200 msec could be obtained easily in the 135-days-of-gestation lamb but never in the 120-day-old neonatal lamb. Similarly, the heart could not be paced at a cycle interval of 300 msec

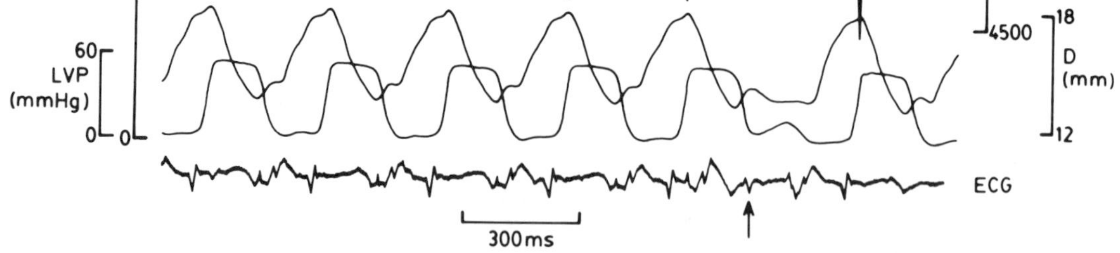

Fig. F.II.11. The force–interval experimental results from a chronically instrumented in utero fetal lamb (134 days' gestation, 15 days after instrumentation) are illustrated: the basic cycle interval, t_0 = 300 msec, and the first test interval, t_1 = 195 msec. The arrow denotes the QRS of the first test systole. The traces from top to bottom are: $\dot{P}$, the first derivative of left ventricular pressure; AoP, aortic pressure; D, left ventricular minor axis dimension; LVP, left ventricular pressure; ECG, electrocardiogram. (Reprinted from Anderson et al[14] with permission.)

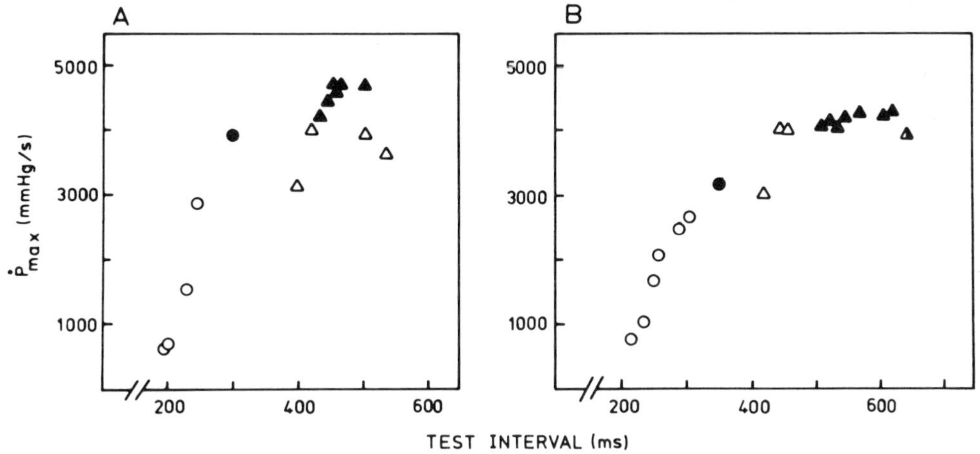

Fig. F.II.12. **A.** The first-stage (circles) and second-stage (triangles) $\dot{P}_{max}$–interval curves for an in utero fetal lamb (136 days' gestation, 14 days postoperation), at a basic interval of t_0 = 300 msec, and for the second-stage experiment, t_1 = 205 msec. Solid symbols denote systoles of equal left ventricular end-diastolic dimension (EDD); open symbols, test systoles with an EDD less than that of the previous regular systole (solid circle). **B.** The first-stage (circles) and second-stage (triangles) $\dot{P}_{max}$–interval curves for the same fetal lamb in (A), studied on the same day at a slower basic cycle interval, t_0 = 350 msec. The second-stage experiment had the same fixed first test interval, t_1 = 205 msec, as in panel A. Solid symbols are for systoles with equal EDD; open symbols represent a EDD less than that of the previous regular systole (solid circle), and the half-solid triangle is from a systole that had an EDD greater than that of the previous regular systole, but $\dot{P}_{max}$ was obtained after left ventricular ejection had begun. (Reprinted from Anderson et al[14] with permission.)

(200 beats per minute) in the 120-day-old neonate without the Wenckebach phenomenon. Sympathetic tone also affects atrioventricular conduction. For example, during an isoproterenol infusion, an extrasystole with a t_1 as short as 160 msec could be obtained as compared to the shortest t_1 of 200 msec during the control state. The spontaneous increases in circulating catecholamine levels at birth and their subsequent fall[35,36] may explain the decrease in refractory period and conduction time that occurs in the first few hours following delivery and their gradual return to the prenatal values over the subsequent neonatal days.

3) The same general relationship between the duration of t_1 and that of t_0 existed at all the ages studied; the shortest values of t_1 were obtained at the shortest t_0 (ie, the faster the heart was paced, the earlier the extrasystole could be introduced).

4) Marked alterations in diastolic ventricular filling, and so ventricular end-diastolic volume, occur with the changes in pacing rate and pattern required to carry out the evaluation of the force–interval relationship.[14,15] The faster the rate, in general, the smaller the end-diastolic volume of the extrasystole. The later in the pacing pause that the potentiated systole was introduced, the greater was its end-diastolic volume. Consequently, if the effects of the force–interval relationship—eg, post-extrasystolic potentiation—are to be evaluated without complications arising from the Frank-Starling mechanism, end-diastolic volume must be monitored so that systoles with the same end-diastolic volumes can be compared (Figs. F.II.11 and F.II.12). This is essential because of the effect of end-diastolic volume on $\dot{P}_{max}$ (see Fig. F.II.6).

When the rate and pattern of stimulation are altered in the fetus and neonate, the complex interaction of the hemodynamic variables is revealed. For example, Figure F.II.11 illustrates the changes brought about by the introduction of an extrasystole. The rise in ventricular pressure induced by the extrasystole prevents the rapid ventricular filling that normally occurs immediately following the regular systole. Then as pressure falls, ventricular diastolic filling begins at a higher ventricular pressure and is more rapid than that prior to the previous regular systole. In this example, the peak extrasystolic pressure does not reach the aortic pressure, yet the minor axis dimension decreases. This may be due in part to fiber rearrangement during this isovolumic systole, but often it is associated with a prominent v wave in the left atrial pressure waveform, suggestive of mitral regurgitation. When the extrasystolic pres-

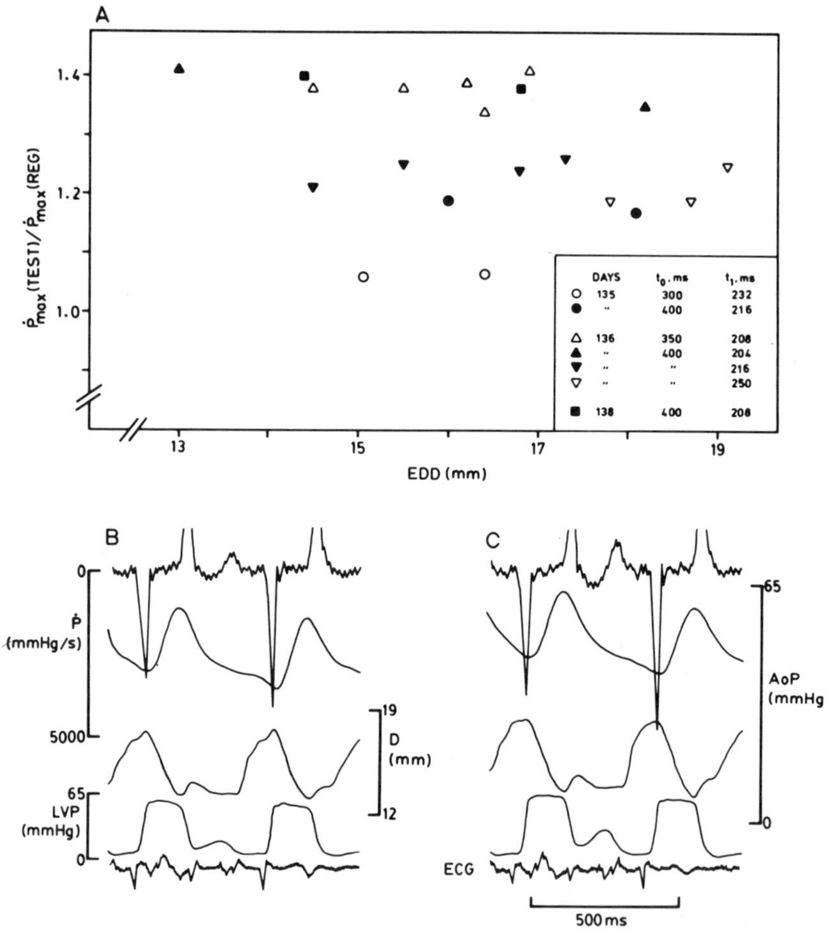

Fig. F.II.13. **A**. The effect of left ventricular end-diastolic dimension (EDD) on the $\dot{P}_{max}$–interval ratio ($\dot{P}_{max}$ of the second test contraction divided by $\dot{P}_{max}$ of the previous regular contraction, both systoles with the same EDD). The ratios obtained at several EDD for each pacing interval are compared for a fetal lamb instrumented at 132 days' gestation. The symbols indicate the day of gestation, the basic pacing interval (t_0), and the timing of the fixed first test interval (t_1). The effect of end-diastolic dimension on post-extrasystolic potentiation (t_0 = 300 msec, t_1 = 205 msec) in a fetal lamb (at 138 days' gestation, instrumented 16 days previously) is shown prior to (**B**) and after (**C**) a left atrial volume infusion. The tracings, from top to bottom, are the following: $\dot{P}_{max}$, first derivative of pressure; AoP, aortic pressure; D, left ventricular minor axis dimension; ECG, electrocardiogram. (Data from Anderson et al.[6])

sure is not sufficient to open the aortic valve and so increase aortic pressure, the aortic diastolic pressure for the post-extrasystolic systole is lower than at the regular rate.

$\dot{P}_{max}$ of the extrasystole is smaller than that of the regular systole, whereas P_{max} of the potentiated systole is greater than that of the regular systole, the latter demonstrating post-extrasystolic potentiation (Fig. F.II.11). The ejection phase characteristics of the post-extrasystolic contraction are also enhanced as the amount and rate of ejection (minor axis shortening) are greater than that of the regular systole. This may be related in part to the lower aortic diastolic pressure; the heart is able to eject more effectively against a lower afterload.[14,38] However, even when aortic diastolic pressure preceding the post-extrasystolic contraction and that of the regular systole are equal, the amount and rate of ejection are still greater in the post-extrasystolic systole. The pulse width for the potentiated systole is, as expected, larger than the systole at the basic rate.

The relationship between the coupling interval (t_1) and the heart's ability to develop pressure $\dot{P}_{max}$; Fig. F.II.12) is similar to the $\dot{F}_{max}$–interval relationship of the isolated muscle: the shorter t_1, the smaller the extrasystole's $\dot{P}_{max}$. As t_1 increases to approach t_0, $\dot{P}_{max}$ rises monotonically to equal $\dot{P}_{max}$ of the previous regular systole.

To describe how this time course of contractility is altered by an extrasystole, a second systole is introduced during the pause following the extrasystole. This post-extrasystolic systole shows a relationship between t_2 and $\dot{P}_{max}$ similar to that found for t_2 and $\dot{F}_{max}$ of the post-extrasystolic contraction in isolated muscle (Fig. F.II.12). That is to say, at the shortest t_2, $\dot{P}_{max}$ has its smallest value, and as t_2 is increased, $\dot{P}_{max}$ rises to a plateau that is in excess of $\dot{P}_{max}$ of the regular systole, demonstrating post-extrasystolic potentiation.

In the chronically instrumented animal a wide variety of rates could be used to evaluate the interaction of heart rate (t_0) and the coupling interval (t_1) on the extent

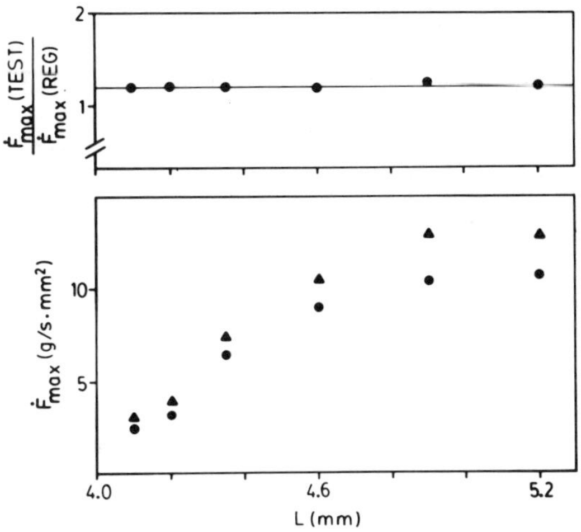

Fig. F.II.14. The upper panel describes the $\dot{F}_{max}$–interval ratio ($\dot{F}_{max}$ of the potentiated test contraction, t_2 = 2,500 msec, following an extrasystole, t_1 = 300 msec, divided by $\dot{F}_{max}$ of the previous regular contraction) as a function of muscle length for an isolated trabeculae carneae from a fetal lamb (126 days' gestation). The lower panel provides the values of $\dot{F}_{max}$ for the test contractions (triangles) and the previous regular contractions (circles). (Reprinted from Anderson et al[6] with permission.)

of post-extrasystolic potentiation. The general relationship between post-extrasystolic potentiation and t_1 and t_0 is the same in both isolated muscle and the intact heart: for the same t_1, the slower the basic rate (the shorter the t_0), the greater the amount of post-extrasystolic potentiation (Fig. F.II.12); for the same t_0, the more premature the extrasystole (the shorter the t_1), the greater the amount of post-extrasystolic potentiation (Figs. F.II.13 and F.II.14).

This complex interaction of t_0 and t_1 and post-extrasystolic potentiation demands that, if the response of the isolated muscle or that of the intact heart is to be compared from one point in development to another, then these pacing parameters must be held constant. This is easily done in isolated muscles, as long as the developmental increase in refractory period is kept in mind by applying extrasystoles with long enough values of t_1 to allow comparisons between muscles from different developmental periods. In the intact animal, the use of the same pacing pattern for two different points of observation is more difficult, since the intrinsic heart rate and the refractory period of the atrioventricular conduction system vary from day to day. Therefore it is essential that a wide range of t_0 and t_1 be used on any given day to ensure that at least some of the usable patterns are the same at different points during development and following different interventions.

In addition to the direct effects of t_0, t_1, and t_2, they also affect the shapes of $\dot{P}_{max}$–interval curves through the Frank-Starling mechanism by their effect on diastolic filling time, and so end-diastolic volume. For example, the end-diastolic volume of the systoles on the rising phase of the curves is (usually) smaller than the end-diastolic volume of the systoles during the plateau phase. Moreover, changing the basic heart rate changes end-diastolic volume; the faster the heart rate, the smaller the end-diastolic volume (Figs. F.II.4 and F.II.8). Consequently, although the shapes of the force–interval curves are similar in the isolated muscle and the intact animal, the responses of the two preparations must be compared with caution.

The effects on $\dot{P}_{max}$ of the interaction between heart rate and end-diastolic volume is dominated by the effect of heart rate over a broad range of rates; despite the fall in end-diastolic volume with an increase in rate, $\dot{P}_{max}$ is still greater at the faster rate (Figs. F.II.8 and F.II.12). However, these results can sometimes mimic those of Kavaler et al[39] and Noble et al,[40] who found that, in the intact adult animal, $\dot{P}_{max}$ changed by only a small amount with a change in rate. Conversely, the results are also in agreement with those of Mahler et al,[22] who demonstrated that, when a pause was introduced to allow the end-diastolic volume to return to that of the lower rate, $\dot{P}_{max}$ was markedly enhanced at the faster rate (Fig. F.II.8).

During those portions of the curves where the end-diastolic volumes of the post-extrasystolic systoles are the same as that of the previous regular systole, the general characteristics of the relationship of the intact animal can be shown to be similar to those found in isolated muscle. These portions of the curves demonstrate that 1) post-extrasystolic potentiation of $\dot{P}_{max}$ is a result of the introduction of the extrasystole and not merely the consequence of a change in ventricular volume, and 2) for some curves, it can be shown that $\dot{P}_{max}$ continues to increase toward a plateau value as t_2 is increased, revealing the time course of contractility that follows an extrasystole. This plateau value, whose systole has the same end-diastolic volume as that of the previous regular systole, is used to obtain the $\dot{P}_{max}$–interval ratio ($\dot{P}_{max}$ of the potentiated systole ÷ $\dot{P}_{max}$ of the regular systole), a descriptor of post-extrasystolic potentiation similar to the $\dot{F}_{max}$–interval ratio of the isolated muscle preparation.

The importance of the effect of ventricular volume on the systoles that are used to obtain the $\dot{P}_{max}$–interval ratio is demonstrated in Figure F.II.12A. The fall in $\dot{P}_{max}$ at the longest t_2 is not a consequence of post-extrasystolic depression (a characteristic seen during exposure of cardiac muscle to a β-sympathomimetic agent, see section II.E), but rather a fall in end-diastolic volume.

Another important hemodynamic variable that can alter $\dot{P}_{max}$, and so the amount of post-extrasystolic potentiation, is aortic diastolic pressure. Note, in Figure F.II.12B, the fall in the second-stage plateau at the longest value of t_2. This was a consequence of aortic diastolic pressure falling to a level that allowed the aortic valve to open and left ventricular ejection to begin before the first derivative of the left ventricular pressure had reached its peak isovolumic value. This blunted the value of $\dot{P}_{max}$. This is most likely to happen when the extrasystole is mechanically ineffective, and the aortic pressure falls below the critical level by the time the post-extrasystolic systole is introduced.

Careful attention to the interaction of the hemodynamic variables and the effects of altering the pacing pattern on the quantitative characteristics of the force–

interval relationship (eg, post-extrasystolic potentiation) allows the magnitude of these changes to be compared from one day to another.

However, two pertinent questions need to be answered before this quantitative approach can be used meaningfully to characterize how the heart changes with development, stress, or birth:

1) Does a change in inotropy alter the characteristics of the force–interval relationship in the heart of the fetus and neonate?

2) Does a change in muscle length or ventricular volume alter these characteristics?

If changes in volume and inotropy alter the amount of post-extrasystolic potentiation for a given pattern of stimulation, then a change in ventricular volume (eg, with birth[15]) could alter post-extrasystolic potentiation, or a concomitant change in inotropy could alter the amount of post-extrasystolic potentiation. This would result in a duplicity of interpretations.

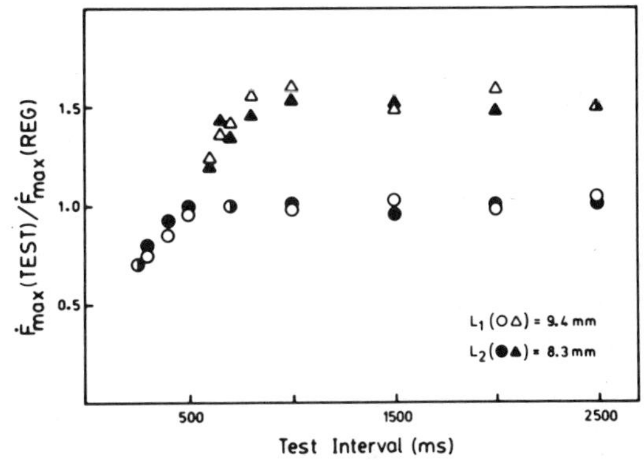

Fig. F.II.15. Effect of muscle length on the normalized force–interval curves. $\dot{F}_{max}$ of the test contraction divided by $\dot{F}_{max}$ of the previous regular contraction is described as a function of the test interval, t_1 or t_2, for an isolated moderator muscle bundle from a fetal lamb at 136 days' gestation. The first-stage results are circles, and the second-stage results are triangles. The curves were obtained at two different muscle lengths; the longer length, L_1 (open symbols), and the shorter length, L_2 (solid symbols). Basic pacing interval, t_0 = 3,000 msec, and for the second-stage curve the fixed first test interval, t_1 = 275 msec. (Data from Anderson et al[6].)

D. Effects of Length on the Force–Interval Relationship

1. In vitro

When the isolated fetal muscle length is changed, the qualitative characteristics of the relationship remain the same (see Fig. F.II.14). Although a change in muscle length alters the peak tension, it has no effect on either the force–interval ratio or the shapes of the force–interval curves that describe the dynamic beat-to-beat changes in contractility (Fig. F.II.15). Stated differently, these results are comparable with the following relationship:

$$\dot{F}_{max} = F(R,P) \times F(L)$$

The function that describes how contractility changes from beat-to-beat [F (R,P)] has the same solution for a given pattern of stimulation at every muscle length, and this solution is scaled upward or downward by a change in muscle length. The effect of length is described by F (L). Thus, the function that describes the Frank-Starling relationship can be separated from the function that describes the effects of a change in rate and pattern of stimulation or inotropic state by making the $\dot{F}_{max}$-interval ratio.

$$\dot{F}_{max}\text{–interval ratio} = \frac{\dot{F}_{maxpot}}{\dot{F}_{maxreg}} = \frac{F(R,P)_{pot}}{F(R,P)_{reg}} \times \frac{F(L)_l}{F(L)_l}$$

$\dot{F}_{maxpot}$, the response of the potentiated contraction; $\dot{F}_{maxreg}$, the response of the regular contraction; $F(R,P)_{pot}$, the solution of F(R,P) for the potentiated contraction; $F(R,P)_{reg}$, the solution of F(R,P) for the regular contraction; $F(L)_l$, the solution of F (L) for a given length, l. By making the ratio, a unitless value is obtained (Fig.

F.II.10) and the Frank-Starling effect eliminated.

This equation also describes the results obtained in isolated myocardium of the adult rabbit, dog, and cat.[26,35,42]

2. In vivo

The complete force–interval experiment involves varying t_1 and t_2. This, in turn, varies ventricular diastolic filling time and thus end-diastolic volume. The variations in end-diastolic volume from one beat to the next could make it difficult to test for the dependence of the force–interval relationship on ventricular volume. For example, when left ventricular volume is increased by a volume infusion, $\dot{P}_{max}$, aortic pressure, end-diastolic pressure, the amount of systolic shortening, and the percent fractional shortening are increased (see Figs. F.II.5, 6, and 13; see also section II.A). Fortunately, on the plateau portion of $\dot{P}_{max}$–interval curves, the end-diastolic volumes of potentiated systoles are constant over a fairly wide range of t_2 and are equal to the end-diastolic volume of the previous regular systole. For this range of times, the effects of a change in volume on the force–interval relationship can be examined in the intact animal.

The relationships of the $\dot{P}_{max}$–interval curves over this range are the same before and after a volume infusion. In other words, although $\dot{P}_{max}$ increases, the ratio of $\dot{P}_{max}$ of the potentiated systole to $\dot{P}_{max}$ of the previous regular systole ($\dot{P}_{max}$–interval ratio) remains constant (the end-diastolic volume of the regular and potentiated systoles being equal). The constancy of the $\dot{P}_{max}$–interval ratio over a range of end-diastolic volumes is illustrated in Figure F.II.13. This demonstrates that if t_0 and t_1 are kept constant,the $\dot{P}_{max}$–interval ratio does not change from one ventricular volume to another.

Thus, the force–interval relationship in the in vivo preparation from the developing heart is separable from, and therefore independent of, the Frank-Starling mechanism.

E. Effect of Inotropy on the Force–Interval Relationship

The classical definition of an inotropic intervention is a maneuver that changes the contractile strength at constant muscle length (or ventricular volume). We have adopted here a more modern definition of inotropy, which is based on the force–interval relationship. The basis for this definition is much more sensitive than the old one, and it provides the framework for classifying the effects of inotropic agents and the inotropic state of the myocardium. The rationale and justification for this definition are reviewed elsewhere.[3] For our present purposes, we focus on the inotropic action of sympathomimetic agents (eg, isoproterenol), since sympathetic tone undergoes developmental changes and figures prominently in the adaptation to the stress of birth.[15,36,37]

1. In vitro

Unlike the effect of a change in muscle length, an inotropic intervention alters the shape of the force–interval curves and the amount of potentiation. For example, in the adult myocardium, isoproterenol increases the slope of the initial portions of both the first- and second-stage curves and brings the plateaus of the curves closer together (Fig. F.II.16).[43] At higher concentrations of isoproterenol the curves become biphasic and, ultimately, the second-stage curves can "droop" below the first-stage curves, producing "post-extrasystolic depression" (Fig. F.II.16). These effects are blocked competitively by practalol or propranolol.[43] These results demonstrate that the function describing the relationship between the rate and pattern of stimulation and contractility (a solution of which produces these curves) must contain (ie, depend upon) inotropy.

The effects of an inotropic agent on the force–interval relationship have clear developmental implications: if during the control state no developmental differences in the relationship are revealed, inotropic agents may, and probably will, reveal de-

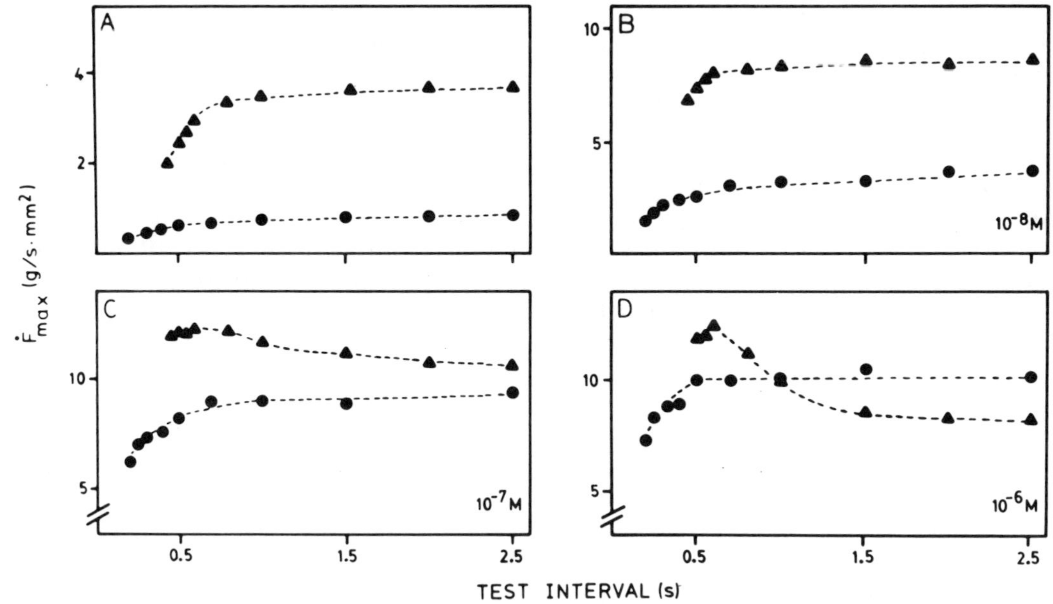

Fig. F.II.16. Effects of isoproterenol on the force–interval relationship of an adult rabbit papillary muscle. The results from the first-stage (circles) and second-stage (triangles; t_1 = 200 msec) experiments prior to (**A**) and during exposure to 10^{-8} M (**B**), 10^{-7} M (**C**), and 10^{-6} M (**D**) isoproterenol. During exposure to 10^{-7} M and 10^{-6} M isoproterenol the second-stage curves were biphasic; ie, they "drooped." This characteristic is not seen in the rabbit in the first three weeks of life.

velopmental differences in myocardial performance.

If the force–interval relationship is considered (see above) to be comparable to a description of contractility, inotropic agents do expose developmental differences in contractility. For example, when isolated muscle from the puppy or from the lamb heart is exposed to isoproterenol or norepinephrine, the decrease in potentiation (the fall in the $\dot{F}_{max}$–interval ratio) depends upon age (Fig. F.II.17)[34]; the fall in the ratio increases with age. This occurred despite the absence of any developmental effect when $\dot{F}_{max}$ or peak tension (at the basic rate) was taken as the response.[34]

The effects of inotropic agents on the shapes of the $\dot{F}_{max}$–interval curves at different ages further reveal these developmental changes in myocardial contractility. The force–interval curves of fetal lambs and neonatal puppy myocardium remain monotonic, even in the highest concentration of isoproterenol or norepinephrine, whereas adult sheep or the two- or three-month-old puppy myocardium produces biphasic curves (see above; Fig. F.II.16). The presence of different sympathomimetic effects on contractility at differ-

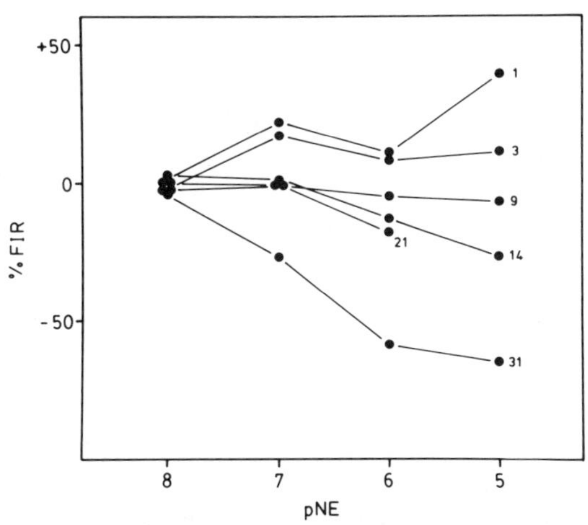

Fig. F.II.17. The norepinephrine (NE) dose–response curves, expressed as a percent change in the force–interval ratio from control (FIR), were obtained from a litter of puppies. The numbers to the right of the curves are the puppies' ages.

ent developmental periods provides us with a tool with which to explore when during development the myocardium achieves adult-like properties and in what sequence. This information can then be used to explore and test for the underlying mechanisms that produce these differences. For example, are there developmental changes in the number of the α- and β-receptors, or in the proportion of the receptors? Does the intracellular messenger or some other step in the transduction process change with development? From such studies a better understanding of how these agents bring about a change in contractility can be achieved.

These developmental differences may also have great significance in the treatment of low cardiac output in the ill premature or full-term infant. When should a sympathomimetic agent be used, which one, and at what dose? Furthermore, these

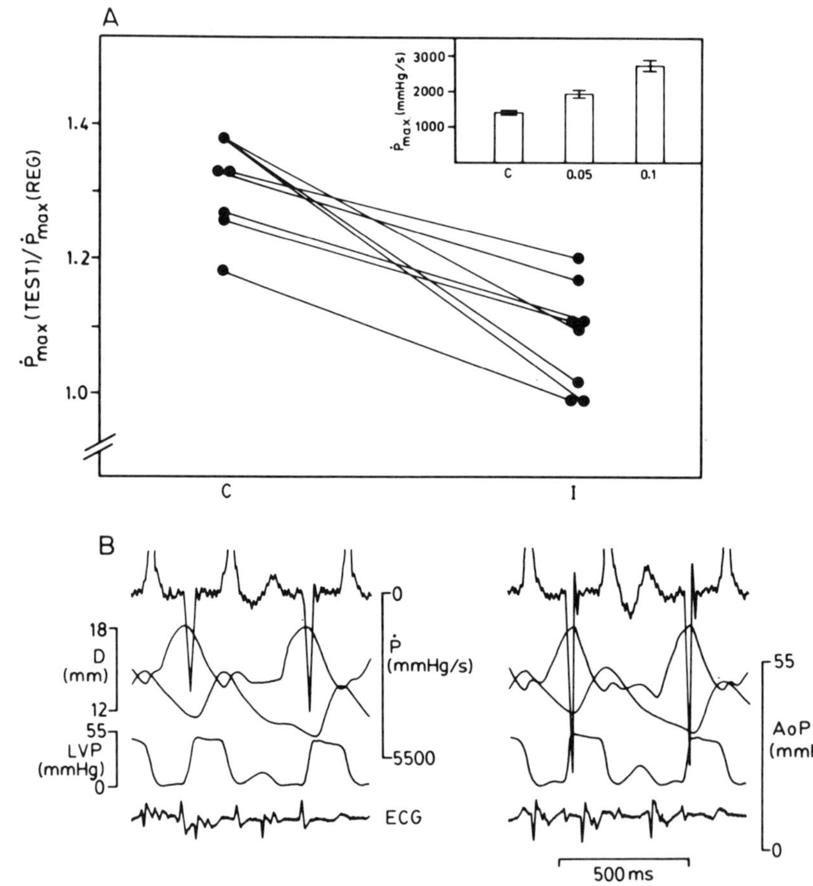

Fig. F.II.18. **A.** The effect of isoproterenol on the $\dot{P}_{max}$–interval ratio is described for six fetal lambs. The solid circles above C were obtained, in the absence of isoproterenol; those in the presence of isoproterenol are above the I. The three lines drawn from the top circle indicate the responses of one lamb to three different doses of isoproterenol. The higher the infusion dose, the lower the ratio. **B.** The response to an extrasystole (t_0 = 300 msec, t_1 = 210 msec) for a fetal lamb (139 days' gestation, instrumented 17 days previously) during the control state and in response to an infusion of isoproterenol, 0.02 μg/kg/min, on the same day. The tracings from top to bottom are the following: Ṗ, first derivative of pressure; D, left ventricular minor axis dimension; AoP, aortic pressure; LVP, left ventricular pressure; ECG, electrocardiogram. (Data from Anderson et al.[6])

developmental changes reveal the power of the force–interval relationship as a tool in dissecting developmental changes in contractility and so discovering the mechanisms of cardiac function.

2. In vivo

The enhancement of the intact heart's inotropic state at a constant rate—eg, during an isoproterenol infusion—is demonstrated by the increase in $\dot{P}_{max}$, the amount of systolic shortening, and the percent fractional shortening (Figs. F.II.6 and F.II.18). A study of the force–interval relationship also demonstrates the effect of this inotropic agent; the $\dot{P}_{max}$–interval ratio falls (Fig. F.II.18). High doses of isoproterenol (eg, 0.05 μg/kg/min) abolish post-extrasystolic potentiation of $\dot{P}_{max}$ and of the amount and rate of ventricular ejection (Fig. F.II.18). These effects of isoproterenol on the $\dot{P}_{max}$–interval ratio are not altered by a change in end-diastolic volume. [Additional effects of fetal isoproterenol infusion are noted: the rate of ventricular diastolic filling is increased and, in general, ventricular end-diastolic volume is increased (Fig. F.II.6). These effects may be due to a redistribution of systemic output, a fall in pulmonary vascular resistance, or a combination of these.]

Thus, as in isolated muscle, the force–interval relationship of the intact animal satisfies two major criteria for an index of contractility: the amount of potentiation for a given rate and pattern of stimulation is not altered by a change in ventricular volume, whereas exposure to an inotropic agent does alter significantly the amount of potentiation. This insensitivity of the force–interval relationship to a change in ventricular volume is of special importance because of the large and acute changes in left ventricular volume that occur with birth (Fig. F.II.7). It ensures that a change in the $\dot{P}_{max}$–interval ratio with birth is due to a change in contractility and is unrelated to the Frank-Starling mechanism.

This relationship, as described by the $\dot{P}_{max}$–interval ratio, has been used successfully in the child[31] to demonstrate a difference in contractility between normal and hypertrophied ventricular myocardium when, at a constant rate, no other descriptor successfully demonstrated a difference; children with left ventricular hypertrophy had significantly higher $\dot{P}_{max}$–interval ratios. Furthermore, the shape of the $\dot{P}_{max}$–interval curves of these children was qualitatively different from those of the child in heart failure.[31] Just as in the presence of a β-agonist, the curves from the child with congestive heart failure were biphasic, demonstrating a droop in the second-stage curves. These results reassure us that the force–interval relationship can be used as a basis for an index of contractility.

III. EFFECTS OF DEVELOPMENT ON CONTRACTILITY

It is assumed frequently that contractility or inotropic state is enhanced with development. Certainly, in view of the developmental changes in other myocardial properties, the likelihood that changes in contractility occur with development seems high; transverse tubules are absent in the fetal heart and then are acquired rapidly in the neonate,[44] and developmental changes in mitochondrial metabolism are also significant.[45] For example, oxygen consumption per milligram protein in the presence of ADP (state 3 respiration) is higher than that of the adult, mitochondria uncoupled by DNP have a higher oxygen consumption in the fetus and newborn than in the adult, and myocardial mitochondria have a significantly greater cytochrome C oxidase activity in the fetus and newborn than in the adult. Also, norepinephrine concentration and adrenergic innervation of the heart undergo marked developmental increases.[46]

Despite all of these developmental changes, there are no developmental changes in the force per cross-sectional area from the fetal to the adult heart (correcting for differences in the amount of contractile material per cross section of myocardium[47]). Furthermore, glycerinated muscles from the fetus and the adult generate the same tensions at equal sarcomere lengths.[48] This apparent absence of developmental differences in contractility brings to mind certain studies of isolated myocardium where normal and hypertrophied myocardium were compared and no difference in force-generating ability was found.[26,49] In these studies when the force–interval relationship was used, significant differences between normal and hypertrophied myocardium were found to exist; post-extrasystolic potentiation was increased in hypertrophy.[46] Seeking a corollary, the same investigators evaluated the force–interval relationship at different stages of development.

The evaluation of post-extrasystolic potentiation (as described by the $\dot{F}_{max}$–interval ratio and the $\dot{P}_{max}$–interval ratio) demonstrated a developmental increase in post-extrasystolic potentiation (Fig. F.II.19).[33,34] These developmental studies, unlike others that sought developmental

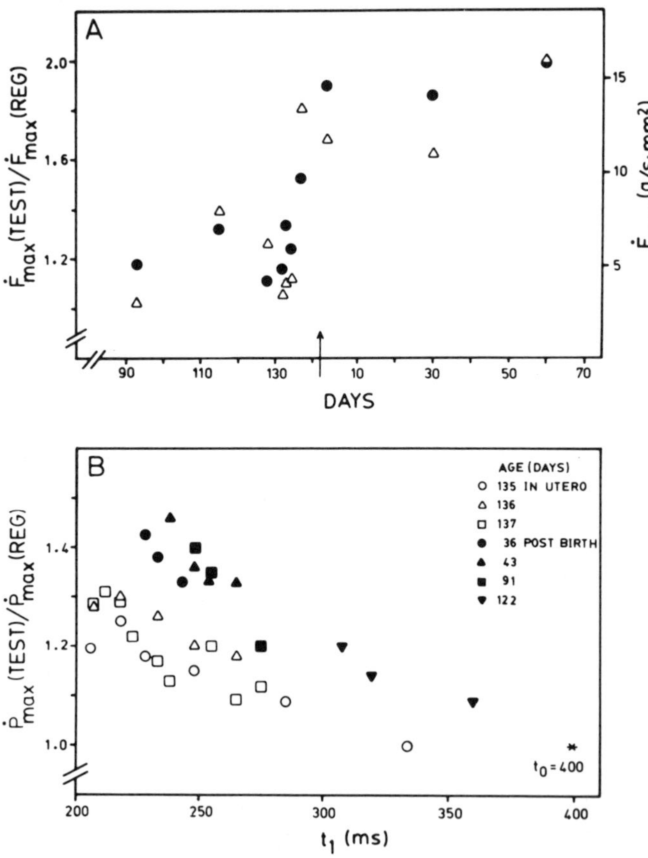

Fig. F.II.19. **A**. $\dot{F}_{max}$–interval ratios (circles) and $\dot{F}_{max}$ (triangles, the maximum rate of rise of force) obtained from isolated ventricular trabeculae from sheep hearts as a function of gestational age (left of arrow) and age following birth (right of arrow). $\dot{F}_{max}$–interval ratio: $\dot{F}_{max}$ of the post-extrasystolic contraction ÷ $\dot{F}_{max}$ of the previous regular contraction, the extrasystolic interval being the same for each ratio. **B**. The $\dot{P}_{max}$–interval ratios (FIR) obtained from a lamb instrumented in utero at 124 days of gestation as a function of the extrasystolic interval (t_1). The older the animal, the greater the $\dot{P}_{max}$–interval ratio for any given t_1. The ratios obtained in the first days following birth are not plotted, but they fell initially below those obtained at gestational ages of 135, 136, and 137 days (open symbols), and then gradually returned to that level by 7–15 days of life and then rose (closed symbols), above the fetal values. (Data from Anderson et al.[33])

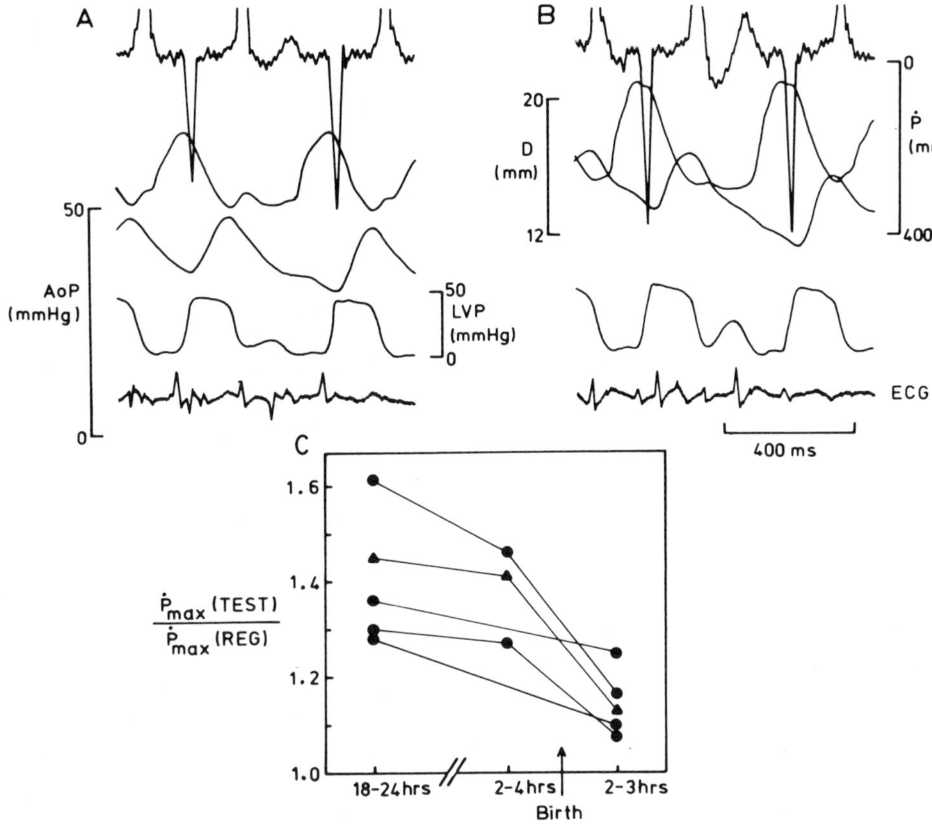

Fig. F.II.20. **A.** Data from a lamb prior to delivery. The first derivative of left ventricular pressure ($\dot{P}$), minor axis dimension (D), aortic pressure (AoP), left ventricular pressure (LVP), and electrocardiogram (ECG) are illustrated from the top of the panel downward. The heart was paced at a constant cycle interval (300 msec) with pauses in the pacing during which an extrasystole and a post-extrasystolic systole were elicited. The QRS complexes of the extrasystoles are denoted by an arrow. **B.** The response of the same lamb as a neonate. The basic pacing interval and the timing of the extrasystole (t_1 = 205 msec) are unchanged in panels A and B. **C.** The $\dot{P}_{max}$–interval ratio [the maximum rate of rise of left ventricular pressure of the potentiated systole ($\dot{P}_{max}$ Test) ÷ $\dot{P}_{max}$Reg of the previous regular systole at the basic pacing interval, both systoles having equal end-diastolic dimensions] from five fetal lambs (18–24 hours prior to delivery; F) and as neonates (N). Ratios for three of the lambs were obtained 3–4 hours prior to delivery (F′). Each lamb's values are connected by a line. The symbols represent the basic pacing intervals: circles, 300m msec; triangles, 350 msec. (Data from Anderson et al.[15])

differences using the force–interval relationship,[18,29] only compared responses obtained at the same rate and pattern of stimulation. In isolated myocardium a sudden large change in the amount of post-extrasystolic potentiation occurred in the last two weeks of gestation (Fig. F.II.19). A plateau level of potentiation was achieved in the first few days of neonatal life and remained constant through development. Similarly, in the intact chronically instrumented fetal lamb, an increase in post-extrasystolic potentiation took place with development. However, as discussed later (see section IV), a fall and rise in post-extrasystolic potentiation occurred in the hours and days that followed delivery (Figs. F.II. 19 and F.II.20).

The increase in post-extrasystolic potentiation with development suggests that the change in the inotropic state of the heart that occurs with development is similar to that which occurs in the presence of mild to moderate hypertrophy. These findings support the concept that growth and development of the heart are modulated by the same mechanisms that the heart uses to respond to pathologic states in which the work of the heart is increased—eg, valvular stenosis.[31] In other words, just as cell size is increased by either growth or by hypertrophy, contractility is induced to change in the same manner and direction by both the normal process of development and the abnormal process of hypertrophy.

IV. EFFECTS OF BIRTH

The effect of birth on the left ventricle provides us with an example of how the developing heart alters ventricular volume, heart rate, and inotropic state to adapt to a change in work load. The physiologic transformation that the fetus undergoes when it becomes a neonate is a subject that is fascinating to all who are interested in growth and development. Certainly changes in left ventricular dynamics must occur in view of the increase in left ventricular output with birth (170 ml/kg/min in the fetus[16] to 400 ml/kg/min in the neonate[10,17]). Few studies have described how the fetal left ventricle of the chronically instrumented fetus adapts to birth. This is technically a difficult problem because it requires that the animals undergo instrumentation several days before birth so that the heart has time to recover from the acute effects produced by the extensive instrumentation. This is essential in that the fetal response to surgery includes the use of the three mechanisms that may be brought into play with birth: 1) heart rate, 2) end-diastolic volume (and so stroke volume), and 3) inotropy.

In the transition from fetal to neonatal life the heart rate increases. In a study by Comline and Silver,[50] the heart rate of the chronically instrumented lamb was shown to increase in the first few minutes of life from a fetal range of 140–170 beats/min to as high as 250–300 beats/min. By one to two hours of age, when the neonatal arterial pH and pCO_2 have become normal, the neonatal heart rate is still sig-

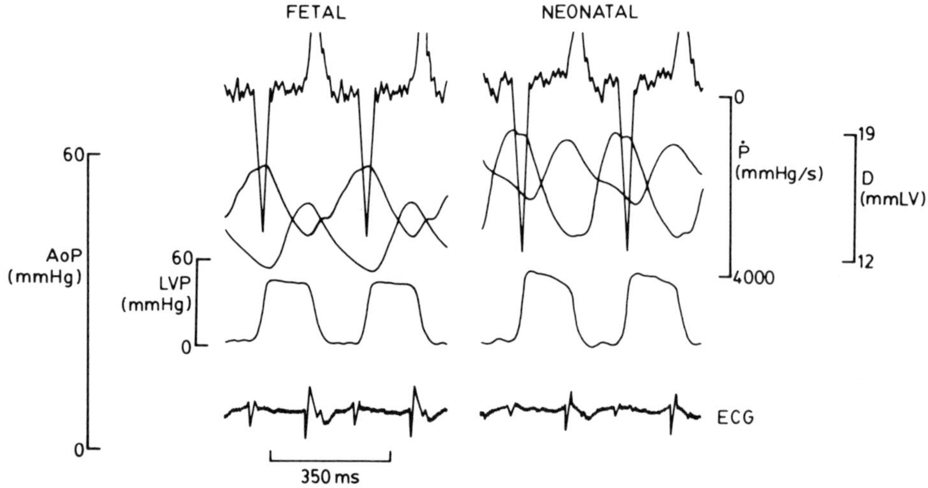

Fig. F.II.21. A comparison of a chronically instrumented fetal lamb's data to its neonatal data. In each panel, the data appear in the following order, from the top of the illustration downward: first derivative of ventricular pressure ($\dot{P}$); minor axis dimension (D), aortic pressure (AoP), left ventricular pressure (LVP), and electrocardiogram (ECG). The pacing interval is the same in both panels (300 msec). (Data from Anderson et al.[15])

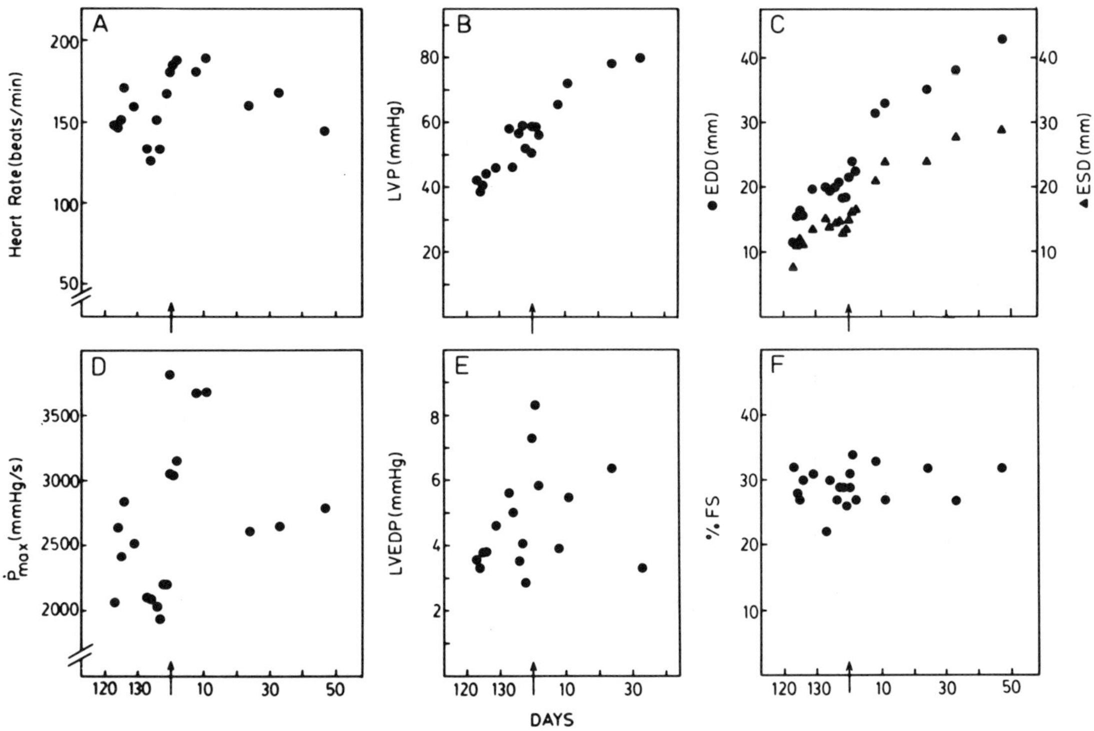

Fig. F.II.22. The effect of development on heart rate (**A**), peak left ventricular pressure (LVP; **B**), left ventricular end-diastolic (EDD) and end-systolic (ESD) minor axis dimension (**C**), the maximum rate of rise of left ventricular pressure ($\dot{P}_{max}$; **D**), left ventricular end-diastolic pressure (LVEDP; **E**), and percent fractional shortening (%FS; **F**) in a lamb that underwent instrumentation at 121 days of gestation. Delivery (noted by the arrows) was per vagina. Days noted at the left of the arrows are gestational and those noted at the right are neonatal.

nificantly higher than that of the fetus.[15,50] Thus, an increase in heart rate—the mechanism that Rudolph and Heymann describe as the major modulator of fetal cardiac output—is used in the adaptation of the left ventricle to neonatal life.

To confirm that the Frank-Starling mechanism is called upon to adjust to birth, an increase in left ventricular end-diastolic volume must be demonstrated to occur with birth. When left ventricular dimensions are monitored prior to and following birth,[15] the mean end-diastolic dimension, and so left ventricular end-diastolic volume, is shown to increase significantly with birth (Figs. F.II.7 and F.II.21). Although the mean values increase, a wide range of fetal and neonatal values of end-diastolic dimension can be found. In some lambs fetal and neonatal systoles were noted that had equal end-diastolic volumes, so that at times the effect of birth on ventricular function was independent of the Frank-Starling relationship.[15] However, such systoles were uncommon. When $\dot{P}_{max}$ and the ejection characteristics of systoles obtained at the same heart rate were compared, percent fractional shortening, systolic shortening, and $\dot{P}_{max}$ were all found to increase significantly (Fig. F.II.7).

Evidence of a change in end-diastolic volume with birth was revealed not only by a change in end-diastolic dimension but also by the abrupt increase in end-diastolic pressure (Fig. F.II.22E). In all lambs the heart was found to be acutely stiffer with birth, apparently because of an increase in left ventricular diastolic filling.

These changes may explain the observation that a volume infusion in the first week of life does not increase left ventricular output to the same extent that it does in the sixth week of life. The marked displacement to the left on the stroke volume–end-diastolic volume relationship (the Frank-Starling relationship) may limit a further increase in end-diastolic volume or stroke volume in response to a volume challenge.

A portion of the increase in systolic shortening, fractional shortening, and $\dot{P}_{max}$ that is found following birth (when systoles at the same heart rate are compared) could be due to an increase in inotropic state. When fetal and neonatal systoles at the same heart rate and end-diastolic volume are compared, a significant increase in $\dot{P}_{max}$ and, to a lesser extent, percent fractional shortening is found to occur with birth,[15] consistent with an increase in inotropic state. The relatively smaller increase of the ejection phase descriptors may be a consequence of the increase in aortic pressure with birth. An acute increase in aortic pressure decreases the rate and amount of ventricular ejection.[38]

The force–interval relationship also changes with birth; the $\dot{P}_{max}$–interval ratio falls markedly following birth (Fig. F.II.20), revealing an increase in inotropic state. This fall begins three to four hours prior to birth, but the greatest portion of the fall occurs following delivery. The fall in the ratio and the rise in $\dot{P}_{max}$ are the same as those produced by a fetal isoproterenol infusion (Fig. F.II.18). These changes appear to correlate well with the increase in circulating levels of catecholamines that takes place prior to and following birth, and the findings suggest that these inotropic changes result from these increases in catecholamines.

V. SUMMARY

In summary, the function of the fetal left ventricle is modulated by a change in heart rate, ventricular volume, and inotropy. The fetal heart uses all three of these mechanisms to adapt to neonatal life. How these mechanisms would interact in response to other forms of stress is uncertain, although the heart of the normal neonate is capable of further increase in rate, inotropic state, and left ventricular end-diastolic volume.[15] The extensive use of these mechanisms with birth may temporarily compromise the ability of the neonatal heart to respond to additional neonatal stresses.

VI. ACKNOWLEDGMENTS

This work was supported in part by NIH grant HL 20749. Dr. Page A.W. Anderson is the recipient of RCDA HL 00500.

The authors wish to thank Mrs. Annette Oakeley and Miss Nancy Halpern, for without their assistance the contents of this chapter would have been markedly reduced.

VII. REFERENCES

1. Frank O. Zur Dynamik des Herz Muskels. Z Biol. 1895; 32:370–447.
2. Starling EH. The Linacre Lecture on the Law of the Heart (Cambridge, 1915, monograph). London: Longmans, Green, 1918.
3. Manring A, Anderson PAW. Cardiac contractility. Crit Rev Bioeng. 1980; 4:165–201.
4. Lakatta EG, Jewell BR. Length-dependent activation: Its effect on the length–tension relation in cat ventricular muscle. Circ Res. 1977; 40:251–257.
5. Huntsman LL, Stewart DK. Length-dependent calcium inotropy in cat papillary muscle. Circ Res. 1977; 40:366–371.
6. Anderson PAW, Manring A, Crenshaw C Jr. Biophysics of the developing heart (II): The interaction of the force–interval relationship with inotropic state and muscle length (preload). Am J Obstet Gynecol. 1980; 138:44–54.
7. Rushmer RF, Smith O, Franklin D. Mechanisms of cardiac control in exercise. Circ Res. 1959; 7:602–627.
8. Heymann MA, Rudolph AM. Effects of increasing preload on right ventricular output in lambs in utero. Circulation. 1973; 48(Suppl IV):37 (143).
9. Kirkpatrick SE, Pitlick PT, Naliboff J, Friedman WF. Frank-Starling relationship as an important determinant of cardiac output. Am J Physiol. 1976; 231:495–500.

10. Klopfenstein HS, Rudolph AM. Post-natal changes in the circulation and responses to volume loading in sheep. Circ Res. 1978; 42:839–845.
11. Rudolph AM, Heymann MA. Circulatory changes during growth in the fetal lamb. Circ Res. 1970; 26:289–299.
12. Romero T, Covell JW, Friedman WF. Comparison of pressure–volume relations of the fetal, newborn and adult heart. Am J Physiol. 1972; 222:1285–1290.
13. Kirkpatrick SE, Covell JW, Friedman WF. A new technique for the continuous assessment of fetal and neonatal cardiac performance. Am J Obstet Gynecol. 1973; 116:963–972.
14. Anderson PAW, Manring A, Crenshaw C Jr. Biophysics of the developing heart (I): The force–interval relationship. Am J Obstet Gynecol. 1980; 138:33–48.
15. Anderson PAW, Manring A, Click KL, Crenshaw C Jr. Biophysics of the developing heart (III): Left ventricular dynamics of the lamb heart: A comparison of the fetus to the neonate. Am J Obstet Gynecol. (in press).
16. Rudolph AM, Heyman MA. Fetal and neonatal circulation and respiration. Annu Rev Physiol. 1974; 36:187–207.
17. Berman W Jr, Musselman J. Myocardial performance in the newborn lamb. Am J Physiol. 1979; 237:H66–H70.
18. Kirkpatrick SE, Naliboff J, Pitlick PT, Friedman WF. The influence of post-stimulation potentiation and heart rate on the fetal lamb heart. Am J Physiol. 1975; 229:318–323.
19. Rudolph AM, Heymann MA. Cardiac output in the fetal lamb: The effects of spontaneous and induced changes of heart rate on right and left ventricular output. Am J Obstet Gynecol. 1972; 124:183–192.
20. Assali NS, Brinkman CR III, Woods JR Jr, Nuwayhid BS, Dandavino A. Ontogenesis of the autonomic control of cardiovascular functions in the sheep. In: Longo, LD, Reneau, PD eds. Fetal and Newborn Cardiovascular Physiology, Vol 1. New York: Garland, 1978: 47–92.
21. Guyton AC. Textbook of Medical Physiology, Philadelphia: Saunders, 1971.
22. Mahler F, Yoran C, Ross J Jr. Inotropic effect of tachycardia and post-stimulation potentiation in the conscious dog. Am J Physiol. 1974; 227:569–575.
23. Huxley AF. Muscle structure and theories of contraction. Prog Biophys. 1957; 7:257–318.
24. Winegrad S. The intracellular site of calcium activation of contraction in frog skeletal muscle. J Gen Physiol. 1970; 55:77–88.
25. Johnson EA, Rowe MJ, Vaughan PL. Quantitative description of the short-term changes in the force of contraction of rabbit papillary muscle with the pattern of stimulation. Aust J Exp Biol Med Sci. 1964; 42:197–208.
26. Anderson PAW, Manring A, Arentzen CE, Rankin JS, Johnson EA. Pressure-inducted hypertrophy of cat right ventricle: An evaluation with the force–interval relationship. Circ Res. 1977; 41:582–588.
27. Blinks DR, Koch-Weser J. Analysis of the effects of changes in rate and rhythm upon myocardial contractility. J Pharmacol Exp Ther. 1961; 134:373–389.
28. Sherlag BJ, Yeh BK, Cranefield PF. Effect of continuous post-extrasystolic potentiation on the acutely failed dog heart. Physiologist. 1964; 7:246.
29. Arcilla RA, Lind J, Zetterquist P, Oh W, Gessner IH. Hemodynamic features of extra-systoles in newborn and older infants. Am J Cardiol. 1966; 18:191–199.
30. Anderson PAW, Manring A, Johnson EA. The force of contraction of isolated papillary muscle: A study of the interaction of its determining factors. J Mol Cell Cardiol. 1977; 9:131–150.
31. Anderson PAW, Manring A, Serwer GA, Benson DW, Edwards SB, Armstrong BE, Sterba RJ, Floyd RD IV. The force–interval relationship of the left ventricle. Circulation. 1979; 60:334–348.
32. Anderson PAW, Manring A, Sommer JR, Johnson EA. Cardiac muscle: An attempt to relate structure to function. J Mol Cell Cardiol. 1976; 8:123–143.
33. Anderson PAW, Manring A, Crenshaw C Jr. Biophysics of the developing heart (IV): Developmental changes in contractility. Circ Res. (in press).
34. Anderson PAW, Manring A, Nassar R. Developmental changes in cardiac contractility. Pediatr Res. 1979; 13:339.
35. Anderson PAW, Rankin JS, Arentzen CE, Anderson RW, Johnson EA. Evaluation of the force–frequency relationship as a descriptor of the inotropic state of canine left ventricular myocardium. Cir Res. 1976; 39:832–839.
36. Eliot JR, Lam R, Leake RD, Hobel CJ, Fisher DA. Plasma catecholamine concentrations in infants at birth. J Pediatr. 1980; 96:311–315.
37. Geis WP, Tatooles GJ, Priola DV, Friedman WF. Factors influencing neuro-hormonal control of the heart in the newborn dog. Am J Physiol. 1975; 228:1685–1689.
38. Mahler F, Ross J Jr, O'Rourke RA, Covell JW. Effects of changes in preload, afterload and inotropic state on ejection and isovolumic phase measures of contractility in the conscious dog. Am J Cardiol. 1975; 35:626–634.
39. Kavaler F, Harris RS, Lee RJ, Fisher VJ. Force–frequency behavior of in situ ventricular myocardium in the dog. Circ Res. 1971; 28:533–544.
40. Noble MIM, Wyler J, Milne ENC, Tranchard D, Bux A. Effect of changes in heart rate on left ventricular performance in conscious dogs. Circ Res 1969; 24:285–295.
41. Wallace AG, Skinner NS Jr, Mitchell JH. Hemodynamic determinants of the maximum rate of rise of left ventricular pressure. Am J Physiol. 1973; 205:30–37.

42. Anderson PAW, Manring A, Johnson EA. The force–frequency relationship: A new basis for an index of cardiac contractility? Circ Res. 1973; 33:665–671.
43. Anderson PAW, Manring A, Johnson EA. Catecholamine effect on the force–interval relationship. Pediatr Res. 1977; 11:386.
44. Legato MJ. Ultrastructural changes during normal growth in the dog and rat ventricular myofiber. In Lieberman M, Sano T, eds. Developmental and Physiological Correlates of Cardiac Muscle. Vol 1. New York: Raven Press, 1976:249–274.
45. Wells RJ, Friedman WF, Sobel BE. Increased oxidative metabolism in the fetal and newborn lamb heart. Am J Physol. 1972; 222:1488–1493.
46. Friedman WF, Poole PE, Jacobowitz D, Seagren SC, Braunwald E. Sympathetic innervation of the developing rabbit heart—Biochemical and histochemical comparisons of fetal, neonatal, and adult myocardium. Circ Res. 1968; 23: 25–32.
47. McPherson RA, Kramer MF, Covell JW, Friedman WF. A comparison of the active stiffness of fetal and adult cardiac muscle. Pediatr Res. 1976; 10:660–664.
48. Friedman WF. The intrinsic physiologic properties of the developing heart. In: Friedman WF, Lesch M, Sonnenblick EH, eds. Neonatal Heart Disease. New York: Grune & Stratton, 1973: 21–49.
49. Spann JF, Buccino RA, Sonnenblick EH, Braunwald E. Contractile state of cardiac muscle obtained from cats with experimentally produced ventricular hypertrophy and heart failure. Circ Res. 1967; 21:341–354.
50. Comline RS, Silver M. The composition of fetal and maternal blood during parturition in the ewe. J Physiol. 1972; 222:233–256.

F. III

Autonomic Control of Fetal Cardiac Activity

Robert N. Wolfson, MD, PhD, Yoram Sorokin, MD, and Mortimer G. Rosen, MD

I. INTRODUCTION

The primary function of the fetal heart is to propel blood to the placental circulation and to deliver blood to fetal tissues at a rate consistent with individual tissue metabolic requirements. These requirements may vary with the stages of fetal development, as well as with fetal activity at any one moment. In this chapter we summarize the characteristics of the fetal circulatory system and our understanding of those factors that regulate cardiac output in this dynamic system.

II. INTRINSIC AUTONOMIC CONTROL

A. Introduction

In the adult, pulmonary and systemic circulations function in series. Therefore right and left ventricular outputs must be equal. In the fetus large communications allow the left and right ventricles to function almost in parallel, and they may be viewed as a single chamber rather than as a sequential system as described for the adult. Because of these cardiovascular communications, a higher fetal heart rate is an absolute prerequisite for adequate distribution of blood.[1] As in the adult, the distribution of blood flow is dynamic and changes with the physiologic needs of the fetus.[1]

B. Cardiac Output

Fetal circulation is characterized by high flow, low vascular resistance, and the relatively passive nature of the umbilical and placental circulations.[1] In fetal sheep,

Cardiac Problems in Pregnancy, pages 365–379

several techniques have been used to measure fetal cardiac output.[2] Fetal cardiac output (as well as fetal heart rate) is high when compared to adult cardiac output.[2–4] Studying several species, Nuwayhid[2,5] found fetal cardiac output to be 2–4 times that seen in the adult.

The high fetal cardiac output may be necessary to support the high fetal oxygen consumption, which is 1.5–2.0 times that of an adult when compared on the basis of body weight.[6] Thus it is possible that increased cardiac output is one mechanism by which the fetus adapts to a low oxygen tension; however, this potential need does not explain the physiology of the process.

Physiologic changes in fetal cardiac output appear to be directly related to changes in fetal heart rate. Rudolph and Heymann[7] measured heart rate and right and left ventricular output in fetal sheep between 0.75 and 0.85 of term gestation. They observed spontaneous increases and decreases in fetal heart rate of greater than 10% of resting level. The increase in fetal heart rate was invariably associated with an increase in both right and left ventricular output, while a decrease in fetal heart rate resulted in a fall in both right and left ventricular output. The causes for these spontaneous fetal heart rate changes were not clear. Although these heart rate changes were often associated with fetal respiratory activity, they were not inhibited when fetal respiratory movements were blocked with succinylcholine, suggesting that the observed changes in fetal heart rate and cardiac output were initiated in the central nervous system and mediated by autonomic reflexes.

Rudolph and Heymann[8] also studied the paced fetal heart in sheep to delineate changes in right ventricular output. They found that cardiac output correlated with fetal heart rate between 150 and 285 beats/min. However, between 285 and 315 beats/min the cardiac output leveled off and thereafter fell with increasing heart rates.

C. Stroke Volume

Intrinsic properties of the myocardium are important determinants of cardiac output. Shortening of the myocardial fibers is related to stroke volume. Myocardial fiber shortening is determined by 1) myocardial fiber length prior to the ventricular contraction (preload), 2) the inotropic state of the myocardium, and 3) the impedance against which the ventricle works (afterload).

1. Preload

The Frank-Starling mechanism states that alterations in end-diastolic fiber length result in changes in the next stroke volume and the force of the next contraction. The greater the amount of blood filling the heart during diastole, the greater the amount ejected during systole. The importance of this mechanism is obvious in the adult, since it maintains the balance between left and right ventricular outputs. However, in the fetus, the role of the Frank-Starling mechanism is not as clear.

Friedman[9] isolated myocardial strips from fetal and adult sheep in order to compare the isometric passive and active length–tension curves. The fetal myocardial strips were quite limited in performance when compared with the adult myocardial strips. Specifically, the isometric force development, extent, and velocity of shortening at any load were reduced in the fetus. At all fetal muscle lengths there appeared to be a reduction in active tension generated by the fetal muscles. In addition, fetal cardiac muscle showed a higher resting tension and reduced compliance when compared to the adult cardiac muscle.

Friedman[9] suggested that these differences may be explained, in part, by age-related changes in myocardial tissue. Fetal myocardial cells were found to have smaller diameters when compared to adult myocardial cells. In addition, the proportion of noncontractile to contractile tissue was significantly higher in the fetus than in adults. A gram of fetal myocardium contained fewer contractile elements than one gram of adult myocardium; thus, taking contractile elements per gram of myocardium into consideration, Friedman found that individual myofilaments in the fetus and the adult are capable of generating similar force. However, as noted per unit area rather than on a weight basis, fetal ventricular muscle generates significantly less force.

As noted earlier, there is some controversy concerning the presence and importance of the Frank-Starling mechanism in the intact fetal heart. Kirkpatrick et al[10] evaluated the importance of the Frank-Starling mechanism in chronically instrumented, unstressed fetal sheep. Left ventricular end-diastolic diameter was used as an indicator of fiber length. They found a close correlation between stroke volume and left ventricular shortening and concluded that the Frank-Starling mechanism was indeed operative in the fetal sheep heart.

In another study Kirkpatrick and Friedman[11] provided additional support for the concept that changes in preload are a fundamental determinant of fetal cardiac output. They used an inflated balloon in the superior vena cava to reduce the left ventricular end-diastolic diameter and left ventricular end-diastolic pressure. An increase in end-diastolic pressure and diameter was achieved with infusion of fetal blood into the left atrium. They found a very close correlation between the extent of shortening of the left ventricular end-diastolic diameter and the end-diastolic pressure. Over the narrow physiologic range of diastolic diameters and pressures, there was an almost linear relationship between the left ventricular end-diastolic diameter and the extent of left ventricular shortening. During fetal respiratory movements, with a stable heart rate, cardiac output was maintained by changes in stroke volume as a result of changes in ventricular filling. In the absence of changes in heart rate, left ventricular cardiac output remained constant over a wide range of respiratory rates.

Anderson et al,[12,13] using isolated myocardial preparations, studied several factors of cardiac contractility. The magnitude of myocardial contractility corresponded to changes in muscle length in accordance with the Frank-Starling mechanism. Nuwayhid et al[5] suggested that as long as the heart maintains its normal rhythm, there is a reciprocal relationship between stroke volume and heart rate.

In the human fetus, studies of cardiac time intervals in the presence of fetal arrhythmias support the operation of the Frank-Starling mechanism in the face of changes in ventricular filling.[14] The fetal cardiac time intervals reflect the electrical and mechanical properties of the conduction system and myocardium. The fetal cardiac time intervals are subdivisions of the cardiac cycle that are delineated by the onset of the QRS complex of the fetal electrocardiogram and the opening and closure of the atrioventricular and semilunar valves detected by Doppler ultrasound. The preejection period reflects the inotropic state of the myocardium[15] and is measured as the interval from the onset of the fetal QRS complex to the opening of the semilunar valves. The ventricular filling time correlates directly with RR interval and is measured as the interval between atrioventricular valve opening and closure. Abrupt prolongation of the RR interval yields an almost equivalent prolongation in the ventricular filling time.[14] Prolongation of the RR interval is associated with abrupt shortening of the preejection period[16] secondary to prolonged ventricular filling, as would be expected if the Frank-Starling mechanism were operative in the human fetus.

In contrast, Rudolph et al[7,8] found that the Frank-Starling mechanism was not as important in maintenance of cardiac output. In chronically instrumented fetal sheep, cardiac output correlated with fetal heart rate. They suggested that the fetal heart can increase cardiac output only by increasing fetal heart rate. Pacing the fetal heart rate over a range of 40–50% above and below the resting fetal heart rate showed parallel changes in cardiac output. Fetal bradycardia was associated with a marked reduction in cardiac output.[7] Increased filling time was not associated with increased cardiac output.

2. Inotropic state of the myocardium

Contraction of the myocardium is initiated when ionic calcium reaches the reactive sites on the myofilaments following excitation and depolarization of the cell membrane. Removal of this calcium results in relaxation. The quantity of ionic calcium delivered to contractile proteins determines the extent of fiber shortening and, therefore, the stroke volume.

In addition to being influenced by calcium, the inotropic state of the myocardium is also modulated by the neurotransmitters acetylcholine and norepinephrine, which are released through autonomically controlled reflexes. Therefore, the anatomic extent and level of function of the autonomic innervation to the heart is important in establishing the inotropic state of the fetal myocardium. As we will describe, early in pregnancy the immaturity of the autonomic innervation precludes its playing a major role in determining the inotropic state of the myocardium. Under these circumstances humoral modulation by adrenal-mediated epinephrine may be the major determinant of myocardial contractility.[17]

Studies in chronically instrumented sheep near term demonstrated that increased frequency of myocardial contraction produced a positive inotropic effect on the fetal heart.[11] This augmentation in contractility was observed in atrial pacing experiments and was not related to adrenergic stimulation. Thus, within normal ranges of fetal heart rate, this appears to be an intrinsic function of the myocardium.

3. Afterload

In studying chronically instrumented fetal sheep, Rudolph et al[8] found that an increase in outflow impedance to the ventricles resulted in an immediate decrease in right ventricular output, stroke volume, and heart rate. When the decreased heart rate was obliterated by blocking the baroreceptor reflex with atropine, the decrease in stroke volume persisted as long as the outflow impedance remained elevated.

D. Heart Rate

1. Origin of the heart beat

The human heart begins to beat approximately 35 days after the onset of the last menstrual period.[18] Robinson and Shaw-Dunn[18] measured the human fetal heart rate between seven and 15 weeks of gestation using M-mode ultrasound techniques. At seven weeks from the last menstrual period the heart rate was 125 beats/min and rapidly increased to 175 beats/min at nine weeks of gestation. The heart rate then gradually decreased to 147 beats/min by 15 weeks of gestation.

Blaney et al[19] recently confirmed these findings and extended the observations to 40 weeks of gestation. They identified a continued decrease in fetal heart rate from 15 weeks, with a minimum of 135 beats/min achieved at approximately 34 weeks of gestation, followed by an increase to 145 beats/min at 40 weeks of gestation. The recent findings of Blaney are somewhat at variance with several earlier studies[20–22] that described a slowing of the fetal heart rate from 160 to 170 beats/min at 15 to 20 weeks of gestation to 140 to 150 beats/min at 40 weeks of gestation, without an observed increase in heart rate during the last six weeks of gestation.

The fetal heart beat originates in the sinoatrial node following spontaneous depolarization of the pacemaker cells. The resting pacemaker cells are characterized by a high intracellular concentration of potassium and a high extracellular concentration of sodium and chloride. Selective permeability of the cell membrane to potassium ions establishes the negative resting potential of the pacemaker cell. Generation of an action potential by the pacemaker cell results from a sequence of changes in cell membrane permeability and, consequently, changes in the resting potential voltage. Sodium and chloride enter the cell while potassium leaves the cell. After the reduction in the resting potential reaches the threshold level, the cell rapidly depolarizes. During repolarization there is an increase in intracellular calcium and potassium and a decrease in intracellular sodium and chloride.

All myocardial cells have the property of rhythmicity. The pacemaker cells of the sinoatrial node depolarize first and determine the rhythm of the fetal heart.

2. Rate control at the cellular level

Heart rate at the cellular level is influenced by many factors, including electrolyte concentrations, temperature, hypoxia, hypercapnia, stretch, and neurotransmitters released by the autonomic nervous system.[23] A lower extracellular potassium concentration produces a faster rate of diastolic depolarization with a resultant increase in heart rate. A higher extracellular calcium concentration yields a lower threshold potential and a decrease in heart rate. An increase in temperature increases the rate of diastolic depolarization and produces a higher heart rate. Stretching of the sinoatrial node, hypoxia, and hypercapnia produce an increase in the rate of diastolic depolarization and an increase in heart rate.

During diastole acetylcholine increases pacemaker cell permeability to potassium. With an increasing flow of potassium to the extracellular fluid, the diastolic resting potential is higher. Acetylcholine slows the rate of spontaneous depolarization and as a result slows the heart rate.

Catecholamines increase the heart rate by reducing the flow of intracellular potassium out of the cell during diastole, with a resultant increase in the rate of membrane depolarization.

Reduction in fetal heart rate mediated by acetylcholine following parasympathetic vagal stimulation develops very rapidly over several heart beats. In contrast, sympathetic stimulation mediated through the catecholamines develops at a relatively slower pace. A more detailed discussion of the biophysics of the developing heart is presented by Anderson and Manring in Chapter F.II.

III. EXTRINSIC AUTONOMIC CONTROL

A. Autonomic Nervous System

1. Parasympathetic development

There is general agreement that in the human after the vagal nerves have sprouted from the hindbrain, neuroblasts migrate down those nerves into the heart, ultimately to become the cardiac plexuses, ganglia, and the postganglionic parasympathetic nerves. Estimation of the time of invasion of the heart by the vagal nerves is controversial but appears to begin around eight weeks of gestation; it is complete in the atria by 12 weeks and in the ventricles by 13 weeks.[24] The first group of ganglion cells, lying between the aorta and pulmonary artery, appear with the nerves at approximately eight weeks. By 13 weeks five distinct groups of ganglia can be demonstrated at the base of the heart.[25] Single nerve fibers penetrate from these ganglia to supply the myocardium. Between 16 and 26 weeks there is gradual invasion of the total atrial epicardial area by ganglia extending from the original five groups and involving the coronary vasculature.[25] This process continues with more extensive distribution of the ganglia until approximately 34 weeks.[26]

Field stimulation of isolated, paced human cardiac muscle has been used to describe preganglionic and postganglionic parasympathetic nerve function. Walker[27] studied fetal specimens between approximately 12 and 20 weeks of gestation. Field stimulation caused release of neurotransmitters from autonomic postganglionic nerves within the myocardium. The inotropic response of the contracting specimen was monitored. The negative inotropic response was enhanced by neostigmine and blocked by atropine, thus indicating that the response was attributed to acetylcholine. Specimens from fetuses less than 15 weeks showed no response, while a consistent inhibitory response occured at approximately 17 weeks or beyond. The absence of inotropic response to field stimulation was not a result of myocardial insensitivity to acetylcholine. Walker[27] demonstrated that as early as 12 weeks fetal myocardial tissue responded to acetylcholine. Gennser and Nilsson[28] also demonstrated myocardial sensitivity to acetylcholine prior to innervation at approximately seven weeks of gestation.

Walker[27] also used nicotine to assess the function of cardiac ganglia. Nicotine is a ganglionic stimulator. Low doses of nicotine had no appreciable inhibitory effect on the fetal myocardium, suggesting that there was an absence of active ganglionic receptor sites in the developing heart. These receptors are the synapses for the parasympathetic preganglionic and postganglionic nerves. Hence it is possible that the vagal ganglia are functionally immature. From these results Walker concluded that vagal transmission to the heart cannot occur before 20 weeks in the human fetus.

It is generally agreed that the inhibitory effect of acetylcholine increases with increasing gestational age in mammalian hearts.[17] As noted, Walker[27] did not demonstrate this in his field stimulation studies between 12 and 20 weeks of gestation. Schifferli,[20] however, did demonstrate an inhibitory trend in the human fetus between 15 and 40 weeks. In this study atropine, in a dosage sufficient to block fetal vagal drive, was given to women during the antenatal period. This resulted in fetal tachycardia along with reduced beat-to-beat variability. The incremental changes in fetal heart rate increased with increasing gestational age and ranged from 5 beats/min at 15 weeks to 20 beats/min at 40 weeks. The postatropine fetal heart rate was consistently near 160 beats/min regardless of gestational age. Schifferli[20] also demonstrated a decreasing trend in fetal heart rate with gestational age from approximately 155 to 130 beats/min, which is consistent with the findings of other authors.[21,22] He therefore concluded that the incremental increase in response to atropine demonstrated increasing vagal tone with fetal development.

The fetal sheep model has yielded extensive information on fetal cardiovascular function. However, in studies describing the autonomic nervous system influence, the findings are sometimes contradictory. Vapaavouri et al[29] assessed the basal level of autonomic activity by quantitating the magnitude of response to selected autonomic blockade. Chronically instrumented fetal sheep between 0.56 and 1.0 of term gestation and neonatal sheep from 2 to 21 days after birth were studied.

Parasympathetic blockade with atropine demonstrated a consistent increase in fetal heart rate at all gestational ages. The incremental increase in heart rate showed an increasing trend up to 0.8 of term gestation. Thereafter the increase in heart rate in response to atropine was unchanged into neonatal life. The threshold dosage of acetylcholine necessary to alter fetal and neonatal heart rate was also shown not to vary with gestational age. Vapaavouri interpreted these data as demonstrating that the change in basal parasympathetic tone was not due to changes in receptor sensitivity, but rather reflected development of parasympathetic control that was complete by approximately 0.8 of term gestation.

Assali et al[30] developed somewhat different conclusions using a similar sheep model. Atropine blockade yielded a consistently increasing basal parasympathetic tone that extended into the neonatal period. The incremental change in heart rate with parasympathetic blockade was consistently less than that produced by sympathetic blockade until the neonatal period. During the neonatal period the incremental change with parasympathetic blockade was greater. Assali interpreted this to demonstrate that 1) parasympathetic tone continues to develop into the neonatal period, 2) sympathetic development precedes parasympathetic development, and 3) sympathetic tone dominates in the fetal period.

In summary, myocardial acetylcholine sensitivity in the human antedates demonstrable innervation by the vagal nerves and postganglionic neurons. Anatomic development of the vagal nerves and postganglionic neurons occurs early in gestation and morphologically resembles that of the neonate by 34 weeks of gestation. Vagal tone appears to increase with gestation. The role of vagal tone in explaining the decrement in fetal heart rate during the period of 15 to 20 weeks of gestation is controversial. Clinical studies support this contention, but pharmacologic in vitro cardiac preparations demonstrate an immature, nonfunctioning parasympathetic ganglion system.

Studies in the fetal sheep generally support those in the human fetus. The finding of sympathetic nervous system predominance, however, is in question, since these studies were carried out in primarily acute preparations where increased levels of catecholamines would be anticipated.

2. Sympathetic development

The anatomic development of the sympathetic nervous system in the fetal heart has been studied for the most part by fluorescent histochemical staining techniques for catecholamines; no thoracic sympathetic fibers to the human fetal heart were demonstrable at ten weeks of gestation.[17] Other studies extended this range of lack of sympathetic neurons from eight to 18 weeks.[31] One group demonstrated weakly fluorescent nerve trunks between ten and 16 weeks in the human fetus.[32]

Fluorescent nerves can be demonstrated at a greater density in atria than in ventricles between 13 and 23 weeks of gestation. These data have prompted the conclusion that humoral sympathetic, rather than neural sympathetic, processes modulate cardiac activity during the first half of human pregnancy.

Field stimulation studies have demonstrated that the positive inotropic response was blocked by propranolol and was enhanced by phenoxybenzamine, which blocks neural uptake of norepinephrine.[27] The more frequent early finding of parasympathetic response than sympathetic response suggested that the parasympathetic or cholinergic nerve supply matures slightly earlier than the sympathetic or adrenergic system.[9]

Reactivity of the human fetal heart to catecholamines has been demonstrated as early as the ninth week of gestation.[17] The human fetal heart is capable of synthesizing norepinephrine as early as 13 weeks of gestation at a rate that shows no change through the twenty-third week.[17] The fetal heart between 12 and 22 weeks is more sensitive to isoproterenol than to norepinephrine,[9] suggesting that the myocardial receptors are beta-adrenergic receptors.

Data supporting humoral, over neural, adrenergic control of the fetal heart in the first half of gestation also came from fetal sheep studies conducted by Friedman,[33] who examined the length–tension relationship of isolated sheep heart muscle. Adult, newborn, and fetal tissues at 0.9 of term gestation were studied under identical conditions. Fetal tissues demonstrated a lower threshold to the inotropic effects of norepinephrine and were threefold more sensitive than the adult to norepinephrine throughout the dose-response curve. In contrast, isoproterenol showed equal responsiveness in adult and fetal tissues. Isoproterenol is a pure beta-agonist and is not taken up and stored in terminal sympathetic nerves. These data indicate that the receptor sensitivity to catecholamines was similar in adult and fetal myocardium. The increased sensitivity of fetal tissues to norepinephrine can be attributed to an immature sympathetic nervous system incapable of inactivating and uptaking norepinephrine, as the adult nervous system can.[33] Similarly, at any concentration of propranolol, the fetal heart rate is more depressed than in the adult, although the beta-blocking action of the drug can be demonstrated to be the same for fetus and adult.[33]

Since the stores of norepinephrine at the terminations of the sympathetic nerves are almost exclusively intracellular, cardiac concentration of norepinephrine in fetal, newborn, and adult myocardium is employed as an index of the magnitude of sympathetic innervation. Friedman[33] found the concentration of norepinephrine to be the lowest in the fetus at 0.9 of term gestation, to be increased in the newborn less than three days old, and to be further increased and approach adult levels after three days of life. Friedman[33] also demonstrated that tyrosine hydroxylase activity, as well as norepinephrine stores, are reduced in the fetal sheep heart. Tyrosine hydroxylase is the rate-limiting enzyme in the synthesis of norepinephrine. Fetal and adult adrenal tissue, however, showed the same level of tyrosine hydroxylase activity and norepinephrine stores. Friedman interpreted this as supporting delayed development of sympathetic innervation rather than immaturity of the enzyme system.

Intrapartum, the human fetus near term was studied for the presence of sympathetic tone by Renou.[34] Following complete parasympathetic blockade by fetal injection of atropine, he infused propranolol in the mother. Within ten minutes of injection of propranolol there was a consistent slowing of the fetal heart rate by approximately 10 beats/minute. Schifferli[20] gave propranolol to eight patients in the last quarter of gestation without preadministration of atropine. He demonstrated significant slowing in only four fetuses, with decrements of 5–10 beats/min. No correlation was found between gestational age and the decrement in fetal heart rate; however, given the sample size this is still inconclusive.

Vapaavouri et al[29] assessed basal sympathetic activity by beta-adrenergic blockade with propranolol and practolol in the fetal sheep between 0.56 and 1 of term gestation and in the neonatal sheep. Fetal heart rate decreased consistently at all ages following beta-blockade. The incremental change in heart rate, and therefore in sympathetic tone, increased significantly after 0.8 of term gestation. Thereafter the incremental change in heart rate leveled off such that the term fetus and the neonate were similar in response. Threshold sensitivity to isoproterenol did not vary with gestational age in the fetus or the neonate. Vapaavouri interpreted these data as demonstrating that the change in basal sympathetic tone was not due to changes in receptor sensitivity, but rather reflected development of sympathetic activity that was delayed compared to parasympathetic activity in the fetus but complete in the neonate.

Assali et al[30] also studied beta-adrenergic blockade in the fetal sheep between 0.43 and 1 of term gestation and in the neonatal sheep. Fetal heart rate consistently decreased in response to beta-blockade with propranolol throughout gestation. The incremental change in heart rate showed an increasing trend and, therefore, increasing sympathetic tone during gestation with no further increase after birth. As noted earlier, the incremental change in heart rate with sympathetic blockade was greater than that produced by parasympathetic blockade until the neonatal period when the reverse was true. Assali interpreted this to indicate that sympathetic activity was dominant in the fetus and matured prior to parasympathetic activity.

In summary, less is known of the function of the sympathetic nervous system in the human fetus than about the parasympathetic nervous system. Anatomically and functionally the sympathetic nervous system appears to develop later than the parasympathetic nervous system; it appears to be immature at birth.

Data on fetal sheep do not in all cases parallel the findings in the human fetus. However, in making such comparisons concerning development of the sympathetic nervous system, it should be understood that the results of sympathetic nerve stimulation in different species support the conclusion that functional adrenergic innervation of the heart develops more rapidly in animals that are relatively independent at birth.[17]

B. Autonomic Reflexes

1. Baroreceptor reflex

The baroreceptor reflex describes an inverse relationship between arterial blood pressure and heart rate that is abolished by parasympathetic blockade with atropine. Recent work by Ismay et al[35] has also demonstrated a less prominent sympathetic component active in the fetal sheep. The reflex is mediated by stretch receptors in the aortic arch and carotid sinuses. Baroreceptor activity has been suggested to explain the decreasing baseline fetal heart rate during the latter half of gestation in the face of increasing arterial blood pressure.

Baroreceptor activity appears as early as 0.6 of term gestation in the fetal sheep.[8] Work by Shinebourn et al[36] in the anesthetized neonatal and fetal sheep between 0.6 and 1 of term gestation demonstrated an increase in reflex sensitivity with gestational age. There was no further increase in baroreceptor sensitivity in the neonatal sheep.

Maloney et al[38] studied the baroreceptor reflex in unanesthetized fetal sheep during the third trimester. Acute increases in blood pressure were induced with phenylephrine. Maloney did not demonstrate an increase in baroreceptor reflex sensitivity with gestational age. The large variance in the data, however, precludes such an assessment.

Ismay et al[35] used phenylephrine to induce acute arterial pressure elevations in chronic fetal sheep preparations between 0.77 and 0.9 of term gestation. Baroreceptor reflex sensitivity was abolished by atropine and increased by propranolol. The identification of a sympathetic component to the baroreceptor response in the fetus is consistent with findings of Pickering et al[37] who showed that baroreceptor activity in man was dependent upon the vagal nerve and inhibited by the cardiac sympathetic nerves. Ismay et al[35] were also unable to demonstrate a correlation between reflex sensitivity and gestational age. However, their use of regression analysis in the face of multiple measures on a limited number of fetal sheep preparations leaves such a conclusion open to question. Thus the relationship of baroreceptor reflex sensitivity and gestational age remains controversial.

2. Chemoreceptor reflex

The role of the systemic arterial chemoreceptors in controlling circulation in the normal fetus is unclear. Both aortic and carotid chemoreceptors are capable of being stimulated from as early as 0.66 of term gestation in the fetal sheep.[3] The carotid chemorecptors appear to be concerned with the control of respiration while the aortic chemoreceptors are involved in the control of circulation. The aortic chemoreceptors operate over a range of oxygen tensions but can be stimulated by changes in pH and carbon dioxide tension. Hypocarbia can abolish the response.[3] Stimulation of the fetal chemoreceptors has been accomplished by induction of maternal hypoxia in acute, anesthetized and, more recently, chronic, unanesthetized fetal sheep preparations. Stimulation of the fetal chemoreceptors in the earlier preparations demonstrated peripheral vasoconstriction and variable changes in the heart rate and blood pressure that could be explained by differing experimental conditions.

In chronic fetal sheep preparation between 0.7 and 1 of term gestation, Walker et al[39] demonstrated that the response to hypoxia was age dependent. In the fetus before 0.8 of term gestation, hypoxia yielded a mild increase in blood pressure and no change in fetal heart rate. For the fetus after 0.8 of term gestation, the response to hypoxia was bradycardia and elevation of blood pressure. Walker also attempted to quantify the relative contributions of the parasympathetic and sympathetic nervous systems by comparing the response of heart rate to cholinergic and adrenergic blockade in the normal and hypoxic fetus. In the fetus before 0.8 of term gestation, both parasympathetic and sympathetic activity were increased during hypoxia without a net change in the fetal heart rate. In the fetus after 0.8 of term gestation, the bradycardia reflected a predominating, increased parasympathetic activity and a sympathetic activity increased over baseline.[39] In the newborn sheep the response to hypoxia was tachycardia mediated synergistically by the sympathetic and parasympathetic nervous systems. Walker attributed these age-dependent responses to maturation of the parasympathetic nervous system with an increasing capacity for vagal influence and a comparatively immature sympathetic nervous system.

Cohn et al[40] examined the circulatory responses to hypoxemia and acidemia in chronic fetal sheep preparations between 0.81 and 0.95 of term gestation. In addition to heart rate, arterial pressure, pH, and oxygen and carbon dioxide tensions, they studied fetal cardiac output, distribution, and absolute organ blood flows during control and hypoxic conditions. During hypoxemia fetal arterial pressure increased and fetal heart rate decreased in a manner similar to that observed by Walker et al.[39] Cardiac output decreased significantly only in those fetuses in which hypoxia was accompanied by acidosis. Fetal body blood flow was decreased; placental flow was maintained; blood flow to the brain, heart, and adrenals increased preferentially; pulmonary, renal, splenic, and gut flows decreased. Acidemia accentuated these changes in flow.

C. Central Nervous System

There is some evidence that fetal central nervous system activity during the latter half of gestation may modify circulatory function in the fetus. The extent of central nervous system control over fetal heart regulation under normal conditions is unknown.

Bernhard and Meyerson[41] found the electrocorticogram from the surface of exposed fetal sheep brain at 0.4 of term gestation to be electrically silent. From 0.46 to 0.6 of term gestation, the fetal cortex exhibited some spontaneous intermittent bursts of activity. After 0.76 of term gestation, the electrocorticogram of fetal sheep demonstrated continuous cortical activity with patterns associated with rapid-eye-movement (REM) and non-REM sleep.

Rosen et al[42,43] recorded the human fetal electroencephalogram during labor after rupture of the membranes and found that the fetal and neonatal electroencephalogram is related to maturity and is unchanged by the normal birth process. With fetal maturation, there is an increase in the faster electroencephalogram frequencies and a progressive diminution in flat electroencephalogram periods.

Dawes et al[44,52] found that a rise in fetal heart rate and fetal blood pressure was associated with REM sleep in chronic fetal sheep preparations. Rudolph and Heymann[7] observed spontaneous changes in fetal heart rate and fetal blood pressure that are present after the inhibition of fetal respiratory movements and suggested that these spontaneous changes may be related to central nervous system activities. Lidocaine infusions into chronic fetal sheep preparations at term produced bursts of high-voltage fetal electrocorticogram activity, associated with marked increases in fetal blood pressure.

Timor-Tritsch et al[45] used transabdominal monitoring of fetal heart rate and its variability, fetal respiratory movement, and fetal body movement for classification of fetal activity into active and quiet periods. These observations suggested the presence of behavioral state cycles (active–quiet) of approximately 62.3 minutes. The active period may include both the equivalent of REM sleep and the awake state. Using the same techniques, they observed a very strong association between fetal movements lasting longer than one second and increases in the fetal heart rate.[46] The fetal heart rate changes had a 1.3-second lag time from the fetal body movement. This suggested a coordinated control of the heart rate and movement, with the stimulus for both originating in the brain. Recently, Dawes et al[47] made similar observations using different criteria and techniques.

Williams et al[48] studied the effect of stimulation of fetal sheep hypothalamic region on the cardiovascular system. Three patterns of cardiovascular response were observed. The most frequent change was a pressor/tachycardia response in fetal sheep from 0.76 to 0.9 of term gestation. This response was mediated by alpha-adrenergic receptors confirmed by blockade by phentolamine. The initial tachycardia was mediated by the beta-adrenergic receptors confirmed by blockade with propranolol. The pressor/tachycardiac response persisted in the newborn sheep, and the response showed a greater increase in the arterial blood pressure than was measured in utero. The second type of response was tachycardia without change in blood pressure. The tachycardia was blocked with propranolol. The third response, pure bradycardia, was blocked with atropine. These experiments suggest potential nervous system pathways connecting the fetal forebrain with the cardiovascular regulatory system.

The importance of the central nervous system in the physiologic control of the fetal heart in normal in utero existence is open to speculation. Integration of several systems, including the central nervous system, seems to provide physiologic control of the fetal heart.

D. Relationship to Respiration

Over 90 years ago Ahlfeld,[49] Weber,[50] and Preyer[51] observed rhythmic movements through the human maternal abdominal wall and ascribed them to fetal breathing activity. Since then the presence of spontaneous fetal breathing movements has been controversial. Recent studies by Dawes et al[44,52] and Merlet et al[53] documented intrauterine fetal breathing movements in chronically catheterized fetal sheep. Boddy and Robinson[54] described chest wall movements in the human fetus using A-mode ultrasound. Duenhoelter and Pritchard [55] documented that radioactive-chromium-labeled erythrocytes were inspired from the amniotic fluid. In the past ten years investigators have reported the characteristics and patterns of fetal breathing in the sheep,[56] in the monkey,[57] and in man.[58–60]

In the monkey, Martin et al[57] described an increase in fetal heart rate variability during fetal breathing episodes. Fetal heart rate baseline was also higher during these episodes than during periods devoid of fetal breathing movements. These investigators found some evidence for a link between fetal breathing and fetal states. In fetal monkeys irregular breathing movements occurred in association with increased fetal heart rate variability, eye, and somatic movements. Active periods (REM sleep) alternated with quiet periods (non-REM sleep), with the latter characterized by a stable fetal heart rate and regular breathing movements.

Fouron et al[61] investigated the cardiovascular changes associated with fetal breathing. In chronically instrumented sheep at term they observed changes in arterial blood pressure, cardiac rate, and rhythm. The initiation of bursts of rapid respiratory movements was associated with a small decrease in both systolic and diastolic pressures. The decrease in blood pressure may relate to changes in intrathoracic vascular bed capacity due to changes in intrathoracic pressure with fetal breathing. The baroreceptor reflex has been hypothesized to play an important role here. The small (less than 10%) decreases in blood pressures are followed by marked (more than 50%) elevations in systolic and diastolic pressures over baseline. These increases are either transitory or continue throughout the burst of fetal breathing. There appears to be a cyclic variation in arterial pressure characterized by lowering of arterial pressures with each inspiration. Fetal heart rate baseline increased during the rapid and irregular fetal breathing movements. The changes in blood pressure and tachycardia may be explained by an increase in sympathetic activity associated with fetal breathing activity. Rudolph and Heymann[7] observed increases in fetal cardiac output and heart rate associated with initiation of fetal breathing movements. They suggested that these changes may be related to changes in electrocortical activity.[7] A fetal respiratory arrhythmia was almost always noted with rapid inspiratory movements. The typical increase in heart rate with inspiration and slowing with expiration was demonstrated. In contrast fetal heart rate and blood pressure were stable during periods of apnea.

Several mechanisms are postulated for the generation of respiratory arrhythmia in the fetus.[23,59] Dalton et al[56] investigated the influence of fetal breathing on heart rate in fetal sheep using an accurately measured RR interval. Fetal breathing was accompanied by an increase in heart rate variability; however, the mean heart rate showed no predictable change. Fetal hypoxia abolished fetal breathing movements and yielded a fall in mean fetal heart rate and an increase in heart rate variability.

Rudolph[62] observed increased superior and inferior vena caval flow during inspiration in fetal sheep. The flow rates were slower with grunting. The magnitude of the change in flow correlated with the synchrony of the fetal breathing and heart beat.

Recently several investigators have reported on the relationship between fetal cardiac activity and fetal breathing in human pregnancy. Timor-Tritsch et al[59,63] recorded fetal breathing movements by placing tocodynamometers on the maternal abdomen. The fetal heart rate was recorded by Doppler ultrasound and the fetal electrocardiogram. Respiratory arrhythmia was documented. Using the same techniques Timor-Tritsch et al[64] documented regular fetal breathing movements in normal term fetuses during quiet activity periods defined as decreased long-term fetal heart rate variability, absence of gross fetal body movements, and a lowered fetal heart rate baseline. In contrast, irregular fetal breathing movements appeared during fetal active periods defined by increased fetal heart rate variability, increased fetal heart rate baseline, and increased duration and frequency of fetal body movements. Junge and Walter[65] found a small association between fetal breathing and fetal activity in the human fetus.

Wheeler et al[66] recorded the fetal heart rate from the fetal electrocardiogram and observed fetal breathing using real-time ultrasound. Fetal breathing was associated with an increase in fetal heart rate variability. The change in mean heart rate was unpredictable. There was no consistent relationship between fetal breathing and fetal activity periods. Fetal respiratory arrhythmia was demonstrable, and heart rate modulations were pronounced during fetal breathing.

Bots et al[67] also used real-time ultrasound to detect fetal breathing and the fetal electrocardiogram to measure fetal heart rate in human pregnancy at term. They observed no increase in heart rate variability during periods of fetal respiratory movements. The results obtained by this group of investigators differ from those obtained by Wheeler et al[66] and Timor-Tritsch et al.[63] It was suggested by Van Geijn[23] that these differences may be explained in part by different methods of data analysis.

Dawes et al[47] used numerical analysis of fetal heart rate patterns in the human fetus at term to investigate the association of fetal heart rate with gross fetal body movements and fetal breathing. Fetal breathing was associated with an increase in short-term (beat-to-beat) fetal heart rate variability. This observed increase in short-term fetal heart rate variability (but not long-term variability) was confirmed by statistical analysis. The magnitude and direction of change in the short-term variability was complexly related to other changes in fetal heart rate (fetal heart rate accelerations and decelerations and fetal heart rate baseline).

IV. REFERENCES

1. Dawes GS. The foetal circulation. In:Foetal and Neonatal Physiology, Vol 8. Chicago: Year Book Medical Publishers, 1968:91–105.
2. Nuwayhid BS. Fetal homeostasis. In: Iffy L, Kaminetzky HA, eds. Principles and Practice of Obstetrics and Perinatology, Vol 11. New York: John Wiley, 1981:269–304.
3. Boddy K. Fetal circulation and breathing movements. In: Beard RW, Nathanielsz PW, eds. Fetal Physiology and Medicine. Philadelphia: W.B. Saunders, 1976:302–308.
4. Rudolph AM. The fetal circulation. In: Congenital Diseases of the Heart, Vol 1 Chicago: Year Book Medical Publishers, 1974:1–16.
5. Nuwayhid B, Brinkman CR III, Su C, Bevan JA, Assali NS. Development of autonomic control of fetal circulation. Am J Physiol. 1975; 228:337–341.
6. Gilbert RD. Venous return and control of fetal cardiac output. In: Longo LD, Reneau DD, eds. Fetal and Newborn Cardiovascular Physiology, New York: Garland Publishers, Inc., 1978:229–316.
7. Rudolph AM, Heymann MA. Cardiac output in the fetal lamb: The effects of spontaneous and induced changes of heart rate on right and left ventricular output. Am J Obstet Gynecol. 1976; 124:183–192.
8. Rudolph AM, Heymann MA. Control of the foetal circulation. In: Foetal and Neonatal Physiology. Proceedings of the Sir Joseph Bancroft Centenary Symposium. Cambridge: Cambridge University Press, 1973:89–111.
9. Friedman WF. The intrinsic physiologic properties of the developing heart. Prog Cardiovasc. Dis. 1972; 15:21–49.
10. Kirkpatrick SE, Pitlick PT, Naliboff J, Friedman WF. Frank-Starling relationship as an important determinant of fetal cardiac output. Am J Physiol. 1976; 231:495–500.
11. Kirkpatrick SE, Friedman WF. Myocardial determinants of fetal cardiac output. In: Long LD, Reneau DD, eds. Fetal and Newborn Cardiovascular Physiology, Vol I. New York: Garland, 1978:370–385.
12. Anderson PAW, Manring A, Crenshaw C. Biophysics of the developing heart I. The force–interval relationship. Am J Obstet Gynecol. 1980; 138:33–43.
13. Anderson PAW, Manring A, Crenshaw C. Biophysics of the developing heart II. The interaction of the force–interval relationship with inotropic state and muscle length (preload). Am J Obstet Gynecol. 1980; 138:44–54.
14. Wolfson RN, Zador IE, Pillay SK. Antenatal human fetal diastoloc time intervals: Ventricular filling time—Relationship to fetal heart rate and gestational age. (manuscript in preparation).
15. Goodlin RC, Girard J, Hallman A. Systolic time intervals in the fetus and neonate. Obstet Gynecol. 1972; 39:295–302.
16. Hawrylyshyn PA, Organ LW, Bernstein A. A new computer technique for continuous measurement of the pre-ejection period in the human fetus: Physiologic significance of pre-ejection period. Am J Obstet Gynecol. 1980;137:801–809.
17. Pappano AJ. Ontogenetic development of autonomic neuroeffector transmission and transmitter reactivity in embryonic and fetal hearts. Pharmacol Rev. 1977; 29:3–32.
18. Robinson HP, Shaw-Dunn J. Fetal heart rates as determined by sonar in early pregnancy. J Obstet Gynaecol. Br Commonw. 1973; 80:805–809.
19. Blaney SR, Chow TTS, Lindahl SA. Assessment of fetal maturity—Another parameter: Different heart rates at varying stages of development. Proc AIUM, New Orleans, Louisiana, 1980.
20. Schifferli PY, Caldeyro-Barcia R. Effects of atropine and beta-adrenergic drugs on the heart rate of the human fetus. In: Boreus L, ed. Fetal Pharmacology. New York: Raven Press, 1973: 259–279.
21. Larks SD, Larks GG. The course of the fetal heart rate during pregnancy. Cardiology. 1972; 57:208–211.
22. Ibarra-Polo AA, Guiloff E, Gomez-Rogers C. Fetal heart rate throughout pregnancy. Am J Obstet Gynecol. 1972; 113:814–818.
23. Van Geijn HP. Studies on Fetal and Neonatal Baseline Heart Rate Variability. Meppel, Netherlands: Krips Repro, 1980.
24. Smith RB. The development of the intrinsic innervation of the human heart between the 10 and 70 mm stage. J Anat. 1970; 107:271–279.
25. Smith RB. Intrinsic innervation of the human heart in foetuses between 70 mm and 420 mm crown–rump length. Acta Anat. 1971; 78: 200–209.
26. Smith RB. The development of autonomic neurons in the human heart. Anat Anz Bd. 1971; 129:70–76.
27. Walker D. Functional development of the autonomic innervation of the human fetal heart. Biol Neonate. 1975; 25:31–43.
28. Gennser G, Nelsson E. Response to adrenaline, acetylcholine and change of contraction fre-

quency in early human foetal hearts. Experientia (Basel). 1970; 26:1105–1107.

29. Vapaavouri EK, Shinebourne EA, Williams RL, Heymann MA, Rudolph AM. Development of cardiovascular responses to autonomic blockade in intact fetal and neonatal lambs. Biol Neonate. 1973; 22:177–188.
30. Assali NS, Brinkmann CR III, Woods JR, Dandavino A, Nuwayhid B. Development of neurohumoral control of fetal, neonatal and adult cardiovascular function. Am J Obstet Gynecol. 1977; 129:748–758.
31. Dail WG, Palmer GC. Localization and correlation of catecholamine-containing cells with adenyl cyclase and phosphodiesterase activities in the human fetal heart. Anat Rec. 1973; 177:265–288.
32. Partanen S, Korkala O. Catecholamines in human fetal heart. Experientia (Basel). 1974; 30:798–799.
33. Friedman WF. The intrinsic physiologic properties of the developing heart. In: Friedman WF, Lesch M, Sonnenblock EH, eds. Neonatal Heart Disease. New York: Grune & Stratton, 1972:21–49.
34. Renou P, Newman W, Wood C. Autonomic control of fetal heart rate. Am J Obstet Gynecol. 1969; 105:949–953.
35. Ismay MJA, Lumbers ER, Stevens AD. The action of angiotension II on the baroreflex response of the conscious ewe and the conscious fetus. J Physiol. 1979; 288:467–469.
36. Shinebourne EA, Vapaavouri EK, Williams EK, Heymann MA, Rudolph AM. Development of baroreflex activity in an anesthetized fetal and neonatal lamb. Circ Res. 1972; 31:710–718.
37. Pickering TG, Gribbin B, Strange Peterson E, Cunningham DJC, Sleigh P. Effects of autonomic blockade on baroreflex in man at rest and during exercise. Circ Res. 1975; 30:177–185.
38. Maloney JE, Cannata J, Dowling MH, Else W, Ritchie B. Baroreflex activity in conscious fetal and newborn lambs. Biol Neonate. 1977; 31:340–350.
39. Walker Am, Cannata JP, Dowling MH, Ritchie BC, Maloney JE. Age-dependent pattern of autonomic heart rate control during hypoxia in fetal and newborn lambs. Biol Neonate. 1979; 35:198–208.
40. Cohn HE, Sacks EJ, Heymann MA, Rudolph AM. Cardiovascular responses to hypoxemia and acidemia in fetal lambs. Am J Obstet Gynecol. 1974; 120:817–824.
41. Bernhard CG, Meyerson BA. Morphological and physiological aspects of the development of recipient functions in the cerebral cortex. In: Foetal and Neonatal Physiology. Proceedings of the Sir Joseph Bancroft Centenary Symposium. Cambridge: Cambridge University Press, 1973:1–19.
42. Rosen MG, Scibetta JJ, Hochberg CJ. Human fetal electroencephalogram III. Pattern changes in presence of fetal heart rate alterations and after use of maternal medications. Obstet Gynecol. 1970; 36:132–140.
43. Rosen MG, Scibetta J, Chik L, Borgstedt A. An approach to the study of brain damage. The principles of fetal electroencephalography. Am J Obstet Gynecol. 1973; 115:37–47.
44. Dawes GS, Fox HE, Leduc BM, Liggins GC, Richards RT. Respiratory movements and rapid eye movements sleep in the fetal lamb. J Physiol. 1972; 220:119–143.
45. Timor-Tritsch IE, Dierker LJ, Hertz RH, Deagan HG, Rosen MG. Studies of antepartum behavioral state in the human fetus at term. Am J Obstet Gynecol. 1978; 132:524–528.
46. Timor-Tritsch IE, Dierker LJ, Zador I, Hertz RH, Rosen MG. Fetal movements associated with fetal heart rate accelerations and decelerations. Am J Obstet Gynecol. 1978; 131:276–280.
47. Dawes GS, Visser GHA, Goodman IDS, Levine DH. Numerical analysis of the human heart rate: Modulation by breathing and movement. Am J Obstet Gynecol. 1981; 140:535–544.
48. William RL, Hof RP, Heyman MA, Rudolph AM. Cardiovascular effects of electrical stimulation of the forebrain in the fetal lamb. Pediatr Res. 1976; 10:40–45.
49. Ahlfeld F. Über Bisher Noch Nicth Beschreibene intrauterine Bewegungen des Kindes, Vol 2. Zweiter Kongress Verh Dtsch Ges Gynaekol. Leipzig: Breithopf un Hartel. 1888:203–210.
50. Weber H. Ueber physiologische Athmungsbewegungen des Kindes im Uterus, Inaugural Dissertation, Universitaet Marburg, 1888.
51. Preyer W. Specialle Physiologie des Embryos. Leipzig: Th. Griebens, Verlag, 1885.
52. Dawes GS, Fox HE, Leduc BM, Liggins GC, Richards RT. Respiratory movements and para doxical sleep in the fetal lamb. J Physiol. 1970; 210:47–48.
53. Merlet C, Hoerter J, Devilleneuve C, Tchobroutsky C. Mise en evidence de mouvements respiratoires chez ce foetus d'agneau in utero au cours du dernier mois de la gestation. CR Hebd Seanc Acad Sci Paris. 1970; 270:2462–2464.
54. Boddy K, Robinson JS. External method for detection of fetal breathing in utero. Lancet. 1971; 2:1231–1233.
55. Duenhoelter JH, Pritchard JA. Human fetal respiration. II. Fate of intra-amniotic hypaque and ^{51}Cr-labeled red cells. Obstet Gynecol. 1974; 43:878–883.
56. Dalton KJ, Dawes GS, Patrick JE. Diurnal, respiratory and other rhythms of fetal heart rate in lambs. Am J Obstet Gynecol. 1977; 127: 414–424.
57. Martin CB, Murata Y, Petrie RH, Parer JT. Respiratory movements in fetal rhesus monkeys. Am J Obstet Gynecol. 1974; 119:939–948.
58. Patrick J, Fetherston W, Vick H, Voegelin R. Human fetal breathing movements and gross

fetal body movements at 34 to 35 weeks gestational age. Am J Obstet Gynecol. 1978; 130:693–699.
59. Timor-Tritsch I, Zador I, Hertz RH, Rosen MG. Human fetal respiratory arrhythmia. Am J Obstet Gynecol. 1977; 127:662–666.
60. Platt LD, Manning FA, Lemay M. Fetal breathing movements: The relationship to fetal condition. Am J Obstet Gynecol. 1978; 132:515–518.
61. Fouron JC, Korcaz Y, Leduc B. Cardiovascular changes associated with fetal breathing. Am J Obstet Gynecol. 1975; 123:868–876.
62. Rudolph AM. Lecture at the Sixth Fetal Breathing Conference, Paris, 1979.
63. Timor-Tritsch IE, Dierker LJ, Hertz RH, Zador I, Rosen MG. Human fetal respiratory movements: A technique for non-invasive monitoring with the use of a tocodynamometer. Biol Neonate. 1979; 36:18–24.
64. Timor-Tritsch IE, Dierker LJ, Hertz RH, Chik L, Rosen MG. Regular and irregular human fetal respiratory movement. Early Hum Dev. 1980; 4/3:315–324.
65. Junge HD, Walter H. Behavioral states and breathing activity in the fetus near term. J Perinat Med. 1980; 8:15–157.
66. Wheeler T, Gennser G, Lindvall R, Murrills AJ. Changes in the fetal heart rate associated with fetal breathing and fetal movement. Br. J. Obstet Gynecol. 1980; 87:1068–1079.
67. Bots RSGM, Jonesma HW, Braat AJHM, Martin CB, DeHaan J. Human fetal breathing movement and heart rate variability. Fifth Conference on Fetal Breathing, Nijmegen, the Netherlands, 1978.

When to Expect Congenital Abnormalities

F.IV

Genetic Causes of Congenital Abnormalities

James H. Moller, MD, and Mary Ella Mascia Pierpont, PhD, MD

Cardiac Problems in Pregnancy, pages 383–418

I. INTRODUCTION

Cardiac abnormalities occur in many genetic diseases. The abnormalities may be present at birth, as in chromosomal conditions and some genetic syndromes, or acquired, as occurs in metabolic storage diseases, neuromuscular disorders, or connective tissue disorders.

This chapter reviews cardiac disease with respect to chromosomal anomalies, and diseases caused by single gene abnormalities. Next, common and uncommon familial disorders without a recognizable pattern of inheritance are considered. Finally, several syndromes that may be of genetic etiology are reviewed. For each condition, emphasis will be placed on etiology, major cardiac findings, and genetic considerations.

II. CHROMOSOMAL PROBLEMS

Many of the recognized chromosomal anomalies are associated with congenital cardiac malformations (Tables F.IV.1 and F.IV.2). There is a degree of specificity of the type of cardiac anomaly for each particular chromosomal anomaly. Thus, by identifying a particular chromosomal abnormality, either by phenotypic expression or by chromosomal karyotyping, important clues about the expected types of cardiac malformation may be obtained.

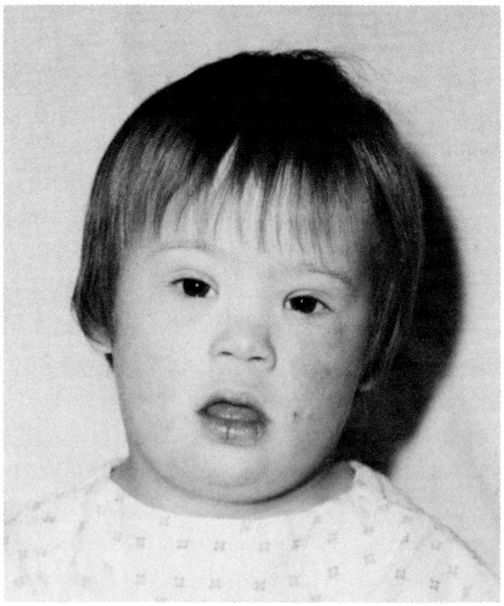

Fig. F.IV.1. Facial appearance of a 2-year-old boy with trisomy 21.

Cultured human lymphocytes normally contain 46 chromosomes, and these can be analyzed by Giemsa or quinacrine banding techniques. Several types of anomalies of chromosomes have been identified: trisomy (the presence of an entire extra chromosome), partial trisomy (presence of an extra portion of a chromosome), deletion (absence of all or a portion of a chromosome), and mosaicism (at least two types of cells, each with a different chromosome content or number). These types of chromosome anomalies can be detected prenatally in amniotic cells obtained by amniocentesis. This may be a useful technique in subsequent pregnancies of parents who have had a child affected by a chromosomal anomaly.

A. Trisomy 21 (Down Syndrome)

Trisomy 21 is the most common autosomal trisomic syndrome and has an overall incidence of one in 660 births. However, incidence is age-dependent, with older mothers having a much greater incidence of infants with trisomy 21. In this syndrome, additional chromosomal material of chromosome 21 is present as: a) an additional chromosome 21 (caused by meiotic nondisjunction, producing 47 chromosomes in each cell), b) translocation of an additional chromosome 21 to another chromosome; or c) mosaic, in which only a proportion of the individual cells have an additional chromosome 21, while the remainder have a normal complement. Chromosomal analysis should always be performed on each patient with features of trisomy 21, since the risk of recurrence of a translocation anomaly is substantially higher than the nondisjunction variety.

Patients with trisomy 21 have a characteristic and recognizable facial appearance, with a flattened nasal bridge, prominent epicanthal folds, and a protruding tongue (Fig. F.IV.1). Other characteristic

TABLE F.IV.1. Common Clinical Findings in Classical Chromosomal Syndromes With Congenital Heart Malformations

	Trisomy 21	Trisomy 18	Trisomy 13	Monosomy X (Turner)	$4p^-$	$5p^-$
General	Varying survival	Early death, failure to thrive	Early death, failure to thrive	Small stature, infertility	Failure to thrive, variable survival	Long survival, cat cry in infancy
Incidence	1:660 (higher with increasing maternal age)	1:3,500, female preponderance	1:7,000, equal sex distribution	1:2,500, females	Less than 1:50,000	1:50,000
Facies and head	"Mongoloid" slant eyes, Brushfield spots, epicanthal folds, protruding tongue	Prominent occiput, low-set ears, micrognathia, abnormal pinnae	Scalp defects, microcephaly, cleft lip/palate, defects of forebrain, low-set ears, microphthalmia	Prominent ears, small mandible, straight lower lip	Microcephaly, prominent glabella, wide nose, coloboma, micrognathia, cleft lip/palate	Microcephaly, moon facies, hypertelorism, high arched palate
Neck and chest	Broad neck, TE fistula	TE fistula, short sternum		Webbed neck, low posterior hairline, shield-shaped chest	Long slender neck, frequent skeletal anomalies	Usually normal
Heart	Malformations in 50%, AV canal, VSD	Malformations in 99%, usually combination of defects	Malformations in 80–90%, VSD, PDA, usually combination of defects	Malformations in 30–35%, coarctation of aorta, aortic stenosis	Malformations in 40–50%, ASD, VSD, PDA	Malformations in 20–25% VSD, PDA, ASD
Abdomen	Duodenal atresia	Renal anomalies	Renal anomalies, hernias	Horseshoe kidney, ovarian dysgenesis, renal anomalies	Renal anomalies	Renal anomalies
Extremities	Clinodactyly, simian lines, hypotonia	Overlapping fingers, rocker bottom feet, talipes equinovarus	Polydactyly, rocker bottom feet	Cubitus valgus, lymphedema in infancy	Long thin limbs, talipes equinovarus	Skeletal malformations rare
Neurological status	Mental retardation, hypotonia	Profound mental and motor retardation	Profound mental and motor retardation	Usually normal intelligence	Profound mental retardation	Profound mental retardation, hypotonia

ASD = atrial septal defect, AV canal = atrioventricular canal, PDA = patent ductus arteriosus, VSD = ventricular septal defect.

syndrome is characterized by microcephaly, defects of the forebrain, central facial anomalies, coloboma, cleft lip, cleft palate, cardiac anomalies, and profound mental and motor retardation. There is marked failure to thrive. Death, usually from infection or cardiovascular disease, occurs in infancy.

Congenital cardiac malformations occur in at least 80% of patients with trisomy 13.[1,9] The most common cardiovascular lesions are ventricular septal defect, patent ductus arteriosus, and atrial septal defect. The most frequent form of cyanotic congenital heart disease in trisomy 13 is tetralogy of Fallot. Both the aortic and pulmonary valves may be bicuspid. Other less frequent cardiovascular lesions are origin of the great vessels from the right ventricle, mitral atresia, and left ventricular outflow obstructive lesions.

Recurrence risk is higher for translocation than nondisjunction, but these and mosaic forms can be detected prenatally by amniocentesis.

D. Turner Syndrome

Turner syndrome is characterized by a specific phenotype and is caused by the deletion of an entire X chromosome. In most patients there are 45 chromosomes, with a normal complement of autosomal chromosomes, but only one X chromosome. However, mosaicism exists in some patients (XX/XO or XO/XY), and others have a structurally abnormal second X chromosome (isochromosome).

The Turner phenotype[10] is characterized by short stature, webbing of the neck (pterygium colli), cubitus valgus, sexual and skeletal infantilism, and cardiovascular malformations. Patients with Turner syndrome have a high incidence of renal anomalies, infertility, and usually intelligence is normal. Lymphedema is noted in some infants (Fig. F.IV.2).

Cardiovascular malformations are present in 30–35% of the cases. Coarctation of the aorta is the most common anomaly, and valvular aortic stenosis occurs much

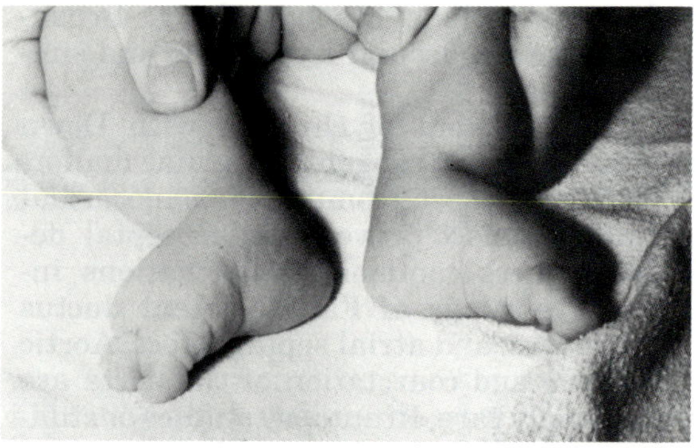

Fig. F.IV.2. Lymphedema of lower extremities in a neonate with Turner syndrome.

less frequently.[11,12] There are occasional cases of the following anomalies: ventricular septal defect, atrial septal defect, patent ductus arteriosus, and dextrocardia. Pulmonary stenosis, common in patients with Noonan syndrome, does not occur in Turner syndrome with XO karyotype. Patients who have mosaic karyotype (45,XO/46,XX) have been described with aortic valvular stenosis, coarctation, or pulmonary stenosis. Hypertension of renal origin occurs in some patients.

When a patient with Turner phenotype is identified, cardiovascular malformation should be sought. Coarctation of the aorta can be identified clinically by decreased pulse amplitude and blood pressure in the lower extremities. Buccal smear (staining of mucosal cells for Barr bodies) will reveal absence or low percentage of Barr bodies. Definitive diagnosis rests with chromosomal analysis. Risk of recurrence in a family is low.

E. $4p^-$ Syndrome

The $4p^-$ syndrome (Wolff-Hirschhorn syndrome) results from the deletion of a substantial portion of the short arm of chromosome 4. In this uncommon chromosomal abnormality, most patients have profound mental retardation and failure to thrive. Many craniofacial abnormalities are present[13]: microcephaly, broad beaked nose, hypertelorism, micrognathia, and occasional cleft lip or palate and coloboma (Fig. F.IV.3). Skeletal anomalies and renal malformations are common. Cardiovascular malformations, most frequently atrial septal defect, occur in 40–50%.[14,15] Ventricular septal defect and patent ductus arteriosus are less frequent. Pulmonary stenosis, dextrocardia, bicuspid aortic valve, and hypoplastic right ventricle have each been reported. The length of survival is extremely variable.

Risk of recurrence is low unless a parent is a balanced carrier for a translocation involving chromosome four. In this situation, recurrence may be 15–25%. Amniocentesis and subsequent chromosomal analysis can detect this anomaly prenatally.

F. $5p^-$ Syndrome

$5p^-$ syndrome (cri du chat) results from deletion of the short arm of chromosome 5. Infants with this syndrome have a shrill cat-like cry that frequently disappears later in childhood. Profound mental retardation is usually present. The most common physical findings are microcephaly, moon facies, and renal abnormalities. Cardiovascular malformations, most commonly ventricular septal defect or patent ductus arteriosus, are found in 20–25%.[16,17]

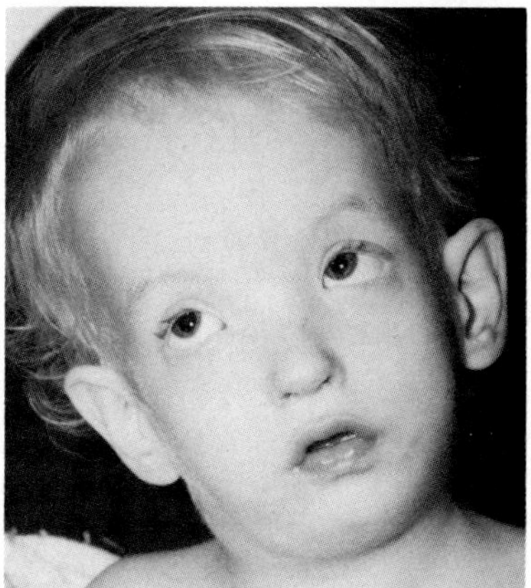

Fig. F.IV.3. Facial appearance of a 2-year-old boy with $4p^-$ syndrome.

Many patients live into adulthood.[18] The risk of recurrence is low, less than 1%, although parents should have karyotypes performed since they may be balanced carriers of a translocation involving chromosome 5. If this is the case, the risk may be increased to 15–25%. Amniocentesis can detect this abnormality prenatally.

G. Trisomy 8

Trisomy 8, one of the less common autosomal trisomic syndromes,[19] is usually present as a mosaic, with only some cells containing an extra chromosome 8. In affected individuals, the shape of the head is unusual, with a prominent forehead, hypertelorism, broad nose, and micrognathia. The neck is short and the trunk long and slender. Other abnormalities include camptodactyly, deep palmar furrows, absent patellae, and renal anomalies. Mild or moderate mental retardation is present in most patients. Cardiovascular abnormalities occur,[20–22] most commonly ventricular septal defect or patent ductus arteriosus.

Risk of recurrence of this disorder is unknown, but amniocentesis can provide prenatal diagnosis for families at risk.

H. Trisomy 9

Trisomy 9 has been reported as a complete trisomy, mosaic, and a partial trisomic condition. These patients have multiple congenital anomalies, the most prominent being microcephaly, low-set ears, hypoplastic ribs, skeletal abnormalities, and profound mental retardation.[23–25] The most common cardiovascular malformations are ventricular septal defect and patent ductus arteriosus. Other malformations reported have included double-outlet right ventricle, variant of atrioventricular canal defect (two leaflets to tricuspid valve), and dextroposition of the heart. Life-span is frequently shortened; risk of recurrence is unknown.

I. 13q⁻ Syndrome

In the 13q⁻ syndrome varying portions of the long arm of chromosome 13 are deleted. As a result the clinical features vary. Most patients have mental retardation, microcephaly, hypertelorism, and broad nasal bridge. When large amounts of genetic material are deleted from chromosome 13, other features, including aplasia or hypoplasia of thumbs and ocular abnormalities such as coloboma and retinoblastoma, are present.[26]

Cardiovascular malformations occur in 10–25% of patients.[27] The most frequent congenital cardiac anomaly is ventricular septal defect, but atrial septal defect, narrowing of the coronary ostia, single ventricle with mitral atresia, and ventricular septal defect with overriding aorta have been reported. The incidence of cardiac disease is difficult to determine because, although cardiac murmurs are mentioned in reports, the underlying cardiac disorder has not been clearly defined.

Risk of recurrence of 13q⁻ syndrome is unknown, but if a parent is a balanced carrier of a translocation of chromosome 13, the risk may be as high as 15–25%.

J. Trisomy 22

Trisomy 22, an uncommon cytogenetic abnormality, usually occurs in the full trisomic state rather than as a mosaic.[28–30] Growth retardation, microcephaly, micrognathia, and mental retardation are common. Other features have not been clearly defined since so few patients have been reported. Cardiovascular abnormalities are present in most patients. The most common conditions are atrial septal defect, ventricular septal defect, and patent ductus arteriosus. Persistent left superior vena cava, aberrant subclavian artery, and tricuspid atresia with hypoplastic right ventricle have each been reported. Risk of recurrence is unknown.

K. Partial Trisomy 22

The cat-eye syndrome results from partial trisomy of chromosome 22. The extra chromosomal material consists of the short arm and a portion of the long arm of chromosome 22. This syndrome is more common in females. Physical features include coloboma of the iris, anal atresia, severe mental retardation, genitourinary abnormalities, microcephaly, and micrognathia.[31,32]

Thirty percent to 40% of the patients have congenital cardiac malformations, usually complex forms of cyanotic heart disease.[33,34] Total anomalous pulmonary venous return, tetralogy of Fallot, and single ventricle with total anomalous pulmonary venous return have been described. Coarctation of the aorta, patent ductus arteriosus, ventricular septal defect, and atrial septal defect have also been reported. The severity of the cardiac condition usually shortens the life-span, with many patients dying in the first year of life.

Recurrence risks of cat-eye syndrome depend on whether either parent is a balanced translocation carrier. If so, risk is increased.

L. XXXXY Syndrome

The XXXXY syndrome is an uncommon chromosomal anomaly with 49 chromosomes, 44 autosomes, and five sex chromosomes. Most patients are phenotypically males, but some have ambiguous genitalia. Most have moderately severe mental retardation, epicanthal folds, low-set ears, short webbed neck, and radioulnar synostosis.[35]

Approximately 15% have cardiac anomalies, almost always patent ductus arteriosus.[36] Rare malformations reported include atrial septal defect, pulmonary stenosis, and anomalous right coronary artery. Recurrence risk is unknown.

III. SINGLE GENE ABNORMALITIES

In this section, many types of syndromes are discussed. Each has a recognizable pattern of inheritance due to the effects of a single gene. Transmission of a genetic disorder by a single gene may be through several patterns: autosomal dominant, autosomal recessive, sex-linked recessive, and sex-linked dominant.

Diseases caused by single gene defects may be diagnosed by their somatic features. In each of the diseases discussed in this section, the cardiac anomalies are fairly specific for the disease. These cardiac anomalies may be congenital or acquired due to disturbances in metabolic pathways, muscle, connective tissue, or nervous tissue.

A. Causes of Congenital Heart Disease

In this section several syndromes without metabolic abnormality are discussed in which cardiac disease is a prominent feature.

1. Holt-Oram syndrome

In Holt-Oram syndrome, skeletal anomalies of the arms are associated with congenital cardiac anomalies.[37] The syndrome is inherited as an autosomal dominant trait displaying a high degree of penetrance (ie, heterozygous individuals manifest the phenotype). The skeletal abnormalities vary in severity. In all patients the thumbs are abnormal, being absent, hypoplastic, bifid, finger-like, or triphalangeal (Fig. F.IV.4). Other malformations range from subtle (syndactyly) to severe (phocomelia). Commonly the radius is absent or hypoplastic.

Congenital cardiac anomalies are common, but in some affected individuals only skeletal abnormalities are present.[38] The most common congenital cardiovascular malformation in Holt-Oram syndrome is secundum atrial septal defect and less frequently ventricular septal defect.[39] Occasionally other abnormalities, including ostium primum atrial septal defect, patent ductus arteriosus, and persistent left superior vena cava, have been reported. Hypoplasia of peripheral blood vessels has also been reported.

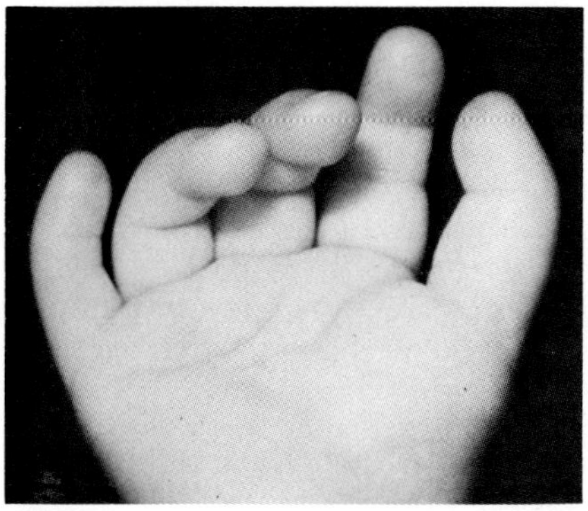

Fig. F.IV.4. Finger-like right thumb in an infant with Holt-Oram syndrome.

In some patients the electrocardiograms show abnormal atrioventricular conduction and bradycardia. In addition, in those with secundum atrial septal the usual pattern of terminal conduction delay in the right anterior chest leads is not found.

Since this disorder is inherited as an autosomal dominant condition, an affected parent has a 50% risk of affected offspring. Unaffected individuals are not carriers.

2. Ellis-van Creveld syndrome

Ellis-van Creveld syndrome, a rare autosomal recessive condition, is also called chondroectodermal dysplasia. The hair, nails, teeth, oral cavity, bones, and heart are involved. The disorder has been identified in many ethnic groups, including French, Italian, English, Scottish, Irish, Dutch, and blacks, but is most concentrated in inbred populations such as the Amish of Pennsylvania.[40,41]

The major clinical finding of Ellis-van Creveld syndrome is short-limbed dwarfism. The trunk is of normal length, but long bones do not grow normally. There is metaphyseal thickening, and the long bones do not achieve a normal length. The shortening is more marked distally. Postaxial polydactyly is common. Hypoplastic and dystrophic fingernails and toenails are frequently present. Oral manifestations include accessory labiogingival frenula, commonly associated with a serrated mandibular alveolar process. The teeth may be malformed and the enamel hypoplastic. Other ectodermal abnormalities are hypotrichosis and fine texture of the hair.

Congenital cardiac abnormalities, commonly atrial septal defect or single atrium, occur in 50% of the patients.[42,43] Less frequent anomalies include ventricular septal defect, primum atrial septal defect with cleft mitral valve or cleft tricuspid valve, atrioventricular canal, single ventricle with atrial septal defect, and total anomalous pulmonary venous return, either isolated or in combination with other cardiac anomalies.

Generally, affected individuals are born to carrier parents. Risk for other affected siblings is 25%. Occurrence of this disorder is rare outside inbred populations.

3. Syndromes associated with prolonged QT interval

In two hereditary syndromes, prolongation of the QT interval, often associated with T wave abnormalities, occurs. These patients are prone to ventricular arrhythmias, syncope, and sudden death.

a. Jervell and Lange-Nielsen syndrome (cardioauditory syndrome) This syndrome, characterized by deafness, cardiac conduction abnormalities, and syncopal episodes, is inherited as an autosomal recessive trait.[44] Deafness is congenital, profound, and symmetrical. Syncopal attacks begin in infancy and may occur infrequently or as often as daily. At least 50% of patients die during a syncopal attack, presumably from ventricular fibrillation. In addition to the prolonged QT interval, the T waves are large and show an abnormal axis, indicating an abnormality of ventricular repolarization. The use of digitalis, propranolol, and cardiac pacemakers has been described, but the data are insufficient to indicate the long-term success of each of these three forms of treatment.

b. Romano-Ward syndrome (long QT syndrome without deafness) In this autosomal dominant condition, prolonged QT interval is associated with syncopal episodes, but not with deafness.[45] At least 50% of patients die before adolescence due to syncopal episodes. In addition to prolonged QT interval and large T waves, the U waves are prominent. Treatment is with digitalis, propranolol, and/or pacemaker, but the long-term results are yet to be determined.

4. Kartagener syndrome

Kartagener syndrome, an autosomal recessive disease, consists of situs inversus, including dextrocardia, bronchiectasis, and sinusitis.[46] A wide phenotypic variation may occur within a sibship. The situs inversus may be complete or incomplete and, despite the associated dextrocardia, congenital cardiac anomalies are uncommon.

Recent studies[47] provide understanding of the respiratory problems and the frequent occurrence of infertility among males with this syndrome. Defective or ineffective ciliary action has been found in sperm of males with Kartagener syndrome and subsequently described in respiratory mucous membranes. There is slow or absent mucociliary transport, and absence of dynein arms in cilia. Other anomalies of cilia, including deficient or extra microtubules, are also found. Because of the defective cilia, the mucociliary clearance mechanism functions inadequately and chronic pulmonary disease of bronchi and sinuses results.

Because of the abnormal findings of the cilia, the name "immobile-cilia syndrome" has been developed. The relationship between the ciliary abnormality and the tendency for situs inversus is unknown, but the concurrence may suggest that genes controlling formation of cilia and determining situs are linked. Layton has given an explanation for the various types of situs.[48] Situs solitus is determined by a dominant gene that normally controls situs solitus. His studies suggest that when this gene is absent visceral situs, whether situs solitus, situs inversus, or situs ambiguous, is determined in a random fashion.

5. Noonan syndrome

Noonan syndrome (also known as male Turner syndrome, Turner phenotype with normal karyotype, XX or XY Turner phenotype, and Ullrich syndrome) was first described by Noonan.[49]

Noonan syndrome is probably inherited as an autosomal dominant trait, but with variable expression. For example, some individuals have severe congenital heart abnormalities and mild facial abnormalities, while others have marked facial manifestations and no cardiac disease. Chromosomal analysis in patients with Noonan syndrome has shown either a normal XX or XY karyotype.

The syndrome includes the following features: short stature, ocular hypertelorism, low-set ears, flat nasal bridge, ptosis, short and webbed neck, cubitus valgus, normal chest configuration, abnormal dermatoglyphics, and congenital heart disease. Not every affected individual has each of these characteristics, so there is a wide range of expression.

Cardiac malformations occur in 50% of individuals with Noonan syndrome. The most common is pulmonary valvular stenosis, usually secondary to a dysplastic pulmonary valve.[50,51] Atrial septal defect may coexist with the pulmonary stenosis. Much less frequent congenital cardiac anomalies include aortic stenosis, ventricular septal defect, tetralogy of Fallot, Ebstein anomaly, supravalvular pulmonary stenosis, and pulmonary arterial branch stenosis. In recent years, hypertrophic obstructive cardiomyopathy has been reported in patients with Noonan syndrome.[52,53] Patients with this cardiac problem may be asymptomatic or develop symptoms with progression of the obstruction.

The electrocardiograms of most patients with Noonan syndrome are unusual and characteristic. The QRS axis is superiorly directed in the frontal plane, usually between $-60°$ and $-120°$. This is particularly unusual in patients with pulmonary stenosis in which right axis deviation is expected. The echocardiograms may show eccentric ventricular hypertrophy of the superior portion of the anterior wall, the septum, and the diaphragmatic portion of the left ventricle (Fig. F.IV.5). The eccentric ventricular hypertrophy may be hemodynamically significant, and may be a variation of hypertrophic obstructive cardiomyopathy.

On chest x-ray films the heart size usually appears normal and, unlike typical valvular pulmonary stenosis, poststenotic dilation of the pulmonary trunk is not present. Right ventriculograms show a dysplastic, thickened pulmonary valve.

6. Leopard syndrome

Leopard is an acronym for the common associated features of *l*entigines, *e*lectrocardiographic abnormalities, *o*cular hypertelorism, *p*ulmonary stenosis, *a*bnormal genitalia, *r*etardation of growth, and *d*eafness (sensorineural).[54,55] Leopard syndrome is believed to be inherited as an autosomal dominant with variable expressivity, so affected individuals have wide variation in phenotype. Many of the features resemble Noonan syndrome.

Lentigines are small dark brown spots which in Leopard syndrome are widely distributed but concentrated over the trunk (Fig. F.IV.6). They may be present at birth or develop subsequently. Most patients with the Leopard syndrome, however, do not have lentigines. Electrocardiographic abnormalities include a superiorly oriented QRS axis ($-60°$ to $-120°$), and occasionally complete heart block or

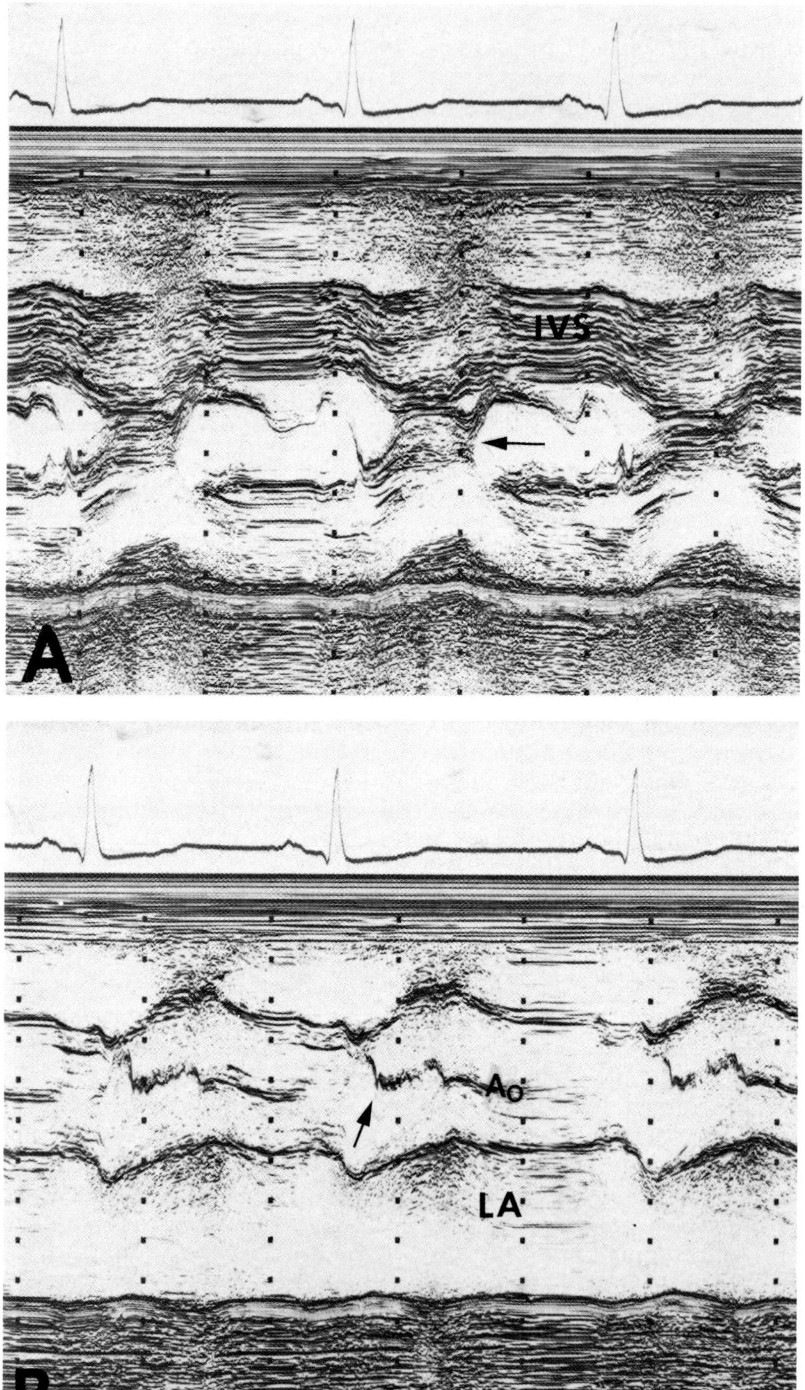

Fig. F.IV.5. Echocardiograms in 18-year-old male with Noonan syndrome. **A.** Recorded through body of left ventricle. Thickened interventricular septum (IVS). Systolic anterior motion of mitral valve (arrow). **B.** Recorded through root of aorta (Ao). Systolic flutter of aortic valve (arrow). LA = left atrium.

complete bundle branch block. The ocular hypertelorism is often associated with triangular-shaped face, ptosis, and low-set ears. Cardiovascular anomalies are common,[56] and pulmonary valvular stenosis due to a dysplastic valve is the most frequent malformation. There may be hypertrophic cardiomyopathy of the interventricular septum resulting in subaortic stenosis and subpulmonary stenosis.[57]

Hypospadias and cryptorchidism are common. Growth retardation occurs in 85% of the patients, with most being below the third percentile for both height and weight. Neurosensory deafness occurs in only 15%.

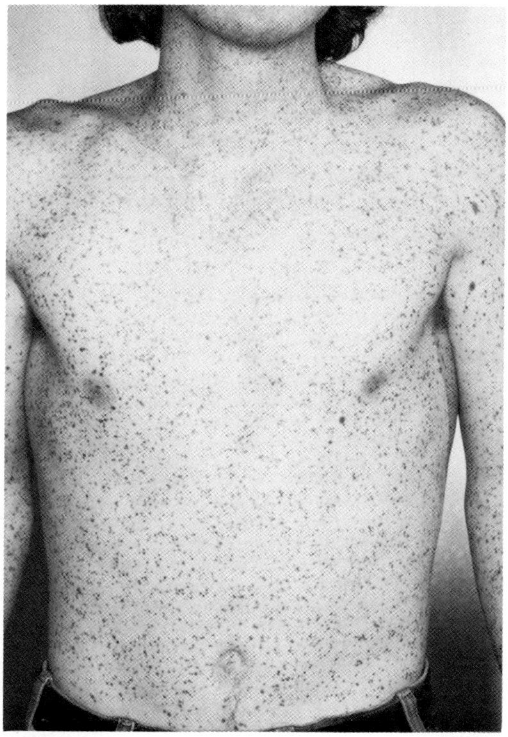

Fig. F.IV.6. Lentigines in 19-year-old male with Leopard syndrome.

B. Metabolic Diseases That Affect the Heart

Metabolic diseases that involve the heart have a number of features in common: they are a) generalized disorders that affect many organ systems; b) progressive; c) caused by the deficiency of an enzyme that allows metabolic products to accumulate in tissues including the heart; d) usually inherited as an autosomal recessive trait or a sex-linked recessive trait; and e) identifiable by biochemical tests that characterize the compounds that accumulate in tissue, and by assay revealing the specific enzyme deficiency.

1. Glycogen storage disease

Although numerous types of glycogen storage diseases have been described, and each may be associated with cardiac abnormalities, in most types cardiac changes are minimal and unimportant, except in type II (Pompe disease) and type III (Cori disease).

a. Pompe disease This disease is transmitted as an autosomal recessive trait. There is absence of lysosomal α-1,4-glucosidase, an enzyme that is concentrated in muscle tissue, but present in smaller amounts in other organs. As a result of the enzymatic deficiency, glycogen accumulates in most tissues, but principally in cardiac and skeletal muscle.[58] As myofibrils are replaced by glycogen, myocardial contractility decreases and myocardial mass increases.

Muscular weakness, cardiac failure, and hepatomegaly are present at birth or develop in early infancy. Ejection murmurs may be present, and cardiomegaly is invariable and massive.[59] Death occurs in the first year of life from congestive cardiac failure. There is no specific treatment.

The electrocardiogram and echocardiogram are diagnostic. The former shows tremendously large QRS complexes (up to 25 mV) and a pattern of either left or biventricular hypertrophy (Fig. F.IV.7). ST and T wave changes in the left precordial leads and a shortened PR interval are common.

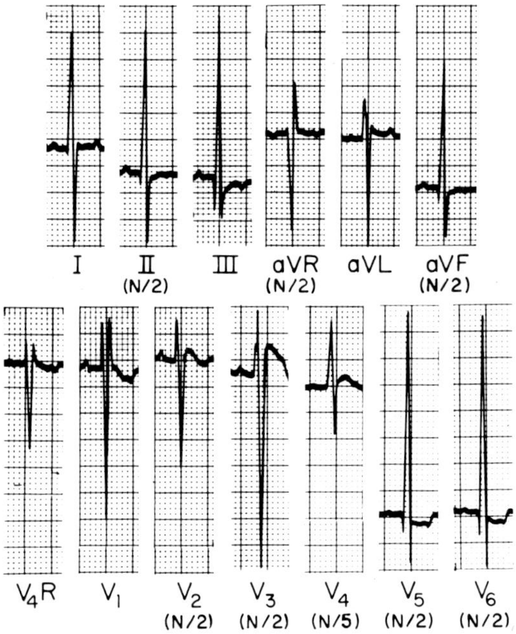

Fig. F.IV.7. Electrocardiogram. Glycogen storage disease type II. Seven-month-old infant. Large QRS voltages. Several leads recorded at half standardization (N/2) and lead V_4 at one-fifth standardization (N/5). Left ventricular hypertrophy. T waves inverted in left precordial leads. (From Moller and Neal,[60] with permission.)

The echocardiogram shows a greatly thickened interventricular septum and posterior left ventricular wall.[61] Findings of muscular subaortic stenosis may be observed.

Diagnosis can be made by demonstrating absence of the enzyme in leukocytes. Prenatal diagnosis is possible by assay of the enzyme in cells from amniotic fluid.

b. Cori disease (limit dextrinosis) This results from a deficiency of amylo-1,6-glucosidase and is inherited as an autosomal recessive trait. Clinical features resulting from the storage of glycogen are a) retarded growth, b) tendency to obesity, c) moderate cardiomegaly,[59] d) yellowish skin, and e) wide-based swinging gait. The disease follows a benign course unless cardiac involvement is extensive. Even with cardiomegaly, the cardiac exam and electrocardiogram are often normal, but sensitivity to anesthesia and cardiodepressive drugs may be present.

2. Mucopolysaccharidoses

The mucopolysaccharidoses include a varied group of inherited metabolic disorders characterized by the accumulation of mucopolysaccharides (glycosaminoglycans). Each type of mucopolysaccharidosis is due to lysosomal deficiency of enzymes involved in mucopolysaccharide metabolism. The severity of the diseases varies, but most are progressive. Since mucopolysaccharides are an important component of connective tissue, the mucopolysaccharide accumulates in multiple organ systems.

Diagnosis of the exact mucopolysaccharidosis rests on identification of excessive amounts of urinary mucopolysaccharide and the measurement of specific enzymatic deficiencies.

a. Hurler syndrome (MPS-IH) This is an autosomal recessive disease that results from deficiency of α-L-iduronidase, which is important in degradation of both dermatan and heparan sulfate. The features include progressive coarsening of facial features (Fig. F.IV.8), hepatosplenomegaly, joint stiffness, kyphosis, umbilical and inguinal hernias, small stature, enlarged head, corneal clouding, and mental retardation. Death usually occurs before 10 years.

Although the heart is usually involved, in only half of the patients is clinical evidence of cardiovascular problems present.[62] A murmur of mitral insufficiency may be heard, and occasionally there is one of aortic insufficiency. Hypertension is common, presumably from renal involvement. The heart is often enlarged, and cardiac failure commonly is the cause of death.

Cells of many tissues have large, clear vacuoles of mucopolysaccharides and are called "gargoyle cells." Any layer of the heart may be involved, the most striking changes occurring in the coronary arteries and the valves.[63,64] Coronary arterial in-

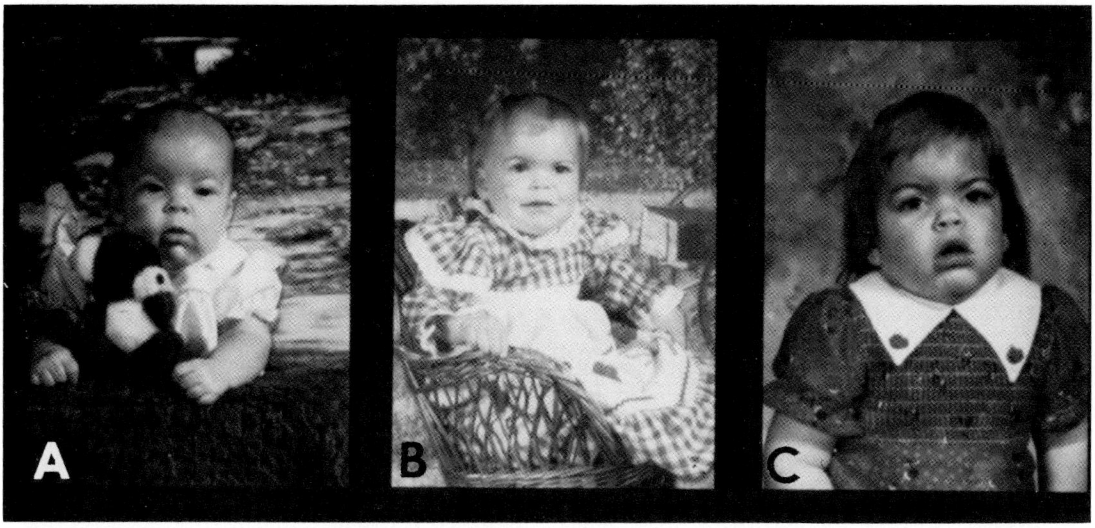

Fig. F.IV.8. Serial photographs showing progressive coarsening of facial features in a young girl with Hurler syndrome. A. 2.5 months; B. 17 months; and C. 36 months.

volvement occurs in 20% of patients. Mucopolysaccharides accumulate in the intima, and less commonly in the media. This, together with fibroblastic proliferation causes coronary arterial narrowing. Histologic evidence of myocardial infarction is, however, uncommon.

Valvular involvement is most frequent in the mitral valve and less frequent in the aortic and tricuspid valves. The mitral valve shows thickening and shortening of the chordae tendineae, yielding either mitral stenosis or insufficiency (Fig. F.IV.9). The aortic valve leaflets may also be thickened.

Diagnosis of Hurler disease can be established by assay of leukocytes for α-L-iduronidase. Prenatal diagnosis can be performed with assay of cultured amniotic cells for α-L-iduronidase and also by finding impaired degradation of acid mucopolysaccharides in amniotic cells.

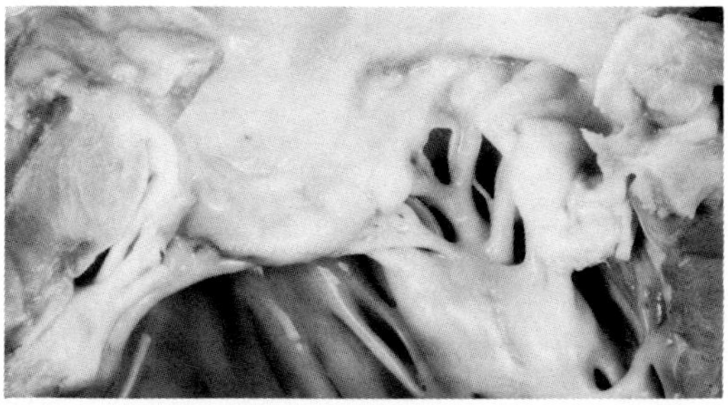

Fig. F.IV.9. Papillary muscle and adjacent portion of mitral valve from a patient with Hurler syndrome. Thickened valve leaflets and chordae tendineae.

b. Hunter syndrome (MPS II) This is an X-linked recessive disease with clinical and cardiac findings similar to those in Hurler syndrome (MPS-IH), except that corneal clouding does not occur and survival is longer. The disease results from a deficiency of iduronate sulfatase, and both dermatan and heparan sulfate are excreted in the urine. Storage of mucopolysaccharides occurs throughout the body. Clinically both mild and severe forms of Hunter syndrome have been described that cannot be differentiated biochemically, but are possibly allelic mutations.

As in Hurler syndrome, cardiac disease is manifest in valvular and coronary arterial changes and is the usual cause of death.[65]

Prenatal diagnosis can be on cultured amniotic cells by mucopolysaccharide accumulation technique and by direct assay for the deficient enzyme.

c. Sanfilippo syndrome (MPS III) Mental retardation is the striking feature of Sanfilippo syndrome and, although skeletal and somatic features are present, they are mild. Corneal clouding does not occur, and cardiac involvement is uncommon. Herd and associates[66] have described a young child with Sanfilippo syndrome who required valve replacement for severe mitral insufficiency.

Three types of Sanfilippo syndrome exist, each being an autosomal recessive trait. In type A, heparan N-sulfatase is deficient, and in type B, N-acetyl-α-glucosaminidase is absent. Both of these enzymatic deficiencies lead to accumulation of heparan sulfate. Type C has a deficiency of acetyl CoA-α-glucosaminide-N-acetyltransferase. Prenatal diagnosis by enzymatic analysis of cultured amniotic cells is possible for types A and B.

d. Scheie syndrome (MPS-IS) This autosomal recessive disease results from a deficiency of α-L-iduronidase, the same enzyme that is deficient in Hurler syndrome. The disease is characterized by severe corneal clouding, deformity of the hands, normal intelligence, aortic valvular disease, but few other somatic abnormalities. Hepatosplenomegaly is not present, growth is normal, and the facies are normal or slightly coarse. The pathologic changes in the aortic valve are similar to those seen in Hurler syndrome and are related to mucopolysaccharide deposition in the valvar cusps. Aortic insufficiency or stenosis is generally mild, and the disease is associated with a normal life-span.

Diagnosis can be made by demonstration of urinary excretion of mucopolysaccharide and subsequent measurement of α-L-iduronidase activity in leukocytes. Discrimination between Hurler syndrome and Scheie syndrome is generally made on the basis of the clinical course, and it is likely that these two syndromes are caused by allelic forms of a single gene.

e. Morquio syndrome (MPS IV) This is an autosomal recessive disease due to deficiency of 6-sulfo-N-acetylhexosaminide sulfatase, leading to excess urinary excretion of keratan sulfate, a substance usually present only in cartilage, the nucleus pulposus, and the cornea. Corneal clouding is present. The striking findings are marked skeletal anomalies leading to severe dwarfism. Frequently there is an associated complication of cervical myelopathy that may lead to quadraplegia. Many affected patients have genu valgum, short thorax, pectus excavatum, and characteristic facies.

Cardiac involvement has consisted mainly of aortic valvular disease—either stenosis or, more commonly, insufficiency. Many patients survive to the third to fifth decade, usually succumbing to cardiorespiratory failure.

f. Maroteaux-Lamy syndrome (MPS VI) An autosomal recessive trait, Maroteaux-Lamy results from deficiency of 4-sulfa-N-acetylgalactosaminide sulfatase (arylsulfatase B) and leads to excessive urinary excretion of dermatan sulfate and storage of mucopolysaccharides.

Affected individuals may have facial and other features like Hurler syndrome, but generally normal intelligence. At least three forms have been reported: mild, intermediate, and severe. In mildly affected patients, life-span may be near normal, but severely affected individuals may not survive childhood.

Murmurs of aortic stenosis[67] or mitral insufficiency have been described, and cardiac failure may develop, depending on the severity of the valvular lesion. Diagnosis is obtained by enzymatic assay, and prenatal diagnosis after amniocentesis is possible.

3. Mucolipidoses

The mucolipidoses represent a heterogeneous group of biochemical disorders characterized by accumulation of excessive amounts of mucopolysaccharides, sphingolipids, and glycolipids in visceral and connective tissue cells. Unlike mucopolysaccharidoses, excess mucopolysaccharides are not found in the urine. This group of disorders includes mucolipidoses types I, II, III, IV, mannosidosis, and fucosidosis. These biochemical disorders are rare, and information about cardiac involvement is incomplete. Some information about cardiac involvement is available for mucolipidosis II, mucolipidosis III, mannosidosis, and fucosidosis.

a. Mucolipidosis II (I-cell disease) In mucolipidosis II, somatic features similar to Hurler syndrome are evident at birth. Infants have coarse facies, thoracic deformities, dysostosis multiplex, retarded psychomotor development, and recurrent respiratory infections. Inherited as an autosomal recessive trait, it results from lysosomal deficiency of a large number of enzymes involved in the metabolism of mucopolysaccharides and various lipid compounds. The deficient enzymes include β-galactosidase, N-actyl-β-galactosaminidase, β-glucuronidase, α-mannosidase, and α-L-iduronidase. Increased levels of these enzymes are found in serum, cerebrospinal fluid, and urine, suggesting an abnormality in their transport into lysosomes.

The heart shows myocardial infiltration by stored lipid compounds and thickening of the cardiac valve leaflets and chordae tendineae, particularly of the mitral valve.[68]

b. Mucolipidosis III Mucolipidosis III is characterized by a claw hand deformity, severe dysostosis multiplex, markedly short stature, corneal clouding, and progressive bone deformity, most apparent in the hands, hips, elbows, and shoulders. All patients have mental retardation. This autosomal recessive disorder is characterized by intracellular deficiency and elevated serum levels of the same enzymes found in mucolipidoses II.

Information on cardiovascular abnormalities in mucolipidoses III is limited. In a number of patients, murmurs of aortic or mitral valvular diseases are found. Most commonly aortic insufficiency is diagnosed.[69] Pathologic confirmation is not available.

c. Mannosidosis Mannosidosis is a generalized storage disorder causing many features found in the mucopolysaccharidoses, but the level of mucopolysaccharides in the urine is normal. Elevated levels of mannose-containing compounds are present in various tissues, and a deficiency of the lysosomal enzyme α-mannosidase can be demonstrated. Inheritance follows an autosomal recessive pattern. The clinical features include coarsening of the facies, hepatosplenomegaly, and psychomotor retardation. Most of the patients manifest severe deafness.

Autopsy studies of a patient who died at the age of 3½ years revealed lysosomal deposition of mannose-containing compounds in the myocardium, endocardium, cardiac valves, and conduction system. In addition, electrocardiograms from several patients with mannosidosis have revealed shortened PR intervals (Fig. F.IV.10).[70,71]

d. Fucosidosis In fucosidosis, the enzyme α-L-fucosidase is deficient and fucose accumulates. This is inherited as an autosomal recessive trait. Infantile, juvenile, and adult forms have been described, indicating a spectrum of severity and manifestations. Most patients have recurrent infections, loss of muscular

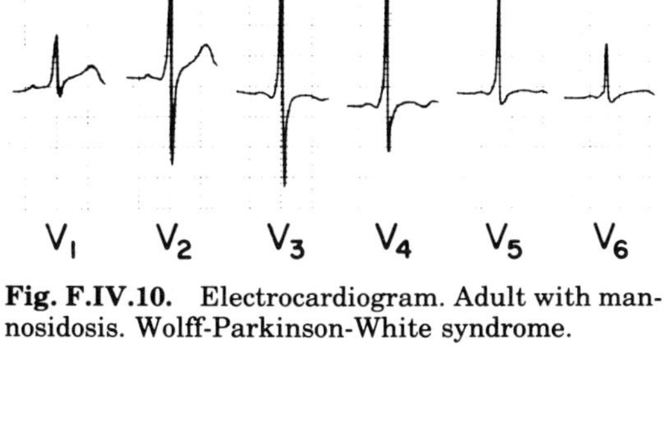

Fig. F.IV.10. Electrocardiogram. Adult with mannosidosis. Wolff-Parkinson-White syndrome.

strength, mental retardation, dysostosis multiplex, and progressive neurological deterioration.

Cardiac disease has been manifested by cardiac enlargement, rhythm disturbances, and electrocardiographic changes.[72] Autopsy studies have demonstrated infiltration of myocardial fibers by fucose.[72,73]

4. Sphingolipidoses

There are many disorders due to deficiency of enzymes necessary for sphingolipid degradation. The compounds that accumulate in tissues have a common chemical core consisting of a long chain aminoalcohol called sphingosine, which is attached by an amide linkage to a long chain fatty acid to form a ceramide. Different sphingolipids are due to the various polar groups linked to the C-1 primary hydroxyl group of sphingosine.

Among the disorders included as sphingolipidoses are Farber disease, Niemann-Pick disease, Gaucher disease, Krabbe disease, metachromatic leukodystrophy, Fabry disease, Tay-Sachs disease, Sandhoff disease, and G_{M1} gangliosidosis. Information on cardiac involvement in these disorders is limited, and only Fabry, Gaucher, Niemann-Pick, and the gangliosidoses will be discussed.

a. Fabry disease This is an X-linked disorder in which the enzyme α-galactosidase is deficient and neutral glycosphingolipids (ceramide-trihexosides) accumulate, particularly in endothelial, perithelial, and smooth muscles of the vascular system. Lesser amounts accumulate in the reticuloendothelial, connective, and myocardial tissues and in the autonomic nervous system.

Fabry disease is characterized by typical skin lesions (angiokeratomas located between umbilicus and knees), excruciating episodes of pain, hypohidrosis, renal failure, lymphedema of the legs, and corneal opacities.

Cardiac involvement increases with age, occurring as a result of renal hypertension, coronary arterial involvement, and infiltration of the myocardium and valves with large amounts of the Fabry lipid.[74] With age, the ventricular walls and interventricular septum become greatly thickened (Fig. F.IV.11) and the valves, principally the aortic and mitral valves, show thickening and nodularity. Interchordal hooding of the mitral valve may be associated with mitral regurgitation.

Clinical manifestations of cardiac involvement include anginal chest pain, myocardial infarction, congestive cardiac failure, and cardiomegaly. Murmurs of mitral insufficiency or aortic stenosis may be present.[74] The electrocardiogram characteristically shows a short PR interval[75] and also signs of myocardial infarction, ventricular hypertrophy, ST-T wave changes, and dysrhythmias. In adult patients with this disease, the echocardiogram shows ventricular myocardial thickening.

Diagnosis can be made by showing the deficiency of the enzyme or by analyzing tissue for the Fabry lipids. Prenatal diagnosis by enzymatic assay of amniotic cells is possible.

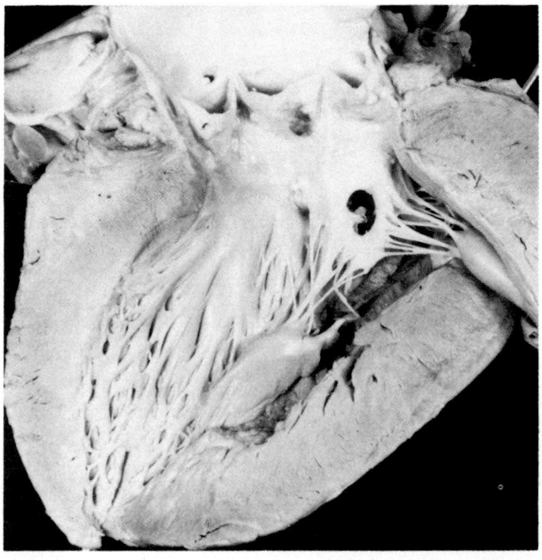

Fig. F.IV.11. Fabry's disease. Left ventricle and aortic root. Thickened left ventricular free wall. Perforation of anterior leaflet of mitral valve secondary to bacterial endocarditis. Nodularity of aortic valve.

b. Gaucher disease Gaucher disease is inherited as an autosomal recessive trait causing a deficiency of glucocerebrosidase. As a result, glucocerebrosides accumulate, primarily in reticuloendothelial cells. This is the most frequently occurring sphingolipidosis and is variable in severity and course. It has been divided into three types: I—chronic nonneuropathic (adult); II—acute neuropathic (infantile); and III—subacute neuropathic (juvenile). In each type the spleen, liver, and bone marrow are infiltrated with glucocerebroside, leading to hepatosplenomegaly, leukopenia, anemia, and bleeding disorders. In types II and III the central nervous system is involved, causing spasticity and regression of motor function.

Constrictive pericarditis has been described in Gaucher disease,[76,77] but it is not life-threatening. The pulmonary capillaries and lymphatics may be infiltrated with glucocerebrosides, causing pulmonary hypertension.[78]

Diagnosis rests upon enzymatic determination or tissue analysis. Prenatal diagnosis can be made from cultured amniotic cells.

c. Niemann-Pick disease This autosomal recessive disease caused by deficiency of sphingomyelinase, leads to accumulation of sphingomyelin. Sphingomyelin accumulates in lysosomes, forming large foam cells in many organs, particularly the liver, spleen, bone marrow, lungs, and nervous system. The foam cells may be found in the heart, and cardiac dysfunction was the cause of death in one patient. Endocardial fibroelastosis has been reported.[79]

Several variant forms of Niemann-Pick disease are known: infantile, juvenile, chronic, adult, or Nova-Scotian variant. In some of these, deficiency of sphingomyelinase can be detected. Prenatal diagnosis of at least the infantile form is possible.

d. Gangliosidoses The gangliosidoses are diseases of glycosphingolipid metabolism caused by intracellular deficiency of various lysosomal hydrolases causing deposition of gangliosides in various tissues. Gangliosides are sphingolipids with at least one sialic acid residue. Diseases result from the accumulation of either G_{M1} gangliosides or G_{M2} gangliosides. For each of the gangliosidoses, inheritance is as an autosomal recessive trait.

i. G_{M1} gangliosidoses

G_{M1} gangliosidoses can be divided into two major types, but other unusual variants with different clinical presentations and phenotypes have been described.

(a) G_{M1} gangliosidosis type I Patients with G_{M1} gangliosidosis type I (infantile generalized gangliosidosis) present within the first two months of life. The major features are coarse facial features, marked bony involvement, enlarged liver and spleen, and progressive mental and motor deterioration. Most die by three years of age. The disease is caused by a deficiency of β-galactosidase. Autopsies have revealed cardiomegaly and foamy histiocytes in the myocardium.[80] Diffuse thickening and nodularity of the mitral valve leaflets occurs. The aortic and mitral valve leaflets are infiltrated by histiocytes containing lipid material. Coronary arterial occlusion by atheromatous-like material and cells with foamy cytoplasm has been reported.[81]

(b) G_{M1} gangliosidosis type II G_{M1} gangliosidosis type II has a later onset and is considered the juvenile variant. The enzyme β-galactosidase is deficient. The disease becomes symptomatic at about 1 year of age. There is progressive developmental regression. Skeletal deformities and enlargement of the liver and spleen are not prominent. Death usually occurs by age 4 to 5 years. The viscera reveal infiltration by foamy histiocytes.

Several other forms of G_{M1} gangliosidosis have been described, but too few patients are reported to classify them as major types of G_{M1} gangliosidosis.

abnormalities,[99] but no consistent pattern. Asymmetric septal hypertrophy and systolic anterior movement of the mitral valve have been described, but a recent study showed concentric left ventricular hypertrophy and abnormal diastolic relaxation.

D. Connective Tissue Diseases

In connective tissue diseases, formation of connective tissue is defective. Cardiac abnormalities occur in a number of connective tissue disorders involving cardiac valves and major arteries. Evidence of cardiac involvement usually develops during childhood rather than being present from birth.

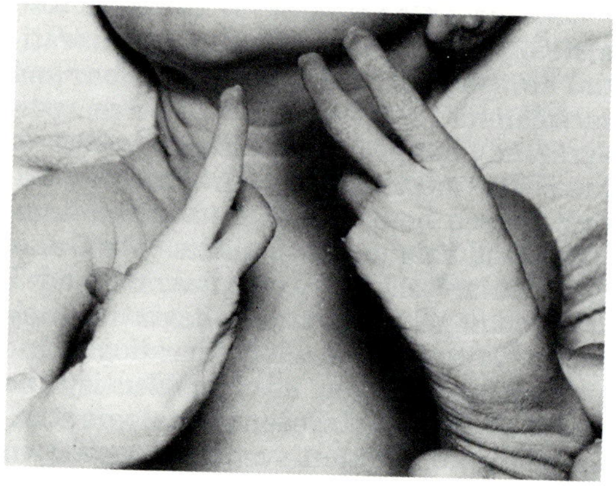

Fig. F.IV.16. Arachnodactyly. Neonate with Marfan syndrome.

1. Marfan syndrome

This autosomal dominant condition is assumed to be an error of protein metabolism, particularly with collagen and elastin. Although involvement is widespread, the major clinical manifestations occur in the heart, eye, and skeletal tissues.[100]

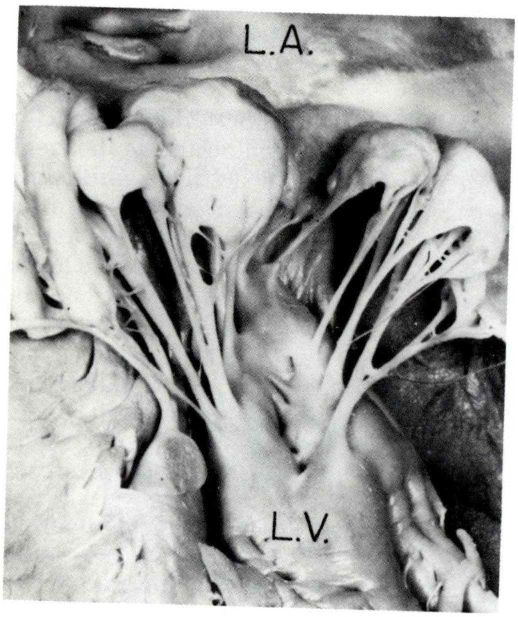

Fig. F.IV.15. Mitral valve. Marfan syndrome. Elongated chordae tendineae. Marked hooding of mitral valve leaflets. Left atrium (LA) and left ventricle (LV). (From Grondin et al,[102] with permission.)

Sixty percent of affected children[101] have cardiac involvement, but the severity and form are variable. The leading cause of death in patients with Marfan syndrome is from cardiac complications. Mitral valve prolapse is the most common cardiac problem in infants and children. Pathologic, auscultatory, and echocardiographic features of mitral valve prolapse are frequently found. The elongated chordae tendineae (Fig. F.IV.15) allow the mitral valve leaflets to prolapse into the left atrium during systole, particularly during mid and late portions. Mitral regurgitation may be severe and lead to congestive cardiac failure. The aorta is also commonly involved, with aneurysmal dilatation of the ascending aorta characteristically involving the aortic root and aortic sinuses. (This can be easily recognized by echocardiography, and the aortographic appearance is diagnostic.) Aortic regurgitation may develop. Involvement of the ascending aorta by a process of cystic medial necrosis is associated with the serious, usually fatal complication of dissecting aneurysm.

Subluxation of the ocular lenses, present in up to 80% of cases, is bilateral and rarely progressive. The lens is usually dislocated superiorly. Since the zonules remain intact, the eye can accommodate, but is myopic.

Several skeletal manifestations are found, including dolichostenomelia, arachnodactyly (Fig. F.IV.16), scoliosis, pectus excavatum, pes planus, lax joints, and high arched palate.

Recognition of the Marfan syndrome is important in order to counsel individuals or parents regarding genetic implications of the disease.[103] In involved individuals, life expectancy is reduced,[104] principally because of cardiac complications. Women with Marfan syndrome should be advised of an added risk of cardiac complications during pregnancy.

2. Contractural arachnodactyly

Contractural arachnodactyly is an autosomal dominant disease that may be confused with Marfan syndrome[105] because the involved patients have arachnodactyly, kyphoscoliosis, pectus excavatum or carinatum, and are taller than normal. But their joints, instead of showing the laxity of Marfan syndrome, have contractures. Characteristically the ears are "crumpled" due to flat top of the helix and antihelix and partial obliteration of the concha. The eyes, heart, and intelligence have usually been normal, but one case with mitral valve prolapse and dilated aortic sinuses has been described.[106]

3. Homocystinuria

Homocystinuria, an autosomal recessive disorder with more than one variant, must be considered in the differential diagnosis of Marfan syndrome, since its skeletal and ocular anomalies are quite similar. The disease results from an inborn error of methionine metabolism, deficiency of cystathionine synthetase.[107] Diagnosis can be established by discovery of increased plasma methionine and homocystine and increased urinary homocystine.

Skeletal anomalies[108,109] include: genu valgum, pes cavus, pectus excavatum or carinatum, arachnodactyly, scoliosis, kyphosis, and dolichostenomelia. Ectopic lenses are common, but they are displaced downward and accommodation is affected. Mild or moderate mental retardation is common. Characteristically the hair is light-colored or prematurely gray.

Thrombosis of medium-sized arteries or veins is a common circulatory problem and may lead to cerebral vascular accident, myocardial infarction, or renal hypertension.

Recognition of this disease is important in order to distinguish it from Marfan syndrome, which has a different prognosis, complications, and inheritance. Following administration of vitamin B_6, half of patients with homocystinuria show decrease in plasma concentration of homocystine and improvement of clinical manifestations, including mental retardation.

4. Ehlers-Danlos syndrome

Ehlers-Danlos is a name applied to a group of at least seven separate conditions, each with distinct clinical and genetic patterns.[110] In common, these conditions have joint laxity and friable, hyperelastic skin. Genetic patterns of autosomal dominant, autosomal recessive, and X-linked recessive have been described for the individual conditions.

Cardiovascular abnormalities are common[111] and include tortuosity and occasional rupture of systemic arteries.[112] Mitral valve prolapse is common.[113] Cardiac anomalies are found in about 20% of patients, including congenital malformations and acquired valvular insufficiency.

E. Neurocutaneous Syndromes That Affect the Heart

A number of diseases are grouped as neurocutaneous syndromes or phakomatoses. These may be inherited as a single gene trait. Commonly, there is a tendency to form benign tumors that involve principally the skin, eye, and nervous system. Two of these syndromes with cardiovascular manifestations are tuberous sclerosis and neurofibromatosis.

It appears to be inherited as a dominant trait. We have observed one family in which the only three offspring had the condition, and each died before six months of age.[133]

E. Cardiomyopathy (Exclusive of Asymmetric Septal Hypertrophy)

The cardiac manifestations of several conditions discussed in this chapter are those of a cardiomyopathy. There remain, however, instances in which more than one member of a family has clinical features and pathologic findings of a cardiomyopathy. In these patients the mode of inheritance appears to be autosomal dominant,[134] and in our experience they have a poor prognosis. Undoubtedly these patients represent a heterogeneous group of conditions that will be more fully understood as further biochemical and ultrastructural studies are performed.

V. UNCOMMON FAMILIAL PROBLEMS WITH POSSIBLE MULTIFACTORIAL INHERITANCE

In most (80–90%) instances of congenital heart disease, no etiologic factor or cause can be found. Studies of familial incidence have been carried out to determine if genetic factors may play a role. In a study from our institution the incidence of congenital cardiac malformations was greater than expected in siblings of children with a congenital cardiac malformation. At our institution[135] the overall incidence of affected siblings is 1.4%, compared to an expected rate of 0.77%. The incidence of 1.7% in later-born siblings[135] is similar to the 1.8% reported by Mori,[136] but less than the 2.8% reported by Nora and associates.[137]

The latter workers reported that the incidence in siblings corresponds closely to the square root of the incidence of the individual lesion in the general population, suggesting a multifactorial inheritance. They, however, included all cases of cardiac malformations in siblings, not just those that were identical, which may account for their reported higher incidence. No data are available to indicate statistical differences in recurrence rate for concordant or discordant lesions.

The incidence of congenital heart disease in parents of affected children[135] was only 0.6%, perhaps because of reduced life expectancy of patients with congenital cardiac malformations. The total incidence of congenital cardiac malformations in offspring of affected parents is perhaps 3%. The concordance rate for the cardiac malformation is closer between parent and child than between siblings (perhaps 30%). If a second child is affected, the recurrence risk is 5–10%, or 10–20% if a parent is also affected.

VI. RECOGNIZABLE SYNDROMES WITHOUT IDENTIFIED GENETIC PATTERN

In this final section, several easily recognizable syndromes are presented. In none has a clearly defined genetic pattern been found. Perhaps future studies will uncover their etiology.

A. DiGeorge Syndrome

The DiGeorge syndrome is a developmental complex that includes deficiency of the thymus and parathyroid glands, abnormal facies, and malformations of the heart and great vessels. Early in embryologic development, anomalous development of the derivatives of the third and fourth pharyngeal pouches occurs causing hypoplastic or aplastic thymus and parathyroid glands.[138] As a result, deficiency in cellular immunity and increased susceptibility to serious infections and severe hypocalcemia and seizures occur.

Congenital cardiovascular disease is present in most patients with DiGeorge syndrome[139–141] (80–90%). The most common cardiovascular malformations (Table F.IV.3) involve either vascular structures

TABLE F.IV.3. Congenital Cardiovascular Malformations in 76 Patients With DiGeorge Syndrome

Interruption of the aortic arch	20
Tetralogy of Fallot	18
Truncus arteriosus	11
Right aortic arch	16
Anomalous right subclavian artery	5
Anomalous left subclavian artery	1
Cervical aorta	1
Double aortic arch	1
Pulmonary stenosis	1
Transposition of the great vessels with pulmonary atresia	1
Double-outlet right ventricle	1

derived from the fourth aortic arch, including interruption of the aortic arch, right aortic arch, and anomalous right subclavian artery, or abnormalities of conotruncal differentiation such as tetralogy of Fallot and truncus arteriosus. Less frequent abnormalities are cervical aorta, double aortic arch, pulmonary stenosis, double-outlet right ventricle, and transposition of the great vessels. Two patients with tetralogy of Fallot had absent pulmonary valve. In infants with abnormalities of the aortic arch or conotruncus, the presence of hypocalcemia should alert the physician to this diagnosis.

The prognosis for an infant with DiGeorge syndrome and cardiac failure is poor. Most die because of congenital cardiac disease at less than 1 month of age. With age, the immunologic deficiency becomes less serious and may be corrected by thymic transplantation. One familial recurrence of the syndrome has been reported.

Perhaps abnormal perfusion of the fourth aortic arch during embryogenesis causes a failure of development or early regression of a transitional blood supply to the precursors of the third and fourth pharyngeal pouches. This compromised circulation leads to hypoplasia or absence of the thymus and parathyroids, which ordinarily develop later in fetal life.

B. Oculoauriculovertebral Dysplasia (Goldenhar Syndrome)

Oculoauriculovertebral dysplasia is another developmental complex of unknown origin. Most patients have ocular abnormalities (epibulbar dermoids, coloboma, or unilateral microphthalmia), ear anomalies (microtia or preauricular tags and blind fistulas), and vertebral defects (hemivertebrae or abnormal ribs). Cardiovascular malformations occur in 15–47% of patients with Goldenhar syndrome.[142–144] The most common cardiac malformation is tetralogy of Fallot, often with a right aortic arch. Pulmonary blood flow may be severely reduced. Ventricular septal defect, either isolated or coexisting with other abnormalities, is the second most common malformation. Patent ductus arteriosus, pulmonary stenosis, and abnormalities of the aortic arch have been reported. Other more complicated cardiovascular lesions, including pulmonary atresia, transposition of the great vessels with AV canal, and vascular ring, have been described.

Patients with Goldenhar syndrome may have associated pulmonary hypoplasia. Dextroposition of the heart because of marked hypoplasia of the right lung has been observed in several cases. Because of pulmonary hypoplasia, severe pulmonary hypertension may develop in association with a cardiac condition permitting a left-to-right shunt. Commonly, the hypoplastic lung occurs on the same side as the major facial anomalies.

C. Rubenstein-Taybi Syndrome

This is a syndrome without chromosomal anomaly or defined mode of inheritance. It is characterized by broad thumbs and toes and facial anomalies.[145] Other anomalies of digits include clinodactyly, overlapping digits, and duplicated phalanges. Facial abnormalities include antimongoloid slant of palpebral fissures, broad nasal bridge, beaked nose, prominent forehead, and heavy eyebrows and lashes. Small head circumference, large and delayed closure of fontanelles, and mental retardation occur and may be profound. Stature is small. Cardiac anomalies have been found in about a quarter of the patients, particularly patent ductus arteriosus and ventricular septal defect.

D. Radial Dysplasia

In radial dysplasia a spectrum of anomalies may exist, ranging from hypoplasia of first metacarpal and thumb, hypoplasia or absence of the radius, or absence of both the radius and ulna. These may occur either unilaterally or bilaterally.

Genetic counseling about radial dysplasia must consider its association with a number of conditions, including Holt-Oram syndrome, Fanconi anemia, thrombocytopenia, trisomy 13, trisomy 18, and Vater syndrome. Isolated radial dysplasia has been reported as both a dominant and a recessive trait. Rarely has a familial incidence of congenital heart disease been reported with radial dysplasia.

The more severe the radial anomaly, the greater the likelihood of congenital heart disease. Cardiac anomalies[146,147] include ventricular septal defect, dextrocardia, patent ductus arteriosus, coarctation of the aorta, and pulmonary stenosis.

VII. REFERENCES

1. Warkany J, Passarge E, Smith LB. Congenital malformations in autosomal trisomy syndromes. Am J Dis Child. 1966; 112:502–517.
2. Greenwood RD, Nadas AS. The clinical course of cardiac disease in Down's syndrome. Pediatrics. 1976; 58:893–897.
3. Park SC, Mathews RA, Zuberbuhler JR, Rowe RD, Neches WH, Lenox CC. Down syndrome with congenital heart malformation. Am J Dis Child. 1977; 131:29–33.
4. Tandon R, Edwards JE. Cardiac malformations associated with Down's syndrome. Circulation 1973; 47:1349–1355.
5. Chi TPL, Krovetz LJ. The pulmonary vascular bed in children with Down syndrome. J Pediatr. 1975; 86:533–538.
6. Weber FM, Sparkes RS. Trisomy E(18) syndrome: Clinical spectrum in 12 new cases, including chromosome autoradiography in 4. J Med Genet. 1970; 7:363–366.
7. Jue KL, Lockman LA, Edwards JE. Anomalous origins of pulmonary arteries from pulmonary trunk ("crossed pulmonary arteries") observation in a case with 18 trisomy syndrome. Am Heart J. 1966; 71:807–812.
8. Kurieu VA, Duke M. Trisomy 17-18 syndrome: Report of a case with diffuse myocardial fibrosis and review of cardiovascular abnormalities. Am J Cardiol. 1968; 21:431–435.
9. Hodes ME, Cole J, Palmer CG, Reed T. Clinical experience with trisomies 18 and 13. J Med Genet. 1978; 15:48–60.
10. Lemli L, Smith DW. The XO syndrome: A study of the differentiated phenotype in 25 patients. J Pediatr. 1963; 63:577–588.
11. VanderHauwaert LG, Fryns JP, Dumonlin M, Logghe N. Cardiovascular malformations in Turner's and Noonan's syndrome. Br Heart J. 1978; 40:500–509.
12. Nora JJ, Torres FG, Sinha AK, McNamara DG. Characteristic cardiovascular anomalies of XO Turner syndrome, XX and XY phenotype, and XO/XX Turner mosaic. Am J Cardiol. 1970; 25:639–641.
13. Miller OJ, Breg WR, Warburton D, Miller DA, deCapoa A, Allerdice PW, Davis J, Klinger HP, McGilvray E, Allen FH Jr. Partial deletion of the short arm of chromosome No. 4 ($4p^-$). Clinical studies in five unrelated patients. J Pediatr. 1970; 77:792–801.
14. Fernandes BJ, Gardner HA, Bedard YC. The $4p^-$ syndrome—an autopsy study. Hum Pathol. 1980; 11:683–685.
15. Guthrie RD, Aase JM, Asper AC, Smith DW. The $4p^-$ syndrome. A clinically recognizable chromosomal deletion syndrome. Am J Dis Child. 1971; 122:421–425.
16. Miller OJ, Warburton D, Breg WR. Deletions of group B chromosomes. In: Bergsma D, ed. Phenotypic Aspects of Chromosomal Aberrations, Part V. Baltimore: Williams & Wilkins for The National Foundation—March of Dimes. BD:OAS 1969; 5(5):100–105.
17. Taylor AI. Patau's, Edwards' and cri du chat syndromes: A tabulated summary of current findings. Dev Med Child Neurol. 1967; 9:78–86.
18. Breg WR, Steele MW, Miller OJ, Warburton D, deCapoa A, Allderdice PW. The cri du chat syndrome in adolescents and adults: Clinical findings in 13 older patients with partial deletion of the short arm of chromosome No. 5 ($5p^-$). J Pediatr. 1970; 77:782–791.
19. Pfeiffer RA. Trisomy 8. In: Yunis JJ, ed. New Chromosomal Syndromes. New York: Academic Press, 1975:197–217.
20. Crandall BF, Bass HN, Marcy SM, Glovsky M, Fish CH. The trisomy 8 syndrome. Two additional mosaic cases. J Med Genet. 1974; 11:393–398.
21. Cassidy SB, McGee BJ, vanEys J, Nance WE, Engel E. Trisomy 8 syndrome. Pediatrics 1975; 56:826–831.

22. Caspersson T, Lindsten J, Zech L, Buckton KE, Price WH. Four patients with trisomy 8 identified by the fluorescence and Giemsa banding techniques. J Med Genet. 1972; 9:1–7.
23. Bowen P, Ying KL, Chung GSH. Trisomy 9 mosaicism in a newborn infant with multiple malformations. J Pediatr. 1974; 85:95–97.
24. Haslam RHA, Broske SP, Moore CM, Thomas GH, Neill CA. Trisomy 9 mosaicism with multiple congenital anomalies. J Med Genet. 1973; 10:180–184.
25. Feingold M, Atkins L. A case of trisomy 9. J Med Genet. 1973; 10:184–187.
26. Taylor AI. Dq⁻, Dr and retinoblastoma. Humangenetik. 1970; 10:209–217.
27. Adams MS. Palm-prints and a ring D chromosome. Lancet. 1965; 2:494–495.
28. Gustavson KH, Hitrec V, Santesson B. Three non-mongoloid patients of similar phenotype with an extra G-like chromosome. Clin Genet. 1972; 3:135–146.
29. Zellweger H, Ionasescu V, Simpson J, Burmeister L. The problem of trisomy 22. A case report and a discussion of the variant forms. Clin Pediatr. 1976; 15:601–618.
30. Hirschhorn K, Lucas M, Wallace I. Precise identification of various chromosomal abnormalities. Ann Hum Genet. 1973; 36:375–379.
31. Bühler EM, Mehes K, Müller H, Stalder GR. Cat-eye syndrome, a partial trisomy 22. Humangenetik. 1972; 15:150–162.
32. Petersen RA. Schmid-Fraccaro syndrome ("cat's eye" syndrome). Partial trisomy of G chromosome. Arch Ophthalmol. 1973; 90:287–291.
33. Gerald PS, Davis CD, Say B, Wilkins J. Syndromal associations of imperforate anus: The cat-eye syndrome. In: Bergsma D, ed. G.I. Tract Including Liver and Pancreas. Huntington, New York: Robert E. Krieger for The National Foundation—March of Dimes. BD:OAS 1972; 8(2):79–84.
34. Freedom RM, Gerald PS. Congenital cardiac disease and the "cat-eye" syndrome. Am J Dis Child. 1973; 126:16–18.
35. Nora JJ, Nora AH. Genetics and Counseling in Cardiovascular Diseases. Springfield, Illinois: Charles C Thomas, 1978:40–41.
36. Karsh RB, Knapp RF, Nora JJ, Wolfe RR, Robinson A. Congenital heart disease in 49, XXXXY syndrome. Pediatrics. 1975; 56: 462–464.
37. Holt M, Oram S. Familial heart disease with skeletal malformations. Br Heart J. 1960; 22:236–242.
38. Gall JC Jr, Stern AM, Cohen MM, Adams MS, Davidson RT. Holt-Oram syndrome: Clinical and genetic study of a large family. Am J Hum Genet. 1966; 18:187–200.
39. Smith AT, Sack GH Jr, Taylor GJ. Holt-Oram syndrome. J Pediatr. 1979; 95:538–543.
40. Feingold M. Ellis-van Creveld syndrome. Clin Pediatr. 1966; 5:431–436.
41. DaSilva EO, Janovitz D, Da Albuquerque SC. Ellis-van Creveld syndrome: Report of 15 cases in an inbred kindred. J Med Genet. 1980; 17:349–356.
42. Lynch JI, Perry LW, Takakuwa T, Scott LP III. Congenital heart disease and chondroectodermal dysplasia. Report of two cases, one in a negro. Am J Dis Child. 1968; 115:80–87.
43. Engle MA, Ehlers KH. Ellis-van Creveld syndrome with asymmetric polydactyly and successful surgical correction of common atrium. In: Bergsma D, ed: Skeletal Dysplasias, Part IV. Baltimore: Williams & Wilkins for The National Foundation—March of Dimes, BD:OAS 1969; 5(4):65–67.
44. Jervell A, Lange-Nielsen F. Congenital deafmutism. Functional heart disease with prolongation of the Q-T interval and sudden death. Am Heart J. 1957; 54:59–68.
45. Garza LA, Vluk RL, Nora JJ, McNamara DG. Heritable Q-T prolongation without deafness. Circulation. 1970; 41:39–48.
46. Kartagener M. Zur pathogenese der bronchiertascen. I. Mitteilung bronchiectasien bei situs viscerum inversus. Beitr Klin Erforsch Tuberk Lungenkr. 1933; 83:489.
47. Eliasson R, Mossberg B, Camner P, Afzelius BA. The immotile-cilia syndrome. A congenital ciliary abnormality as an etiologic factor in chronic airway infections and male sterility. N Engl J Med. 1977; 297:1–6.
48. Layton WM Jr. Random determination of a developmental process: Reversal of normal visceral asymmetry in the mouse. J Hered. 1976; 67:336–338.
49. Noonan JA. Hypertelorism with Turner phenotype: A new syndrome with associated congenital heart disease. Am J Dis Child. 1968; 116:373–380.
50. Celermajer JM, Bowdler JD, Cohen DH. Pulmonary stenosis in patients with the Turner phenotype in the male. Am J Dis Child. 1968; 116:351–358.
51. Siggers DC, Polani PE. Congenital heart disease in male and female subjects with somatic features of Turner's syndrome and normal sex chromosomes (Ullrich's and related syndromes). Br Heart J. 1972; 34:41–46.
52. Hirsch HD, Gelband H, Garcia O, Gottlieb S, Tamer DM. Rapidly progressive obstructive cardiomyopathy in infants with Noonan's syndrome. Report of two cases. Circulation. 1975; 52:1161–1165.
53. Phornphutkul C, Rosenthal A, Nadas AS. Cardiomyopathy in Noonan's syndrome. Report of 3 cases. Br Heart J. 1973; 35:99–102.
54. Gorlin RJ, Anderson RC, Blaw M. Multiple lentigines syndrome. Am J Dis Child. 1969; 117:652–662.
55. Gorlin RJ, Anderson RC, Moller JH. The Leopard (multiple lentigines) syndrome revisited. In: Bergsma D, ed. BD:OAS 1971; 5(7): 110–115.

56. Kraunz RF, Blackmon JR. Cardiocutaneous syndrome continued. N Engl J Med. 1968; 279:325.
57. Somerville J, Bonham-Carter RE. The heart in lentiginosis. Br Heart J. 1972; 34:58–66.
58. Huijing F, vanCreveld S, Losekoot G. Diagnosis of generalized glycogen storage disease (Pompe's disease). J Pediatr. 1963; 63:984–987.
59. Hohn AR, Lowe CU, Sokal JE, Lambert EC. Cardiac problems in the glycogenoses with specific reference to Pompe's disease. Pediatrics. 1965; 35:313–321.
60. Moller JH, Neal WA. Heart Disease in Infancy. New York: Appleton-Century-Crofts, 1981:277.
61. Rees A, Elbl F, Minhas K, Solinger R. Echocardiographic evidence of outflow tract obstruction in Pompe's disease (glycogen storage disease of the heart). Am J Cardiol. 1976; 37:1103–1106.
62. Krovetz LJ, Lorincz AE, Schiebler GL. Cardiovascular manifestations of the Hurler syndrome. Hemodynamic and angiocardiographic observations in 15 patients. Circulation. 1965; 31:132–141.
63. Okada R, Rosenthal IM, Scaravelli G, Lev M. A histopathologic study of the heart in gargoylism. Arch Pathol. 1967; 84:20–30.
64. Renteria VG, Ferrans VJ, Roberts WC. The heart in the Hurler syndrome. Gross, histologic and ultrastructural observations in five necropsy cases. Am J Cardiol. 1976; 38:487–501.
65. Schieken RM, Kerber RE, Ionasescu VV, Zellweger H. Cardiac manifestations of the mucopolysaccharidoses. Circulation 1975; 52: 700–705.
66. Herd JK, Subramanian S, Robinson H. Type III mucopolysaccharidosis: Report of a case with severe mitral valve involvement. J Pediatr. 1973; 82:101–104.
67. Wilson CS, Mankin HT, Pluth JR. Aortic stenosis and mucopolysaccharidosis. Ann Intern Med. 1980; 92:496–498.
68. Martin JJ, Leroy JG, Farriaux JP, Fontaine G, Desnick RJ, Cabello A. I-cell disease (mucolipidosis II). A report on its pathology. Acta Neuropathol. 1975; 33:285–305.
69. McKusick VA, Neufeld EF, Kelly TE. The mucopolysaccharide storage disease. In: Stanbury JB, Wyngaarden JB, Fredrickson DS, eds. The Metabolic Basis of Inherited Disease, 4th Ed. New York: McGraw-Hill, 1978:1282–1307.
70. Desnick RJ, Sharp HL, Grabowski GA, Brunning RD, Quie PG, Sung JH, Gorlin RJ, Ikonne JU. Mannosidosis: Clinical, morphologic, immunologic, and biochemical studies. Pediatr Res. 1976; 10:985–996.
71. Mehta J, Desnick RJ. Abbreviated PR interval in mannosidosis. J Pediatr. 1978; 92:599–601.
72. Durand P, Philippart M, Barrone C, DellaCella G. A new glycolipid storage disease. Pediatr Res. 1967; 1:416.
73. Durand P, Barrone C, DellaCella G. Fucosidosis. J Pediatr. 1969: 75:665–674.
74. Desnick RJ, Blieden LC, Sharp HL, Hofschire PJ, Moller JH. Cardiac valvular anomalies in Fabry disease. Clinical, morphologic, and biochemical studies. Circulation. 1976; 54:818–825.
75. Mehta J, Tuna N, Moller JH, Desnick RJ. Electrocardiographic and vectorcardiographic abnormalities in Fabry's disease. Am Heart J. 1977; 93:699–705.
76. Benbassat J, Bassan H, Milwidsky H, Sacks M, Groen JJ. Constrictive pericarditis in Gaucher's disease. Am J Med. 1968; 44:647–652.
77. Harvey PKP, Jones MC, Anderson EG. Pericardial abnormalities in Gaucher's disease. Br Heart J. 1969; 31:603–606.
78. Roberts WC, Fredrickson DS. Gaucher's disease of the lung causing severe pulmonary hypertension with associated acute recurrent pericarditis. Circulation. 1967; 35:783–789.
79. Westwood M. Endocardial fibroelastosis and Niemann-Pick disease. Br Heart J. 1977; 39:1394–1396.
80. Landing BH, Silverman FN, Craig JM, Jacobi MD, Lahey ME, Chadwick DL. Familial neurovisceral lipidosis. Am J Dis Child. 1964; 108:503–522.
81. Hadley RN, Hagstrom JWC. Cardiac lesions in a patient with familial neurovisceral lipidosis (generalized gangliosidosis). Am J Clin Pathol. 1971; 55:237–240.
82. Rodriquez-Torres R, Schneck L, Kleinberg W. Electrocardiographic and biochemical abnormalities in Tay-Sachs disease. Bull NY Acad Med. 1971; 47:717–730.
83. Blieden LC, Desnick RJ, Carter JB, Krivit W, Moller JH, Sharp HL. Cardiac involvement in Sandhoff's disease: Inborn error of glycosphingolipid metabolism. Am J Cardiol. 1974; 34:83–88.
84. Sanyal SK, Leung RKF, Tierney RC, Gilmartin R, Pitner S. Mitral valve prolapse syndrome in children with Duchenne's progressive muscular dystrophy. Pediatrics. 1979; 63:116–123.
85. Mahoney MJ, Haseltine FP, Hobbins JC, Banker BQ, Caskey CT, Golbus MS. Prenatal diagnosis of Duchenne's muscular dystrophy. N Engl J Med. 1977; 297:968–973.
86. Zellweger H, Antonik A. Newborn screening for Duchenne muscular dystrophy. Pediatrics. 1975; 55:30–34.
87. Roses AD, Roses MJ, Miller SE, Hull KL Jr, Appel SH. Carrier detection in Duchenne muscular dystrophy. N Engl J Med. 1976; 294:193–198.
88. Pickard NA, Gruemer HD, Verrill HL, Isaacs ER, Robinow M, Nance WE, Myers EC, Goldsmith B. Systemic membrane defect in the proximal muscular dystrophies. N Engl J Med. 1978; 229:841–846.
89. Jackson CE, Strehler DA. Limb-girdle mus-

cular dystrophy: Clinical manifestations and detection of preclinical disease. Pediatrics. 1968; 41:495–502.

90. Baldwin BJ, Talley RC, Johnson C, Nutter DO. Permanent paralysis of the atrium in a patient with facioscapulohumeral muscular dystrophy. Am J Cardiol. 1973; 31:649–653.
91. Dodge PR, Gamstorp I, Byers RK, Russell P. Myotonic dystrophy in infancy and childhood. Pediatrics. 1965; 35:3–19.
92. Josephson ME, Caracta AR, Gallagher JJ, Damato AN. Site of conduction disturbances in a family with myotonic dystrophy. Am J Cardiol. 1973; 32:114–118.
93. Kennel AJ, Titus JL, Merideth J. Pathologic findings in the atrioventricular conduction system in myotonic dystrophy. Mayo Clin Proc. 1974; 49:838–842.
94. Prystowsky EN, Pritchett ELC, Roses AD, Gallagher J. The natural history of conduction system disease in myotonic muscular dystrophy as determined by serial electrocardiographic studies. Circulation. 1979; 60:1360–1364.
95. Perloff JK. Cardiomyopathy associated with heredofamilial neuromyopathic diseases. Modern Concepts Cardiovasc Dis. 1971; 40:23–26.
96. VanderHauwaert LG, Dumoulin M. Hypertrophic cardiomyopathy in Friedreich's ataxia. Br Heart J. 1976; 38:1291–1298.
97. Gach JV, Andriange M, Franck G. Hypertrophic obstructive cardiomyopathy and Friedreich's ataxia. Report of a case and review of literature. Am J Cardiol. 1971; 27:436–441.
98. Novick R, Adams P Jr, Anderson RC. Cardiac manifestations of Friedreich's ataxia in children. Lancet. 1955; 75:62–65.
99. St. John Sutton MG, Olukotun AY, Tajik AJ, Lovett JL, Giuliani ER. Left ventricular function in Friedreich's ataxia. An echocardiographic study. Br Heart J. 1980; 44:309–316.
100. Pyeritz RE, McKusick VA. The Marfan syndrome: Diagnosis and management. N Engl J Med. 1979; 300:772–778.
101. Phornphutkul C, Rosenthal A, Nadas AS. Cardiac manifestations of Marfan syndrome in infancy and childhood. Circulation. 1973; 47:587–596.
102. Grondin CM, Steinberg CL, Edwards JE. Dissecting aneurysm complicating Marfan's syndrome (arachnodactyly) in a mother and son. Am Heart J. 1969; 77:301–306.
103. Payvandi MH, Kerber RE, Phelps CD, Judisch GF, El-Khoury G, Schrott HG. Cardiac, skeletal and ophthalmologic abnormalities in relatives of patients with the Marfan syndrome. Circulation. 1977; 55:797–802.
104. Murdoch JL, Walker BA, Halpern BL, Kuzma JW, McKusick VA. Life expectancy and causes of death in the Marfan syndrome. N Engl J Med. 1972; 286:804–808.
105. Hecht F, Beals RK. "New" syndrome of congenital contractural arachnodactyly originally described by Marfan in 1896. Pediatrics 1972; 49:574–578.
106. Gruber MA, Graham TP Jr, Engel E, Smith C. Marfan syndrome with contractural arachnodactyly and severe mitral regurgitation in a premature infant. J Pediatr. 1978; 93:80–82.
107. Gerritsen T, Waisman HA. Homocystinuria, an error in the metabolism of methionine. Pediatrics. 1964; 33:413–420.
108. Carson NAJ, Dent CE, Field CMB, Gaull GE. Homocystinuria. Clinical and pathological review of ten cases. J Pediatr. 1965; 66:565–583.
109. Kennedy C, Shih VE, Rowland LP. Homocystinuria: A report in two siblings. Pediatrics. 1965; 36:736–741.
110. McKusick VA. Multiple forms of Ehlers-Danlos syndrome. Arch Surg. 1974; 109:475–476.
111. Antani J, Srinivas HV. Ehlers-Danlos syndrome and cardiovascular abnormalities. Chest. 1973; 63:214–217.
112. Lees MH, Menashe VD, Sunderland CO, Morgan CL, Dawson PJ. Ehlers-Danlos syndrome associated with multiple pulmonary artery stenoses and tortuous systemic arteries. J Pediatr. 1969; 75:1031–1036.
113. Brandt KD, Summer RD, Ryan TJ, Cohen AS. Herniation of mitral leaflets in the Ehlers-Danlos syndrome. Am J Cardiol. 1975; 36:524–528.
114. Lagos JC, Gomez MR. Tuberous sclerosis: Reappraisal of a clinical entity. Mayo Clin Proc. 1967; 42:26–49.
115. Tsakraklides V, Burke B, Mastri A, Runge W, Roe E, Anderson R. Rhabdomyomas of heart. A report of four cases. Am J Dis Child. 1974; 128:639–646.
116. Neal WA, Knight L, Blieden LC, Bessinger FB Jr, Edwards JE. Congenital rhabdomyoma of heart simulating tricuspid atresia. Am Heart J. 1975; 89:514–520.
117. Moller JH, Neal WA. Heart Disease in Infancy. New York: Appleton-Century-Crofts, 1981:114.
118. Fenoglio JJ Jr, McAllister HA Jr, Ferrans VJ. Cardiac rhabdomyoma: A clinicopathologic and electron microscopic study. Am J Cardiol. 1976; 38:241–251.
119. Kaufman RL, Harmann AF, McAlister WH. Family studies in congenital heart disease IV: Congenital heart disease associated with neurofibromatosis. In Bergsma D, ed. The Cardiovascular System, Part XV. Baltimore: Williams & Wilkins for The National Foundation—March of Dimes. BD:OAS 1972; 8(5):92–95.
120. Neiman HL, Mena E, Holt JF, Stern AM, Perry BL. Neurofibromatosis and congenital heart disease. Am J Roentgenol. 1974; 122:146–149.
121. Rosenquist GC, Krovetz LJ, Haller JA Jr, Simon AL, Bannayan GA. Acquired right ventricular outflow obstruction in a child with neurofibromatosis. Am Heart J. 1970; 79:103–108.
122. Garcia RE, Friedman WF, Kaback MM, Rowe

RD. Idiopathic hypercalcemia and supravalvular aortic stenosis. Documentation of a new syndrome. N Engl J Med. 1964; 271:117–120.
123. Jue KL, Noren GR, Anderson RC. The syndrome of idiopathic hypercalcemia of infancy with associated congenital heart disease. J Pediatr. 1965; 67:1130–1140.
124. Jones KL, Smith DW. The Williams elfin facies syndrome. A new perspective. J Pediatr. 1975; 86:718–723.
125. Underhill WL, Tredway JB, D'Angelo GJ, Baay JEW. Familial supravalvular aortic stenosis. Comments on the mechanisms of angina pectoris. Am J Cardiol. 1971; 27:560–565.
126. Schmidt RE, Gilbert EF, Amend TC, Chamberlain CR Jr, Lucas RV Jr. Generalized arterial fibromuscular dysplasia and myocardial infarction in familial supravalvular aortic stenosis syndrome. J Pediatr. 1969; 74:576–584.
127. Henry WL, Clark CE, Epstein SE: Asymmetric septal hypertrophy (ASH): The unifying link in the IHSS disease spectrum. Observations regarding its pathogenesis, pathophysiology, and course. Circulation 1973; 47:827–832.
128. Clark CE, Henry WL. Epstein SE. Familial prevalence and genetic transmission of idiopathic hypertrophic subaortic stenosis. N Engl J Med. 1973; 289:709–714.
129. ten Cate FJ, Hugenholtz PG, van Dorp WG, Roelandt J. Prevalence of diagnostic abnormalities in patients with genetically transmitted asymmetric septal hypertrophy. Am J Cardiol. 1979; 43:731–736.
130. Maron BJ, Lipson LC, Roberts WC, Savage DD, Epstein SE. "Malignant" hypertrophic cardiomyopathy: Identification of a subgroup of families with unusually frequent premature death. Am J Cardiol. 1978; 41:1133–1140.
131. Lynch HT, Mohiuddin S, Moran J, Kaplan A, Sketch M, Zencka A, Runco V. Hereditary progressive atrioventricular conduction defect. Am J Cardiol. 1975; 36:297–301.
132. Sarachek NS, Leonard JJ. Familial heart block and sinus bradycardia. Classification and natural history. Am J Cardiol. 1972; 29:451–457.
133. Davachi F, McLean RH, Moller JH, Edwards JE. Hypoplasia of right ventricle and tricuspid valve in siblings. J Pediatr. 1967; 71:869–874.
134. Kariv I, Kreisler B, Sherf L, Feldman S, Rosenthal T. Familial cardiomyopathy. A review of 11 families. Am J Cardiol. 1971; 28:693–706.
135. Anderson RC: Fetal and infant death, twinning and cardiac malformations in families of 2,000 children with and 500 without cardiac defects. Am J Cardiol. 1976; 38:218–224.
136. Mori K, Ando M, Takao A. Genetic aspects of congenital heart disease. Jpn Circ J. 1973; 37:35–39.
137. Nora JJ, McGill CW, McNamara DG. Empiric recurrent risks in common and uncommon congenital heart lesions. Teratology. 1970; 3:325–329.
138. Robinson HB Jr. DiGeorge's or the III–IV pharyngeal pouch syndrome: Pathology and a theory of pathogenesis. Perspect Pediatr Pathol. 1975; 2:173–206.
139. Freedom RM, Rosen FS, Nadas AS. Congenital cardiovascular disease and anomalies of the third and fourth pharyngeal pouch. Circulation. 1972; 46:165–172.
140. Finley JP, Collins GF, DeChadarévian JP, Williams RL. DiGeorge syndrome presenting as severe congenital heart disease in the newborn. Can Med Assoc J. 1977; 116:635–640.
141. Moerman P, Goddeeris P, Lauwerijns J, VanderHauwaert LG. Cardiovascular malformation in DiGeorge syndrome (congenital absence of hypoplasia of the thymus). Br Heart J. 1980; 44:452–459.
142. Greenwood RD, Rosenthal A, Sommer A, Wolff G, Craenen J. Cardiovascular malformations in oculoauriculovertebral dysplasia (Goldenhar syndrome). J Pediatr. 1974; 85:816–818.
143. Friedman S, Saraclar M. The high frequency of congenital heart disease in oculo-auriculovertebral dysplasia (Goldenhar's syndrome). J Pediatr. 1974; 85:873–874.
144. Shokeir MHK. The Goldenhar's syndrome. A natural history. In: Bergsma D, ed. Annual Review of Birth Defects, 1976. New York: Alan R. Liss, Inc. for The National Foundation—March of Dimes. BD:OAS 1977; 13(3):67–83.
145. Rubenstein JH, Taybi H. Broad thumbs and toes and facial abnormalities. Am J Dis Child. 1963; 105:588–608.
146. Carroll RE, Louis DS. Anomalies associated with radial dysplasia. J Pediatr. 1974; 84:409–411.
147. Harris LC, Osborne WP. Congenital absence or hypoplasia of the radius with ventricular septal defect: Ventriculo-radial dysplasia. J Pediatr. 1966; 68:265–272.

F.V

Infectious Causes of Congenital Abnormalities

Edwin G. Brown, MD, and Eugene Ainbender, MD

I. INTRODUCTION

Heart abnormalities are among the most common congenital malformations of the newborn infant. Heart defects occur approximately four to eight times in every 1,000 live births.[1–3] Quite simply, congenital heart malformations are inherited or caused by environmental factors or a combination of the two. The role of heredity and environment in relation to congenital heart defects has been extensively reviewed.[1–5]

Infection as a cause of congenital heart abnormalities (malformations or lesions acquired in utero),[6] is the subject of this chapter.

II. EVIDENCE FOR AN INFECTIOUS ETIOLOGY OF CONGENITAL HEART ABNORMALITIES

In 1941, Gregg described the association of maternal rubella contracted during pregnancy with the triad of cataracts, deafness, and congenital heart defects.[7] This important observation was soon confirmed by others.[8] Gregg's discovery, the isolation of rubella virus,[9,10] and the development of serological techniques that were used during the 1964 rubella epidemic in the United States helped to establish beyond doubt that congenital heart defects can be of infectious origin.

Cardiac Problems in Pregnancy, pages 419-431

It is interesting that during the 40 years since Gregg's description of the teratogenicity caused by maternal rubella, little evidence has been found that any other infection is responsible for congenital heart defects.

Bacterial, mycotic, and parasitic infections involving the mother and fetus have not proved to be a cause of congenital heart abnormalities. Moreover, the infection they cause is frequently overwhelming or interferes so severely with organogenesis that fetal death and abortion result. For example, Vibrio fetus[11,12] (Vibrio is now known as Campylobacter fetus) and Salmonella typhi[13] infections often are followed by intrauterine death and abortion.

In addition to rubella, a number of other viral illnesses contracted by the mother in the first trimester of pregnancy adversely affect the fetus. A primary maternal infection with vaccinia virus can cause a lethal fetal infection.[14] Maternal measles is associated with an increased incidence of fetal malformation and perinatal death.[15,16] The information on varicella and mumps viruses is confusing. In one prospective study it was concluded that mumps and varicella had no obvious harmful effects on the fetus,[17] yet in maternal varicella, cases of fetal teratogenesis without heart defects have been reported.[18] In mumps, one study[19] demonstrated increased fetal mortality without heart disease, whereas others[20-22] implicated maternal mumps infection as a cause of fetal and newborn endocardial fibroelastosis (EFE). This association of EFE with mumps virus has been questioned by others.[23]

An increased number of congenital heart defects (significantly larger than the control group) has been identified following pregnancies complicated by coxsackie B virus infection,[24] and the majority of the malformations are persistent ductus arteriosus and ventricular septal defect. These facts suggest that coxsackie B viruses are cardiovascular teratogens.

Cytomegalovirus (CMV) is known to infect the fetus, but CMV as a cause of cardiovascular abnormalities is a moot question. There is no consistent pattern to the cardiac defects, and most infants with congenital CMV infection have normal hearts. Indeed, it is unlikely that CMV is a cardiovascular teratogen.

Respiratory viruses such as influenza have no viremic phase; therefore, infection of the fetus is not likely to occur. In one study, no congenital heart defects were found following an outbreak of maternal influenza.[17]

Before the eighth to tenth week of gestation, heart defects caused by an infectious agent are the result of a disturbance of organogenesis (congenital malformation). After that time heart development is essentially complete, and an infection can damage normally developed tissue (lesion).

According to Dudgeon,[25] four criteria should be satisfied before an infection contracted during pregnancy is accepted as the cause of a congenital defect. The criteria he uses are set forth in Table F.V.1.

TABLE F.V.1. Criteria Used to Establish a Causal Relationship Between a Maternal Infection and Congenital Defects *

Clinical	Each infection tends to produce a syndrome or repetitive pattern of clinical manifestations.
Epidemiological	The same manifestations should be observed with the same agent following maternal illness in different countries.
Virological	Persistence of the infective agent in fetal tissues and evidence of a chronic infective state after birth.
Immunological	Persistence of antibody in the child after the normal decline of maternal antibody; presence of antibody in the IgM fraction.

*After Dudgeon JA[18] by permission of the authors and W.B. Saunders Company.

As a cause of congenital heart malformations, it appears that rubella is the only infection that truly satisfies Dudgeon's criteria. Although only a small portion of the total number of congenital heart defects can be related directly to rubella virus infection during pregnancy, this small fraction of cases provides the basis for further discussion because, theoretically, it is possible to prevent maternal viral infections and thereby eliminate at least one cause of congenital heart disease.

III. A PATHWAY TO FETAL INFECTION AND MALFORMATION

Only viral infections (specifically those known to be associated with congenital heart abnormalities) will be discussed since few other infectious agents have been implicated in congenital heart disease. The pathogenesis of viral infection in the fetus has been reviewed,[26] and only a brief discussion of the events leading to fetal infection and damage follows. A schematic diagram of the pathogenesis of these events is shown in Figure F.V.1.

A. Susceptibility of the Gravid Female to Infection

1. Socioeconomic factors

Age and social status are important in the contracting of rubella and CMV infection. Individuals from lower socioeconomic strata usually live in crowded urban areas and frequently develop immunity to infectious diseases early in childhood. In industrial countries, only 5 to 20% of women in their childbearing years are susceptible to rubella.[27,28] By contrast, 25 to 75% of the same population of women in certain tropical island communities are susceptible.[29] Also, most women who enter the childbearing period have had CMV infection (30–60%).[30] A correlation between the standard of living and number of children who acquire CMV infection has been noted. In Tanzania, almost 91% of infants and children between the age of six months and 14 years have antibody to cytomegalovirus.[31]

2. Genetic–viral interaction

There are certain populations where asympomatic mothers who carry hepatitis B antigen do not readily transmit infection vertically to their offspring.[32–35] However, 40% of infants born to Taiwanese mothers who carry hepatitis B antigen become persistent carriers.[36]

Rubella virus may infect more easily cells that contain HLA1 or the combination of HLA1 and HLB8 antigens. A statistically significant increase in antigens HLA1, HLA3 and HLB5, HLB8 has been found in infants who have congenital rubella infection.[37,38] In Japan congenital rubella infection is rare.[39,40] Perhaps it is because HLA1 and HLB8 antigens are not present in the Japanese.

The susceptibility of any population to viral infection certainly is influenced by geographic location, age of the inhabitants, sanitation, housing, population density, nutrition, personal hygiene, racial and genetic characteristics, and possibly other factors. Any research into the pathogenesis of congenital heart abnormalities or other fetal defects believed to be caused by an infectious agent will require careful analysis of these important variables.

B. Maternal Resistance to Infection

The development of cell-mediated immunity may be important in the recovery from virus infections that infiltrate the plasma membranes of the cells they infect.[41] However, during pregnancy, some maternal cell-mediated immune responses are depressed. Heterologous sera from pregnant women depress the phytohemagglutinin transformation of lymphocytes from healthy nonpregnant women.[42–44] Of greater interest, this suppressive action on maternal lymphocyte transformation is further enhanced by fetal serum.[45] This suggests that the immune inhibitory factor in maternal serum might be derived from the fetopla-

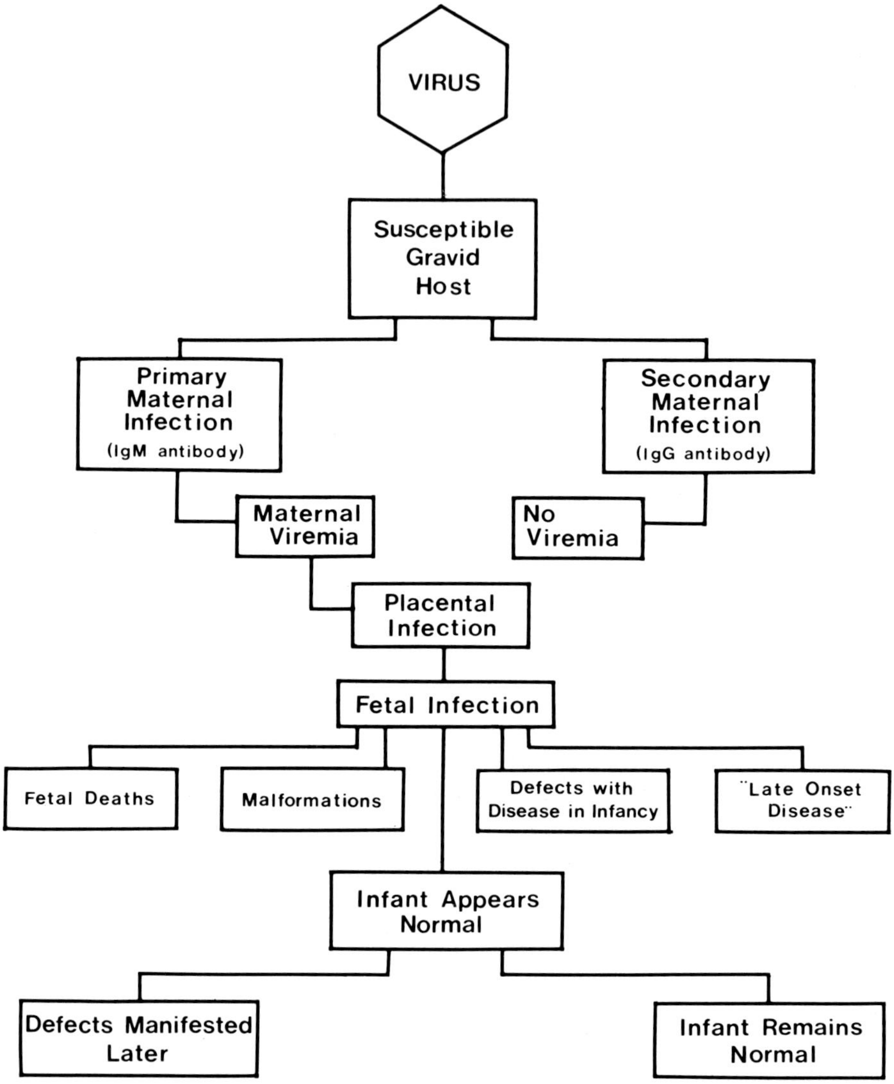

Fig. F.V.1. Pathogenesis of viral invasion of the fetus showing the spectrum of fetal damage that may result. Drawn after Catalano and Sever.[26]

cental unit. Aside from the obvious importance in preventing rejection of the fetus, suppression of the maternal cell-mediated immunity could enhance the severity of maternal illness. Thus, there is a greater potential for infection of the fetus and metabolic injury to the maternal–fetal complex as a result of fever and other toxic manifestations of the disease.

C. Placental Resistance to Infection

Although infections ascending into the amniotic sac from the vagina or cervix are known to occur, most intrauterine viral infections result from transplacental hematogenous dissemination of the virus. Since the placenta is a fetal organ, there is no reason to assume that it should possess any defense mechanisms (immunologic or otherwise) significantly different from the fetus. The placenta does synthesize interferon, and placental tissues under certain conditions in vitro, when challenged with rubella virus, produce large concentrations of this substance. However, cell cultures of other fetal tissues produce less interferon.[46,47] The exact significance of this difference is unknown, but it indicates that there may be an antiviral function of the placenta independent of the fetus.

Any resistance imposed by the placenta might well depend upon the time the infection occurs during gestation. Placental infection has been documented in 85% of maternal rubella exposures occurring in the first eight weeks of gestation; fetal infection was demonstrated in only 50% of these preganancies.[48] A higher isolation rate of virus from both placenta and fetus has been achieved by others.[49,50] In early gestation, the placenta does not appear to act as a significant barrier to fetal infection. After the tenth week of gestation, however, isolated placental infection is three to six times more common than fetal infection.

Specific IgG antibodies are found in the maternal blood shortly after a viral infection, but they are not normally transferred to the fetus by the placenta in any substantial amount before 16 to 20 weeks gestation.[51] Even in the case of chronic rubella infection, the transfer of immune substances across the placenta matures normally.[52] Therefore, the fetus cannot directly benefit from maternal antibody formation. Moreover, some viruses grow and survive in fetal tissues because they propagate from cell to cell through intracellular connections and do not leave the confines of the cell membrane.[53] Since there is no exposure to the plasma, these viruses cannot be inactivated by humoral antibodies. It seems that the placenta offers little more resistance to infection than a weak physical barrier, especially during the early stages of gestation when the fetus is most vulnerable to injury.

D. Fetal Resistance to Infection

Immunoglobulin production depends upon the development of B (bursa equivalent) cells of the lymphocyte population. Cells containing surface-bound immunoglobins—IgM, IgG, IgA, and IgD—are found only in the liver during early gestation, and it is not until after 14 to 15 weeks that they are found in other organs (spleen and blood).[54]

About the eighth week of gestation, primitive stem cells enter the thymus and diffentiate into thymocytes (T cells). By 12–13 weeks, the fetal T lymphocytes, or cellular immune system, become immunocompetent.[55]

During the early stages of development of the fetal humoral immune system, circulatory antibody levels remain low, even when there is a large concentration of rubella virus.[51] This may be because an inadequate number of cells produce antibody or because the cells are not capable of making sufficient antibody before infection overwhelms the developing fetus and severely stresses its metabolic functions. Likewise, if a viral infection occurs before the T cells proliferate, a specific tolerance of cell-mediated immune responses might occur.

It appears that following successful invasion of the mother by a virus during early gestation, placental and fetal immune systems are not completely able to prevent spread of virus into the fetal tissues. Chronic infection can result and interfere with organogenesis.

E. Teratogenesis

Generalized vasculitis of the placenta and the fetus (as found in rubella) is an attractive hypothesis to explain the genesis of some types of congenital heart malformations. Obliterative angiopathy affecting capillaries and larger blood vessels of the placenta and fetus is apt to cause disturbed morphogenesis, impaired nutrition, and retarded fetal growth.

Rubella virus has been associated with disseminated damage of systemic and pulmonary blood vessels. Varying degrees of sclerosis and stenosis of these vessels occur.[56] One of the chief abnormalities is a deficiency of elastic tissue within the walls of the pulmonary and systemic arteries. There is also intimal thickening of these vessels.[57] Moreover, where elastic tissue is deficient, the amount of intimal proliferation is greatest. In the ductus arteriosus both smooth muscle and elastic tissue are reduced in content.[58]

Elastic tissue fibers form in the ground substance surrounding cells of the media.[59] Fine thread-like aldehyde fuchsin fibers have been identified at approximately 6½ weeks gestation.[60] The cells from which these fibers seem to take their origin resemble smooth muscle cells more than fibroblasts.[61] It is possible that rubella virus (in this instance) interferes with elastic tissue formation in pulmonary and systemic arteries, and this is probably the event responsible for further changes in these vessels. Eventually this causes vascular stenosis and alteration of the hemodynamics.

Angiopathy of the microcirculation can cause thrombosis and disseminated intravascular coagulopathy. If this occurs in the placenta and fetus, blood flow to any developing organ system is reduced or curtailed. Hypoxia and malnutrition are manifested or death results. Depending on the time the insult occurs, organogenesis is arrested or slowed until sufficient circulation is reestablished, permitting improved metabolism.

Immune complexes are known to form during the course of hepatitis B infection; they can damage the kidney and cause nephritis.[62] In the same way viruses could injure the heart. In patients who have EFE, cellular immunity has been demonstrated with the mumps skin test antigen, but humoral antibodies rarely are found.[21] A similar immune response was noted following the intradermal inoculation of immune complexes into the guinea pig.[63] Intrauterine mumps virus infection in humans could result in the formation of viral-antibody complexes. It is possible that EFE is the result of tissue damage caused by immune complexes, but no evidence is yet available to suggest or exclude this possibility.[64]

A functional circulatory system is established by the fourth week of gestation, and the ventricular septum is completely developed by the eighth week. In the meantime, the common atrial canal is being closed by growth of the septum primum and septum secundum. It is during this time that interference with maturation of the heart by any of the mechanisms described above could result in one or more cardiovascular abnormalities. In congenital rubella, certain types of heart malformations relate closely to the time of infection during gestation[65]; the onset of pulmonary artery stenosis is between 30 and 90 days gestation; ventricular septal defects, between 16 and 47 days gestation; and injury to the ductus arteriosus, between 25 and 62 days gestation.

IV. INFECTIOUS AGENTS WITH AN ESTABLISHED OR PROBABLE ROLE AS CARDIOVASCULAR TERATOGENS

A. Rubella

Rubella infection is distributed throughout the world and is most prevalent during the spring months. Fever, an exanthem (usually of three days duration), preauricular adenopathy, and arthritis, especially of the smaller peripheral joints, are the common clinical manifestations.

The virus replicates throughout the body a week or longer before illness begins. Specific antibodies are detected in maternal blood during the course of the disease. Within a week or two, the peak concentration of hemagglutination inhibition (HI) antibodies is observed. Shortly thereafter, neutralizing and fluorescent antibody titers rise.[66,67] Complement-fixing (CF) antibodies appear more slowly and do not attain a peak concentration before four to eight weeks (occasionally as long as five to six months) following disease.[67] To document a rubella infection, knowledge of the rubella antibody titers prior to pregnancy is helpful. If there is no information in this regard it is necessary to measure serially the various antibodies mentioned above, and it may be necessary to determine if they are of the gamma M type. Before a therapeutic abortion is considered, every effort should be made to document serologically that the woman's rubella-form rash was truly caused by a rubella infection.

Knowledge of the teratogenic effects of this virus has grown considerably since its isolation in 1962[9,10] and the rubella epidemic in the United States in 1964. For all practical purposes, rubella has become the prototype of malformations induced by infectious agents.

The frequency and type of defects that occur following maternal rubella infection depend upon the gestational age of the conceptus.[48,68] Eighty-five percent of infants who are infected in the first eight weeks after maternal rubella have detectable congenital defects by age one to four years. The incidence of detectable defects is 52% for nine to 12 weeks, approximately 16% for 13 to 20 weeks, and few or none after 20 weeks.[69]

Intrauterine growth retardation (small-for-dates infant) was the most common characteristic of congenital rubella-infected infants born during the years 1962 to 1964. On normal growth curves, 60% fell below the tenth percentile and 90% below the fiftieth percentile.[70] Also, intrauterine growth retardation seldom existed without associated defects. In fact, the mean birth weight of infants exposed to rubella who have no demonstrable malformations fell into the normal percentiles. In contrast, mean birth weight and head circumference were lower in infected infants with defects.[71]

The incidence of cardiovascular abnormalities varies from 60 to 100%.[26] Most of these malformations are of the acyanotic type. A list of the diseases is found in Table F.V.2. In one evaluation of 37 patients, 34 (92%) had cardiovascular malformation limited to the great vessels and ductus arteriosus, and the remainder had complex intracardiac defects [72]; 28 had pulmonary artery abnormalities with persistent ductus arteriosus (PDA); and six had isolated pulmonary artery disease. Although not a frequent finding, hypoplasia of the aortic isthmus was observed. The pulmonary artery malformations consisted of hypoplasia of the branches, supravalvular stenosis of the main pulmonary artery, pulmonary valvular stenosis, and pulmonary valvular atresia. One-third of all patients developed congestive heart failure, and 13 (approximately ⅓) underwent cardiothoracic surgery. Clearly, there is a significant morbidity associated with the cardiovascular abnormalities. Pulmonary artery disease constitutes an important component of the cardiovascular malformations found in the rubella syndrome. Pulmonary artery involvement with and without PDA has been observed.[73–77] Persistent ductus arteriosus was the only cardiovascular defect found in eight of 12 low birth weight

TABLE F.V.2. Cardiovascular Abnormalities Reported With Congenital Rubella Infection

*Persistent ductus arteriosus (PDA)
*Pulmonary artery lesions and PDA
*Pulmonary artery lesions
1. Valvular stenosis
2. Hypoplasia and stenosis of the branches
3. Supravalvular stenosis
4. Valvular atresia
Hypoplasia of the aortic isthmus
Coarctation of the aorta
Aortic stenosis
Renal artery stenosis
? Cerebrovascular stenosis
Atrial septal defect
Ventricular septal defect
Tetralogy of Fallot
Tricuspid atresia
Truncus arteriosus
Transposition of the great vessels
Endocardial cushion defect
Complex lesions with asplenia
Myocarditis

*The most frequently observed defects.

infants who had other stigmata of congenital rubella. Of the remaining four patients, two had pulmonary valvular stenosis and two had peripheral pulmonary artery stenosis.[78]

Extracardiac malformations involving the renal arteries have also been observed.[79,80] Renal artery stenosis with systemic hypertension was noted in 13 cases.[80]

In 47 infants with congenital rubella, ten had electrocardiographic evidence of ischemic myocardial disease. These changes were found at birth or within the first ten days of life. Seven had active disease in the neonatal period, and four died. Postmortem examination showed myocarditis compatible with viral disease. Damage to the heart and great vessels caused by rubella appears to be confined to the first trimester, but the virus can be present and destroy myocardial tissue for some time after birth.[81] Seven other infants with electrocardiographic evidence of myocardial damage have been reported.[74] This type of lesion could account for cardiac arrest and heart failure in infants who have no evidence of structural heart abnormalities.

In congenital rubella, malformations of the heart and other organs are almost invariably associated with fetal growth retardation. Conventional[82] and real-time ultrasound scanning[83] can be used to assess fetal growth during the first trimester with relatively good accuracy. This is done by measurement of the fetal crown-rump length (CRL). The fetus grows rapidly during the first trimester; thus, significant retardation of growth will become evident by CRL measurement. Retardation of fetal growth and serological evidence of maternal rubella infection support a diagnosis of fetal infection and probable malformations of the heart and other organs. It may be that ultrasonic and serological assessment of the pregnant woman with rubella will permit the obstetrician and hospital committees on abortion to provide the mother and father with better advice concerning the termination of a pregnancy. However, the clinical importance of the combined use of these techniques remains to be evaluated.

It is also possible to detect valvular disease, large septal defects, and abnormalities of rhythm with real-time ultrasound scanning, but the chance of demonstrating structural defects in early pregnancy (before 20 weeks) is probably not very great.

As suggested before, it is theoretically possible to prevent congenital rubella. As Horstmann stated,[27] "It becomes obvious that problems associated with the prevention of rubella are unique in that the major concern of immunization is not the vaccinee per se, but rather the future fetus." Can immunization of children increase and maintain immunity of the population sufficient to protect the fetus from maternal rubella infection?

According to the United States National Registry of Congenital Rubella Syndrome, cases of congenitally acquired rubella have decreased steadily since 1969. The trend of decreasing disease is encouraging because it began along with the administration of the rubella vaccine.[84,85] However, immune responses following rubella vaccination differ from those acquired naturally[86]; it will be important to observe if infants and children who are vaccinated maintain rubella immune status during their childbearing years.

B. Cytomegalovirus

The clinical manifestations of congenital CMV range from "silent" infection to severe disease in the fetus and newborn. Severe infection includes hepatomegaly, jaundice, splenomegaly, petechiae, chorioretinitis, and cerebral calcifications. There are, of course, malformations involving the cardiovascular system. These are listed in Table F.V.3. Unlike rubella, there is no consistent pattern to the heart abnormalities and no evidence to show that they are quantitatively or qualitatively different from heart defects found in the normal population. Indeed, the same cardiovascular teratogenicity dem-

TABLE F.V.3. Cardiovascular Abnormalities Reported With Congenital CMV Infection

Atrial septal defect
Ventricular septal defect
Enlarged ductus arteriosus
Arterial abnormalities with hyperplasia of the elastica
Tetralogy of Fallot
Anomalous pulmonary venous return
Mitral stenosis
Accessory semilunar fold of the foramen ovale

onstrated in congenital rubella is not evident. This casts considerable doubt on congenital CMV as a true cardiovascular teratogen.

C. Coxsackieviruses (Enteroviruses)

Infection with these viruses is quite common; often the illness is subclinical and infection goes unrecognized. However, coxsackie B virus can cause myocarditis and meningocephalitis in the newborn infant whose mother acquires intrauterine infection late in pregnancy.[87,88] Moreover, there is evidence to suggest that infection contracted early in pregnancy causes heart malformations.[89]

One large prospective study[90] has systematically made a serological search for selected maternal enteroviral infections associated with congenital anomalies, particularly congenital heart disease.[24] Sera from 22,935 women were collected.[90] Of this group, sera from 630 mothers with abnormal infants and 1,164 control sera were studied for evidence of maternal infection during the first trimester of pregnancy. They were evaluated for evidence of coxsackieviruses B1–5 and A9 and echoviruses 6 and 9. Coxsackievirus B3 and B4 infections were associated with cardiovascular defects. Analysis of the coxsackievirus B1–5 group indicated an overall association with congenital heart defects; also, the likelihood of cardiovascular abnormalities increased when the mother was infected with two or more coxsackieviruses. Serological evidence of infection occurred often without obvious maternal illness. This lends support to the contention that asymptomatic maternal viral infections may cause congenital heart defects. The heart malformations found during the study[24,90] are listed in Table F.V.4). Persistent ductus arteriosus and VSD were the most common. Although the defects encountered in infants whose mothers had coxsackie B virus infection are similar to those in children with congenital heart disease without maternal infection, the incidence of heart malformation was found to be more than double the rate expected in the normal population.[24]

This study[24] suggests an etiological role of the coxsackie B viruses as cardiovascular teratogens; however, it can be questioned on the following points: first, the infectious agent has never been isolated from the fetal tissues, nor has fetal antibody production to the viruses been confirmed; second, since enteroviral infection is most common during the summer and fall, the largest number of infants who have malformations would be born in the spring and summer. In fact, 19 of 26 infants with defective hearts were born during the months of June through November, which means that the first trimester was in the late fall and winter. It is significant, however, that infants in this study who had heart defects also had intrauterine growth retardation, which suggests an infectious etiology associating coxsackie B virus with the heart abnormalities.[90]

TABLE F.V.4. Cardiovascular Abnormalities Reported Following Coxsackievirus Infections During Pregnancy

*Ventricular septal defect
*Persistent ductus arteriosus
Atrial septal defect
Aortic stenosis
Aortic atresia
Tricuspid atresia
Transposition of the great vessels
Tetralogy of Fallot

*The most frequently observed defects.

At present there does not seem to be sufficient mortality or morbidity of mother or fetus to suggest the development of a vaccine program for coxsackieviruses. Besides, the antigenic heterogeneity of the coxsackie B viruses would severely hamper the development of such a program.

D. Mumps

Gestational mumps associated with fetal and newborn EFE has been the subject of considerable debate, and this issue presently is not resolved.

Several investigators reported that a large number of children with EFE demonstrated a positive skin test to mumps antigen (cutaneous delayed hypersensitivity).[20,21,22,91] Also, frequently there was a history of maternal exposure to infection with mumps virus during pregnancy. This relationship was further supported by an experiment wherein mumps virus introduced into a chick embryo produced a heart lesion similar to human encocardial fibroelastosis.[92] Others have not been able to confirm the relationship between EFE and delayed hypersensitivity to mumps.[23,93,94] Those who support this argument believe that the mumps skin test is nonspecific. They further suggest that a positive skin test is the result of cross-reactivity with parainfluenza virus or other proteins that have antigenic sites similar to mumps virus. Also, they claim and have demonstrated that patients with EFE have only a weakly positive mumps skin test.

To explain the lack of humoral antibody in the fetus and newborn infant following maternal mumps infection or exposure, an experiment was performed in rhesus monkeys.[95] In them, intrauterine infection was caused by injection of mumps virus into the mother during the first third of gestation. Replication of the virus in the fetal and placental tissues occurred, but only for one week. It was thought that the virus disappeared because of transplacental passage of maternal 7S neutralizing antibody. Pregnant monkeys develop both delayed hypersensitivity responses and neutralizing antibody to mumps after experimental infection. Four infant monkeys that survived to term had delayed hypersensitivity but no humoral antibody. These experimental data might explain the observation of the absence of humoral antibody to mumps in a number of Eskimo children (without EFE or other defects) who were born on a remote island in the Bering Sea during a mumps epidemic.[64]

Recent experience in several large medical centers indicates that the diagnosis of primary EFE has not been made as frequently as in the previous decade, and mumps during pregnancy has become rare. It would appear that the rather interesting controversy over the possible relationship between EFE and gestational mumps will never be resolved. The performance of a carefully controlled prospective study would take too long to be of any practical use.

It is to be hoped that the immunization of children with mumps vaccine will prevent maternal mumps infection in those who will become pregnant in the future. Investigators who believe that fetal EFE is associated with maternal mumps infection should therefore see a reduction in the number of infants who have primary EFE. The reduced number of cases of primary EFE (anecdotal information) observed in the past decade might be related to such a reduction in gestational mumps infection; perhaps the proponents of mumps-associated EFE were correct.

V. CONCLUSIONS

Infections caused by bacteria, parasites, and mycotic agents have not proved to be cardiovascular teratogens. The rubella virus, however, fulfills all the criteria of Dudgeon and is a cardiovascular teratogen. Very possibly the coxsackie B viruses will be added to this list in the future. Although mumps is suspiciously associated with primary EFE, there are not enough cases of mumps infection during pregnancy in the United States to examine this relationship further. Undoubtedly, as serological and virologic techniques are used more frequently during pregnancy, other viruses will prove to be cardiovascular teratogens. Fortunately rubella infection of the pregnant woman is now unusual, probably the result of immunization programs. However, in the occasional early gestational infection with rubella, serological and ultrasound techniques should permit the diagnosis of maternal–fetal disease.

Heart abnormalities should be suspected following a viral infection associated with intrauterine growth retardation. With greater experience in the use of real-time ultrasound scanning, the in utero diagnosis of heart malformations will be made more frequently.

VI. REFERENCES

1. Campbell, M. Causes of malformations of the heart. Br Med J. 1965; 2:895–904.
2. McKeown T, Record RG. Malformations in a population observed for five years after birth. In: Wolstenholme GEW, O'Connor CM, eds. Ciba Foundation Symposium on Congenital Malformations. Boston: Little, Brown and Company, 1960:5.
3. Kerrebijn KF. Incidence in infants and mortality from congenital malformations of the circulatory system. Acta Paediatr Scand. 1966; 55:316–320.
4. Higgins ITT. The epidemiology of congenital heart disease. J Chronic Dis. 1965; 18:699–721.
5. Shaw RF. The relative role of heredity and environment in congenital heart disease. Lancet. 1965; 85:519–524.
6. Mims CA. Pathogenesis of viral infections of the fetus. Prog Med Virol. 1968; 10:194–237.
7. Gregg NM. Congenital cataract following German measles in the mother. Trans Ophthalmol Soc Aust. 1941; 3:35–46.
8. Swan C, Tostevin AL, Moore B, Mayo H, Black GHB. Congenital defects in infants following infectious diseases during pregnancy. Med J Aust. 1943; 2:201–210.
9. Parkman PD, Buescher EL, Artenstein MS. Recovery of rubella virus from army recruits. Proc Soc Exp Biol Med. 1962; 111:225–230.
10. Weller TH, Neva FA. Propogation in tissue culture of cytopathic agents from patients with rubella-like illness. Proc Soc Exp Biol Med. 1962; 111:215–225.
11. Eden AN. Perinatal mortality caused by Vibrio fetus. J Pediatr. 1966; 68:297–304.
12. Willis MD, Austin WJ. Human Vibrio fetus infection. Report of two dissimilar cases. Am J Dis Child. 1966; 112:459–462.
13. Hicks HT, French H. Typhoid fever and pregnancy, with special reference to foetal infection. Lancet. 1905; 1:1491–1493.
14. Enthwhistle DM, Bray PT, Lawrence KM. Prenatal infection with Vaccinia virus. Br Med J. 1962; 2:238–239.
15. Hill AB, Doll R, Galloway TM, Hughes JP. Virus diseases in pregnancy and congenital defects. Br J Prev Soc Med. 1958; 12:1–7.
16. Siegel M. Congenital malformations following chickenpox, measles, mumps, and hepatitis. JAMA. 1973; 226:1521–1524.
17. Manson MM, Logan WPD, Loy RM. Rubella and other virus infections during pregnancy. Rep Publ Hlth Med Subj No. 101. London: Ministry of Health, 1960.
18. Hanshaw JB, Dudgeon JA, eds. Viral Diseases in the Fetus and Newborn. Philadelphia: W.B. Saunders Co., 1978:200–201.
19. Siegel M, Fuerst HT, Peress NS. Comparative fetal mortality in maternal virus diseases. A prospective study on rubella, measles, mumps, chickenpox and hepatitis. N Engl J Med. 1966; 274:768–771.
20. Noren GR, Adams P Jr, Anderson RC. Positive skin test reactivity to mumps virus antigen in endocardial fibroelastosis. J Pediatr. 1963; 62:604–606.
21. St. Geme JW Jr, Noren GR, Adams P Jr. Proposed embryopathic relation between mumps virus and primary endocardial fibroelastosis. N Engl J Med. 1966; 275:339–347.
22. Shone JD, Muñoz AS, Manning JA, Keith JD. The mumps antigen skin test in endocardial fibroelastosis. Pediatrics. 1966; 37:423–429.
23. Gersony WM, Katz SL, Nadas AS. Endocardial fibroelastosis and the mumps virus. Pediatrics. 1966; 37:430–434.
24. Brown GC, Evans TN. Serologic evidence of coxsackievirus etiology of congenital heart disease. JAMA. 1967; 199:183–187.
25. Dudgeon JA. Infective causes of human malformations. In human malformations. Br Med Bull. 1976:77–83.
26. Catalano LW, Sever JL. The role of viruses as causes of congenital defects. Annu Rev Microbiol. 1971; 25:255–282.
27. Horstmann DM. Rubella: The challenge of its control. J Infect Dis. 1971; 123:640–654.
28. Witte JJ, Karchmer AW, Case G, Hermann KL, Abrotyn E, Kassanoft I, Neill JS. Epidemiology of rubella. Am J Dis Child. 1969; 118:107–111.
29. Dowdle WR, Ferreira W, Gomes LFD, King D, Kourany M, Madalengoitia J, Pearson E, Swanston WH, Tosi HC, Vilches AM. WHO collaborative study on the sero-epidemiology of rubella in Caribbean and Middle and South American population in 1968. Bull WHO. 1970; 42:419–422.

30. Hanshaw JB. Congenital and acquired cytomegalovirus infection. Pediatr Clin North Am. 1966; 13:279–293.
31. Krech UH, Jung M, Jung F. Cytomegalovirus infections of man. Basel: S. Karger, 1971:1–5.
32. Schweitzer IL, Mosley JW, Ashcaval M, Edwards VM, Overby LB. Factors influencing neonatal infection by hepatitis B virus. Gastroenterology. 1973; 65:277–283.
33. Papaevangelou G, Kremartinou T, Prevedourakis C, Kaskarelis D. Hepatitis B antigen and antibody in maternal blood, cord blood, and amniotic fluid. Arch Dis Child. 1974; 49:936–939.
34. Schweitzer IL, Dunn AEG, Peters RL, Spears RL. Viral hepatitis B in neonates and infants. Am J Med. 1973; 55:762–771.
35. Skinhøj P, Sandemann H, Cohn J, Mikkelson M, Olesen H. Hepatitis associated antigen (HAA) in pregnant women and their newborn infants. Am J Dis Child. 1972; 123:380–381.
36. Stevens CE, Beasley, RP, Tsui J, Wy-Chan L. Vertical transmission of hepatitis B antigen in Taiwan. N Engl J Med. 1975; 292:771–774.
37. Honeyman MC, Menser MA. Ethnicity is a significant factor in the epidemiology of rubella and Hodgkin's disease. Nature. 1974; 251:441–442.
38. Honeyman MC, Dorman DC, Menser MA, Forrest JM, Guinan JJ, Clark P. HL-A antigens in congenital rubella and the role of antigens 1 and 8 in the epidemiology of natural rubella. Tissue Antigens. 1975; 5:12–18.
39. Kono R, Hibi M, Hayakawa Y, Ishii K. Experimental vertical transmission of rubella virus in rabbits. Lancet. 1969; 1:343–347.
40. Best JM, Banatvala JE, Bowen JM. New Japanese rubella vaccine: Comparative trials. Br Med J. 1974; 3:221–224.
41. Allison AC. Interactions of T and B lymphocytes and macrophages in recovery from virus infections. Proc R Soc Med. 1973; 66:1151–1160.
42. Thong YH, Steele RW, Vincent MM, Hensen SA, Bellanti JA. Impaired in vitro cell-mediated immunity to rubella virus during pregnancy. N Engl J Med. 1973; 289:604–606.
43. Purtilo DT, Hallgren HM, Yunis EJ. Depressed maternal lymphocyte response to phytohaemagglutinin in human pregnancy. Lancet. 1972; 1:769–771.
44. Finn R, St. Hill CA, Govan AJ, Ralfs IG, Gurney FJ. Immunological responses in pregnancy and survival of fetal homograft. Br Med J. 1972; 3:150–152.
45. St. Hill CA, Finn R, Denye V. Depression of cellular immunity in pregnancy due to a serum factor. Br Med J. 1973; 3:513–514.
46. Banatvala JE, Potter JE, Webster MJ. Foetal interferon responses induced by rubella virus. In: Elliot K, Knight J, eds. Intrauterine Infection (Ciba Foundation Symposium 10). Amsterdam: Associated Scientific Publishers, 1973: 77–79.
47. Banatvala JE, Potter JE, Best JM. Interferon response to sendai and rubella viruses in human foetal cultures, leukocytes and placental cultures. J Gen Virol. 1971; 13:193–201.
48. Alford CA Jr, Neva FA, Weller TH. Virologic and serologic studies on human products of conception after maternal rubella. N Engl J Med. 1964; 271:1275–1281.
49. Thompson KM, Tobin JO. Isolation of rubella virus from abortion material. Br Med J. 1970; 1:264–266.
50. Rawls WE, Desmyter J, Melnick JL. Serological diagnosis and fetal involvement in maternal rubella. JAMA. 1968; 203:627–631.
51. Alford CA, Blankenship WJ, Straumfjord JV, Cassady G. The diagnostic significance of IgM-globulin elevations in newborn infants with chronic intrauterine infections. Birth Defects. 1968; 4(7):5–19.
52. Alford CA Jr. Studies on antibody in congenital rubella infections. 1. Physiochemical and immunologic investigations of rubella-neutralizing antibody. Am J Dis Child. 1965; 110: 455–463.
53. Mims CA. Factors in the mechanism of persistence of viral infections. Prog Med Virol. 1974; 18:1–14.
54. Lawton AR, Self KS, Royal SA, Cooper MD. Ontogeny of B-lymphocytes in the human fetus. Clin Immunol Immunopathol. 1972; 1:84–93.
55. Carr MC, Stiles DP, Fudenberg HH. Dissociation of responses to phytohaemagglutinin and adult lymphocytes in human foetal lymphoid tissues. Nature [New Biol]. 1973; 241:279–281.
56. Singer DB, Rudolph AJ, Rosenberg HS, Rawls WE, Bonivk M. Pathology of the congenital rubella syndrome. J Pediatr. 1967; 71:665–675.
57. Campbell PE. Vascular abnormalities following maternal rubella. Br Heart J. 1965; 27:134–138.
58. Campbell M. Place of maternal rubella in the aetiology of congenital heart disease. Br Med J. 1961; 1:691–696.
59. Karner HE, Cox J. Electron microscope study of developing chick embryo aorta. J Ultrastruct Res. 1960; 4:420–454.
60. Frankel HH, Bernick S, Patek PR, Edmondson HA, Peters RL, Paule WJ. Elastic membranes of the developing human aorta. Arch Pathol. 1963; 76:474–483.
61. Paule WJ. Electron microscopy of the newborn rat aorta. J Ultrastruct Res. 1963; 8:219–235.
62. Nydegger UE, Miescher PA. Detection and clinical implication of circulating immune complexes in hepatitis B virus infection. In: Bianchi L, Gerok W, Sickinger K, Stadler GA, eds. Virus and the Liver. Lancaster, England: MTP Press Limited. 1980:183–195.
63. Uhr JW, Salvin SB, Pappenheimer AM Jr. Delayed hypersensitivity. II. Induction of hypersensitivity in guinea pigs by means of antigen-antibody complexes. J Exp Med. 1957; 105: 11–24.
64. Aase JM, Noren GR, Reddy DV, St. Geme JW Jr. Mumps-virus infection in pregnant women and the immunologic response of their offspring.

N Engl J Med. 1972; 286:1379–1382.
65. Ueda K, Nishida Y, Oshima K, Shephard TH. Congenital rubella syndrome: Correlation of gestational age at time of maternal rubella with type of defect. J Pediatr. 1979; 94:763–765.
66. Plotkin SA. Rubella virus. In: Lennette EH, Schmidt NJ, eds. Diagnostic Procedures for Viral and Rickettsial Infection. 4th Ed. New York: American Public Health Association, 1969:364–413.
67. Lennette EH, Schmidt NJ. Neutralization, fluorescent antibody and complement fixation tests for rubella. In: Friedman H, Prier JE, eds. Rubella. Springfield, Illinois: Charles C Thomas Co., 1973:18–32.
68. Alford CA Jr., Kanich LS. Cogenital rubella: A review of the virologic and serologic phenomena occurring after maternal rubella in the first trimester. South Med J. 1966; 59:745–748.
69. Peckham CS. Clinical and laboratory study of children exposed in utero to maternal rubella. Arch Dis Child. 1972; 47:571–577.
70. Cooper LZ, Green RH, Krugman S, Giles JP, Mirick GS. Neonatal thrombocytopenia purpura and other manifestations of rubella contracted in utero. Am J Dis Child. 1965; 110:416–427.
71. LeJarraga H, Peckham CS. Birthweight and subsequent growth of children exposed to rubella infection in utero. Arch Dis Child. 1974; 49:50–54.
72. Hastreiter AR, Joorabchi B, Pujatti G, van der Horst RL, Pataesil G, Sever JL. Cardiovascular lesions associated with congenital rubella. J Pediatr. 1967; 71:59–65.
73. Rowe RD. Maternal rubella and pulmonary artery stenosis. Report of eleven cases. Pediatrics. 1963; 32:180–185.
74. Korones SB, Ainger LE, Monif GRG, Roane J, Sever JL, Fuste F. Congenital rubella syndrome: Study of 22 infants. Myocardial damage and other new clinical aspects. Am J Dis Child. 1965; 110:434–440.
75. Liggins GC, Phillips LI. Rubella embryopathy. An interim report on a New Zealand epidemic. Br Med J. 1963; 711–713.
76. Sperling DR, Verska JJ. Rubella syndrome. Cardiovascular manifestations and surgical therapy in infants. Calif Med. 1966; 105:340–344.
77. Franch RH, Gay BB. Congenital stenosis of the pulmonary artery branches. Am J Med. 1963; 35:512–529.
78. Starkova O, Ebrahim S. Personal Communication. Cited by Marshall WC. The clinical impact of congenital rubella. In: Elliot K, Knight J, eds. Intrauterine Infections. Ciba Foundation Symposium 10. Amsterdam: Associated Scientific Publishers, 1973:3–22.
79. Menser MA, Dorman DC, Reye RDK, Reid RR. Renal-artery stenosis in the rubella syndrome. Lancet. 1966; 1:790–792.
80. Esterly JR, Oppenheimer EH. Intrauterine rubella infections. In: Rosenberg HS, Bolande RP, eds. Perspectives in Pediatric Pathology, vol 1 Chicago: Year Book Medical Publishers. 1973: 313–338.
81. Ainger JE, Lawycr NG, Fitch CW. Neonatal rubella myocarditis. Br Heart J. 1966; 28:691–697.
82. Robinson HP, Fleming JEE. A critical evaluation of sonar "crown-rump length" measurements. Br J Obstet Gynaecol. 1975; 82:702–710.
83. Adam AH, Robinson HP. An evaluation of realtime scanning in the first trimester of pregnancy. In: Bennet MJ, Campbell S, eds. Real Time Ultrasound in Obstetrics. London: Blackwell Scientific Publications, 1980:39–48.
84. Krugman S, Katz SL. Rubella immunization: A five year progress report. N Engl J Med. 1974: 290:1375–1376.
85. Modlin JF, Brandling-Bennet DA. Surveillance of the congenital rubella syndrome: 1969–1973. J Infect Dis. 1974; 130:316–318.
86. Ogra PL, Kerr-Grant D, Umana G, Dzierba J, Weintraub D. Antibody response in serum and nasopharynx after naturally acquired and vaccine-induced infection with rubella virus. N Engl J Med. 1971; 285:1333–1339.
87. Kibrick S, Benirschke K. Acute aseptic myocarditis and meningoencephalitis in the newborn child infected with coxsackie virus group B, type 3. N Engl J Med. 1956; 255:883–889.
88. Kibrick S, Benirschke K. Severe generalized disease (encephalohepatomyocarditis) occurring in the newborn period and due to infection with coxsackie virus, group B: Evidence of intrauterine infection with this agent. Pediatrics. 1958; 22:857–875.
89. Fruhling L, Korn R, Lavillaureix J, Surjus A, Foussereau S. La myo-endocardite chronique fibroelastique du nouveau ne et du nourisson (fibro-elastose). Ann Anat Pathol. 1962; 7: 227–303.
90. Brown GC, Karunas RS. Relationship of congenital anomalies and maternal infection with selected enteroviruses. Am J Epidemiol. 1972; 95:207–217.
91. Vosburgh JB, Diehl AM, Liu C, Laver RM, Fabiyi A. Relationship of mumps to endocardial fibroelastosis. Am J Dis Child. 1965; 109:69–73.
92. St. Geme JW Jr., Peralta H, Farias E, Davis CWC, Noren GR. Experimental gestational mumps virus infection and endocardial fibroelastosis. Pediatrics. 1971; 48:821–826.
93. Guntheroth WG. Endocardial fibroelastosis and mumps. Pediatrics. 1966; 38:309.
94. Chen SC, Thompson MW, Rose V. Endocardial fibroelastosis: Family studies with special reference to counseling. J. Pediatr. 1971; 79: 385–392.
95. St. Geme JW Jr, Peralta H, Van Pelt LF. Intrauterine infection of the rhesus monkey with mumps virus: Abbreviated viral replication in the immature fetus as an explanation for split immunologic recognition after birth. J Infect Dis. 1972; 126:249–256.

F.VI

Metabolic Causes of Congenital Abnormalities

Fredda Ginsberg-Fellner, MD

I. INTRODUCTION

Although the etiology of congenital heart disease in most cases is unknown, increasing information is accumulating concerning roles for various drugs, infections, nutritional disturbances, and hypoxia. Such environmental factors may be responsible for up to 10% of neonatal cardiovascular malformations, while 75% of such abnormalities are produced by unknown factors.[1] Even when known maternal disease is associated with the development of congenital heart disease, the exact mechanisms causing maldevelopment of the fetal heart remain to be elucidated. The heart begins to take shape during the second intrauterine week, and the ventricular

Cardiac Problems in Pregnancy, pages 433–453

system is fully developed by the eighth week.[2] Thus, radical alterations and the effects that result in their production must occur between the second and eighth intrauterine weeks. However, later alterations in cardiac muscle, which must be differentiated from congenital heart disease in the perinatal period, have also been reported.[3–7] Many different metabolic factors have been described as affecting cardiac development. Their roles depend not only on the type of agent but also on its actual concentration, the specific time the fetus is exposed to the agent, and the gene type of the host.[8] Among metabolic teratogens, the roles of various body nutrients have been most carefully explored. Within this group, the effects of elevated blood glucose levels are now being intensively investigated.

II. DIABETES MELLITUS IN PREGNANCY

Diabetes mellitus in pregnancy is a very common disease. White reported a prevalence of one insulin-dependent diabetic per 1,000 pregnancies,[9] North et al reported a rate of 2.7 diabetics per 1,000 pregnancies (based on review of birth certificates) in New York State from 1958 to 1969,[10] and the collaborative perinatal study reported 5.6 cases per 1,000.[11,12] In addition, the latter study found an additional 7.5 gestational diabetics (White class A[13]—ie, women not known to have diabetes prior to pregnancy who develop glucose intolerance during pregnancy but revert to normal postpartum) per 1,000 pregnancies. This most complete survey then suggests that at least 13 of each 1,000 pregnancies (1.3%) are complicated by diabetes mellitus. Table F.VI.1 shows White's classification of diabetes mellitus in pregnancy,[13] which is used by most investigators to correlate the severity of the disease with both maternal and fetal morbidity.

A. Congenital Heart Disease and Morbidity in Infants of Diabetic Mothers

In 1937 Hurwitz and Irving were the first to report cardiac enlargement in an infant of a diabetic mother.[14] They also observed an increased amount of glycogen in the myocardium. In 1946 Miller reported two cases of congenital heart disease among 19 consecutive autopsies on infants born to diabetic mothers, one cor biventriculare with hypoplasia of the aorta, and one bicuspid pulmonary valve.[15] White reported a 17% prevalence of congenital anomalies in 2,147 diabetic pregnancies (almost all in insulin-dependent women) followed at the Joslin clinic from 1924 to 1974; 61% of these abnormalities resulted in perinatal death.[16] The most common lesion noted was interventricular septal defect. Navarrete et al studied 152 women without known diabetes in Mexico City, who delivered mal-

TABLE F.VI.1. Classification of Diabetes in Pregnancy*

Class	Description
A	Gestational or chemical diabetic; asymptomatic
B	Overt diabetes, onset after age 20, duration less than ten years
C	Overt diabetes, onset before age 20, duration ten to 20 years
D	Overt diabetes, duration more than 20 years or onset before age ten, benign retinopathy
E[a]	Calcified pelvic vessels
F	Nephropathy (proteinuria, azotemia)
R	Malignant (proliferative) retinopathy (retinitis proliferans)

*After White.[13]
[a]This classifications is not generally employed in current practice.

formed infants from 1964 to 1967[17]; 68% had abnormal standard or triamcinolone glucose tolerance tests three to eight weeks after delivery versus only 3.3% of a control group of 60 women. In addition, eight of 13 mothers of infants with cardiac abnormalities displayed abnormal carbohydrate tolerance. In 1964 Pedersen et al presented data demonstrating a significant difference of total, major, fatal, and multiple anomalies in infants of diabetic women.[18] Eight hundred fifty-three such infants were compared to 1,212 infants from a high-risk population; 6.4% of the 853 had anomalies, compared to 2.1% in the control group. Of the perinatal deaths, 12.2% were attributable to fatal malformations. In class F mothers, where vascular disease is most prominent, 16.7% had infants with congenital abnormalities. Kucera retrospectively reviewed data from 1945 through 1965[19]; 4.8% of 7,101 infants of diabetic mothers had congenital malformations.

An increased prevalence of anomalies has also been found in infants of Pima Indians in southern Arizona, who have the highest prevalence of diabetes so far reported.[20] Of 247 Pima Indian women studied, 87 had diabetes, 28 were borderline diabetics, and 132 were nondiabetics. Medical records of 1207 children of these women (96.3% of their offspring) were reviewed and included children born to mothers who now had overt diabetes but who had previous deliveries when they were not yet diabetic. Anomaly rates were 19.1% in infants of overt diabetics, 3.5% in prediabetics and 3.9% in nondiabetics. Congenital heart disease accounted for 33% of anomalies in infants of overt diabetics, 16% in prediabetics, and 26% of nondiabetic pregnancies. In the diabetics, one aortic stenosis, one atrial septal defect, and one undiagnosed lesion in a child who died at age one month of congestive heart failure were found. Early onset of diabetes (before age 25) was associated with an increased prevalence of anomalies, but paternal diabetes had no influence. Rowland et al reviewed a series of 470 Caucasian infants of diabetic mothers followed at the Joslin Clinic before 1973 and found a 4% incidence of proved congenital heart disease.[21] Transposition of the great arteries ($n = 4$), ventricular septal defect ($n = 3$), and coarctation of the aorta ($n = 3$) were found in ten cases, or more than half. Two patients had atrial septal defects. Single examples of isolated patent ductus arteriosus, aortic stenosis, tricuspid atresia, anomalous left coronary artery, mitral stenosis, and truncus arteriosus were also present. These authors found no relationship between gestational influences of maternal disease, including vascular complications and duration, on the development of the cardiac disease. Driscoll et al reported the postmortem findings in 95 of 104 infants of diabetic mothers in a cohort of 721 live-born infants delivered in Boston between 1940 and 1956.[22] Fourteen of 95 had congenital heart disease. The majority of such women had received exogenous estrogens and progestins. The occurrence of congenital malformations was not correlated with the severity or duration of the diabetes.

Gabbe and colleagues have carefully studied both gestational and insulin-dependent pregnant diabetics.[23,24] At Los Angeles County Women's Hospital between 1970 and 1972, 261 class A diabetics and 166 women in classes B–F were evaluated, representing 1.5% of all deliveries. The perinatal mortality rate was 19/1,000 in class A diabetics and 80/1,000 in classes B–F, which is significantly higher ($P < .005$). During the same interval total perinatal mortality was 32/1,000, which is not significantly different (although somewhat higher) than that noted in the gestational diabetics. In an expanded study of 260 class B–F diabetic women, where more careful follow-up was performed, the perinatal mortality rate fell to 46 per 1,000, which is still increased from the normal of 24 per 1,000.[24] Three infants (of 12) who died had congenital heart disease, including two cases of ventricular septal defect and one case of coarctation of the aorta. In 1977, in an extensive review on congenital malformations in infants of diabetic mothers, however,

Gabbe concluded that he was unable to identify the mechanisms underlying the production of such defects.[25]

Most studies agree that cardiac abnormalities constitute the largest group responsible for the two- to threefold increase in congenital abnormalities noted in infants of diabetic mothers.[26–32] Thus, Day and Insley surveyed 205 cases.[26] One hundred and seventeen of these mothers were on insulin at the time of conception. Fifty-seven women were diagnosed during pregnancy, and 31 were known to be diabetic prior to pregnancy but were treated by either diet or oral antidiabetic agents at the time of conception. The largest number of abnormalities (15%) was found in infants whose mothers were insulin-dependent at the time of conception. Of these, four (representing 34 per 1,000) had abnormalities of the cardiovascular system, and thus constituted the largest group. Lesions seen included two persistent ductus arteriosus, one cor triloculare, and one single atrium with a common atrioventricular canal and anomalous systemic venous drainage. A control group, at the same time, had only 2.8 cardiovascular abnormalities per 1,000 neonates. Unlike other reported series, these authors could not relate the development of abnormalities to the length of the disease, the age of onset, the maternal age, or the presence of vascular disease. An apparent effect of increasing parity was noted, and whether this could be related to poor diabetic control with succeeding pregnancies is unknown. Levin and Kanarek,[27] in a five-year study of live-born infants at the Queen Victoria Memorial Hospital in Johannesburg, found 141 children with congenital heart disease among 21,810 live births (0.65%), but they felt that this prevalence might be too low. The five most common lesions, ventricular septal defect (34.8%), patent ductus arteriosus (17.7%), coarctation of the aorta (11.4%), ventricular septal defect with pulmonary stenosis (7.8%), and atrial septal defect (3.5%), accounted for 75% of all cardiac abnormalities. Sixty-one diabetic or prediabetic mothers were found in these series, and four (7%) gave birth to an infant with cardiac problems, including one coarctation and one ventricular septal defect. Other investigators have reported that the chances of an affected infant with congenital heart disease being born to a diabetic mother varied from one in 39 to 1 in 57,[28,29] with great vessel disease being predominant. Thus, transposition of the great vessels occurs 45 times more frequently among diabetic mothers.[30] Soler and co-workers, in 1976,[31] reported congenital malformations in a series of 701 infants born to diabetic mothers between 1950 and 1974 in Birmingham, England. They found that patients belonging to White class A did not have an increased prevalence of infants with congenital malformations, while the remaining classes had a greater incidence. They found an overall incidence for anomalies of 8.1% (3 to 4 times higher than in their normal control population), with 3.8% being lethal. Nonfatal cardiac abnormalities included two atrial septal defects, two patent ductus arteriosus, one congenital heart block, one tetralogy of Fallot, and two no definitive diagnosis, while the fatal abnormalities included four transpositions of the great vessels, four ventricular septal defects, and two cor triloculares with multiple cardiac defects. In two of seven sets of twins, both infants had malformations. Five additional women each had two children with congenital abnormalities, and a third had three infants with such abnormalities. The risk for congenital malformations was similar for White classes B–F, but the risk for fatal anomalies was twice as high in classes C–F as in class B. Thus, abnormalities of the cardiovascular system occurred in 2.3% of the diabetic infants versus 0.21% in a control group. The Joslin Clinic also recently reported the pregnancy outcome in 147 diabetic women, 71% of whom were insulin-dependent for more than ten years.[32] A 14% incidence of birth defects was found, with 9% being major and 5% being minor. One woman with class B diabetes had an infant with a ventricular septal defect. A class D woman had a child with severe cardiac anomalies and hypoplastic lungs. Two infants with ventricular septal defects and two with patent ductus arteriosus were also noted in this group.

As improvements in the care of the pregnant diabetic occurred, the prevalence of congenital anomalies increased to account for 40% of perinatal deaths.[33] As the general health of women with insulin-dependent diabetes mellitus diagnosed in childhood (White classes C–R, indicating onset prior to age 20 or duration longer than ten years) improves, even more pregnancies may be expected in such women. Until recently the blood glucose levels in women with diabetes during pregnancy were probably nowhere near normal levels. Data accumulated until 1978–1980, therefore represent women in whom it can be reasonably assumed that elevated blood glucose concentrations were present throughout the period of embryogenesis, as well as during the rest of the pregnancy.

Several possible pathogenic mechanisms, including hyperglycemia, hypoglycemia, insulin, uterine and placental vascular compromise (leading to altered fetal nutrition and/or oxygenation), and chromosome changes, have been invoked as possible mechanisms to explain the increased prevalence of congenital abnormalities in infants of diabetic mothers.[34] Reid proposed that certain fetal cells might be especially sensitive to fluctuating glucose levels.[35] During periods of hyperglycemia, glycolysis would predominate, while reversion to euglycemia would rapidly reduce the rate of glycolysis, widening the energy gap. However, to date no mechanisms have been conclusively demonstrated.

However, data now accumulating strongly implicate maternal hyperglycemia per se as the most important etiologic factor[36,37] in the development of fetal malformations. How such changes in maternal metabolism affect organ teratogenesis has not been elucidated. Data in animal models do show a direct effect of high glucose levels; thus, embryo organ cultures to which high concentrations of glucose are added have developmental anomalies, including exencephaly.[38–40] To date, cardiac changes have not been found in these models. In addition, sera from animals in which diabetes was induced by streptozotocin have produced growth retardation in cultured embryos.[41] How hyperglycemia affects organogenesis is still highly speculative. It is now known, for example, that glucosylation of multiple body proteins is increased when glucose concentrations are elevated.[42,43] Such glucosylation might alter intrauterine differentiation and/or maturation of organs. Clearly, the elucidation of mechanisms of action of etiologic agents promoting teratogenesis remains of paramount importance.

B. Blood Sugar Abnormalities, Oral Antidiabetic Agents, and Cardiac Malformations

When the oral hypoglycemic antidiabetic agents were introduced, it was common practice to use tolbutamide or similar drugs in the treatment of mild degrees of carbohydrate intolerance in pregnancy. In addition, women classified as class B diabetics often were on these agents prior to and at the time of conception and therefore continued to take these agents at least during the earlier parts of embryogenesis. In 1960 Larsson and Sterky reported the results of a pregnancy in a 16-year-old treated with tolbutamide throughout her pregnancy.[44] Six weeks before her estimated due date, the patient went into labor spontaneously and gave birth to a premature female infant weighing 1,100 gm, who died 15 minutes later. The child had dextrocardia, complete absence of the atrial septum, and a small ventricular septal defect. The patient had been taking tolbutamide for 1 1/2 years, and prior to the pregnancy she had normal fasting blood glucose concentrations and excreted less than 5 gm of glucose in her 24-hour urine collections. However, during the pregnancy, glycosuria increased to 25 gm per day; in fact, increasing glycosuria first suggested that the patient might be pregnant. Larsen and Sterky then suggested that perhaps tolbutamide should not be used during pregnancy because either the hyper- or the hypoglycemic effects of this drug could produce difficulties. One year later Campbell et al[45] reported that oral hypoglycemic agents were routinely given to about 90% of the prenatal Indian diabetics in Durban, South Africa. Twenty-one women so treated had five fetal losses, and one of the aborted fetuses was grossly malformed. Schiff and co-workers in 1970[46] reported neonatal thrombocytopenia and other congenital malformations associated with administration of tolbutamide during pregnancy. The affected infant, who weighed 3.812 kg at 37 weeks gestation, also had pulmonary congestion consistent with transient pulmonary edema of the neonate, which subsequently regressed. Of 60 mothers in Soler's group on oral hypoglycemic agents, five (8.3%) had infants with congenital defects.[31] One of these was a neonate with transposition of the great vessels born to a mother who took Metaprel® 1.5 gm daily through the 26th week of gestation and then insulin until parturition. A preauricular sinus malformation was found in the neonate of a woman who took Tolinase® 350 mg daily through the 37th week of gestation. These rates were similar to those in an insulin-treated group. Thus, the question of the teratogenicity of tolbutamide remains unanswered. Today, it is common practice for all pregnant diabetics who are taking oral antidiabetic agents to be changed to insulin as soon as they are known to be pregnant. However, in view of the possible risks of the oral agents, it might be wise for all women of childbearing age with diabetes (or at least those planning to have children) to use insulin at all times. It is important to note that antidiabetic drugs, including tolbutamide, have been administered to many animals in experimental studies, but heart abnormalities have not been reported.

C. Blood Glucose Control and the Development of Congenital Heart Disease in Infants of Diabetic Mothers

During the past five years evidence has been rapidly accumulating linking various of the complications of diabetes mellitus with long-term hyperglycemia. The development of a blood test, hemoglobin A_1C[47,48] (glycosylated hemoglobin), which provides a measurement of mean blood glucose levels in a patient during the preceding four to six weeks, enables an estimate of what blood glucose levels are like in any diabetic. Hemoglobin A_1C and (A_1a_1, A_1a_2, and A_1B) are formed by nonenzymatic addition of glucose to the N-terminal valine in the beta chain of human hemoglobin A.[49] In most cases this is an essentially irreversible process such that the glycohemoglobin formed is not destroyed until the red blood cells themselves are destroyed. Since in most circumstances the life-span of red blood cells is approximately 120 days (and the half-life is about 60 days), significant changes in hemoglobin A_1C can be demonstrated by repeating these tests every four to eight weeks. Early studies demonstrated a rise in hemoglobin A_1C in the third trimester of pregnant, normal subjects compared with the nonpregnant population, possibly related to the increased new red cell mass at that time.[50] Subsequent studies show that, in most diabetics, glycohemoglobin levels decline as pregnancy progresses.[51] This is not surprising in view of the fact that the normal body glucose levels in women also decline during pregnancy, such that the normal mean fasting blood sugars average 60 mg/dl and two-hour postprandial concentrations are between 80 and 87 mg/dl.[52] In addition, as hemoglobin A_1C has a decreased reactivity to 2,3-diphosphoglycerate and an increased affinity for oxygen, its decreased concentration may be a maternal compensatory mechanism to increase oxygen delivery to the fetus.[53] Furthermore, the motivation for controlling blood sugar levels is more apt to be present during pregnancy than at other times. It is only during the past two or three years that serious attempts at maintaining normoglycemia during diabetic pregnancies have been made. Pioneer programs at various centers have shown an overall improvement in fetal morbidity and mortality as well as in the development of congenital abnormalities. In a small study of 50 patients with insulin-dependent diabetes, Jovanovic et al failed to find any congenital abnormalities.[54] However, the number expected in such a small group, is one or less, and thus these data are not statistically significant. However, some earlier data also support the importance of normoglycemia in pregnancy in decreasing the prevalence of congenital anomalies. Drury summarized his experiences in treating 328 insulin-dependent diabetic women during 649 pregnancies.[55] In the later years, he aimed at maintaining fasting blood glucose levels below 100 mg/dl and postprandial levels below 120 mg/dl. Two injections of insulin per day were used. Hypoglycemic coma developed at least once during 41 pregnancies. Thirty-eight infants survived and were normal, and the remaining three died long after the hypoglycemic episode. Eleven infants had congenital malformations. Karlsson and Kjellmer analyzed diabetic pregnancies in Sweden from 1961 to 1970.[56] Perinatal mortality declined from 23.6% in the group whose mean blood sugar level was greater than 150 mg/dl to 15.3% in the group whose mean was 100–150 mg/dl, to 3.8% in the group whose mean was less than 100 mg/dl. The fetal malformation rate was increased threefold in those with long-standing diabetes with or without vasculopathy and was also related to mean blood glucose levels, with a rate of 3.8% in those whose mean blood glucose was below 100 mg/dl. It is important to note that the glucose levels were obtained, for the most part, after the 30th week of gestation. Jervell at al reported the results of a regimen of close metabolic and obstetric control in the second and third trimesters in 234 pregnant diabetics in Oslo from 1970 to 1977.[57] Perinatal mortality was 4.3%, and 5.5% had anomalies. Six cases of congenital heart disease occurred, with two each born to mothers in White's classes, C, D, and F. Recent studies at Mount Sinai Hospital (New York) reveal four cases of congenital abnormalities during the past two years in more than 200 pregnancies, 80% of them in gestational diabetic mothers.[58] The four congenital abnormalities included two in infants born to women with gestational diabetes and two delivered of insulin-dependent diabetic mothers. This prevalence of cardiac abnormalities is somewhat increased from the rate in the normal population of eight cases per 1,000. However, it is to be stressed that these women in general were not treated until well after the first trimester of pregnancy. A national collaborative study involving five centers is now in progress in which attempts are being made to normalize blood glucose levels prior to pregnancy and at earlier stages of pregnancy in insulin-dependent diabetic mothers. This might be useful, as attested to by the recent retrospective study of Miller et al[36] from the Joslin Clinic and the Boston Lying-In Hospital. They examined the medical records of all pregnant insulin-requiring diabetics who were followed at the Joslin Diabetes Clinic and the Boston Hospital for Women from April 1977 until April 1980 to ascertain which women had initial hemoglobin A_1C levels measured at the first clinic visit before 14 weeks of gestation. All the infants were examined by one of the authors or an associate at birth and at discharge from the hospital, and follow-up information was obtained from the nurse or the infant's pediatrician between three and 16 months after birth to elicit anomalies that were not found on the initial examination. One hundred and sixteen subjects met all criteria and were included in the study. Thirty-eight were White class B, 32 class C, nine D, 26 class D (benign retinopathy), six class R (proliferative retinopathy), and five class F (diabetic nephropathy). Each cardiac diagnosis was confirmed by cardiac catheterization, echocardiography, or autopsy. The assays for hemoglobin A_1C included the labile reversible component of glycosylated hemoglobin, which is dependent on the blood glucose at the time of sampling.[59] Thus these absolute values may be somewhat increased over values obtained by other investigators. As shown in Table F.VI.2, 15 of the 116 insulin-dependent diabetic women who were studied in the first trimester were delivered of infants with major congenital abnormalities. Eight infants had congenital heart defects, three of which were fatal. Mean initial hemoglobin A_1C levels were significantly higher in the group delivering infants with anomalies. The mean hemoglobin A_1C concentration in women with major anomalies was 9.5 ± 1.0% (SD) versus 8.4 ± 1.6% ($P < .01$) at initial sampling, which occurred at a mean of 10.2 ± 2.2 weeks in those with major anomalies and at 9.3 ± 1.8 weeks in those with no anomalies; the latter was a nonsignificant difference. Concomitantly, although the mean blood sugars were increased at the A_1C sampling time, being 207 ± 83 mg/dl versus 186 ± 76 mg/dl, these were not significant. Interestingly, the mean, 9.7%, for the women delivering children with cardiac abnormalities was higher than the mean for all other anomalies combined. Although more anomalies occurred in mothers with diabetic microangiopathy than in those without, the differences were also not significant. This is the first conclusive study where significant numbers of glycosylated hemoglobin measurements were obtained very early in pregnancy. The incidence and type of anomalies in this survey were similar to those studied in other surveys of diabetic pregnant women. Pedersen reported a strong negative association between insulin reactions in the first trimester, which theoretically would be associated with improved blood glucose control and the incidence of anomalies.[60] Leslie et al observed in 1978 that three of five women with elevated hemoglobin A_1C values in the first trimester had infants with major congenital abnormalities, while no malformations occurred in 20 women with lower A_1C values.[37] However, this too was an extremely small study. Thus, the prospective studies of tight diabetic control in the first trimester of pregnancy and possibly prior to conception are awaited with great interest in that it may finally be possible to show that such blood glucose control, as measured by hemoglobin A_1C levels, is associated with the first significant reported reduction in congenital heart disease in offspring. It is of interest that women with elevated A_1C levels were found in the group being followed by the Joslin Clinic, which has been the proponent of tight blood glucose control in the first trimester.[61] Our studies revealed that the first trimester is the time when blood glucose levels are most likely to be elevated. In our class B–F diabetics, mean A_1C levels of 10.0% decrease by the 16th week of gestation to 4.5% in the majority of our

TABLE F.VI.2. Congenital Heart Disease in Offspring of Diabetic Mothers Related to Blood Glucose Control*

Anomaly	White class	Initial maternal hemoglobin A_1C (%)[a]
Transposition of great arteries	B	10.0
Ventricular septal defect	R	11.0
Atrial septal defect	D	9.3
Tetralogy of Fallot	F/R	9.0
Single ventricle[b]	C	10.2
Ventricular-septal defect	C	8.1
Single ventricle, mitral valve atresia, pulmonic stenosis[b]	B	11.3
Hypoplastic left heart[b]	B	8.7

*From Miller et al.[36]
[a]Normal nondiabetic range <6%.
[b]Fetal or neonatal death.

patients.[62] Higher A_1C levels were seen throughout pregnancy in mothers who had infants with congenital abnormalities. Programs aimed at tight blood glucose control during pregnancy now include early ascertainment of pregnancy by use of basal body temperatures[63] and detection of dates of ovulation,[64] sequential chorionic gonadotropin levels every month in patients at risk for pregnancy or desirous of becoming pregnant,[65] home blood glucose monitoring, which enables self determination of capillary blood glucose concentrations several times per day,[66–68] strict diet,[69] careful observation and education, and multiple insulin doses (in some centers, three or four doses of combined intermediate and short-acting insulin or just short-acting insulin alone are used).[70,71] In addition, mini-pumps for constant subcutaneous administration of basal insulin doses and bolus amounts prior to meals have been employed in experimental protocols.[72] The goal of improved blood glucose control in diabetic women during pregnancy thus is probably obtainable in a majority of patients if sufficient education and a team approach are used. Not only should improved control affect the development of various abnormalities in patients, but also it has been shown by many groups to be associated with a decrease in the amount of fetal macrosomia and other neonatal problems.[54,58]

D. Insulin and Possible Congenital Malformations

Insulin is the key metabolic signal for fuel storage in the fed state, while in the fasted state, relatively lower concentrations of insulin and glucagon are the signals for fuel mobilization.[73] In pregnancy, other hormones and nutritional factors also affect the metabolic state. Glucose levels are normally maintained within very narrow limits, returning to baseline values rapidly. In times of metabolic need the organism tries to maintain protein stores, to conserve nitrogen, and switches to primarily using fat as fuel. This has been described by Frankel et al as accentuated catabolism in the basal state and faciliated anabolism in the fed state.[74] Chomette administered insulin to rabbits of several breeds on days 6–11 in pregnancy.[75] Treatment was followed by hypoglycemic convulsions. Ectopia cordis was found in many of these animals. However, a direct role on the fetus for maternal insulin itself is unlikely since insulin does not cross the human placenta,[76] and thus many of the effects attributed to insulin may reflect extreme hypoglycemia. In this regard, Wicks demonstrated fetal defects in offspring of women who received insulin shock treatment early in pregnancy.[77]

Careful analysis of the data from the collaborative perinatal project by regression analysis found that only the duration of diabetes in women who received insulin therapy had effects on congenital anomalies.[11,12,28] Insulin reactions, ketoacidosis, blood sugar greater than 200 mg/dl, or insulin therapy did not appear to have any effect. However, this does not prove that insulin and/or blood sugar levels have no relationship, since most data suggest that the longer a person has diabetes, the greater the chances are that the patient will have increasing periods of hyperglycemia. In addition, malformations in this study were divided based on the diabetic state of the father. None of the malformation indices for the "father only" diabetic category were significantly different from the respective incidences where neither parent was diabetic. Thus, there was an incidence of major malformations of 0.09% if the father only was diabetic, 17% if the mother only was diabetic, and 0.08% if neither was diabetic out of a total number of 51,803 pregnancies.

The teratogenic effects of maternal diabetes are such that the resulting malformations are generally distributed throughout the organ systems and occur in multiple rather than in single forms, suggesting that the teratogenic agents must have their effects in the early stages of embryonic development. They therefore do not relate to insulin administration alone, which orignally appeared to neither increase nor decrease the malformation risk. However, this is at variance with the finding that insulin prevents the increased occurrence of congenital malformations induced in pregnant mice. Lichtenstein et al reported abnormalities in offspring of white rats given large doses of protamine zinc insulin (PZI) during pregnancy.[78] These experiments were stimulated by reports that insulin injected into developing eggs produced malformations in chick embryos.[79] Seven to eight units of PZI given subcutaneously each day as a single dose appeared to be the maximum amount tolerated by rats weighing more than 150 gm. Insulin was injected daily throughout the gestation period beginning on the second day of pregnancy or earlier. Ninety-six rats produced 783 fetuses. Abnormalities were found only in that the weights of the insulin-treated rats were smaller and there were mild skeletal deformities. In contrast, Horii and collaborators[80] showed that congenital malformations could be prevented in alloxan-diabetic mice by providing insulin in physiologic doses. In mice, although skeletal abnormalities can be produced, treatment with insulin does not result in any cardiac malformations. Thus, it is probably safe to conclude that insulin per se is not a teratogen to the developing cardiac system in animals or in man, even if hypoglycemia (and the risk for this is somewhat increased by new programs for improved blood glucose control during pregnancy) is added as a risk factor. Apparently, decreases in oxygen production or other mechanisms involved in hypoglycemia within the mother do not result in cardiac malformations in the infant. Possibly this is related to the fact that although the mother may be hypoglycemic, the blood glucose levels required for development in the fetuses are still maintained, and it is well known that fetuses are able to function well at low blood glucose concentrations.[81] Since teratogenesis often reflects cell death, very low blood sugar levels could contribute to the development of anomalies. However, no satisfactory studies in humans are available. In addition, none of the anomalies produced in animals were cardiac in nature.

E. Cardiomyopathies in Infants of Diabetic Mothers

In the perinatal period, symptoms of cardiomyopathies, including cardiomegaly, cyanosis, and pulmonary congestion, are difficult to distinguish from those of congenital heart disease. Such differential diagnosis is of importance since prognosis and treatment are drastically different. In infants of diabetic mothers, since both congenital heart disease and cardiomyopathies occur with increased frequency, both entities should be carefully considered in the evaluation of the infants. In 1943 Miller and Wilson first reported six infants of diabetic mothers with enlarged hearts, on x-ray films, and the cardiac enlargement took variable lengths of time to return to normal.[3] Wolfe and Way[4] summarized the features of cardiomyopathies in infants of diabetic mothers. At birth, cardiorespiratory distress must often be differentiated from congenital heart disease. Respiratory difficulty may be secondary to idiopathic respiratory distress syndrome, which occurs with increased frequency in these infants (up to 25%) and to persistence of the fetal circulation. Radiographic evidence of cardiomegaly and/or clinical features suggesting congestive heart failure may occur in 50% or more of infants of diabetic mothers. The cardiomegaly may be secondary to the increased prevalence of hypoglycemia, hypocalcemia, birth asphyxia, and hyperviscosity common in such infants. Hypertrophy and hyperplasia of myocardial cells was shown by Naeye in the hearts of such infants.[82] In a careful study of 28 infants of diabetic mothers, Wolfe and Way[4] found 12 infants with cardiomegaly and tachypnea of unknown etiology. Echocardiographic dimensions and function indicated that ten of the 12 had a mild nonobstructive cardiomyopathy with a modest increase in interventricular septal size and diminished left ventricular function. The other two had murmurs and echocardiographic patterns characteristic of obstructive hypertrophic cardiomyopathy. In such patients symptoms may last for several months. Seven other infants had rapidly reversible (within 72 hours) congestive cardiomyopathies. Two of 28 infants had congenital heart disease.

Way et al described 11 infants of diabetic mothers who had signs of congestive heart failure and cardiorespiratory distress.[5] Most developed symptoms during the first week of life, and nine had systolic ejection murmurs, with the harsher murmurs noted in the obstructive form of the hypertrophic cardiomyopathy. Ten of 11 infants had cardiomegaly. One had a normal electrocardiogram, four had right ventricular and six, left ventricular, hypertrophy. All infants had thickening of the interventricular septum on echocardiogram, an in three of them there was systolic anterior motion of the mitral valve leaflet. Five infants had cardiac catheterizations, and three of them had significant gradients across the subaortic region. Four others had mild-to-moderate elevations of pulmonary arterial pressures. Follow-up evaluations were performed between three and 40 months of age. By one month of age, all infants were asymptomatic, and chest radiographs became normal by three to 20 months. Echocardiograms showed regression or return to normal of septal hypertrophy and decreasing murmurs. The etiologies of these septal changes still are unknown, but roles for catecholamines, nerve growth factor, insulin, and growth hormone have all been suggested.

Three infants with hypertrophic obstructive cardiomyopathy with features of suboaortic stenosis were also described by Gutgesell et al, who suggested that digitalis and diuretics are contraindicated because outflow obstruction is increased.[6] Propranolol, however, may be used. Breitweser et al described one infant with nesidioblastosis and five of 18 infants of diabetic mothers who had septal hypertrophy on echocardiograms[7]; all were hyperinsulinemic. They found no correlation between the presence of this hypertrophy and hypocalcemia, polycythemia, or birth asphyxia. However, all had profound hypoglycemia. They then suggested that insulin is important in the developing heart since the heart is rich in insulin receptors and contains marked insulin-degrading capacity. Furthermore, as disproportionate thickening of the interventricular septum is found in the normal developing human heart,[83] the lesions noted may be secondary to an exaggeration of the normal developmental process.

III. OTHER POSSIBLE TERATOGENS

A. Thyroid Hormones

The fetal placental unit does not participate to any great extent in the maternal thyroid economy. Irreversible developmental consequences of athyrosis in the offspring of euthyroid mothers, as well as the birth of normal infants to hypothyroid mothers, attest to the relative independence of maternal and fetal thyroid hormone pools.[84–86] Triiodothyronine apparently cannot cross the placenta very rapidly, and neither can thyroxin.[87] Iodine is thought to be rapidly transferred[88] as are thyronine analogs such as DIMIT (3′,5′, dimethyl 5-isopropylthyronine, which has one-fifth the activity of thyroxin).[89] Thyroid stimulating hormone apparently also does not traverse the placenta, while the thyrotropin-releasing hormone (TRH) does.[90] Long-term maternal ingestion of large doses of T_3 (up to 300 μg every 24 hours) has resulted in inconsistent and incomplete fetal T_4 suppression near term.[91] The long-acting thyroid stimulating hormone (LATS) does cross the placenta.[92] Hyperthyroidism with an incidence of one to two cases per 1,000 pregnancies is the second most common endocrinopathy of pregnancy, with Graves disease being the most common cause of hyperthyroidism.[93] Propylthiouracil (PTU), the drug most commonly used for hyperthyroidism, appears to be transferred into the fetal circulation less readily than other compounds such as Tapazole.[94] Congenital anomalies have been reported to be increased in mothers treated with PTU. Mujtaba and Burrow[95] summarized the results of PTU and methimazole therapy to 21 hyperthyroid women during 26 pregnancies. Five children had congenital abnormalities, including one born with aortic atresia. This child, whose mother received 50 mg of PTU daily during pregnancy, which maintained her in the euthyroid state, weighed 2,795 gm at birth. A sib of this child, however, did not have any cardiovascular abnormalities despite the fact that the mother received 100–300 mg of PTU daily during that pregnancy. Forty years ago the first effects of hypothyroidism in pigs were demonstrated wherein every case had a persistent foramen ovale.[96] Hyperthyroidism in animals, however, has not resulted in any cardiac abnormalities. The presence of autoimmune thyroiditis, with antimicrosomal and/or antithyroglobulin antibodies (particularly common in infants of women with insulin-dependent diabetes mellitus)[97] may also produce transient abnormalities in thyroid function in the infants. Hyperthyroidism can also be associated with abnormalities in glucose metabolism, such that hyperglycemia is present, which can contribute, as previously described, to the development of cardiac abnormalities.

B. Steroid Hormones

Cushing syndrome and its clinical and biochemical manifestations may be remarkably exacerbated by pregnancy and may be associated with prematurity and stillbirth.[98] Metabolic insults to the infant may reflect a more general insult, related possibly to hyperglycemia. In the presence of unrecognized Addison disease and hypocortisolemia, hypoglycemia may develop. In addition, in a large study of Long-Evans female rats that were subjected to various doses of hydrocortisone administered subcutaneously for seven days during the first, second, or third weeks of pregnancy, no malformations that could be attributed to this treatment were revealed.[99]

C. Estrogens

To date, estrogens have not definitely been linked with the development of cardiac malformations. However, the use of estrogen and progesterone in managing pregnant diabetics,[100] as previously advocated by White, may be associated with an increased prevalence of transposition of the great vessels.[101]

D. Possible Role of Islet Cell Antibodies and Insulin Antibodies

Over the past several years it has been demonstrated that type I insulin-dependent diabetes mellitus is associated with a high prevalence of circulating pancreatic cytoplasmic and surface islet cell antibodies.[102–104] These antibodies are present in close to 100% of insulin-dependent diabetics at the time of diagnosis, with a gradual decrease in their prevalence with increased duration of diabetes leading to a prevalence of between 10 and 30% five years after diagnosis of the disease. Those patients who have such antibodies for long periods often have associated other autoimmune diseases, particularly thyroiditis and/or an increased incidence of antithyroglobulin and antimicrosomal antibodies.[105] We recently reported the presence of such islet cell antibodies[106,107] in 10–20% of women diagnosed as having gestational diabetes as well as in our insulin-dependent population. Fifty percent of infants of islet cell antibody-positive mothers also have such antibodies. Other workers have corroborated these findings.[108,109] The relationship of these antibodies to other abnormalities in these infants is unknown at this point. Two of four infants born with congenital heart disease at Mount Sinai Hospital (New York) have such antibodies, but it is not clear if they are involved in this teratogenesis. Since these antibodies (as well as insulin-binding antibodies) are of the IgG class and thus traverse the placenta, they may well produce pancreatic damage. In addition, other organ-specific cytotoxic antibodies are often found in diabetics, and Volkova and Maysky have claimed that some developmental anomalies are associated with organ-specific antibodies.[110] Obviously, prospective studies are required to determine whether any of these cytotoxic antibodies could be important in the development of congenital heart disease.

E. Hyperphenylalaninemia

Table F.VI.3 summarizes reported congenital heart disease in a survey of 123 women known to have elevated phenylalanine levels.[111] Seventeen percent of mothers had phenylalanine concentrations greater than or equal to 20 mg/dl, 19% had values of 16–19 mg/dl, and 8% had values of 11–15% mg/dl. Twelve percent had one or more offspring with congenital heart disease. No mothers with phenylalanine levels below 10 mg/dl, however, had offspring with cardiac defects. The frequency of congenital heart disease among the 348 offspring of these 123 mothers showed a similar pattern of increase relative to the mother's blood phenylalanine level, as compared with a frequency of eight per 1,000 for a general like population. Among 36 offspring with cardiac malformations, seven (19%) had tetralogy of Fallot, four (11%) had ventricular septal defects, three (8%) had coarctation of the aorta, two (6%) had patent ductus arteriosus, and one each (3% each) had a single ventricle or an atrial septal defect. Eighteen had unspecified lesions. The rates for specific lesions are similar to the rates expected among children with congenital heart disease in the general population, except for tetralogy of Fallot, which occurred at almost 5 times the expected frequency of 4%. Thirty-four pregnancies occurred in women to whom a low phenylalanine diet was adminstered during pregnancy, which reduced the blood phenylalanine concentrations from 20 mg/dl or greater to between 4 and 12 mg/dl. In four of 11 pregnancies treated during the first trimester, congenital heart disease still occurred, and it also occurred in two of 16 treated during the second trimester; however, it did not occur in any of the four first treated in the third trimester. Only three patients were treated prior to conception, and no congenital abnormalities occurred in their offspring. If the data are sorted, then the high frequency of congenital heart disease occurred in offspring of mothers whose phenylalanine concentration was 11 mg/dl or greater, suggesting that a teratogenic effect occurred during the first gestational trimester. Since no other congenital anomalies appeared with increased frequency in these offspring, this is an unusual pattern in human teratogenesis where multiple effects usually occur. It is also conceivable that phenylalanine has a specific interaction with the embryonal heart. Future studies are therefore warranted in this area.

TABLE F.VI.3. Maternal Hyperphenylalaninemia and Congenital Heart Disease in Offspring*

	Maternal phenylalanine levels (mg/dl)			
	≧20	16–19	11–15	3–10
Affected in terms of mothers at risk	13/77 (17%)	3/16 (19%)	1/13 (8%)	0/17 (0%)
Affected total number of infants	27/225 (12%)	7/46 (15%)	2/33 (6%)	0/44 (0%)

*From Lenke and Levy.[111]

F. Vitamin Deficiencies

To date significant studies have been performed only in animal models,[112] and it remains unclear whether those data can be extrapolated in any ways to humans. About two decades ago, it first became possible to produce congenital malformations experimentally in animals by dietary deficiencies in the pregnant animal. Obviously, this is superior to previous studies, which produced congenital malformations in lower classes of animals, since the prenatal maternal–offspring relationship is not as similar as it would be in other mammals.

1. Deficiency of vitamin A

In 1933 Hale reported the results of feeding a vitamin A-deficient diet to a registered New Jersey pig starting at four months of age.[113] Five and one-half months later the animal was bred, and after the first month of pregnancy she was given small doses of cod liver oil, which contains vitamin A and prevents destruction of the fetus. In the first litter of 11, all were eyeless and two had ectopic eyes. Many other types of abnormalities occurred in these animals, including cardiac defects. However, this diet probably also lacked riboflavin, panthothenic acid, nicotinic acid, and vitamin B_{12}. The young vitamin-deficient rats had underdeveloped heart muscle that retained its spongy fetal structure. Cardiovascular malformations were analyzed by Wilson et al,[114] who found a large number of aortic arch anomalies of various types such as supernumerary, absent, ectopically arising, and transposed vessels. The heart was subject to two types of abnormalites, incomplete interventricular septum and general retardation of myocardial development, giving the wall of the heart a highly fetal spongy appearance. Many of the cardiovascular anomalies observed in rats closely simulated malformations observed in many other animals. Of interest, the heart anomalies were more frequent in the offspring of females who were supplemented with vitamin A at various times during pregnancy. This was interpreted as being the result of salvaging young that would otherwise have perished. These observations were further interpreted to indicate that the teratogenic influence of vitamin A deficiency presumably was exerted during the process of organogenesis rather than on differentiating tissues. Vitamin A deficiency in pregnant rabbits, however, failed to result in the development of cardiac abnormalities.[115]

2. Deficiency of riboflavin

In 1940 Warkany and Nelson reported that deficiency of riboflavin produced congenital malformation in the offspring of rats.[116] They placed 60–65-day-old Long-Evans female rats on riboflavin-deficient diets containing various levels of galactoflavin, a riboflavin antimetabolite. Anomalies produced included defects of the interventricular septum of the heart and of the aortic arch pattern.[117] With this type of antimetabolite therapy, the deficiency could be shortened, and four days of deficiency was shown to produce only cardiovascular malformations. Similar data have also been described in mice.[118]

3. Deficiency of vitamin B_{12} and folic acid

Vitamin B_{12} deficiency has been shown to produce serious tissue anomalies in the heart, liver, and spleen in rats.[119] Evans and co-workers extensively studied the effects of induction of deficiency of folic acid in rats by using the antagonist X-methyl folic acid. Depending on the days that the antagonist was administered, various abnormalities occurred, including some of the cardiovascular system. They also placed female rats on a folic acid-deficient diet containing no antagonists from 21 to 64 days before breeding and continuing through gestation and induced, among other abnormalities, those in the heart.[120] Nelson et al found cardiovascular anomalies in pregnant female rats treated from day 7 to 8½ by employing an experimental folic acid-deficient diet for various periods during the first week (14 days) of gestation. Afterwards, the females were transferred to a folic acid-supplemented diet for the remainder of gestation.[121] If treatment was performed from day 8 to 9½, cardiovascular defects predominated. A small number of cardiovascular defects was noted when the animals were treated from day 9 to 10½. The abnormal mothers maintained on the deficient diets from day 9 to 11 showed more abnormalities and a moderate incidence of cardiovascular anomalies. No cardiac malformations were produced when the treatment was begun after day 11 of gestation. The extensive work of Nelson showed that treatment from day 7 to 9 results predominantly in cardiac malformation and from day 9 to 11, predominantly in vascular defects. The abnormalities incurred included interventricular septal defects, patent ductus arteriosus, double or right aortic arch, absence of ductus arteriosus, aberrant origin of great arteries, and other variations in the pattern of arteries derived form the embryonic arches. Many of these malformations are similar to those reported in vitamin A deficiency. However, the folic acid deficiency-induced malformations could be prevented by supplementation with this vitamin as late as day 10 of gestation, whereas the vitamin A-induced malformations were not prevented when vitamin A was given on day 9. Thus, temporal differences may exist in requirements for different vitamins, at least in animals.

4. Deficiency of pantothenic acid

Evans and Nelson et al used pantothenic acid antagonists such as x-methypanthothenic acid and sodium omega methyl pantothenate in Long-Evans rats to produce transient deficiencies of the vitamin.[122] They produced defects of the interventricular septum of the heart and of the aortic arch. In addition, it was found that folic acid deficiency itself could produce a secondary pantothenic acid deficiency.

5. Deficiency of vitamin E

Cheng and Thomas produced congenital malformations in Sprague-Dawley rats using a vitamin E-deficient diet from weaning to maturity and supplementation with the vitamin at various times during pregnancy.[123] Dextrocardia was found when the deficient diet was given during the first eight days of gestation and then the vitamin itself was introduced between days 9 and 12. Deficiencies of choline produce similar results.

G. Other Nutrient Deficiencies

Deficiencies of choline and vitamin K have failed to produce congenital malformations in mice and rats, and deficiencies of thiamine and niacin have failed to produce any cardiac abnormalities. Likewise, defects of vitamin D, vitamin C, and essential fatty acids have not been reported to produce cardiac anomalies in animals.[112]

H. Deficiencies in Amino Acids

Deficiencies in amino acids have not been shown to cause congenital abnormalities. Likewise, fasting during various periods of pregnancy has not resulted in cardiac abnormalities. Amino acid antagonists, including 6-mercaptopurine and azaserine, which produce various congenital abnormalities in animals, have not to date resulted in cardiac abnormalities.[112]

I. Hypervitaminosis A

Giroud and Martinet gave 60,000 IU of vitamin A to rats per day orally for three successive days, starting at five or six different periods in gestation.[124] They found that 11% of animals had abnormalities of the cardiovascular system, distributed equally between abnormalities of the aortic arch arteries and those of the heart.

J. Alcohol Ingestion

The complete fetal alcohol syndrome originally described by Lemoin et al,[125] and and later by Ulleland[126] and Jones et

TABLE F.VI.4. Cardiac Malformations in the Fetal Alcohol Syndrome*

	Number	Percent of total
Patients with cardiac malformations	31	41
Additional patients with functional murmurs	12	16
Cardiac lesions		
Ventricular septal defects		
Simple VSD (1 with mesocardia)	15	
VSD + subpulmonary and subaortic stenosis	1	
VSD + aortic regurgitation	1	
VSD + coarctation	1	
VSD + coarctation + small LV + mitral	1	
VSD + 2° ASD	1	
Total	20	26
Tetralogy of Fallot	4	5
Secundum atrial septal defect	3	4
Peripheral pulmonary artery stenosis	2	3
Double outlet right ventricle and pulmonary atresia	1	
Dextrocardia (with VSD)	1	
Patent ductus arteriosus and 2° pulmonary hypertension	1	
Cor pulmonale	1	

VSD = ventricular septal defect; LV = left ventricle; ASD = atrial septal defect.
*From Sanders et al.[129]

al,[127] includes poor intrauterine and postnatal growth, microcephaly, motor and mental retardation, small palpebral fissures, hypoplastic philtrum, anteverted nostrils, and mid-facial hypoplasia. In 1979 Hoberman[128] demonstrated a minor hemoglobin component in the blood of alcoholics. This glycosylated hemoglobin, which is distinct from hemoglobin A_1C as well as from other previously described glycosylated hemoglobins, appears to form via 5-deoxy-D-xyulose-1-phosphate and hemoglobin A. This compound is formed in a reaction between acetaldehyde, the first product of alcohol oxidation and dihydroxyacetone phosphate. Like hemoglobin A_1C's relation to blood glucose levels over the preceding four to eight weeks, this glycosylated hemoglobin appears to reflect a dose-time record of alcohol consumption. Thus it will be useful in establishing the time course, and perhaps the alcohol dose, required for various teratogenic effects.

To date the number of reported cases of the fetal alcohol syndrome exceeds 600. Recently Sandor et al described the cardiac findings in 76 patients (69 were children ages birth to 18 years of North American Indian mothers) with documented features of this syndrome.[129] The cardiac assessment consisted of physical examination, chest radiograph, ECG, and echocardiography. Cardiac catheterization was performed when indicated hemodynamically or when the clinical diagnosis was in doubt. As shown in Table F.VI.4, 41% of patients had cardiac lesions, and an additional 16% had functional murmurs of either the basal ejection or left sternal border early systolic type. Ventricular septal defects were the most common lesions. Earlier reviews reported transient murmurs and atrial septal defects to be the most frequent cardiac lesions (25–50%).[130–131] Loser and Majewski reported the cardiac catheterization findings in 16 of 56 patients.[132] Atrial septal defects were found in ten of 16, ventricular septal defects in three, and there was one case each of mild idiopathic hypertrophic subaortic stenosis, atrioventricular canal, and aplasia of the right pulmonary artery.

The wide spectrum of cardiac malformations suggests a nonspecific teratogenic effect of alcohol or its metabolites.

The exact prevalence of the fetal alcohol syndrome, particularly in its partial forms, is unknown, but estimates range from one to five per 1,000 live births.

IV. SUMMARY

Various metabolic agents appear to be of great importance in the pathogenesis of congenital heart disease. As particular malformations cannot be produced after certain stages of development have passed, the time of exposure to such metabolic teratogens is crucial. Some agents may only act acutely and produce specific malformations only at particular embryologic stages. Other agents are chronic (? glucose) and act at various times when the embryo is sensitive to them. For example, since vitamins act as prosthetic groups for enzymes important in various metabolic activities, and if these enzymes are important in embryonic development, then absence of the vitamins may result in interruption of biochemical sequences. Thus, although it would be impossible to mimic the effects of the exaggerated deficiencies or excesses of various nutrients in the human pregnancy, it is possible that even minor degrees of excesses or deficiencies, particularly if more than one is present, might act synergistically to induce certain abnormalities. Obviously, the genetic pool itself must be important, but its contribution is even more difficult to investigate. The ongoing studies of the teratogenic influences of maternal hyperglycemia may elucidate, for the first time, prototypic biochemical and cellular mechanisms responsible for alterations in the metabolism and signals of specific cell types, which must underly the development of abnormalities found in congenital heart disease. Such descriptions would then provide the basic data required for designing protocols for the prevention and/or amelioration of such anomalies. Finally, although metabolic factors such as those associated with diabetes mellitus may be important etiologically in only a small number of infants with congenital heart disease, they potentially can be controlled. Thus, if they are implicated in any neonate, future pregnancies of this mother can be more carefully monitored and appropriately controlled.

V. ACKNOWLEDGMENTS

This work was supported in part by NIH grant HD 11583.

VI. REFERENCES

1. Congenital malformations of the heart—Incidence and etiology. In: Rowe RD, Freedom RM, Mehrizi A, Bloom KR eds. Neonate with Congenital Heart Disease, 2nd Ed. Philadelphia: W.B. Saunders, 1981:110–135.
2. General principles. In: Nadas AS, ed., Pediatric Cardiology, 2nd Ed. Philadelphia: W.B. Saunders, 1963:339–365.
3. Miller HC, Wilson HM. Macrosomia, cardiac hypertrophy, erythroblastosis and hyperplasia of the islands of Langerhans in infants born to diabetic mothers. J Pediatr. 1943; 23:251–266.
4. Wolfe RR, Way GC. Cardiomyopathies in infants of diabetic mothers. Johns Hopkins Med J. 1977; 140:177–180.
5. Way GL, Wolfe RR, Eshaghpour E, Bender RI, Jaffe RB, Ruttenberg HD. The natural history of hypertrophic cardiomyopathy in infants of diabetic mothers. J Pediatr. 1979; 95: 1020–1025.
6. Gutgesell HP, Mullins CE, Gillette PC, Speer M, Rudolph AJ, McNamara DG. Transient hypertrophic subaortic stenosis in infants of diabetic mothers. J Pediatr. 1976; 89:120–125.
7. Breitweser JA, Meyer RA, Sperling MA, Tsang RC, Kaplan S. Cardiac septal hypertrophy in hyperinsulinemic infants. J Pediatr. 1980; 96:535–539.
8. Simpson JL. Genetics of diabetes mellitus (DM) and anomalies in offspring of diabetic mothers. Semin Perinatol. 1978; 2:383–394.
9. White P. Pregnancy and diabetes, medical aspects. Med Clin North Am. 1965; 49:1015–1024.
10. North AF Jr, Mazumdar S, Logrillu VM. Birthweight, gestational age and perinatal deaths in 5,471 infants of diabetic mothers. J Pediatr. 1977; 90:444–447.
11. Niswander KR, Gordon M. The collaborative perinatal study of the National Institute of Neurological Disease and Stroke. The women and their pregnancies. Philadelphia: W.B. Saunders, 1972:239–245.

12. Chung CS, Myrianthopoulos NC. Factors affecting risks of congenital malformations: II Effects of maternal diabetes. Birth Defects 1975; 11 (10):23–37.
13. White P, Koshy P, Duckers J. The management of pregnancy complicating diabetes and of diabetic mothers. Med Clin North Am. 1953; 37:1481–1496.
14. Hurwitz D, Irving FC. Diabetes and pregnancy. Am J Med Sci. 1937; 194:85–92.
15. Miller HC, The effect of diabetic and prediabetic pregnancies on the fetus and newborn infant. J Pediatr. 1946; 29: 455–461.
16. White P. Diabetes mellitus in pregnancy. Clin Perinatol. 1974; 1:331–347.
17. Navarrete VN, Torres IH, Rivera IR, Shor UP, Gracia PM. Maternal carbohydrate disorder and congenital malformations. Diabetes. 1967; 16:127–130.
18. Mølsted-Pedersen L, Tygstrup I, Pedersen J. Congenital malformations in newborn infants of diabetic women: Correlation with maternal diabetic vascular complications. Lancet. 1964; 1:1124–1126.
19. Kucera J. Rate and type of congenital anomalies among offspring of diabetic women. J Reprod Med. 1971; 7:61–70.
20. Comess LJ, Bennett PH, Burch TA, Miller M. Congenital anomalies and diabetes in the Pima Indians of Arizona. Diabetes. 1969; 18: 471–477.
21. Rowland TW, Hubbell JP, Nadas AS. Congenital heart disease in infants of diabetic mothers. J Pediatr. 1973; 83:815–820.
22. Driscoll SG, Bernirschke K, Curtis GW. Neonatal deaths among infants of diabetic mothers. Am J Dis Child 1960; 100:818–835.
23. Gabbe SG, Nestman JH, Freeman RK, Anderson GV, Lowenschen RI. Management and outcome of class A diabetes. Am J Obstet Gynecol. 1977; 127:465–469.
24. Gabbe SG, Nestman JH, Freeman RK, Goebelsmann UT, Lowensohn RI, Nochimson P, Cetrulo C, Quilligan EJ. Management and outcome of pregnancy in diabetes mellitus, classes B to R. Am J Obstet Gynecol. 1977; 129: 723–728.
25. Gabbe SG, Congenital malformations in infants of diabetic mothers. Obstet Gynecol Survey. 1977; 32:125–132.
26. Day RE, Insley J. Maternal diabetes and congenital malformation. Survey of 205 cases. Arch Dis Child. 1976; 51:935–938.
27. Levin SE, Kanarek KS. The incidence of congenital heart disease in Johannesburg. A 5 year study of liveborn infants at the Queen Victoria Maternity Hospital. S Afr Med J 1973; 47:1855–1858.
28. Mitchell SC, Sellman AH, Westphal MC, Park J. Etiologic correlates in a study of congenital heart disease in 56,109 births. Am J Cardiol. 1971; 28:653–657.
29. Rubin A, Murphy DP. The frequency of congenital malformations in the offspring of nondiabetic and diabetic individuals. J Pediatr. 1958; 53:579–585.
30. Rowe RD, Mehrizi A. The Neonate with Congenital Heart Disease. Philadelphia: W.B. Saunders, 1968:411.
31. Soler NG, Walsh CH, Malins JM. Congenital malformations in infants of diabetic mothers. Q J Med. 1976; 45:303–313.
32. Kitzmiller JL, Cloherty JP, Younger MD, Tabatabail A, Rothchild SB, Sosenko I, Epstein MF, Singh S, Neff RK. Diabetic pregnancy and perinatal morbidity. Am J Obstet Gynecol. 1978; 131:565–580.
33. Dundon S, Murphy A, Ratery J, Drury MI. Infants of diabetic mothers. J Irish Med Assoc. 1974; 67:371–375.
34. Simpson JL. Genetics of diabetes mellitus and anomalies in offspring of diabetic mothers. In: Merkatz IR, Adam PAJ eds. The Diabetic Pregnancy: A Perinatal Prospective. New York: Grune & Stratton, 1979:235–247.
35. Reid RA. Diabetes and congenital abnormalities. Lancet. 1970; 1:1030.
36. Miller E, Hare JW, Cloherty JP, Dunn PJ, Gleason RE, Soeldner JS, Kitzmiller JL. Elevated maternal hemoglobin A_1C in early pregnancy and major congenital anomalies in infants of diabetic mothers. N Engl J Med. 1981; 304:1331–1334.
37. Leslie RDG, Pyke DA, John PM, White JM. Haemoglobin A_1 in diabetic pregnancy. Lancet. 1978; 2:958–959.
38. Cockroft DL, Coppola PT. Teratogenic effects of excess glucose on head-fold rat embryos in culture. Teratology 1977; 16:141–146.
39. Sadler TW. Effects of maternal diabetes on early embryogenesis II hyperglycemia induced exencephaly. Teratology. 1980; 21:349–356.
40. Cockroft DL, Freinkel N, Phillips LS, Shambaugh GE. Metabolic factors affecting organogenesis in diabetic pregnancy. Clin Res. 1981; 29:577A (abstrt).
41. Sadler TW. Effects of maternal diabetes on early embryogenesis. I. The teratogenic potential of diabetic serum. Teratology. 1980; 21:339–347.
42. Brownlee M, Vlassara H, Cerami A. Measurement of glycosylated amino acids and peptides from urine of diabetic patients using affinity chromatography. Diabetes. 1980; 29:1044–047.
43. Cohen MP, Urdanivia E, Surma M, Wu VY. Increased glycosylation of glomerular basement membrane collagen in diabetes. Biochem Biophys Res Commun. 1980; 95:765–769.
44. Larsson Y, Sterky G. Possible teratogenic effects of tolbutamide in pregnant prediabetics. Lancet. 1960; 2:1424–1426.
45. Campbell GD. Possible teratogenic effects of tolbutamide in pregnancy. Lancet. 1961; 1:891–892.
46. Schiff D, Aranda JV, Stern L. Neonatal thrombocytopenia and congenital malformations as-

sociated with administration of tolbutamide to the mother. J Pediatr. 1970; 77:457–458.
47. Bunn HF, Haney DN, Kamin S, Gabbay KH, Gallop PM. The biosynthesis of human hemoglobin A_1C; slow glycosylation of hemoglobin in vivo. J Clin Invest. 1976; 57:1652–1659.
48. Koenig RJ, Peterson CM, Jones RL, Saudek C, Lehrman M, Cerami A. Correlation of glucose regulation and hemoglobin A_1C in diabetes mellitus. N Engl J Med 1976; 295:417–420.
49. Bunn HF, Haney DN, Gabbay KH. Further identification of the nature and linkage of the carbohydrate in hemoglobin A_1C. Biochem Biophys Res Commun. 1975; 67:103–109.
50. Peripheral blood erythrocyte counts and cell indices, Part II: Normal values for pregnant women. In: Altman PL, Katz DD, eds. Human Health and Disease, Vol 2. Bethesda: Federation of American Societies for Experimental Biology, 1977: 153.
51. Vintzileos AM, Thompson JP. Glycohemoglobin determinations in normal pregnancy and in insulin-dependent diabetics. Obstet Gynecol. 1980; 56:435–439.
52. Mintz D, Skyler J, Chez R. Diabetes mellitus and pregnancy. Diabetes Care. 1978; 1:49–63.
53. Bunn HF, Briehl RW. The interation of 2,3-diphosphoglycerate with various human hemoglobins. J Clin Invest. 1970; 49:1088–1095.
54. Jovanovic L, Peterson C, Saxena B, Yusoff M, Saudek C. Feasibility of maintaining normal glucose profiles in insulin-dependent pregnant diabetic women. Am J Med. 1980; 68:105–112.
55. Drury MI. Diabetes mellitus and pregnancy: The nine month experiment. Postgrad Med J. 1979; 55(Suppl 2):36–39.
56. Karlsson K, Kjellmer I. The outcome of diabetic pregnancies in relation to the mother's blood sugar level. Am J Obstet Gynecol. 1972; 112:213–220.
57. Jervell J, Moe N, Skjaeraasen J, Blystad W, Egge K. Diabetes mellitus and pregnancy management and results at Riks-hospitalet, Oslo, 1970–1977. Diabetologia. 1979; 16:151–155.
58. Franklin BH, Mark EM, Nechemias C, Hausknecht RU, Ginsberg-Fellner F. Macrosomia in infants of pregnant diabetics with near-normal glucose control in the third trimester. Diabetes. 1981; 30 (Suppl 1):4A.
59. Goldstein DE, Peth SB, England JD, Hess RL, DaCosta J. Effects of acute changes in blood glucose on HbA_1C. Diabetes. 1980; 29:623–628.
60. Pedersen J, Mølsted-Pedersen L, Anderson B. Assessors of fetal perinatal mortality in diabetic pregnancy. Diabetes 1974; 23:302–305.
61. Joslin EP, Root HF, White P, Marble A. The Treatment of Diabetes Mellitus, 10th Ed. Philadelphia: Lea & Febiger, 1959.
62. Franklin BH, Mark EM, Horlick MNB, Witt ME, Sudzin H, Nechemias C, Hausknecht RU, Ginsberg-Fellner F. Factors in the macrosomia of gestational diabetes. in preparation.
63. Davajan V, Mishell DRJ Jr. Evaluation of the infertile couple. In: Mishell DR Jr, Davajan V eds. Reproductive Endocrinology, Infertility and Contraception. Philadelphia: F.A. Davis Co., 1979:315.
64. Morgan CA, Cooke ID. A comparison of the competitive protein binding assay and the radioimmunoassay for plasma progesterone during the normal menstrual cycle. J Endocrinol. 1972; 54:445–451.
65. Saxena BB, Hasan SH, Haour E, Schmidt-Gollwitzer M. Early diagnosis of pregnancy. Science. 1974; 184:793–795.
66. Sonksen PH, Judd S, Lowy C. Home monitoring of blood glucose: New approach to management of insulin-dependent diabetic patients in Great Britain. Diabetes Care. 1980; 3:100–107.
67. Skyler JS, Lasky IA, Skyler DL, Robertson EG, Mintz DH. Home blood glucose monitoring as an aid in diabetes management. Diabetes Care. 1978; 1:150–157.
68. Walford S, Allison SP, Gale EAM, Tattersall RB. Self-monitoring of blood glucose: Improvement in diabetic control. Lancet. 1978; 1:732–735.
69. Committee on Maternal Nutrition: Maternal Nutrition and the Course of Pregnancy. Washington, D.C.: National Research Council/National Academy of Sciences, 1970.
70. Jovanovic L, Peterson CM. Management of the insulin-dependent diabetic woman. Diabetes Care. 1980; 3:63–68.
71. Skyler JS, O'Sullivan MJ, Robertson EG, Skyler DL, Holsinger KK, Lasky IA, McLeod AGW, Burkett G, Mintz DH. Blood glucose control during pregnancy. Diabetes Care. 1980; 3:69–76.
72. Pickup JC, Keen H, Parsons JA, Alberti KGMM, Rowe AS. Continuous subcutaneous insulin infusion: Improved blood glucose control and intermediary metabolic control in diabetics. Lancet. 1979; 1:1255–1257.
73. Felig P. Body fuel metabolism and diabetes mellitus in pregnancy. Med Clin North Am. 1977; 61:43–66.
74. Freinkel N, Metzger B, Nitzan M, et al. Facilitated anabolism in late pregnancy: Some novel maternal compensations for accelerated starvation. In: Malaisse WJ, Pirart J, eds. Proceedings VIII Congress of the International Diabetes Federation. Amsterdam: Excerpta Medica, 1974.
75. Chomette G. Entwicklungsstorungen nach insulin schock beim trachtiger Kaninchen. Beitr Pathol Anat. 1955; 115:439–451.
76. Adam PAJ, Teramo K, Raiha N, et al. Human fetal insulin metabolism early in gestation: Response to acute elevation of the fetal glucose concentration and placental transfer of human insulin I-131. Diabetes. 1969; 18:409–413.
77. Wickes IG. Fetal defects following insulin coma therapy in early pregnancy. Br Med J. 1954; 2:1029–1030.

78. Lichtenstein H, Guest GM, Warkany J. Abnormalities in offspring of white rats given protamine zinc insulin during pregnancy. Proc Soc Exp Biol Med 1951; 78:398–402.
79. Duraiswami PK. Insulin-induced sketetal abnormalities in developing chickens. Br Med J. 1950; 2:384–390.
80. Horii K, Watanabe G, Ingalls TH. Experimental diabetes in pregnant mice: Prevention of congenital malformations in offspring by insulin. Diabetes. 1966; 15:194–204.
81. Holmberg NG, Kaplan B, Karvonen MJ, Lind J, Malm M. Permeability of human placenta to glucose, fructose and xylose. Acta Physiol Scand. 1956; 36:291–298.
82. Naeye R. Infants of diabetic mothers: A quantitative morphologic study. Pediatrics. 1965; 35:980–988.
83. Maron BJ, Verter J, Kapur S. Disproportionate ventricular septal thickening in the developing normal human heart. Circulation. 1978; 57:520–526.
84. Greeman GW, Gabrielson MO, Howard-Flanders J, Wessel MA. Thyroid dysfunction in pregnancy: Fetal loss and follow-up evaluation of surviving infants. N Engl J Med. 1962; 267:426–431.
85. Kennedy AL, Montgomery DAD. Hypothyroidism in pregnancy. Br J Obstet Gynaecol. 1978; 85:225–230.
86. Lachelin GCL. Myxedema and pregnancy. J Obstet Gynaecol Br Commonw. 1970; 77:77–79.
87. Grumbach MM, Werner SC. Transfer of thyroid hormone across the human placenta at term. J Clin Endocrinol Metab. 1956; 16:1392–1395.
88. Gibson M, Tulchinsky D. The maternal thyroid. In: Tulchinsky D, Ryan KJ eds. Maternal-Fetal Endocrinology. Philadelphia: W.B. Saunders, 1980:121.
89. Burrow GN. Hyperthyroidism during pregnancy. N Engl J Med. 1978; 298:150–153.
90. Espstein MF, Chez RA, Dakes GK, Vaitukaitis JL. Hypothalamic-pituitary control of perinatal prolactin secretion in Macaca mulatta. Endocrinology. 1976; 99:743–751.
91. Raiti S, Holzman GB, Scott RL, Blizzard RM. Evidence for the placental transfer of triiodothyronine in human beings. N Engl J Med. 1967; 277:456–459.
92. Selenkow HA, Birnbaum MD, Hollander CS. Thyroid function and dysfunction during pregnancy. Clin Obstet Gynecol. 1973; 16:66–108.
93. Burrow GN. Thyroid Diseases. In: Burrow GN, Ferris T eds. Medical Complications During Pregnancy. Philadelphia: W.B. Saunders, 1975.
94. Marchant B, Brownlie BEW, Hart DM, Horton PW, Alexander WD. The placental transfer of propylthiouracil, methimazole and carbamazole. J Clin Endocrinol Metab. 1977; 45:1187–1193.
95. Mujtaba Q, Burrow GN. Treatment of hyperthyroidism in pregnancy with propylthiouracil and methimazole. Obstet Gynecol. 1975; 46:282–286.
96. Smith GE. Fetal athyrosis, a study of the iodine requirements of the pregnant sow. J Biol Chem. 1917; 29:215–225.
97. Bottazzo GF, Mann JI, Thorogood M, Baum JD, Doniach D. Autoimmunity in juvenile diabetics and their families. Br Med J. 1978; 2:165–168.
98. Gimes EM, Fayez JA, Miller GL. Cushing's syndrome and pregnancy. Obstet Gynecol 1973; 42:550–556.
99. Gunberg DL. Some effects of exogenous hydrocortisone on pregnancy in the rat. Anat Rec. 1957; 129:133–153.
100. Nora JJ, Nora AH. Birth defects and oral contraceptives. Lancet. 1973; 1:941–943.
101. Levy EP, Cohen A, Fraser FC. Hormone treatment during pregnancy and congenital heart defects. Lancet. 1973; 1:611–614.
102. Lendrum R, Walker G, Cudworth AG, Theophanides C, Pyke DA, Bloom A, Gamble DR. Islet-cell antibodies in diabetes mellitus. Lancet. 1976; 2:1273–1276.
103. Richens ER, Quilley J, Hartog M. Immunologic features of juvenile onset diabetic patients correlated to HLA type. Clin Exp Immunol. 1979; 26:198–204.
104. Irvine WJ, McCallum CJ, Gray RS, Campbell CJ, Duncan LJP, Farquhar JW, Vaughan H, Morris PJ. Pancreatic islet cell antibodies in diabetes mellitus correlated with the duration and type of diabetes, co-existent autoimmune disease and HLA type. Diabetes. 1977; 26:138–147.
105. Bottazzo GF, Florin-Christensen A, Doniach D. Islet cell antibodies in diabetes mellitus with autoimmune polyendocrine deficiencies. Lancet. 1974; 2:1279–1283.
106. Ginsberg-Fellner F, Dobersen M, Mark EM, Nechemias C, Hausknecht RU, Rubinstein P, Notkins AL. Islet cell antibodies in gestational diabetes. Lancet. 1980; 2:362–363.
107. Rubinstein P, Walker M, Krassner J, Carrier C, Carpenter C, Nechemias C, Hausknecht R, Mark EM, Dobersen MJ, Notkins AL, Ginsberg-Fellner F. HLA antigens and islet cell antibodies (ICA) in gestational diabetes (GD). Hum Immunol. (in press).
108. Gamlen TR, Aynsly-Green A, Irvine WJ, et al. Immunological studies in the neonate of a mother with Addison's disease and diabetes mellitus. Clin Exp Immunol. 1977; 28:192–195.
109. Tingle AJ, Lim G, Wright VJ, Dimmick JE, Hunt JA. Transplacental passage of islet cell antibody in infants of diabetic mothers. Pediatr Res. 13:1323–1325, 1979.
110. Volkova LS, Maysky IN. Immunologic interaction between mother and embryo. In: Edwards RG, ed. Immunology and Reproduction. London: International Planned Parenthood Federation, 1969:211–230.
111. Lenke RR, Levy HL. Maternal phenylketonu-

ria and hyperphenylalaninemia. N Engl J Med. 1980; 303:1202–1208.
112. Kalter H, Warkany J. Experimental production of congenital malformations in mammals by metabolic procedure. Physiol Rev. 1959; 39:69–115.
113. Hale F. Pigs without eyeballs. J Hered. 1933; 24:105–106.
114. Wilson JG, Warkany J. Aortic arch and cardiac anomalies in offspring of vitamin A deficient rats. Am J Anat. 1949; 85:113–155.
115. Lamming GE, Salisbury GW, Hays RL, Kendall KA. Effect of incipient vitamin A deficiency on reproduction in the rabbit. II Embryonic and fetal development. J Nutr. 1954; 52:227–239.
116. Warkany J, Nelson RC. Appearance of skeletal abnormalities in the offspring of rats reared on a deficient diet. Science 1940; 92:383–384.
117. Nelson MM, Baird CDC, Wright HV, Evans HM. Multiple congenital abnormalities in the rat resulting from riboflavin deficiency induced by the antimetabolite galactoflavin. J Nutr. 1956; 58:125–134.
118. Kalter H, Warkany J. Congenital malformations in inbred strains of mice induced by riboflavin-deficient galactoflavin-containing diets. J Exp Zool. 1957; 136:531–566.
119. Jones CC, Brown SO, Richardson LR, Sinclair JG. Tissue abnormalities in newborn rats from vitamin B_{12} deficient mothers. Proc Soc Exp Biol Med. 1955; 90:135–140.
120. Evans HM, Nelson MM, Asling CW. Multiple congenital abnormalities resulting from acute folic acid deficiency during gestation. Science. 1951; 114:479.
121. Nelson MM, Wright HV, Asling CW, Evans HM. Multiple congenital abnormalities resulting from transitory deficiency of pteroylglutamic acid during gestation in the rat. J Nutr. 1955; 56:349–369.
122. Nelson MM, Wright HV, Baird CDC, Evans HM. Teratogenic effects of pantothenic acid deficiency in the rat. J Nutr. 1957; 62:395–405.
123. Cheng DW, Thomas BH. Relationship of time of therapy to teratogenicity in maternal avitaminosis E. Proc Iowa Acad Sci. 1953; 60:290–299.
124. Giroud A, Martinet M. Malformations diverses du foetus de Rat suivant les stades d'administration de Vitamin A en exces. C R Soc Biol. 1955; 149:1088–1090.
125. Lemoine P, Harousseau H, Borteyru J-P, Menuet J-C. Les enfants de parents alcooliques; Anomalies observees. Ouest Med. 1968; 25:476–481.
126. Ulleland CN. The offspring of alcoholic mothers. Ann NY Acad Sci. 1972; 197:167–169.
127. Jones KL, Smith DW, Ulleland CN, Streissguth AP. Pattern of malformation in offspring of chronic alcoholic mothers. Lancet. 1973; 1:1267–1271.
128. Hoberman HD. Synthesis of 5-deoxy-D-xyulose-1-phosphate by human erythrocytes. Biochem Biophys Res Commun. 1979; 90:757–763.
129. Sanders GGS, Smith DF, MacLeod PM. Cardiac malformations in the fetal alcohol syndrome. J Pediatr 1981; 98:771–773.
130. Veghely PV, Osztovics M, Kardos G, Leisztner L, Szaszovszky E, Igali S, Imrei J. The fetal alcohol syndrome: Symptoms and pathogenesis. Acta Paediatr Acad Sci Hung. 1978; 19:171–181.
131. Clarren SK, Smith DW. The fetal alcohol syndrome. N Engl J Med. 1978; 298:1063–1067.
132. Loser H, Majewski M. Type and frequency of cardiac defects in embryofetal alcohol syndrome: Report of 16 cases. Br Heart J. 1977; 39:1374–1379.

F.VII

Environmental Causes of Congenital Heart Abnormalities

Kenneth D. Rosenman, MD

I. INTRODUCTION

The etiology of the majority of birth defects is unknown. A dramatic example of this is our inability to explain the cause of the twofold increase in the rate of ventricular septal defects and patent ductus arteriosus over the last decade. Although such a rise, which does not appear to be due to better diagnostic capabilities, points to an environmental cause, the actual precipitating event(s) remains elusive.[1] Even the small percentage of birth defects that appear to be of genetic origin may be initiated by environmental events that cause a gene mutation or a chromosomal aberration. Environmental exposures can be classified by source as due to personal habits (alcohol, cigarettes, medications), occupational exposures (chemicals, metals) or environmental exposures (air, water, food). Exposure to infectious agents that cause congenital heart defects is discussed in Chapter F.V.

Rapid identification of the cause of birth defects is possible when an unusual and clinically apparent defect is induced at a comparably high rate as compared to a low baseline rate. The experience with thalidomide and phocomelia best illustrates this form of recognition. It was this association, uncovered in the early 1960s, that provided the impetus for the current scientific concern that environmental exposures are a major factor in birth defects.

The difficulty in making additional associations between environmental exposure and birth defects is due to the complexity of assessing exposures. Environmentally induced events that cause increases in the relatively common types of birth defects can only be recognized with formal epidemiological studies. In fact, in situations where the environmental agent causes a small increase in a relatively common defect there is no method for uncovering that adverse effect. When an agent causes a relatively large increase from baseline, then comparative interviews of parents of children with and without birth defects (case-control studies), or interviewing pregnant women and assessing the outcome of their pregnancy (prospective studies) may be done. Because there are critical periods in fetal development, not only is it important to assess what a

Cardiac Problems in Pregnancy, pages 455–459

pregnant woman is exposed to during her pregnancy but also to assess the dose and the particular trimester or part of trimester during which she was exposed. Furthermore, exposures prior to the pregnancy during ovarian development and/or exposures of the father that may effect spermatogenesis may be important and need to be assessed. Since it may not be the environmental exposure by itself but an interaction between the exposure and genetically susceptible individuals, information on exposure alone may not reveal causal relationships.

Methodological problems in collecting relevant data from parents with a child who has a birth defect and comparing the findings with information collected from less concerned and motivated control parents who have children without birth defects can lead to inaccurate conclusions. The amount and detail of information needed to draw reliable conclusions makes data collection a formidable task if the study is done prospectively. This is so because very large numbers of women need to be interviewed (ie, in the National Collaborative Perinatal Project 50,000 women were interviewed) to have a sufficient number of birth defects to analyze possible associations.

Because of the difficulties and the expense of assessing the cause of birth defects in humans, animal studies have been used not only to study the mechanisms of teratogenicity but also to uncover teratogenic substances. Extrapolating from animal experiments to humans is complicated by varying species sensitivity. For example, the rat and mouse are relatively insensitive to the effect of thalidomide, whereas the rabbit, monkey, and human are highly sensitive. Whether humans are insensitive to substances that have been shown to be teratogenic in different animal species is not known. The absence of evidence in humans implicating substances that have been shown to be teratogenic in animals may be a result of the methodological difficulties of conducting human epidemiological studies.

A limited number of environmental factors associated with congenital heart defects are discussed in this chapter. Undoubtedly astute physicians, epidemiologists, and toxicologists will uncover additional associations in this relatively new area of investigation.

II. PERSONAL EXPOSURE

The most thoroughly studied associations between environmental exposure and congenital heart disease have been done on the use of medications during pregnancy. The prominent defects associated with the ingestion of thalidomide during pregnancy were phocomelia and amelia (partial and total absence of limbs). However, various case series reported cardiovascular defects to be present in up to 20% of the children born with limb abnormalities. Women taking the medication from the fortieth to the forty-fifth day of pregnancy were the ones most likely to have children with a cardiovascular anomaly. No specific cardiac anomaly predominated.

There have been approximately ten studies examining the relationship between oral contraceptives, hormonal pregnancy tests, and congenital heart defects.[2,3] Most of those studies have shown a small but consistent increase (approximately twice the risk) in congenital heart defects in the offspring of women exposed to hormones during pregnancy. Initial reports indicated a specific association with conal-trunco defects, but follow-up reports have not indicated an increase in any specific anomaly. Investigations have not been able to pinpoint whether it is the estrogen or progesterone or a combination of the two that is the causal agent.

There is one case-control study of women who had children with congenital heart defects that showed that 18% of the mothers of affected children had used dexamphetamine, whereas the drug had been used by 8% of the mothers of normal children.[4] Further studies replicating these results need to be done before any firm conclusions can be drawn.

In studying an association between medication ingestion and congenital heart defects, it is necessary to control for the underlying condition for which the medication was given. For example, the relationship between insulin and congenital heart defects may in fact be an association between maternal diabetes and congenital heart disease. Similarly, an association between antibiotic use during pregnancy and congenital heart defects may actually be an association with the infectious agent for which the antibiotics were prescribed as either specific or nonspecific therapy.[2] The association between the development of congenital heart defects and ingestion of oral contraceptives, however, cannot be explained on this basis, since there is no underlying disease for which oral contraceptives are taken.

Beta-adrenergic drugs cause aortic arch anomalies in chick embryos; and the more beta-andrenergic activity a drug has, the higher the rate of anomalies. Propranolol, for example, blocks the development of the aortic arch anomalies. There is no evidence in humans that beta-adrenergic drugs have a similar effect.

Chronic consumption of alcohol during pregnancy has been associated with a syndrome consisting of central nervous system dysfunction, growth deficiencies, and a characteristic cluster of facial abnormalities. Cardiac abnormalities may be present in children with the fetal alcohol syndrome. The frequency of the fetal alcohol syndrome has been reported to between one to two cases per thousand live births and partial expression at three to five cases per thousand live births.[6] The frequency of the syndrome increases with the amount of alcohol ingested. In one study 20% of women who had six drinks or more per day had a child with a major congenital anomaly. Women who drank less than that amount had children with major congenital anomalies 2–3% of the time.[7] In up to 50% of children with the fetal alcohol syndrome, murmurs usually secondary to atrial septal defects are present.[6] In up to 25% of the children a ventricular septal defect, a great vessel anomaly, or the tetrology of Fallot is present.[6] The presence of the typical facies characterized by short palpebral fissures, a hypoplastic upper lip with a thinned vermillion, and a diminished or absent philtrum is indicative of the fetal alcohol syndrome and should raise the suspicion of an associated congenital heart defect.

All studies that have investigated a relationship between cigarette smoking and congenital heart defects have shown no association.[8]

III. OCCUPATIONAL EXPOSURE

A large and increasing number of women work during pregnancy.[9] Surveys have indicated that up to 65% of women work during pregnancy. In a study from the State of New York, where the mother's usual occupation must be reported on the birth certificate, 63% of the mothers who worked during the pregnancy were incorrectly listed as housewives on the birth certificate.[10] Medical providers need to become aware of the work exposures of their pregnant patients both to be able to recognize new associations between occupational exposure and birth defects and to advise women on what exposures to avoid.

Studies of female and male anesthesiologists, nurse anesthetists, operating room nurses, and operating room technicians have generally indicated that women workers or wives of male workers who are exposed to anesthetic agents have an increase in adverse birth outcomes. Spontaneous abortions have been the major type of adverse events noted. At least two studies have also indicated increased rates of congenital heart defects.[11,12] The increase is not limited to any specific anomaly. These investigations have not pinpointed individual anesthetic agents although the absence of an effect in the offspring of male dental workers,[13] who use mainly nitrous oxide, suggests that the adverse fetal effects among operating room personnel may be caused by exposure to halogenated hydrocarbons such as halothane, enflurane, and methoxyflurane. However, female dental workers exposed only to nitrous oxide have increased spontaneous abortions,[13] and nitrous oxide does cause adverse reproductive effects in animal models. It is to be hoped that national programs to promote better work practices that minimize leaks, the introduction of waste anesthetic gas-scavenging systems, and an emphasis on routine equipment maintenance will reduce occupational exposure and its associated adverse health effects.

Azo dyes refer to a large group of dyes that are commonly used in animal models to study the mechanism of formation of congenital heart defects. The same dye causes different anomalies to be increased in various strains of rats. In addition, different dyes from this group have different effects. Azo dyes are also commonly used in industry to color textiles, food, and cosmetics. There have been no studies of women workers or the wives of male workers who are exposed to azo dyes during their production or industrial use. There are approximately 7.8 million pounds of azo dyes produced a year in the United States. The actual number of workers exposed to these substances in industrial settings is not known. In New Jersey approximately 15% of the work force in the organic dye industry are women. At a much lower level, all pregnant women are exposed to these substances in consumer products. Significant exposure to these agents is possible, and further study is imperative.

IV. ENVIRONMENTAL EXPOSURE

Although environmental exposure to a number of agents such as mercury, PCBs, and hexachlorobenzene have been associated with birth defects, none of the abnormalities have included heart defects. There is no evidence that toxins present in air, water, or food are associated with congenital heart defects in humans. Cardiovascular malformations have been described in animal models after exposure to the pesticides 2,4,5,T; carbaryl; malathion; and parathion.

Electrocardiographic and autopsy evidence indicates that infants born and raised at high altitudes retain right ventricular dominance throughout childhood, unlike children at lower altitudes. In studies from the South American Andes, the incidence of patent ductus arteriosus at 4,500–5,000 meters altitude is 30 times that found at sea level.[14] It is suggested that at high altitudes, hypoxia and pulmonary hypertension, which remain as chronic conditions after birth, are causal factors. Unlike the human studies, increased rates of ventricular septal defects have been reported in the offspring of pregnant rats after they were placed in hypoxic atmospheres.

V. REFERENCES

1. Layde PM, Erickson JD, Dooley K, Edmonds LD. Is there an epidemic of ventricular septal defects in the USA? Lancet. 1980; 1:407–408.
2. Rothman K, Fyler DC, Goldblatt A, et al. Exogenous hormones and other drug exposures of children with congenital heart disease. Am J Epidemiol. 1979; 109:433–439.
3. Heinonen OP, Slone D, Monson RR, et al. Cardiovascular birth defects and antenatal exposure to female sex hormones. N Engl J Med. 1977; 296:67–70.
4. Nora JJ, Vargo TA, Nora AA, et al. Dexamphetamine: A possible environmental trigger in cardiovascular malformations. Lancet. 1970; 1:1290–1291.
5. Hodach RL, Hodach AE, Fallon JF, et al. The role of β-adrenergic activity in the production of cardiac and aortic arch anomalies in chick embryos. Teratology. 1975; 12:33–45.
6. Clarren SK, Smith DW. The fetal alcohol syndrome. N Engl J Med. 1978; 298:1063–1067.
7. Ouellette EM, Rosett HL, Rosman NP, et al. Adverse effects on offspring of maternal alcohol abuse during pregnancy. N Engl J Med. 1977; 297:528–530.
8. Landesman-Dwyer S, Emmanul I. Smoking during pregnancy. Teratology. 1979; 19:119–126.
9. Hendershot GE. Pregnant workers in the United States. Advance data from Vital and Health Statistics of the National Center for Health Statistics, Vol II. Hyattsville, Maryland: The National Center for Health Statistics, 1977.
10. Carucci PM, Prasad S. A comparison of mothers' occupations reported on live birth certificates and on a survey questionnaire. Pub Health Rep. 1979; 94:432–437.
11. Pharoah POD, Alberman E, Doyle P. Outcome of pregnancy among women in anesthetic practice. Lancet. 1977; 1:34–36.

12. Occupational disease among operating room personnel: A national study. Anesthesiology. 1974; 41:321–340.
13. Cohen EN, Brown BW, Wu ML, et al. Occupational disease in dentistry and chronic exposure to trace anesthetic gases. Am J Dent Assoc. 1980; 101:21–31.
14. Penazda D, Arias-Stella J, Sime F, et al. The heart and pulmonary circulation in children at high altitudes. Pediatrics. 1964; 34:568–582.

Noninvasive Evaluation of the Fetal Heart

F.VIII

The Doppler Effect

Joyce Newman, MD, PhD

I. INTRODUCTION

Fetal heart rate monitoring, the counting of the fetal heart rate, is in wide use today. The principle sounds simple enough, but, in fact, requires extremely complex technology. A signal must be detected, free of artifact, and it must be counted. The counted signals must be related one-to-one to the actual heart beat.[1] All this involves many steps of electronic processing. It is hoped that presenting some of the basic methodology will provide the reader with sufficient information to appreciate the advantages, as well as the limitations, of the different means of monitoring, and also the artifacts that may be introduced by the equipment itself.

There are basically three different principles that may be used to detect the heart rate. The first involves the acoustic vibrations associated with each heart cycle. These can be heard with a stethoscope or amplified with a microphone—a technique called phonocardiography. The second principle is the detection of electrical signals—ie, electrocardiography. The third principle is the detection of the motion of the heart valves via the Doppler effect.

Phonocardiography has many disadvantages. There is a great deal of noise that interferes with the signal, and the signal is often lost during the contractions. Sensitive microphones have been developed that conform to the maternal abdomen and are designed to pick up those frequencies associated with fetal heart sounds. Most fetuses produce one to two audible heart sounds per cycle. Computer logic is used to eliminate the interval between S_1 and S_2 so that only one sound is counted for each cycle. A great deal of interfering noise is produced from bowel sounds, maternal pulsatile vessels, etc.

Cardiac Problems in Pregnancy, pages 463–473

These are reduced by filtering and computer logic circuits, but quite often an acceptable tracing cannot be produced.[2,3] Therefore, this method is not in widespread use today and has been surpassed by the two other methods.

Doppler shift ultrasonography is the most common noninvasive method in use today for measuring the fetal heart rate[2] and is discussed at length in this chapter. Electrocardiography is described in Chapter F.IX.

II. THE DOPPLER PRINCIPLE

Consider a source emitting sound waves at a particular frequency, f. (Frequency is the number of cycles per second and is the same as pitch.) If an observer is stationary relative to the source, he will hear the same frequency, f. However, if the source is moving relative to the observer, the observed frequency will be different. Only motion parallel to the line between the source and the observer has this effect. Motion perpendicular to the line between source and observer does not cause a frequency change.*

If f is the frequency of the source, V the speed of the source relative to the observer, U the speed of sound in the medium, and α the angle between the velocity of the source and the line between the source and observer, then to first order the change in frequency, Δf, is given by:

$$\Delta f = \frac{fV \cos \alpha}{U}$$

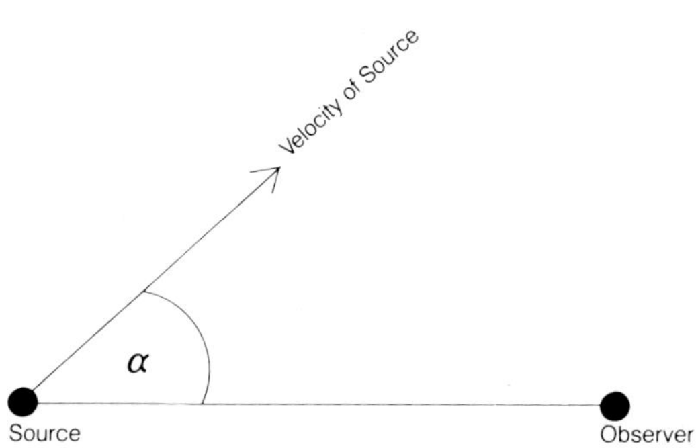

The frequency increases if the source approaches the observer (pitch is higher) and decreases if the source recedes (pitch is lower). There are examples of this in everyday life: the change in pitch of an ambulance siren or train whistle as it approaches and the use of radar to check automobile speeds. This principle is also used to measure the velocity of stars (see Fig. F.VIII.1).

When used for fetal monitoring, a low power high-frequency sound wave is projected. The sound waves are reflected from moving targets in the fetus's circulatory system. The reflected sound waves are detected by a receiver,[4] and any shift in frequency is detected. The sounds we hear from these instruments are not true sounds but are artificially created when a frequency shift is detected.[2]

The term ultrasound refers to sound waves with a frequency range between 18 thousand and 15 million cycles per second.[1] (This is above the audible range.) The production and detection of these waves makes use of the piezoelectric effect.[1] Certain crystals, such as quartz, have the property that when an alternating electrical voltage is applied across the crystal, the crystal responds by vibrating and producing sound waves (the transducer). Also, when a sound wave is set up in these crystals an alternating electrical potential is set up (the receiver). Therefore, a sound signal can be converted to an electrical signal and vice versa. The transducers and receivers of all ultrasound equipment contain these crystals.

The penetration distance of ultrasound waves decreases with frequency and increases with power. Resolution is better at high frequencies. A compromise is reached and most equipment uses a signal of about 2 megahertz (1 Hertz = 1 cycle/second) and a power of 2–5 milliwatts/cm^2. The Doppler shift is usually of the order of a few hundred Hertz and this is easily detected.[1]

*At very high velocities requiring a relativistic treatment, transverse Doppler effects do exist. Transverse effects would not be detected at the velocities relevant to this discussion and so are correctly neglected.

Ultrasound waves are pressure waves, not electromagnetic waves like light. Nevertheless, they have some very similar properties. At interfaces part of the wave is transmitted and part is reflected.

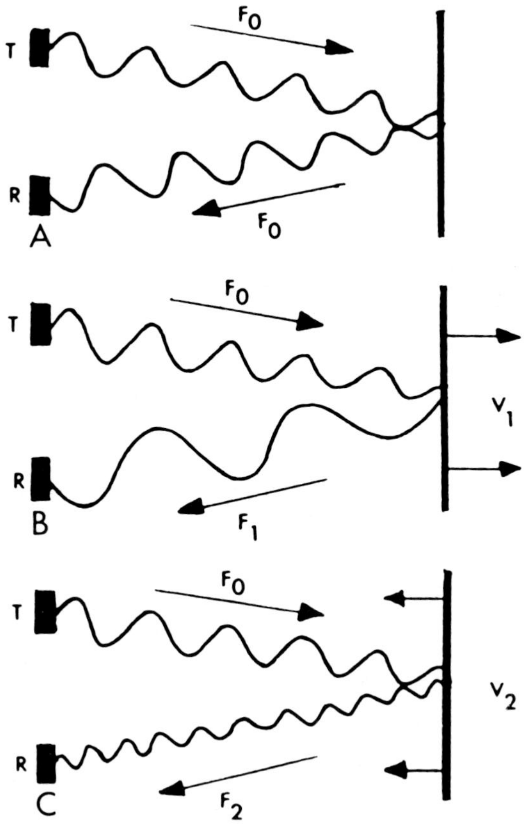

Fig. F.VIII.1. Doppler effect transducer contains a transmitting crystal and a receiving crystal. These quartz crystals make use of the piezoelectric phenomenon that enables mechanical and electrical energy to be interconverted. They are easily damaged mechanically or by excessive heat or moisture. Transmitting crystal T sends a beam of sound at a frequency of F_0 (usually about 2 MHz) toward a reflecting surface. Stationary surface reflects the sound at the same frequency (**A**). If the reflector is moving away from the transmitter at velocity V_1 (**B**) the received sound is heard by the receiver as a lower frequency (F_1). If the reflecting surface is moving toward the receiving crystal at velocity V_2 (**C**) the reflected sound is heard as a higher frequency F_2. (Figures F.VIII.1, 7, and 8 are by permission from Klapholz H. Techniques of fetal heart rate monitoring. Semin Perinatol. 1978; 2:119–129.)

Ultrasound waves obey the same laws of reflection and refraction (Snell's law) that light waves do, and they can be focused. Use is made of these properties in the design of various types of ultrasound equipment. Scanners, such as those used in echocardiography or B-mode scanning have to detect the amplitude and the time of arrival of the sound echoes. However, to reiterate, the fetal heart monitors detect only a frequency shift. If the reflected wave has not been reflected from a moving target, no frequency shift occurs and no signal is recorded. By the same token, reflection from a moving target other than a fetal heart can also produce a signal.

Figure F.VIII.2 is a diagram illustrating the use of a Doppler apparatus, and Figure F.VIII.3 is a block diagram of the electronics. All crystals of the transducer must make contact with the skin for the sound waves to be properly transmitted. Air is a very poor conductor of sound waves. Therefore, a sound-conducting gel is used between the transducer and the skin.[1]

III. COMPONENTS OF THE DOPPLER SIGNAL

The Doppler signal is not one sharp event but is made up of several components, corresponding to the different times of moving events in the cardiac cycle. There is atrial contraction, ventricular contraction, ventricular relaxation, etc. By studying simultaneous electrocardiographic (ECG) recordings, the main components have been identified.[1] They are atrial contraction, atrioventricular (A-V) valve opening, and A-V valve closing. The time between atrial contraction and closure of the A-V valves is approximately the same as the PR interval of the ECG and is relatively constant. This causes the Doppler sounds to resemble heart sounds. (Remember that Doppler sounds are not true sounds but are created electronically and coincide with the moment a frequency shift is detected.)

The opening of the AV valves is heard distinctly only at rates below 140 beats

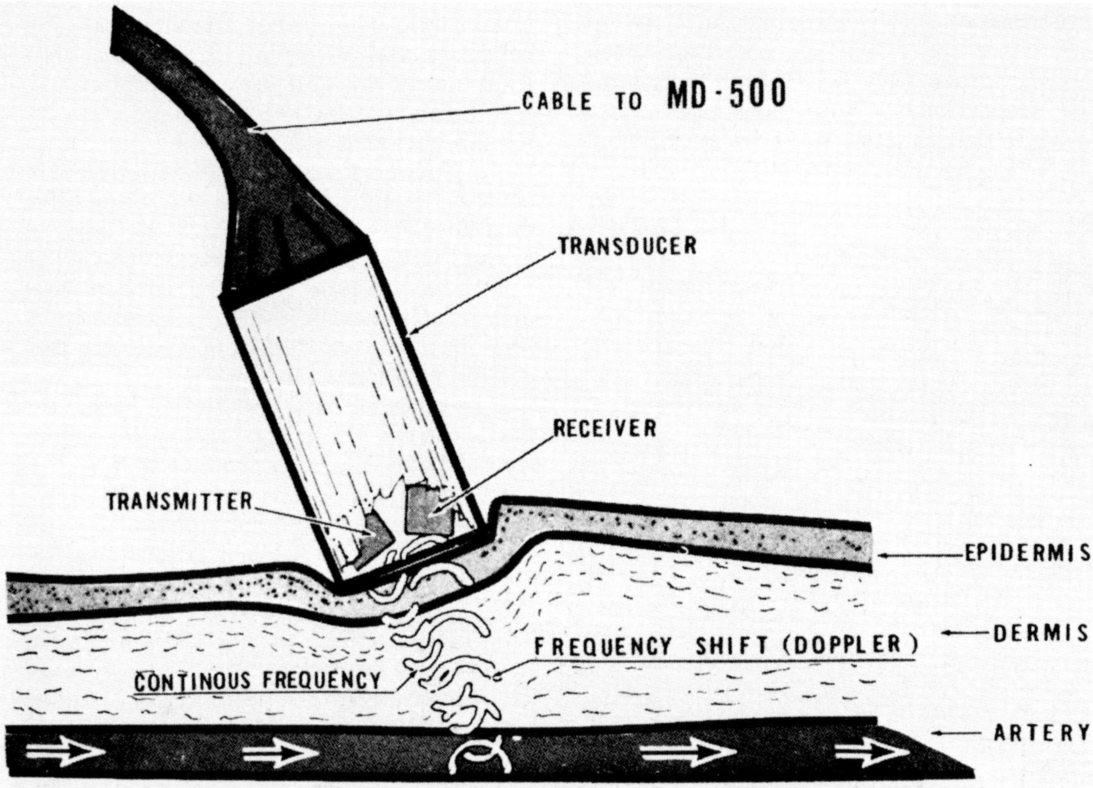

Fig. F.VIII.2. Illustration of the transmission and pick-up of the ultrasound by the transducer. (Figures F.VIII.2, 3, and 6 are by permission from Barton JJ. Evaluation of the Doppler shift principle as a diagnostic aid in obstetrics. Am J Obstet Gynecol. 1968; 102:563–567.)

per minute. This sometimes gives the effect of a gallop rhythm but of course has no pathological significance. As the rate increases the signal from the opening of the AV valve merges with that from the atrial contraction. However, at lower rates the signal from AV valves opening is sometimes a cause of double counting[1] (see Figs. F.VIII.4 and F.VIII.5).

IV. ADVANTAGES OF DOPPLER COUNTING

The main advantage is that it is a noninvasive method that can be used as early as ten weeks from the last menstrual period. At ten weeks the successful pickup rate is 37%; at 12 weeks, 82%; at 14 weeks, 97%; and from 16 weeks and up, virtually 100%[4] (see Fig. F.VIII.6). Therefore, when compared with abdominal fetal ECG the Doppler is far more successful in its pickup rate. It is also very easy to use. Usually the difference between maternal and fetal heart rates is such that there is no difficulty in distinguishing between them. Occasionally, however, a signal from a pulsing maternal pelvic vessel is misinterpreted as a fetal rate (see Fig. F.VIII.7)[2].

V. PROBLEMS WITH DOPPLER MONITORING

Since the fetus moves it is hard to keep a beam of sound continuously aimed at a mitral valve. The transmitted beam is therefore made broad enough to reflect from the entire heart. The various parts of the heart move at different times and at different rates. This yields a signal that is made up of several components (this point has already been discussed). In addition to the atrial contractions and A-V valve closing and opening, occasionally signals from aortic and pulmonary valve motions are picked up. All of these components change in clarity. The important point is that, because of all these components, there is no certainty of timing. There is no sharply defined time of onset corresponding to each beat as there is an R wave in an ECG. Therefore, and this point must be emphasized, the variability on a Doppler recording cannot be used as a reliable index of beat-to-beat change. In most equipment the last three beats are averaged, and the updated average is displayed on a beat-to-beat basis.[2,5]

Besides the fetal heart, there are other moving objects that can reflect the sound waves and cause false signals. These include bowels, maternal vessels, and maternal and fetal movements.[6]

Counting can sometimes be difficult because 1) the amplitude of the reflected signal may vary by a factor of 50 within a short time, 2) the components of the Doppler signal vary with rate and fetal position, and, as has already been pointed out, 3) there is no unique point to count.

In every system, there is a minimum level signal below which the count is unreliable. In fact, a weak reflected wave is the main cause of unreliable tracings and sometimes gives false deceleration patterns. Such weak reflections are most likely to occur during labor. Some causes of a weak signal are 1) fetus descends out of range, 2) maternal obesity, 3) pushing, and 4) fetal position.[1] Strong signals are those reflected from fast-moving, large, flat targets perpendicular to the beam and mov-

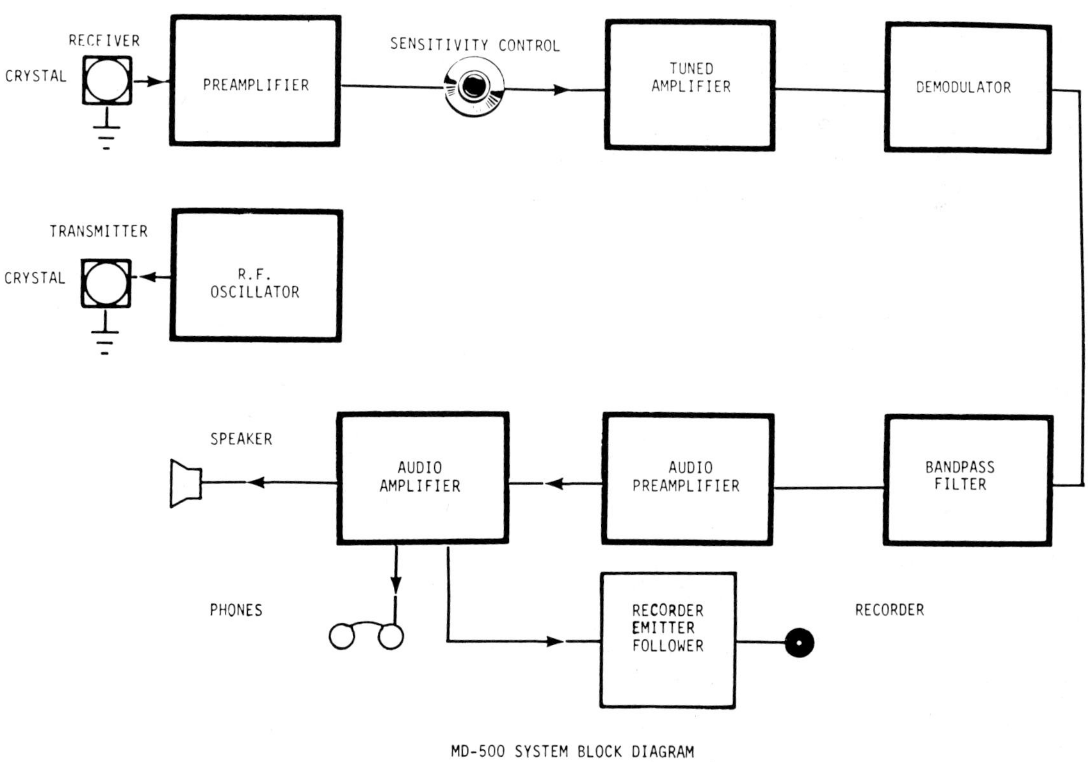

Fig. F.VIII.3. System block diagram of the ultrasound apparatus.

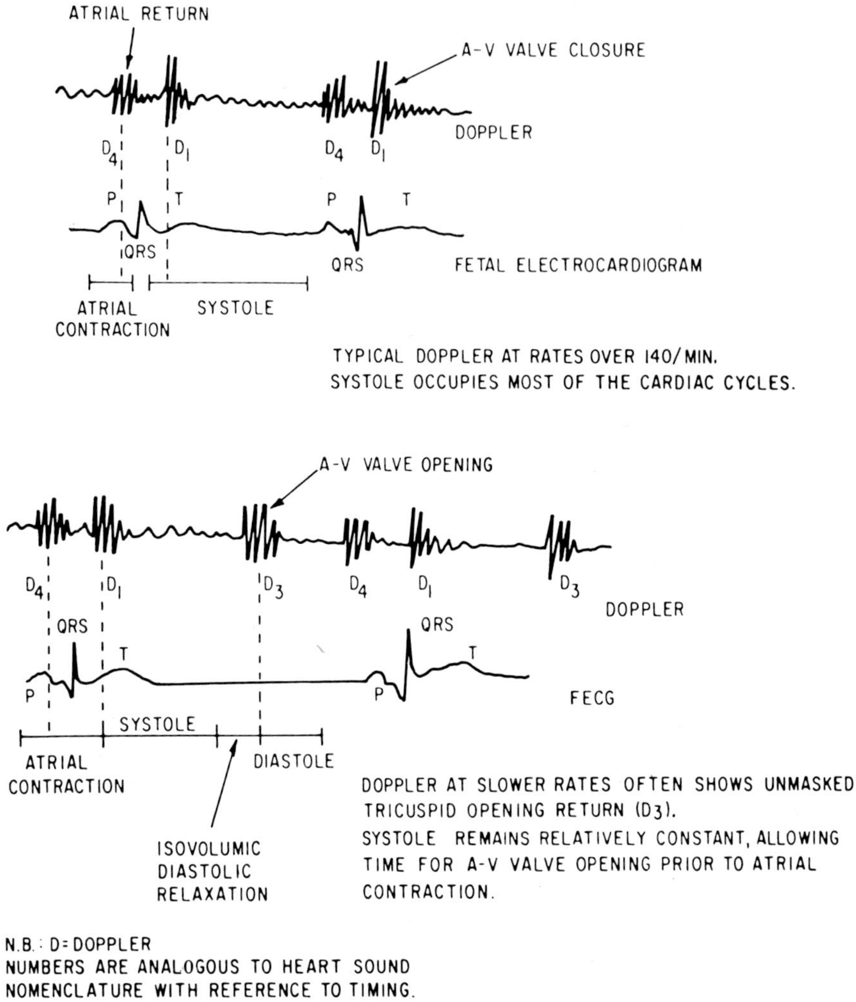

Fig. F.VIII.4. Components of Doppler-detected fetal heart motion. (Figures F.VIII.4, 5, and 9 are by permission of the publisher and the author from Hochberg HM. Fetal monitoring instrumentation. In Clinical Studies in Fetal Monitoring. A Guide for the Users of the Fetasonde 2100.)

ing parallel to it. The AV valves in most fetal positions are usually moving in an anterior-posterior direction. In most fetal positions a good signal is reflected from these valves. However, as the fetus turns, the signal may be lost, or some components of the signal may be lost before others. Certain fetal positions are such that the transducer cannot be properly positioned so that the beam is perpendicular to the valves. A weak signal results.[1]

To minimize errors due to reflections from other moving objects and from the variable detection of the number of components in the heart signal, most instruments make use of a computer logic system. Rate changes greater than a certain percent are rejected as noise. Occasionally, there are logic errors and the machine may half count or double count (see Fig. F.VIII.8).

Another point to be emphasized concerns twins. Two different pieces of Doppler equipment cannot be used reliably on the same patient. The second receiver will pick up transmissions from the first trans-

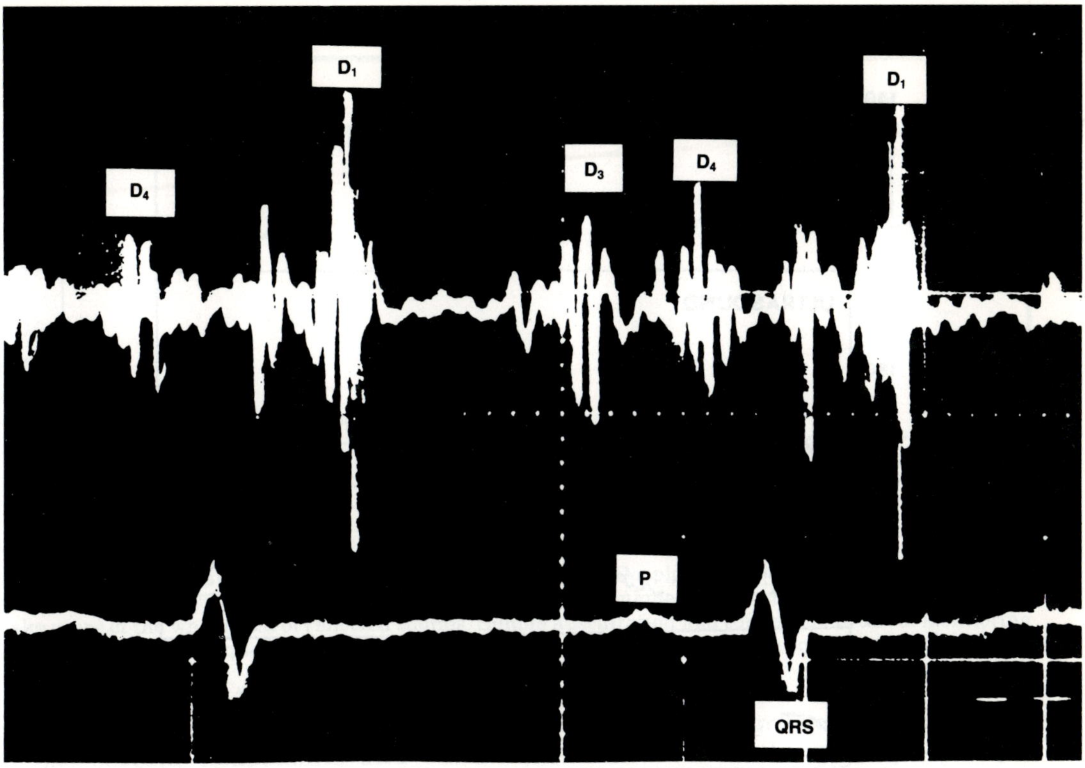

Fig. F.VIII.5. Oscilloscope photograph of Doppler signal from the fetal heart.

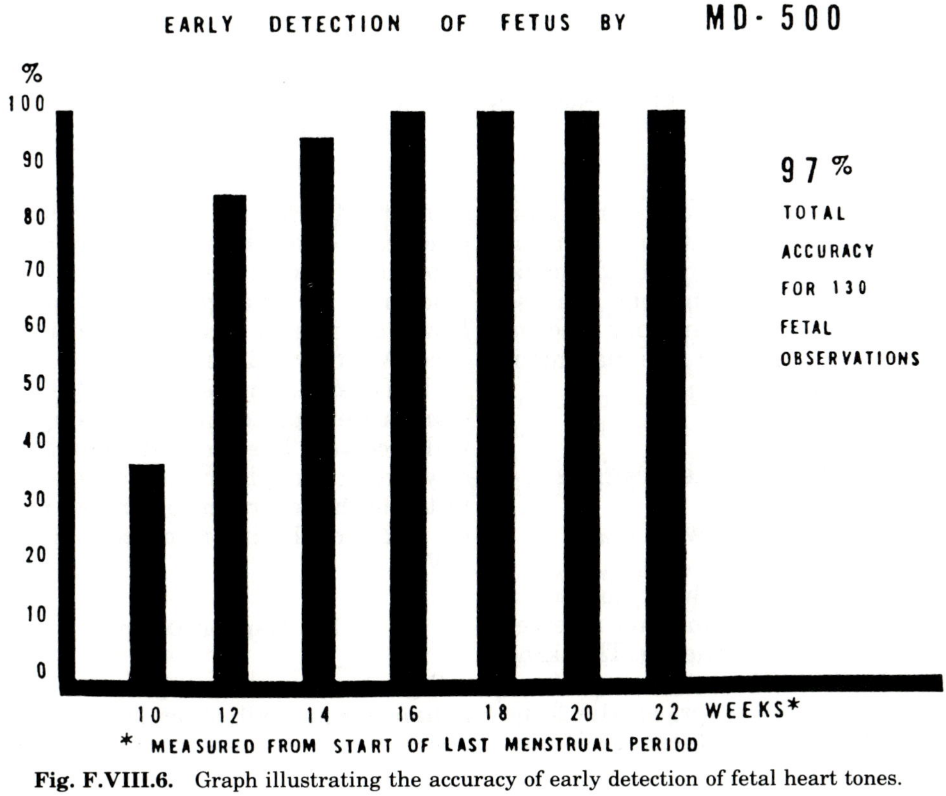

Fig. F.VIII.6. Graph illustrating the accuracy of early detection of fetal heart tones.

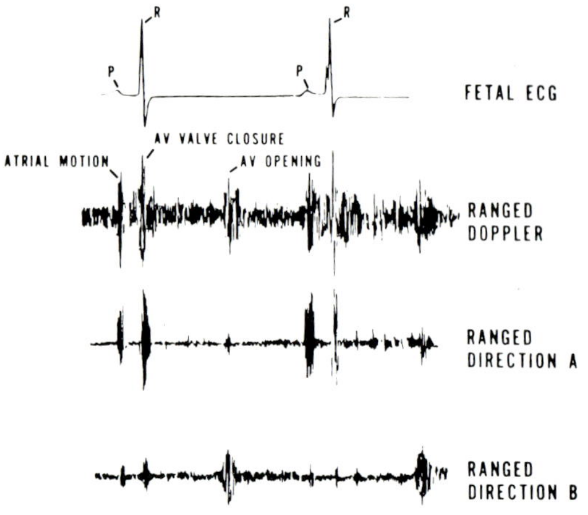

Fig. F.VIII.10. Diagram of the effect of electronic selection of directional Doppler components from a ranged Doppler fetal heart signal. The fetal P is followed by a Doppler signal representing atrial contraction. A complex follows the QRS, which mainly represents AV valve closure but also probably includes semilinear valve opening. If the heart rate is below about 140 beats per minute, the isovolumic diastolic relaxation ends before atrial contraction. Another Doppler component is seen at the lower rates, most likely representing the rapid AV opening at the rapid filling phase of diastole. This is merged with atrial contractions at higher rates. The directional signals (Ranged direction A and B) often separate the Doppler energy from the atrial and AV valve closure events from the AV valve opening. This may indicate that the ranging permits selection of mainly one valve leaflet or that one leaflet produces the highest velocity and energy, rather than there being equal motion of all valve leaflets. (Figures F.VIII.10 and 11 are by permission from Lauersen NH, Hochberg HM, George MED, Tegge CS, Meighan JJ. Technical aspects of ranged directional Doppler: A new Doppler method of fetal heart rate monitoring. J Reprod Med. 1978; 20:77–83.)

the transducer is parallel to these valves. The OA, ROA, LOA, SA, SLA, and SRA positions are usually easy to monitor. Occiput transverse positions are difficult to monitor once the head is engaged, because there is no flat surface parallel to the valves. This position is sometimes better monitored if the patient is on her side. Occiput posterior and sacrum posterior positions put limbs between the transducer and the heart and therefore are associated with a higher incidence of spurious signals.

As the fetus descends in station, Doppler monitoring usually becomes easier because the fetal position does not change as randomly. The transducer may have to be moved to follow the descent. However, when the head is at the introitus and the patient is pushing, the Doppler signal is often lost because the fetal heart is behind the pubic bone. False deceleration patterns may be observed because of the reception of a weak signal.

Fetal movement can produce spurious Doppler signals. This is seen especially at the start of contractions or if the fetus is particularly irritable.

Maternal factors can also affect the quality of the tracing. Obese women are harder to monitor. The distance to the fetus may be greater, and the signal may therefore be weak. Maternal motions can

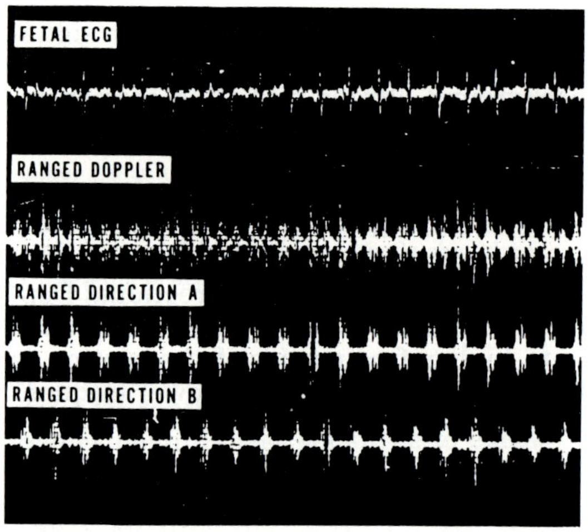

25 mm/sec

Fig. F.VIII.11. Oscillographic recording of simultaneous fetal scalp ECG, bidirectional Doppler, and both directional Doppler signals. The standard bidirectional Doppler (ranged Doppler) shows multiple components with variability in amplitude and predominance and baseline "clutter." Ranged directional Doppler signals show separation of this complicated signal into the distinct components with far less variability and baseline clutter. The voltages are the same scale in all tracings, demonstrating that there is little loss of signal amplitude. The apparent increase in the signal-to-noise ratio and the uniqueness of the directional signals are well demonstrated. Direction A represents atrial contractions and AV, valve closure. Direction B represents AV valve opening.

cause loss of the signal. The more fixed in position the fetus is, the less effect maternal motion has.

VIII. SAFETY

At high intensities ultrasound waves have been noted to cause tissue damage. The injurious effects are related to intensity and exposure time. Initially seen are heating, then vasodilation, then vasoconstriction, cavitation, and tissue destruction. Based upon peripheral nerve studies[4] the upper limit of safety has been set at 1 watt/cm^2. This is over 300 times the intensity used in Doppler instruments. With prolonged exposure at fields exceeding 100 milliwatts/cm^2 cataracts have been produced.[4] This is still an intensity 20–30 times higher than the Doptone. To date, there are no reports of maternal or fetal injuries or chromosome damage at the level of ultrasound intensities used in Doppler equipment.

IX. REFERENCES

1. Hochberg HM. Fetal monitoring instrumentation. Clinical Studies in Fetal Monitoring. A Guide for the Users of the Fetasonde 2100. Cranbury, New Jersey: Roche Medical Electronics, III-1–III-61.
2. Klapholz H. Techniques of fetal heart rate monitoring. Semin Perinatol. 1978; 2:119–129.
3. Klapholz H, Schifrin BS, Myrick R. Role of maternal artifact in fetal heart rate pattern interpretation. Obstet Gynecol. 1974; 44:373–378.
4. Barton JJ. Evaluation of the Doppler shift principle as a diagnostic aid in obstetrics. Am J Obstet Gynecol. 1968; 102:563–570.
5. Lauersen NH, Hochberg HM, George MED, Tegge CS, Meighan JJ. A new technique for improving the Doppler ultrasound signal for fetal heart rate monitoring. Am J Obstet Gynecol. 1977; 128:300–302.
6. De Haan J. Fetal monitoring by physical methods. I. Technical questions. Eur J Obstet Gynecol Reprod Biol. 1973: 3/2:57–66.
7. Lauersen NH, Hochberg HM, George MED, Tegge CS, Meighan JJ. Technical aspects of ranged directional Doppler: A new Doppler method of fetal heart rate monitoring. J Reprod Med. 1978; 20:77–83.

F.IX

Intrauterine Electrocardiography

Joyce Newman, MD, PhD

I. INTRODUCTION

The fetal electrocardiogram was first recorded by Cremer from a maternal abdomen in 1906 shortly after Einthoven developed the string galvanometer.[1,2] Although abdominal fetal electrocardiography was available for many years, its use was limited by electrical noise problems. The maximum amplitude of the fetal R wave from the maternal abdomen is in the range of 10–50 microvolts.[3] This is an amplitude 20–100 times less than the adult R wave. The small amplitude of the fetal R wave was often less than background electrical noise and so not detectable. In order to improve the signal, electrodes have been placed subcutaneously on the maternal abdomen, and also transabdominally into the uterine cavity and into the fetus. These techniques gave adequate recordings but were not very practical. Vaginal and rectal electrodes have also been tried, but with limited success.[4,5] The best method to date is what is referred to as internal monitoring—ie, an electrode placed vaginally directly into the fetal presenting part. The R wave so recorded is several hundred microvolts,[3] and, for reasons to be explained later, maternal disturbances are minimal. Therefore the signal-to-noise ratio is substantially better than with abdominal recordings. However, because this technique requires ruptured membranes, its use is limited to the intrapartum period.[1] It should be pointed out that none of the methods available to record fetal electrocardiograms (ECGs) can give the qualities found in adult electrocardiography.[6]

For many years the widespread use of fetal monitoring was limited by the poor signal-to-noise ratio and the bulk and cost of amplifiers.[2] The invention of semicon-

Cardiac Problems in Pregnancy, pages 475–490

ductors permitted the construction of modern miniature circuits for amplification and also microprocessors.[7] Microprocessors are computers with significant capabilities that occupy a small amount of space. Fetal monitors today have logic circuits and memories that used to be available only on large computers. The use of filtering, amplification, weighted time averaging, and logic circuits has signifi-

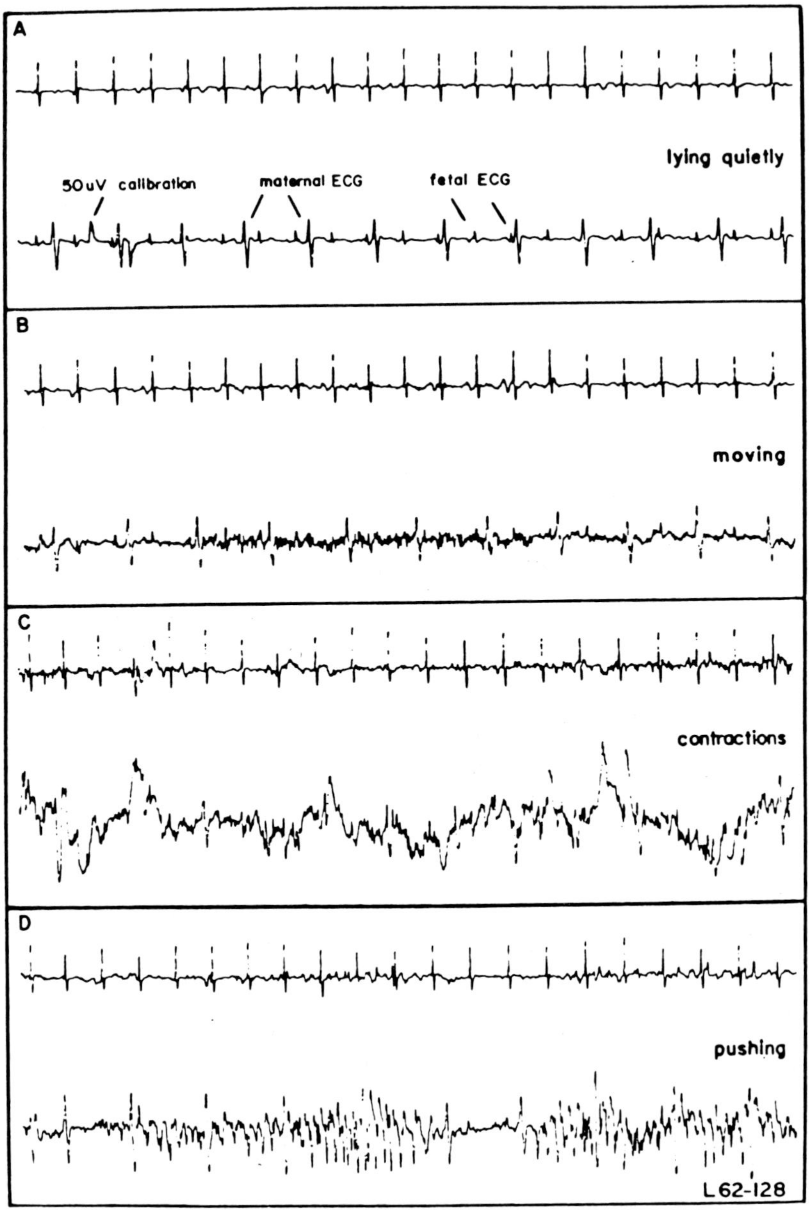

Fig. F.IX.1. A comparison of fetal ECGs recorded with a vaginal electrode (upper tracings) and abdominal electrode (lower tracings). These tracings were made during labor. The better signal-to-noise ratio of the vaginal electrode is apparent. During contractions and "pushing" the fetal ECGs in the lower tracings are obliterated completely by the electromyogram. (Figures F.IX.1 and 8 are by permission from Hon EH. Instrumentation of fetal heart rate and fetal electrocardiography. II. A vaginal electrode. Am J Obstet Gynecol. 1963; 86:772–784.)

cantly improved the signal-to-noise ratio in both abdominal and internal fetal electrocardiography.[3]

Abdominal fetal electrocardiography has also been improved by the minimization of electrode-to-skin impedance, electrodes with small polarization effects, proper shielding and grounding, and electrical isolation from other equipment. Nevertheless, during labor the interference from maternal myometrium and maternal movement is so high that this technique cannot be used (see Fig. F.IX.1).[3] During pregnancy abdominal fetal ECGs have been picked up as early as 11 weeks (see Fig. F.IX.2), but they are not always obtainable.[8] The technique fails about 25% of the time, especially with obesity and polyhydramnios.[7]

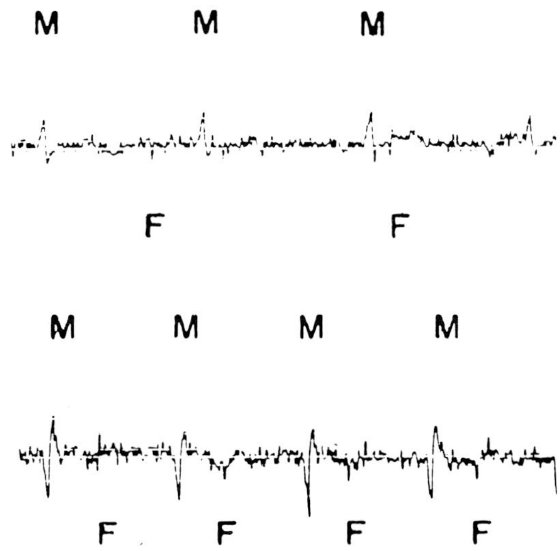

Fig. F.IX.2. The early fetal electrocardiogram. Upper tracing shows two fetal complexes at 11 ½ weeks of embryologic age, with the fetal heart rate about 90 per minute. Lower tracing, also at 11 ½ weeks in another subject, shows several consecutive fetal complexes, with the rate about 100 per minute. (Figures F.IX.2 and 3 are by permission from Larks SD, Dasgupta K. Fetal electrocardiography, with special reference to early pregnancy. Am Heart J. 1958; 56:701–714.)

II. USE OF FETAL ELECTROCARDIOGRAPHY

As experience accumulated it was found that rate had more useful information than waveform.[9] Because the peak of an R wave is so specific in time, R-R time intervals can be measured quite precisely, especially with internal monitoring where the noise level is low. For purposes of measuring heart rate, fetal electrocardiography surpasses all other methods. For measuring instantaneous heart rate and beat-to-beat variability, it is the only method. Doppler measurement and phonocardiography do not have a sufficiently well-defined time of onset. As is well known, rate measurements have proved useful in the detection of fetal distress. Certain fetal cardiac abnormalities have also been detected.[10] Paroxysmal supraventricular tachycardia and paroxysmal atrial flutter have been reported. Congenital heart block may be detected as a persistent bradycardia.[9] Intrauterine dysrythmias are described in more detail in Chapter F.XIII.

The shape of the P, QRS, and T waves in most cases cannot be seen directly because of noise. The amplitude of fetal P and T waves is about 5 microvolts. Skin noise is between 3 and 5 microvolts. Electrical noise adds another 1–2 microvolts. So the P and T waves are usually masked.[2] Some monitors are equipped to electronically average several waveforms.[3] An approximate waveform can then be displayed, which is sometimes helpful for diagnosing congenital abnormalities.

Abdominal ECGs have been used to document fetal life, but other methods such as the Doppler have a better success rate. Abdominal ECGs have been used to document twins (see Fig. F.IX.3). This is best done with two sets of electrodes. The display of two distinct ECGs on one tracing is excellent proof of twins. However, the tracing must be read extremely carefully, and sometimes the noise level prevents the pickup of both signals.[2] People have tried to correlate the direction of the QRS complex with fetal position, but this has not proved valuable.

In summary, at present, fetal electrocardiography has its most important application in rate-related information.

III. THEORETICAL EXPLANATIONS

A. Principle of Electrocardiography

The heart, like all body tissues, is electrically neutral (ie, the positive and negative charges are equal). If an object is electrically neutral and all the charges are uniformaly distributed, then no electrical field will be set up. However, if, in spite of the total charge neutrality, there is an uneven charge distribution, then there will be an electric field which can be detected. The electric field is most simply described via a mathematical quantity called the electric potential. (The electric field is not the same as the potential but can be derived from it.)

The electric potential at a point P is given by:

$$V_P = \sum_i \frac{q_i}{r_i} \tag{1}$$

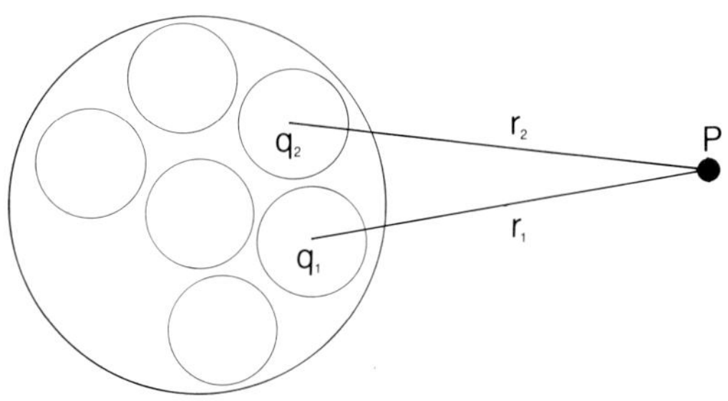

where V is the potential at point P, each q_i is the net charge in the *i*th region, and r_i is the distance from q_i to P. If the object is neutral all of the q_i add up to zero, but the sum of the q_i/r_i may not be zero. The potential at a second point, say Q, would be defined in a similar fashion. If we put an electrode at point P and another at point Q, we can measure the potential difference $V_P - V_Q$. If the charge distribution varies in time, then $V_P - V_Q$ will also vary with time. Preceding each heart beat there is a transient redistribution of electrical charges within the heart. If electrodes are placed at two different points (say on the skin), then transient changes in the potential difference between those points will be measured, and this is what

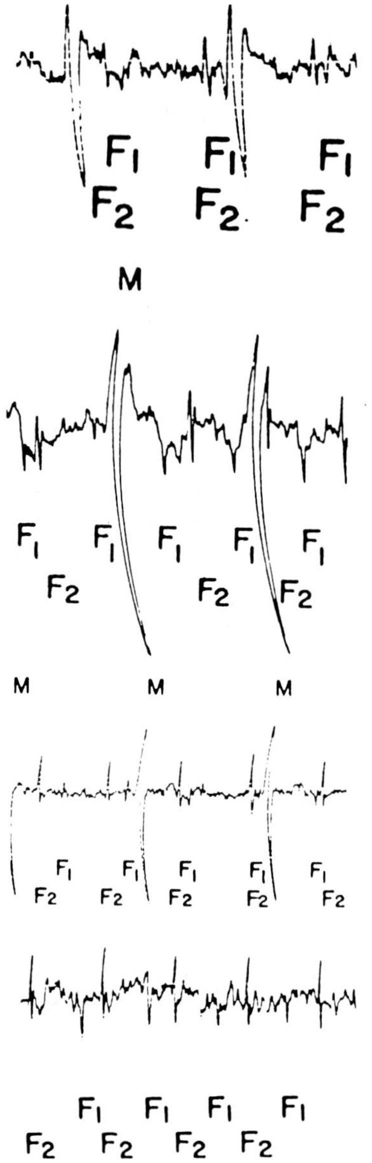

Fig. F.IX.3. The fetal electrocardiogram in multiple pregnancy: four different sets of twins. In each instance the presence of twins was demonstrable radiologically, and viable twins were delivered. In the lowest tracing the original diagnosis of twins was made by the fetal electrocardiogram at 21 weeks.

is displayed in an ECG. Since the signal depends on the distances to the sources, changing the positions of the electrodes changes the signal. Hence, the signal is different in different leads.

It should also be noted that the strength of the signal will depend on the dielectric and conductive properties of the medium through which it is propagated. This fact was left out of Equation 1 for the sake of simplicity but will be referred to later on in the discussion.

Sometimes in discussions of adult ECGs the heart is described as an equivalent dipole. This is not really accurate. However, any charge distribution can be described as a mathematical sum of various multipoles—eg, dipole, + quadripole, + octapole, + . . . 2^n pole, + ... The potential for the dipole term falls off as $1/r^2$, the quadripole term as $1/r^3$, the octapole term as $1/r^4$, and so on. If the distances from the source are large compared to the size of the source, then the higher order terms become unimportant. In those situations the dipole approximation can sometimes be useful.

The physical principles involved in fetal ECGs are the same as those in adult ECGs. However, with fetal monitoring, whether it be internal or external, there are electrical sources in addition to the fetal heart. There are the large signal from the maternal heart and signals from maternal myometrial and skeletal activity. All these must be separated from the fetal signal.

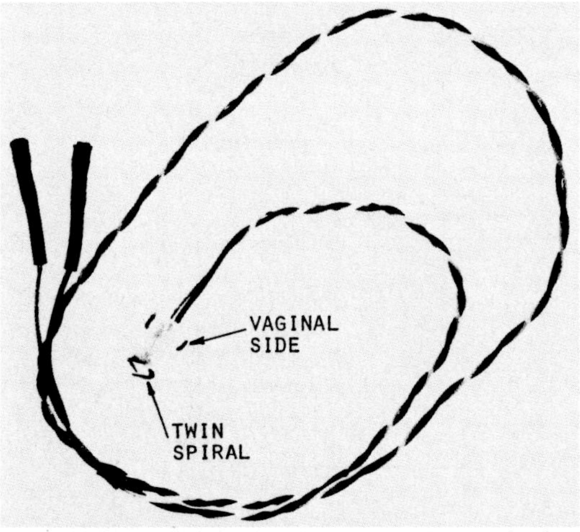

Fig. F.IX.4. Double spiral electrode. View of a double spiral electrode which is composed of stainless steel, with two points that grip and enter the upper layers of the skin. The double spiral electrodes may be easier to insert than the single spiral model. It has been found that the more electrode metal penetrating the skin, the cleaner and larger is the amplitude of signal and the lower the electrical background noise. (By permission of the publisher and the author from Hochberg HM. Fetal monitoring instrumentation. In Clinical Studies in Fetal Monitoring. A Guide for the Users of the Feta sonde 2100.)

B. Elimination of Maternal Signal

The fetal scalp electrode detects the potential difference between the fetal presenting part and the vaginal wall of the mother (see Fig. F.IX.4). One pole is a sharp metal electrode that is placed subcutaneously into the fetal presenting part. The second pole is a piece of metal contacting the vaginal fluid less than 1 cm distant. The distance of 1 cm between the electrodes is so small compared with the distance to the maternal heart that the potential difference due to the maternal signal is almost zero[11,12]; ie,

$$\text{maternal } V_P - V_Q = \frac{q_{mat}}{r_p} - \frac{q_{mat}}{r_Q}$$

$$\text{if } r_P \cong r_Q,\ V_P - V_Q \cong 0$$

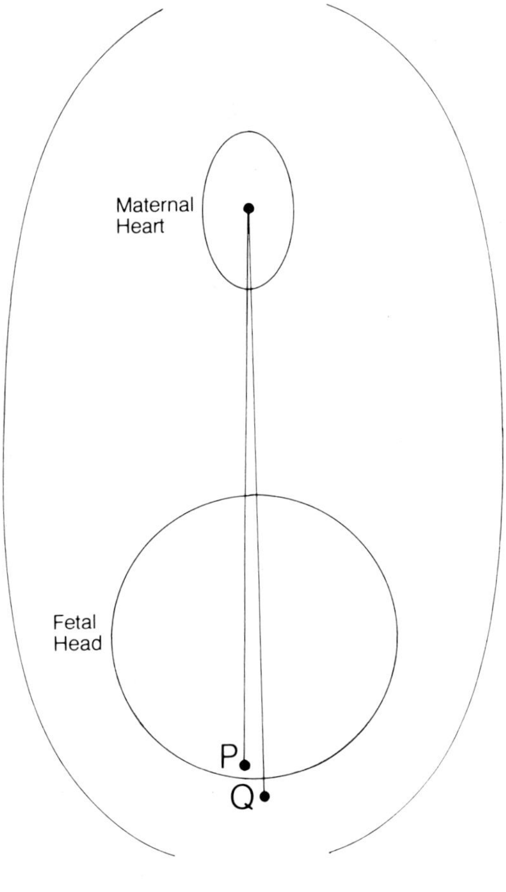

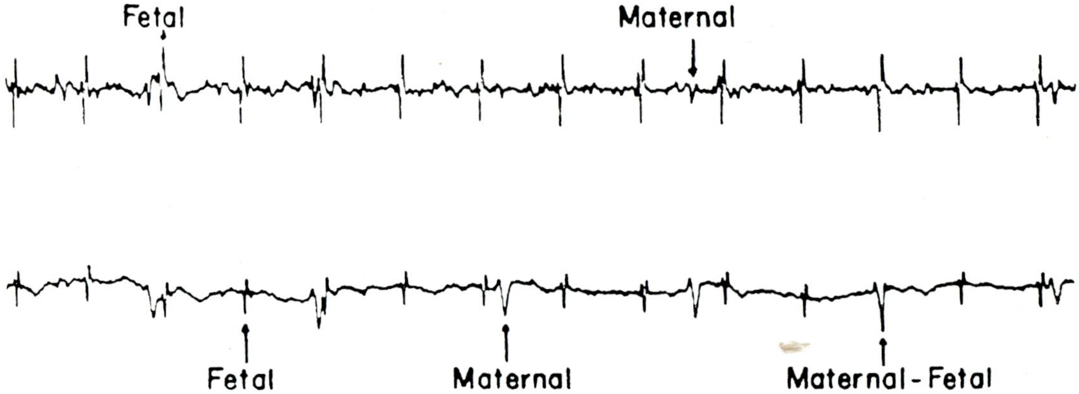

Fig. F.IX.5. Separation of fetal and maternal electrocardiogram. The upper tracing shows attenuation of the maternal ECG and the separation of the fetal ECG for counting. The lower tracing shows the combined maternal and fetal ECGs as they are usually obtained from the mother's abdomen. (By permission from Hon EA. The electronic evaluation of the fetal heart rate. Am J Obstet Gynecol. 1958; 75: 1215–1230.)

The fetal signal, however, is not cancelled since 1) it is closer to the source and 2) the electrodes are separated by the skin resistance of fetal scalp. Both electrodes are connected to a plate on the mother's leg, which is grounded to eliminate interference. The same principle also eliminates myometrial and skeletal muscle signals from the mother.

With external fetal monitoring the separation of the maternal signal is more complicated and depends heavily on elec-

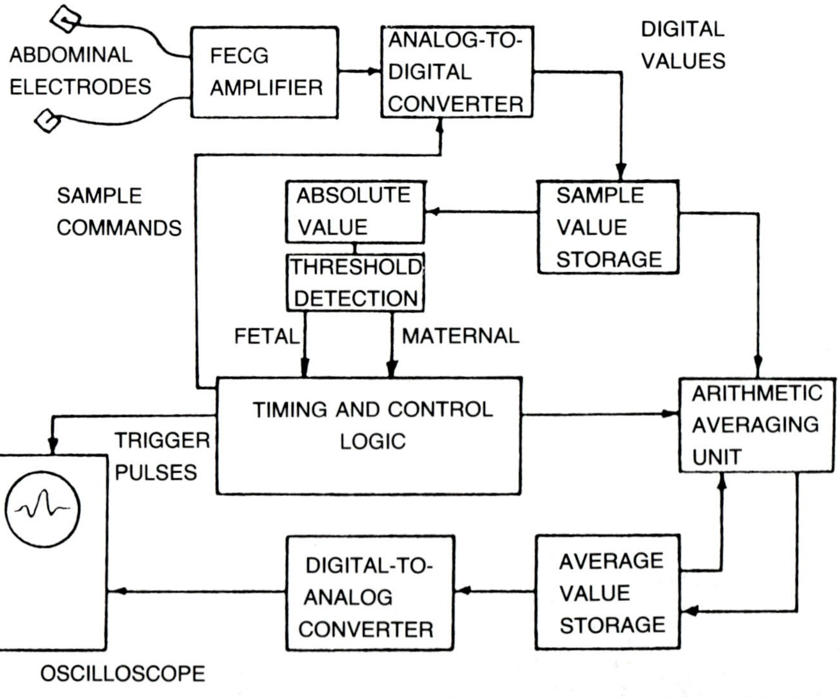

Fig. F.IX.6. Block diagram of new averaging system. (By permission from Rhyne VT. Digital signal enhancement of the fetal electrocardiogram. Am J Obstet Gynecol. 1968; 102:549–555.)

tronic filtering and computer programing circuits. The methods differ depending on the apparatus. In simpler equipment both signals are processed, both signals are displayed, and the record has to be separated manually.[13] In others the maternal signal is separated by rate or amplitude and attenuated electronically, and only the fetal signal is displayed (see Fig. F.IX.5).[3,13] There are two main methods of accomplishing this. The first is called blanking: all signals during the maternal complex are blanked out. By this method, 15% to 20% of fetal signals are lost because they overlap maternal signals.

The second method is subtraction or filtering.[14] This is a fairly complicated technique. The fetal signal has a QRS complex that lasts 30–70 milliseconds, usually about 50 milliseconds. Therefore the fetal signal has frequency components between 2 Hz and 250 Hz (1 Hz equals 1 cycle/sec). The maternal QRS lasts about 85 milliseconds and has a band width from 0.1 Hz to 100 Hz. Therefore, the frequency spectra overlap and preclude simple linear filtering. There is also a large amplitude of low-frequency baseline drift secondary to maternal respiration. This forces a higher low cut-off frequency. There is also a large amount of noise from electrophysiological activity in the vicinity of the electrodes. There is also AC hum (60 Hz) from power lines. Therefore, simple filtering according to frequency would not sufficiently separate maternal and fetal signals, nor would it eliminate noise. Use is made of computer circuitry and memory. The maternal signal is identified and averaged over several complexes. This average maternal signal is then subtracted from each signal. This yields a signal made up of the fetal ECG plus noise. Backward averaging of the fetal signal is then done to eliminate noise (see Figs. F.IX.6 and F.IX.7). The results are 87% in identifying dura-

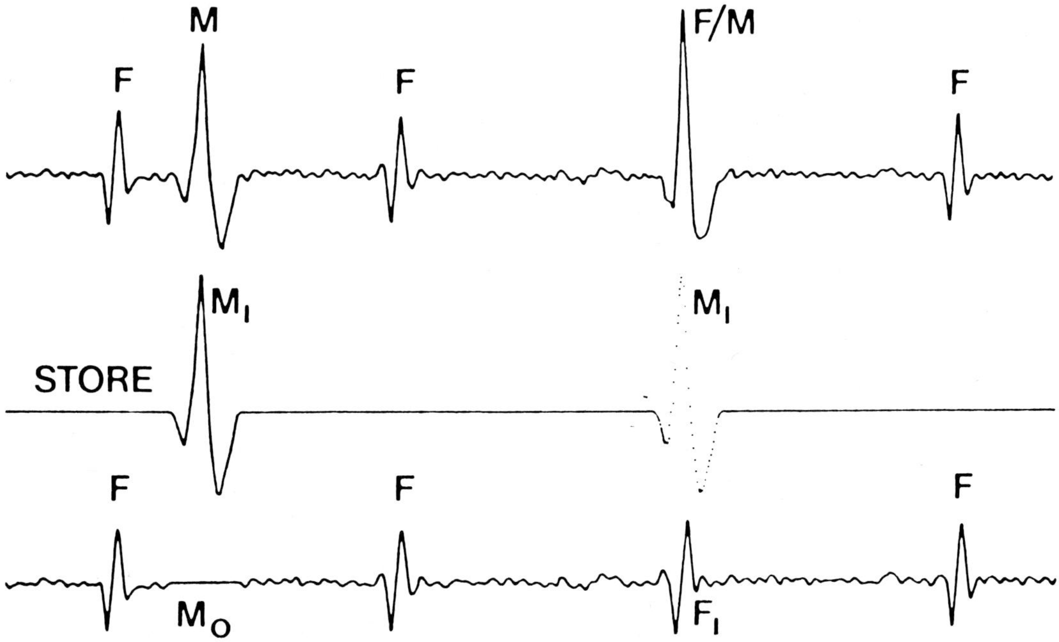

Fig. F.IX.7. The effect of the store and subtractor. The upper record shows the fetal and maternal ECG complexes before processing. The lower record shows the fetal ECG signals after processing by the store and subtractor. Pure fetal complexes (F) pass unchanged. The pure maternal complex (M) is subtracted from itself (M_0) and at the same time is retained by the store (M_1). This last pure maternal complex (held by the store) is subtracted from the combined feto-maternal complex (F/M) to leave the fetal complex (F_1) to appear in the processed recording. (From Wheeler et al. Br J Obstet Gynaecol 1978; 85:12–17, with permission.)

tion and amplitude of fetal QRS. About 60% of the time these complex averaging techniques can reproduce an average P wave and a PR interval.[6]

C. Scheme of Fetal ECG System

All fetal monitors today, both internal and external, involve several steps of elec-

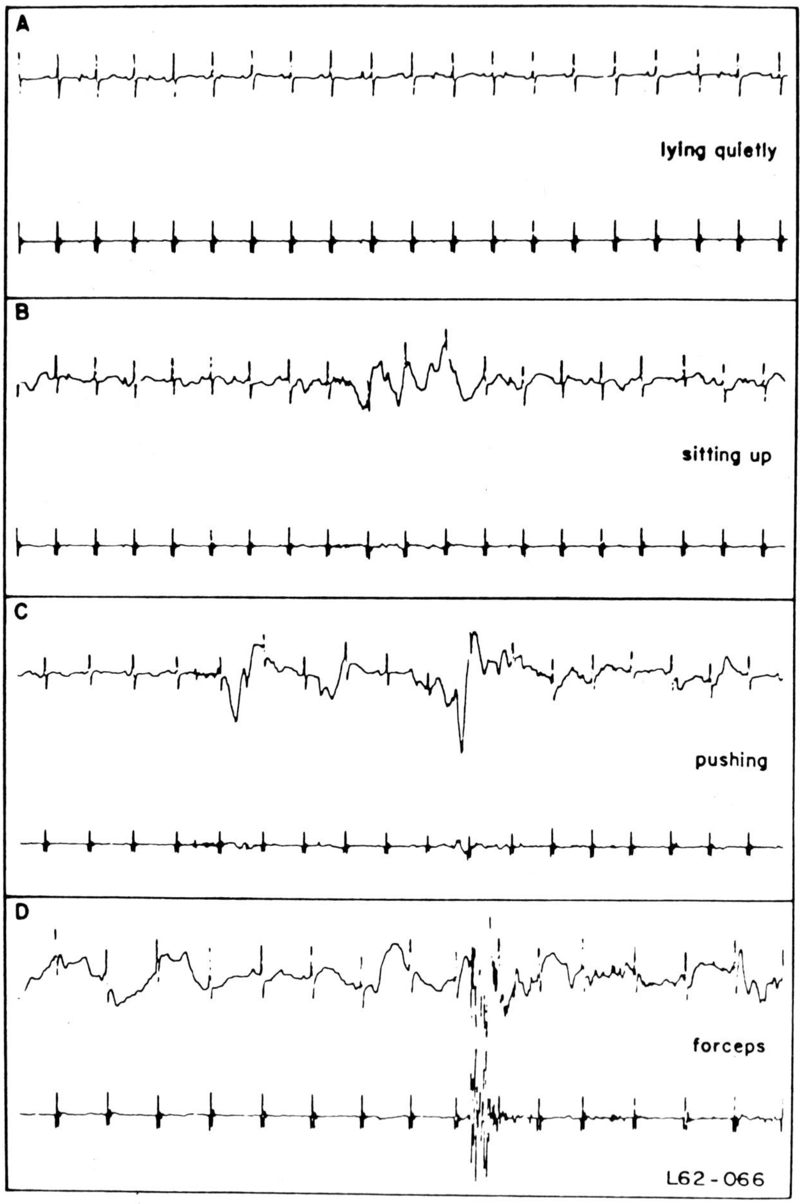

Fig. F.IX.8. Fetal ECGs recorded with a vaginal electrode during labor. Upper tracings in panels **A–D** are fetal ECGs, lower tracings in panels **A–D** are filtered fetal ECGs. **A,** Patient lying quietly. **B,** Patient sitting up. **C,** Patient "pushing" with contractions. Note increase in baseline noise of fetal ECG. Filtered fetal ECG tracings remain clear. **D,** Record made during forceps delivery. Note momentary artifact on both tracings. (By permission from Hon EH. Instrumentation of fetal heart rate and fetal electrocardiography. II. A vaginal electrode. Am J Obstet Gynecol. 1963; 86:772–784.)

tronically processing the input signal in order to improve the signal-to-noise ratio. It is important to understand the basic scheme of this because, although the signal-to-noise ratio is improved, certain distortions can be produced that must be appreciated when interpreting the final signal.

The input signal is the potential difference between two electrodes. This signal is fed into the monitor via a high input impedance to decrease the sensitivity to noise. The mother is grounded via a safety isolated ground wire to prevent the pickup of electrical signals that radiate from other electrical equipment.[11] The input signal is then filtered (Figs. F.IX.8 and F.IX.9) to remove baseline wandering and eliminate certain noise components.[3,7,11,12] The filter accentuates frequency components in the range of 120 Hz.[7] The filtering distorts ST segments and T waves,[11] so these may not be interpreted reliably in the final signal. After filtering, a fixed shape pulse is produced; this is called a trigger pulse, as it triggers other monitor functions.

After filtering, the signal is amplified via an automatic gain control. Occasionally the automatic gain can pick up interference from 60 Hz power lines and produce false arrhythmias.[7] This can be

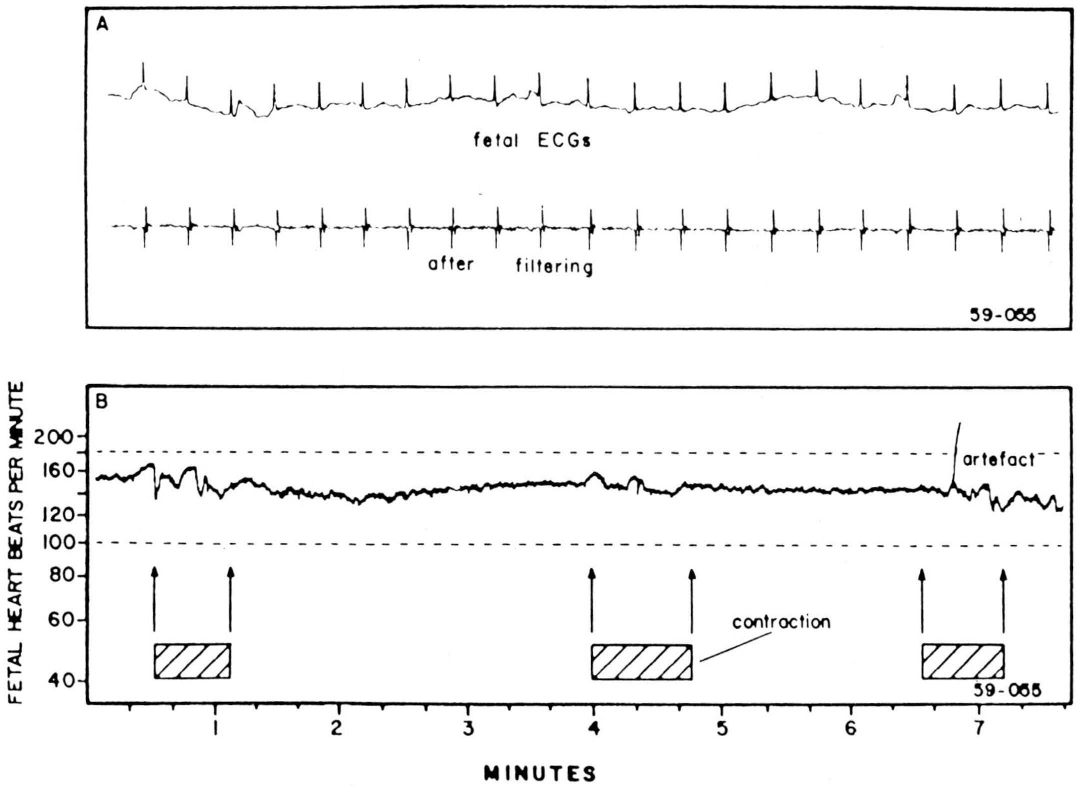

Fig. F.IX.9. A, Fetal ECG tracing from scalp electrode. Note absence of maternal ECG. The upper tracing is the unfiltered fetal ECG; the lower tracing has been filtered preparatory to automatic counting. **B,** A rate-time graph of the fetal heart rate recorded during labor. Note the accurate record through contractions. The above is an unretouched graph made directly from the patient during the second stage of labor with the patient pushing with contractions and was recorded under the usual conditions prevailing in a labor room. The single artifact was associated with extreme movement. Minor movements, such as raising a leg, talking, or drinking, had no effect on the record. (By permission from Hon EH, Hess OW. The clinical value of fetal electrocardiography. Am J Obstet Gynecol. 1960; 79:1012–1023.)

minimized by improving the grounding on the leg plates. There is an R wave detector that detects either the peak of the R wave or the maximum slope of the R wave. The same point must be used for each beat to get an accurate R-R interval. If t is the R-R interval, the instantaneous heart rate is $(1/t) \times 60$. The ease of defining the R-R interval is the main advantage for electrocardiography. The Doppler methods, for example, do not have a sharply defined time of onset and so have a trigger inaccuracy.[15]

After the R-R interval is converted to a rate, it is processed through a logic circuit before being displayed. All monitors today employ some form of logic circuit in order to prevent spurious noise from being counted as a fetal QRS complex. A certain R-R interval is computed and stored in memory for comparison with the following interval. The following interval is accepted only if it does not differ by more than a fixed percentage of the previous interval. Thus rate changes of more than a certain amount are rejected and rates greater than a specific upper limit are rejected. A rate that is too arrhythmic, too rapid, or too slow may be rejected as noise. The benefit is a more noise-free tracing. The disadvantage is that some real arrhythmias may be obscured. On most monitors the displayed ECG has less modification than the rate print-out and is worth looking at when it is suspected that a true arrhythmia is being rejected. In some instruments the logic circuit can be turned off to better demonstrate arrhythmias. This is sometimes referred to as the "pen lift" turned on or off.[3,7,11,13]

To improve the signal-to-noise ratio further, some monitoring systems use coherent time averaging. Averaging improves signal-to-noise ratios, but it also makes the system less sensitive to dynamic changes. Therefore the averages are weighted, with more weight given to recent signals.[16]

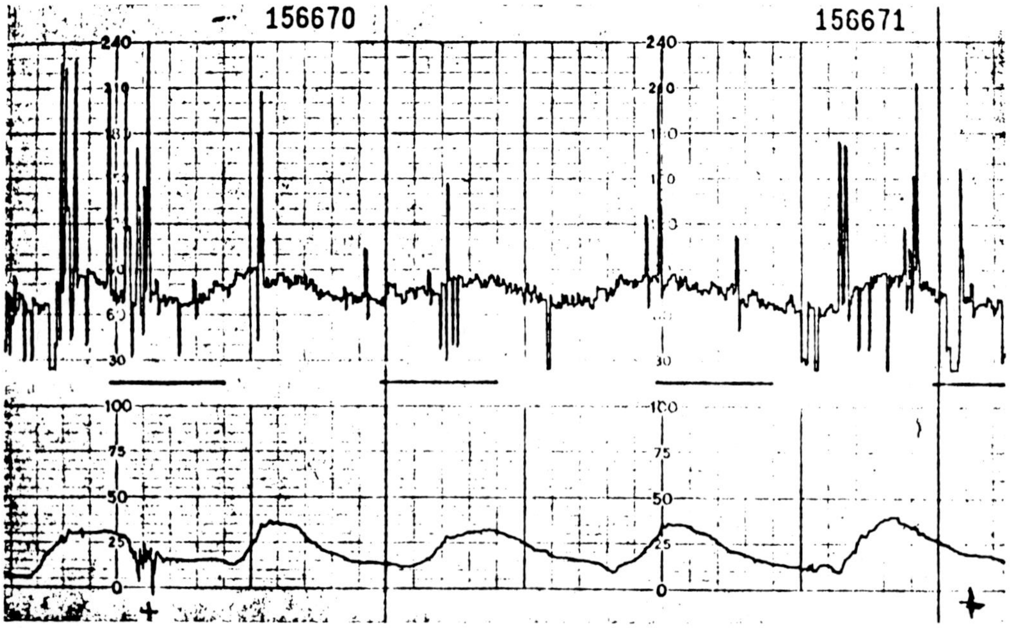

Fig. F.IX.10. The rate on the print-out in beats per minute varies directly with the maternal uterine contractions and coincides with the maternal cardiac rate and pulse. (By permission from Schneiderman CI, Waxman B, and Goodman CJ. Maternal–fetal electrocardiogram conduction with intrapartum fetal death. Am J Obstet Gynecol. 1972; 113:1130–1133.)

IV. FETAL DEATH

In the event of fetal death the internal monitor will sometimes display the maternal ECG[17] (see Fig. F.IX.10). To understand this phenomenon, refer back to how the maternal signal is eliminated from the internal ECG signal. Ordinarily the maternal signal at the fetal electrode and at the electrode in the vaginal fluid is so similar in amplitude that it is cancelled when the potential difference is taken. However, in the event of fetal death the conductivity of the fetal tissue is very different from the surrounding maternal tissue. Therefore the electrode placed subcutaneously in the fetal part sees a much stronger maternal signal than the electrode in the vaginal fluid. The potential difference between the two electrodes thus yields a net maternal signal.

Although this phenomenon is rare, failure to recognize it might result in an incorrect diagnosis of fetal bradycardia and force an unnecessary operative delivery. It should be suspected when 1) no fetal heart is heard with a fetoscope or Doppler; 2) no fetal movements are felt; 3) the rate varies directly with uterine contractions; and 4) a high voltage QRS complex is seen on the oscilloscope. For purposes of emphasis, because the maternal heart rate may vary with contractions, the tracing will often appear to have decelerations or accelerations (see Figs. F.IX.11–14).

To make the diagnosis of fetal death with certainty, the tracing from the internal monitor should be compared with a maternal electrocardiogram as to rate, onset of QRS, and duration of QRS. The fetal QRS duration is half that of the adult.[18]

V. TYPES OF ELECTRODES

A variety of electrodes have been used for internal monitoring. The electrode must pierce the skin and the metal be placed subcutaneously. The greater the amount of metal under the skin, the clearer and larger the fetal signal.[11] The electrode must also have enough mechanical strength so that it does not break easily; it must not become dislodged easily with vaginal ex-

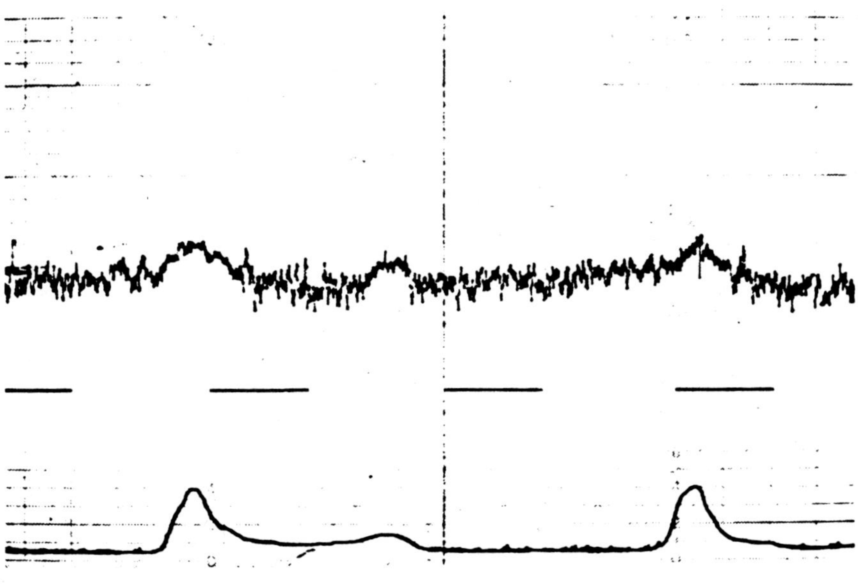

Fig. F.IX.11. Maternal heart rate simulating acceleration patterns. (Figs. F.IX.11–14 are by permission from Odendaal HJ. False interpretation of fetal heart rate monitoring in cases of intrauterine death. S Afr Med J. 1976; 50:1963–1965.)

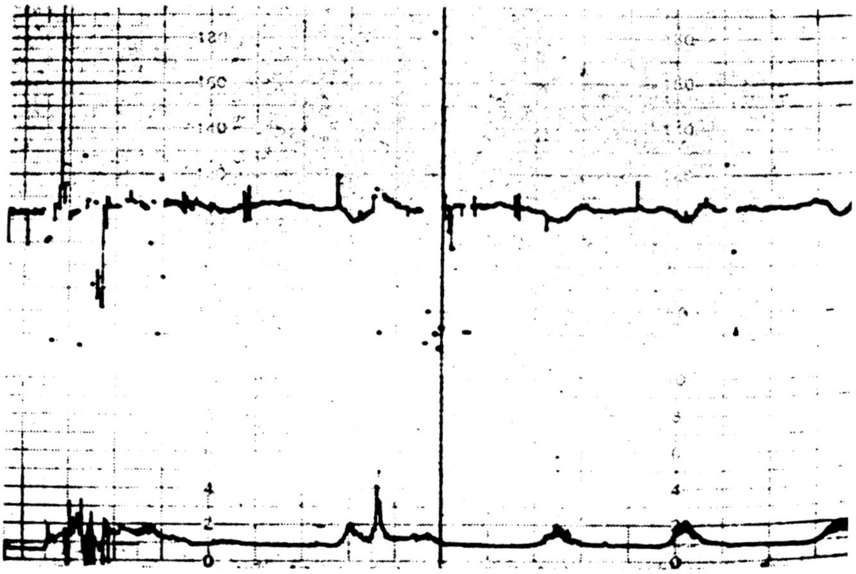

Fig. F.IX.12. Maternal heart rate simulating deceleration patterns.

aminations. Occasionally a dislodged electrode may produce false readings. Also, the electrode must be capable of mass production.

Random fluctuations in the concentration of metallic ions at the electrode–tissue junction can produce artifacts. Electrodes made of Ag/AgCl help stabilize the signal. The silver ion concentration depends upon the chloride ion concentration. The chloride ion concentration of tissues is high and so is relatively constant.[19]

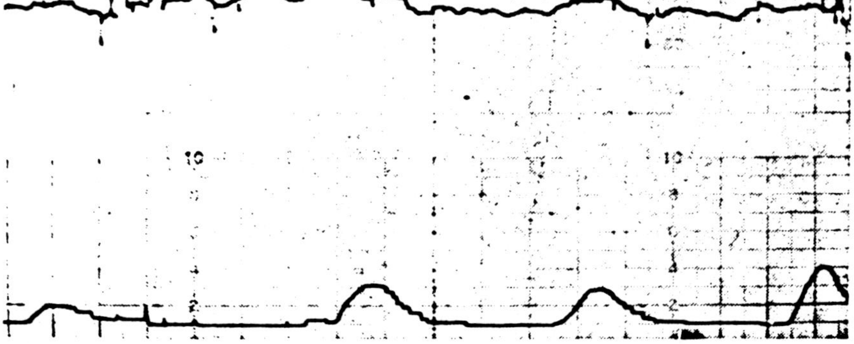

Fig. F.IX.13. Loss of beat-to-beat variations simulated.

However, silver chloride electrodes tend to degenerate in light and are difficult to mass produce. Stainless steel has been found to be adequate for routine use and is easy to mass produce.[11]

The types of electrodes have included clip, needle, hook, and screw types. The clip type of electrode was popular for a while. This was an adaptation of a surgical skin clip. It gave a good signal and was not dangerous to the fetal skin. However, it had to be applied with special forceps and under direct vision, and it was also easily broken. The spiral electrodes have become more popular. They are screwed into the skin of the presenting part, and their application is guided by palpation rather than direct vision. They are therefore easier to apply and can be used at an earlier stage of dilatation than the clip type.[11,24]

VI. COMPLICATIONS OF ELECTRODES

Although rare, complications of scalp electrodes have been reported.

Scalp abscesses have been reported with an incidence between 0.1 and 0.4%.[20,25] Usually they are local and treated with simple drainage. The incidence may be somewhat underestimated because scalp abscesses are often not manifest until post-discharge. Very rarely a scalp abscess can be more serious. Two cases of skull osteomyelitis and sepsis have been reported.[20]

Minor ecchymoses of the fetal scalp have been reported.[12] A case of fetal bleeding occurred when an electrode lacerated a scalp artery.[20] Very rarely, fetal damage can occur, as when an electrode was applied to a fetal eyelid.[20] There is also a report of drainage of cerebrospinal fluid when an electrode was applied over the posterior fontanelle.[21]

VII. SAFETY

All AC-powered equipment has some leakage. Ordinarily skin resistance is high enough to prevent the passage of currents through the body. However, intracavitary catheters, pacemaker wires, etc can provide a pathway that bypasses skin resistance. Imperceptibly small 60 cycle currents passing through the heart via a catheter can prove fatal. These currents

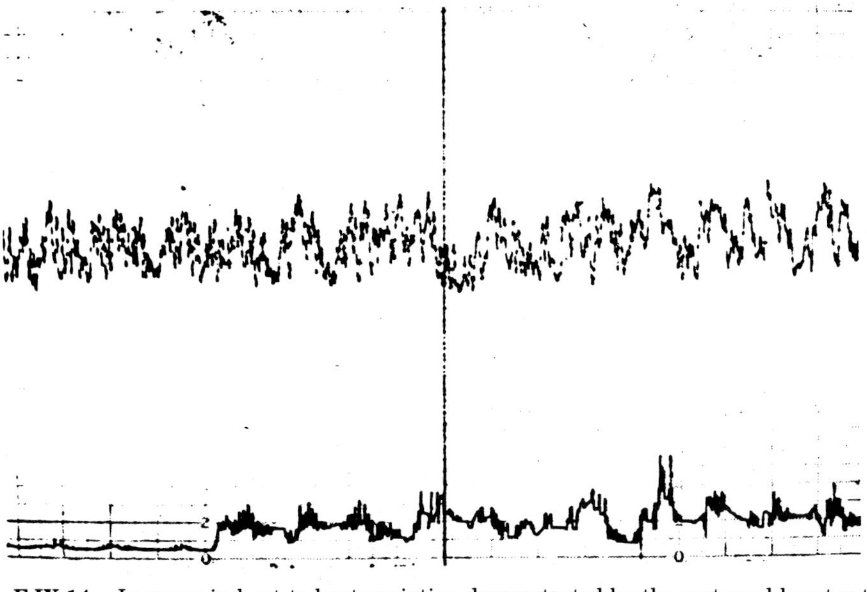

Fig. F.IX.14. Increase in beat-to-beat variation demonstrated by the maternal heart rate.

do not have to come from monitoring equipment but can come from other electrical equipment such as lamps, electric beds, television sets, etc. Contact with a faulty electrical appliance can pass current through the body and out an intracavitary wire to ground. Fetal scalp electrodes can provide such a pathway. For this reason, modern monitoring equipment has built-in protection against accidental electrocutions. The signal has to pass through a disconnection of very high resistance so that more than a few microamperes cannot be passed through the instrument. The signal may be passed by a small radiotransmitter enclosed within the instrument. With such isolation current cannot pass through the patient and through the instrument to ground. Accidental electrocutions are thus prevented.[3,11,19]

VIII. LIMITATIONS OF FETAL ECG INHERENT IN EQUIPMENT DESIGN

As has been mentioned previously, because the signal is filtered, there is distortion of ST segments and T waves. Also, noise filters and computer logic may produce a loss of certain arrhythmias (see Fig. F.IX.15). Abdominal ECG monitors rely extremely heavily on computer logic to disregard the maternal tracing. With a rapid maternal rate and a slow fetal rate a considerable artifact may be introduced by computer logic.[7]

True signals may be obscured by noise (see Fig. F.IX.16). Occasionally the noise is large enough and similar enough to the desired signal that false pathology is interpreted.[11] For example, a pickup from a 60 Hz power line gave a constant heart rate of 150 and no variability (see Fig. F.IX.17). These cases will always give a rate that is a multiple of 30.[22]

Electrical noise arising within the electrode and amplifier system is referred to as parasitic oscillations. These may be mistaken for multiple pregnancies, but the uniform height and rhythm suggest artifact.[2]

It should also be pointed out that different paper speeds can emphasize different aspects of a tracing. Slow paper speeds emphasize beat-to-beat variations, and faster paper speeds emphasize gross rate changes.[23]

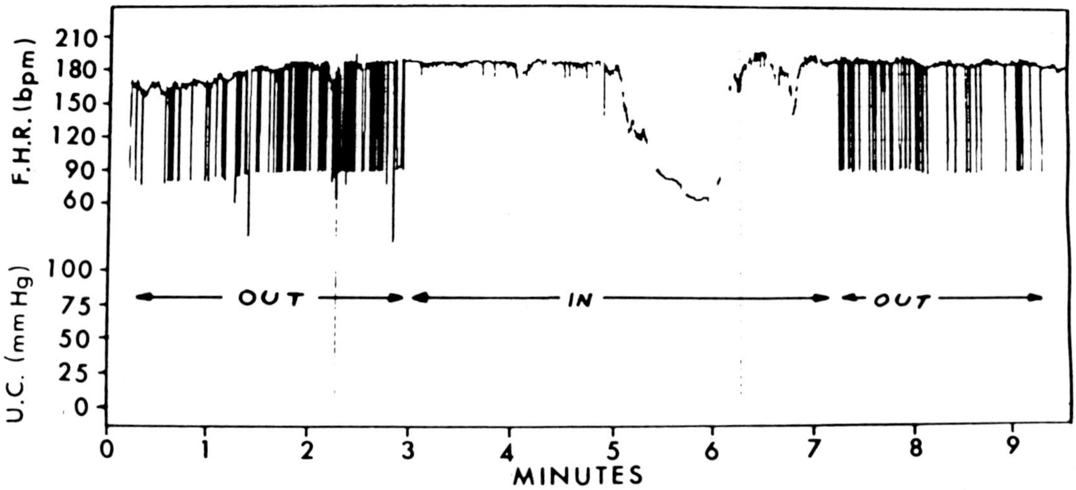

Fig. F.IX.15. Monitor logic has obscured an obvious case of dropped beats. With the "pen-lift" activated (IN) the arrhythmia is completely obscured. When the logic is disabled (OUT) one can clearly see that almost every other heart beat is dropped. This may be either fetal or machine error. Simple auscultation proved this to be a real case of intermittent heart block. Mother was permitted to labor and delivered an infant with Apgar scores of 9 at 1 min and 10 at 5 min. Heart block spontaneously resolved at delivery. (Figures F.IX.15 and 16 are by permission from Klapholz H. Techniques of fetal heart rate monitoring. Semin Perinatol. 1978; 2:119–129.)

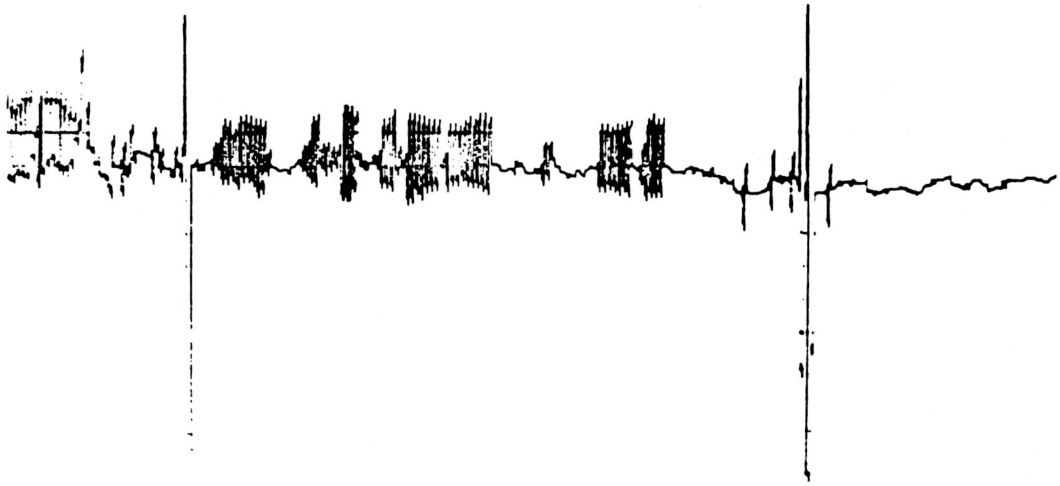

Fig. F.IX.16. Excessive (60-Hz) interference resulting in baseline drift of ECG resulted in above tracing. Reversal of electrode polarity promptly corrected this artifact. Such tracings should also make one think of a fetal arrhythmia. Auscultation of the fetus and reversal of the polarity switch will be diagnostic. Self-reversal is a feature of newer monitors.

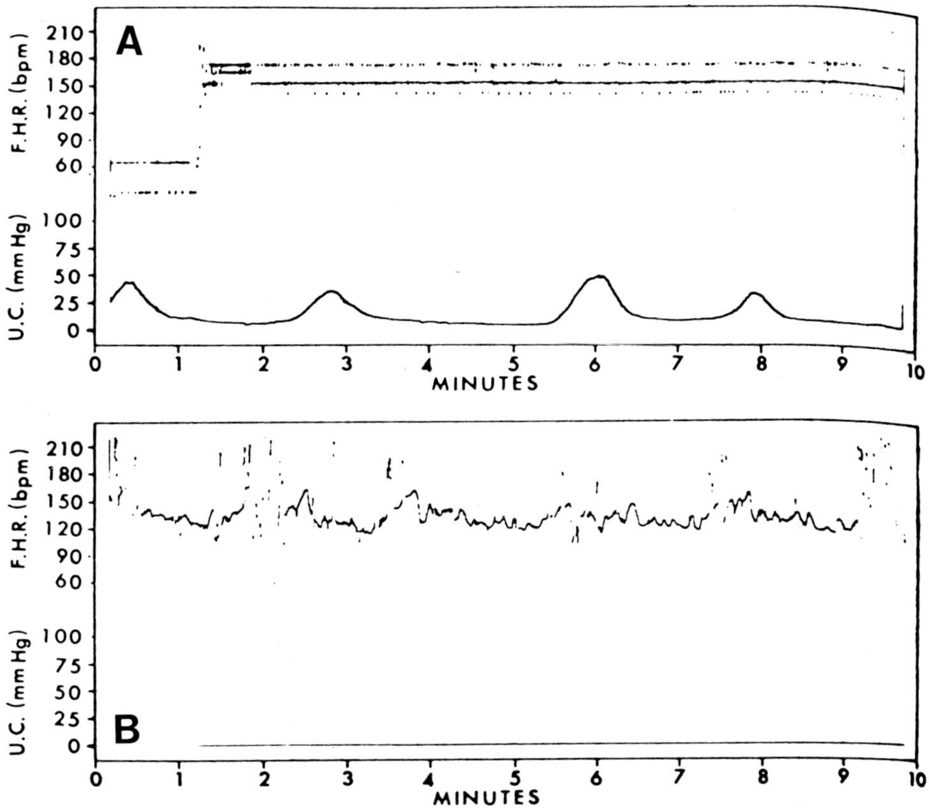

Fig. F.IX.17. Upper graph (**A**): constant fetal heart rate of 150 is shown. Note that there are small "spikes" every few seconds similar to those seen when premature contractions are present. There is no short-term variability. Lower graph (**B**): The same patient, but recorded on a monitor with built-in 60-Hz rejection filtering. This is a perfectly normal recording. (Reprinted with permission from The American College of Obstetricians and Gynecologists. Obstetrics and Gynecology 53:245–247, 1979.)

IX. REFERENCES

1. Cremer M. Über die direkte Ableitung der Aktionströme des menschlichen Herzens von Öesophagus und über das Elektrokardiogramm des Fötus. Munchen Med Wochnschr. 1906; 53:811.
2. Hon EH, Hess OW. The clinical value of fetal electrocardiography. Am J Obstet Gyencol. 1960; 79:1012–1023.
3. Van Bremmel JH, de Haan J, Veth TFL. Instrumentation for obstetrics and gynecology. In: Ray CD, ed. Medical Engineering. Chicago: Yearbook, 1974:548–558.
4. Freidman S, Eckerling B. Fetal electrocardiogram obtained with subcutaneous maternal electrodes. Am J Obstet Gynecol. 1969; 103:1160–1162.
5. Figueroa-Longo JG, Poserio JJ, Alvarez LO, Caldeyro-Barcia R. Fetal electrocardiogram at term labor obtained with subcutaneous fetal electrodes. Am J Obstet Gynecol. 1966; 96:556–564.
6. Behrer MR, Glaeser DH, Cox JR, Woolf RB. Quantification of the fetal electrocardiogram through LINC computer processing. Am J Obstet Gynecol. 1968; 102:537–548.
7. Klapholz H. Techniques of fetal heart rate monitoring. Semin Perinatol. 1978; 2:119–129.
8. Larks SD, Dasgupta K. Fetal electrocardiography, with special reference to early pregnancy. Am Heart J. 1958; 56:701–714.
9. Roche Medical Electronics. Fetal Monitoring in Clinical Obstetrics: An Introduction. Clinical Studies in Fetal Monitoring: A Guide for Users of the Fetasonde 2100. Cranbury, New Jersey: Roche Medical Electronics, I-1–I-7.
10. Klapholtz H, Schifrin BS, Rivo E. Paroxysmal supraventricular tachycardia in the fetus. Obstet Gynecol. 1974; 43:718–721.
11. Hochberg HM. Fetal monitoring instrumentation. In: Clinical Studies in Fetal Monitoring: A Guide for the Users of the Fetasonde 2100. Cranbury, New Jersey: Roche Medical Electronics, III-1–III-61.
12. Hon EH. Instrumentation of fetal heart rate and fetal electrocardiography. II. A vaginal electrode. Am J Obstet Gynecol. 1963; 86:772–784.
13. Hon EH. The electronic evaluation of the fetal heart rate. Am J Obstet Gynecol. 1958; 75:1215–1230.
14. Wheeler T, Murrills A, Shelly T. Measurement of the fetal heart rate during pregnancy by a new electrocardiographic technique. Br J Obstet Gynaecol. 1978; 85:12–17.
15. De Haan J. Fetal monitoring by physical methods. I. Technical questions. Eur J Obstet Gynecol Reprod Biol. 1973; 3/2:57–66.
16. Rhyne VT. Digital signal enhancement of the fetal electrocardiogram. Am J Obstet Gynecol. 1968; 102:549–555.
17. Timor-Tretsch I, Gergely Z, Abramovici H, Brandes JM. Misleading information from fetal monitoring in a case of intrapartum death. Obstet Gynecol. 1974; 43:713–717.
18. Schneiderman CI, Waxman B, Goodman CJ. Maternal-fetal electrocardiogram conduction with intrapartum fetal death. Am J Obstet Gynecol. 1972; 113:1130–1133.
19. Unger FW, Eng P, Goodwin JW. Instrumentation for fetal electrocardiography and intrauterine pressure: A new scalp electrode and radiotelemetry system. Am J Obstet Gynecol. 1972; 112:351–357.
20. Ledger WJ. Complications associated with invasive monitoring. Semin Perinatol. 1978; 2:187–194.
21. Goodlin RC, Harrod JR. Complications of fetal spiral electrodes. Lancet. 1973; 1:559.
22. Klapholtz H. Artifactual fetal heart rate recording secondary to 60-Hz power line interference. Obstet Gynecol. 1979; 53:245–247.
23. Goodlin RC. Comparison of instantaneous fetal heart rate recorders. Obstet Gynecol. 1972; 40:265–267.
24. Hon EH, Paul RH, Hon RW. Electronic evaluation of fetal heart rate. XI. Description of a spiral electrode. Obstet Gynecol. 1972; 40:362–365.
25. Cordero L, Hon EH. Scalp abscess: A rare complication of fetal monitoring. J Pediatr. 1971; 78:533–537.
26. Odendaal HJ. False interpretation of fetal heart rate monitoring in cases of intrauterine death. South Afr Med J. 1976; 50:1963–1965.

F.X

Systolic Time Interval

Yuji Murata, MD

I. INTRODUCTION

Evidence that alterations in the course of the cardiac cycle reflect ventricular function was introduced by Wiggers[1] in 1921 through his animal studies. Following this study Katz and Feil[2] described a technique in human adults to investigate the cardiac intervals, which were defined by electrical and mechanical activities using simultaneous recordings of the phonocardiogram (PCG), central arterial pulse tracing, and electrocardiogram (ECG). More recently, Weissler and his co-workers,[3] using a similar method, proved the clinical applicability and usefulness of systolic time intervals. They demon-

Abbreviations: ECG, electrocardiogram; PCG, phonocardiogram; DCG, Doppler cardiogram; STI, systolic time intervals; EMLT, electromechanical latent time; PEP, preejection period; VET, ventricular ejection time; ICT, isovolumic contraction time; A-V valve, atrioventricular valve; Mc, A-V valve closure; Ao, semilunar valve opening; Ac, semilunar valve closure; Mo, A-V valve opening; FHR, fetal heart rate; LVEDP, left ventricular end-diastolic pressure; CST, contraction stress testing of fetal heart rate; NST, nonstress testing of fetal heart rate; UCG, ultrasound cardiogram.

Cardiac Problems in Pregnancy, pages 491–508

strated that there were differences in left ventricular ejection time between normal individuals and patients with cardiovascular diseases.

The first attempt to measure the systolic time intervals (STIs) of the human fetus was made in 1966 by Persianinov,[4] who reported various fetal cardiac intervals measured from simultaneous recordings of fetal ECG and PCG, both of which were obtained noninvasively through the maternal abdomen. The current technique to determine the fetal STIs using a simultaneous recording of fetal ECG and ultrasound Doppler cardiogram was introduced by Murata et al[5] in 1971. This technique has proved to be accurate and clinically applicable and has been used in the investigation of fetal systolic time intervals.

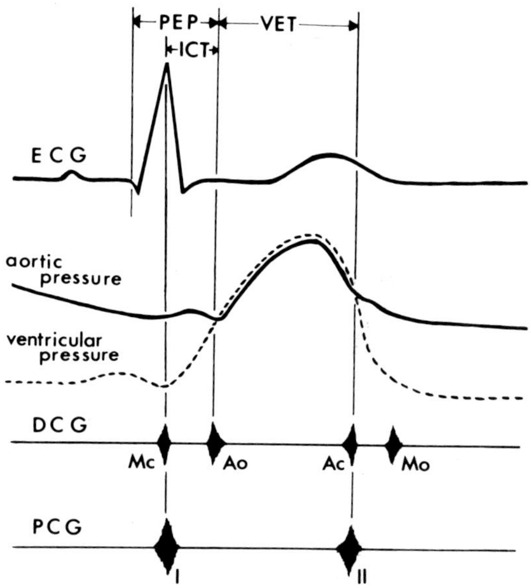

Fig. F.X.1. Electrical and mechanical events occurring during one cardiac cycle. From the top, ECG: electrocardiogram, aortic pressure tracing, intraventricular pressure tracing; DCG: ultrasound Doppler cardiogram; PCG: phonocardiogram. PEP: preejection period; ICT: isovolumic contraction time; VET: ventricular ejection time. Electromechanical latent time can be calculated by substracting the ICT from the PEP. The mechanical systole is a sum of ICT and VET. The total systole is PEP plus VET. Mc, Ao, Ac, and Mo on the DCG are atrioventricular (A-V) valve closure, semilunar valve opening, semilunar valve closure and A-V valve opening, respectively. I and II on the PCG channel indicate the first and second sounds of the heart.

The published data on STIs of human fetuses, as well as laboratory animals under experimental conditions, seem to indicate that the STIs, especially the preejection period (PEP) and the ventricular ejection time (VET), can be useful parameters in determining the functional integrity of the fetal myocardium.

II. DEFINITION OF THE SYSTOLIC TIME INTERVALS

One cardiac cycle contains several intervals that can be defined by the sequentially occurring electrical and mechanical events shown in Figure F.X.1. These individual intervals are called systolic time intervals (STIs) which can be divided into electromechanical STIs or mechanical STIs depending upon the reference points for the measurement of intervals. The electromechanical STI is an interval measured between an electrical event (usually the onset of the Q wave) and a mechanical event. The mechanical events are represented by the sequential movements of the opening and closing of cardiac valves (Mc, Ao, Ac, and Mo). The mechanical STI can be defined by any two mechanical events of the heart during systole.

A. Electromechanical Latent Time (EMLT)

The EMLT is the interval between the onset of ventricular depolarization and the atrioventricular valve (A-V valve) closure (Mc). This is one of the electromechanical STIs. Following the previous cardiac cycle, the A-V valves remain open until the contraction of ventricular muscle begins. Ventricular contraction increases the intraventricular pressure, reversing the pressure gradient from the ventricle to the atrium, promoting valve closure. The EMLT can, therefore, be described as the lag time between the electrical excitation and the onset of mechanical activity of the ventricle.

B. Isovolumic Contraction Time (ICT)

The ICT is a mechanical STI that is defined as the interval between A-V valve closure (Mc) and semilunar valve opening (Ao). At this time the ventricles are normally closed chambers filled with blood. When the myocardium contracts the intraventricular pressure increases without changing the volume of the ventricle (isovolumic contraction). When intraventricular pressure exceeds systemic pressure, the semilunar valves open (Ao) and ejection of the blood into the great vessels commences.

C. Preejection Period (PEP)

The PEP is the sum of two intervals, EMLT and ICT. Therefore, the indicating PEP is the interval from the onset of ventricular depolarization to the beginning of ejection from the ventricle. The PEP has been the most extensively studied electromechanical STI in the fetus, infants, and adults, and it is known to be a sensitive indicator of myocardial performance.

D. Ventricular Ejection Time (VET)

The VET occurs during the ejection of the blood from the ventricle to the great vessels. As soon as ejection starts, the intraventricular pressure equals and supresses the resting (diastolic) pressure and reaches a maximum (systolic) pressure; then it falls. At the point where the intraventricular pressure becomes lower than the systemic pressure (diastolic pressure), the semilunar valve closes (Ac) and the heart enters the diastolic phase. The VET is a representative mechanical STI and has been thoroughly investigated in infants and adults.

E. Mechanical Systole

Mechanical systole is an interval from A-V valve closure (Mc) to similunar valve closure (Ac) during which the ventricle muscle continuously contracts. This phase is a mechanical STI that consists of two other mechanical STIs, the ICT and the VET.

F. Total Systole

Total systole is an electromechanical STI and is the sum of the PEP and the VET. This interval indicates the total time required for the heart to complete the systolic phase.

III. METHOD OF DETERMINATION OF SYSTOLIC TIME INTERVALS

The determination of electromechanical STIs requires an electrocardiogram to identify the onset of myocardial depolarization. By definition, as described previously, electromechanical STIs are to be measured from the onset of ventricular depolarization, which can be identified as the onset of the Q wave on the ECG. By convention, however, many investigators choose the peak of the R wave as a measuring point simply because the R wave is more easily identifiable especially when determination is automated using a computer or other electronic processes.

Although the ECG signal obtained directly from the fetus provides a clear signal and thus is preferable for determination of STIs, this can only be obtained using a scalp electrode following rupture of the amniotic membranes. During the antepartum period, however, satisfactory ECG signals for STI determination can also be recorded in approximately 80% of the patients studied using electrodes placed on the maternal abdomen[6] (Fig. F.X.2). Determination of either electromechanical or mechanical STIs requires information about mechanical events that occur sequentially in a cardiac cycle. Noninvasive methods that have been popular are the phonocardiogram and the ultrasound Doppler cardiogram. Apexcardiograms and carotid tracings are also noninvasive and are favorably used in adult subjects, but obviously neither is feasible for the fetus in utero. Intraventricular pressure curves or central arterial pressure curves can also be used to obtain the necessary information. However, both are invasive techniques requiring catheterization and thus are limited to laboratory experiments on fetal animals.

PCG in conjunction with FECG was employed by Persianinov et al[4] and Goodlin et al[7] in an earlier stage of the investigation for fetal STIs. Based on the assumptions that the first sound in the PCG (S_1) is created by mitral valve closure[8] and the second sound (S_2) by aortic closure[9] the Q-S_1, Q-S_2 and S_1-S_2 are compatible with electromechanical latent time (EMLT), total systole, and mechanical systole, respectively. The simultaneous recording of ECG and PCG, therefore, cannot separately determine the PEP and VET. Furthermore, many investigators have often encountered difficulties in collecting high-quality fetal heart sound consistently through the maternal abdomen.

Conversely, as clinical obstetric practice indicates, an ultrasound Doppler device can usually provide clear signals from the fetal heart during either the antepartum or the intrapartum period. In order to identify the fetal heart valve motions, the original signals must be conditioned through an appropriate band-pass filter. Murata et al reported that the frequency range of 600–2,000 Hz provides the most optimal signals to identify opening and closing movements of the fetal cardiac valves[10] (Fig. F.X.2). The identification of these signals in one cardiac cycle appearing on the filtered Doppler cardiogram has been carried out by means of the frequency spectrogram[11] and fetal UCG.[5] These studies indicated that the four consistent pulsatile signals in one cardiac cycle were from 1) the A-V valve closure (Mc), 2) the semilunar valve opening (Ao), 3) the semilunar valve closure (Ac), 4) and the A-V valve opening (Mo).

In adults, the STIs are predominantly determined in the left ventricle. The cardiac valve movements, therefore, are those from the mitral (M) and aortic (A) valves and can be clearly separated from the tricuspid and pulmonic valves. In the fetus, however, this separation of the signal is impossible by the technique using simultaneous recording of the FECG and Doppler cardiogram. Accordingly, Ac, Ao, Mc, and Mo are presenting closure and opening of the semilunar valve and A-V valve of the fetus, respectively.

Figure F.X.1 and Table F.X.1 demonstrate the critical points of measurement in each systolic time interval as previously defined.

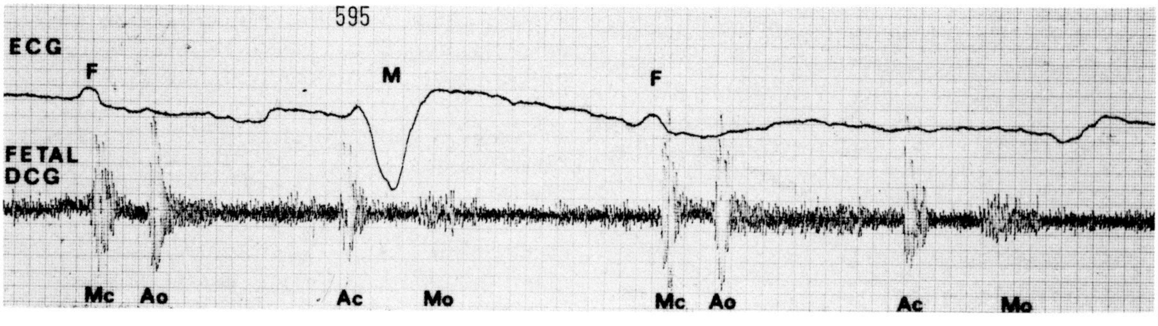

Fig. F.X.2. A simultaneous recording of the abdominal fetal electrocardiogram and fetal Doppler cardiogram. F and M on the ECG indicate fetal and maternal QRS complex obtained through electrodes placed on the maternal abdomen. Mc: atrioventricular (A-V) valve closure; Ao: semilunar valve opening; Ac: semilunar valve closure; Mo: A-V opening. (From Murata et al.[6])

TABLE F.X.1. Definition of Systolic Time Intervals

Systolic time intervals	Physiologic implication	Intervals to be measured	Method to be used
Electromechanical latent time (EMLT)	Delay from ventricular depolarization to onset of mechanical contraction	Q-Mc	ECG & DCG
Isovolumic contraction time (ICT)	Time required for ventricular muscle to increase intraventricular pressure until ejection starts	Mc-Ao	DCG only
Preejection period (PEP)	Time between onset of ventricular depolarization to beginning of ejection	Q-Ao	ECG & DCG
Ventricular ejection time (VET)	Duration of blood ejection from ventricle to great vessel	Ac-Ao	DCG only
Mechanical systole	Total duration of ventricular muscle contraction	Mc-Ac or S_1-S_2	DCG only or PCG only
Total systole	Total time required for heart to complete systole, starting from electrical excitation	Q-Ac or Q-S_2	ECG & DCG or ECG & PCG

IV. PHYSIOLOGY OF SYSTOLIC TIME INTERVALS

The present knowledge of physiologic behavior of the STIs in the fetal cardiac cycle have been derived primarily from findings on laboratory animals, usually chronically instrumented fetal lambs and monkeys, and from minimal observations on human fetuses. In most instances, when the experimental observations were carried out, fetal animals were under physiologic conditions in utero, having recovered from surgical insults and anesthesia, both of which are required for establishing this type of preparation. Some observations, however, were made during or immediately after the surgery on the fetuses, and therefore the interpretation of data must be made with caution because of the potential effects of direct stress from surgery and/or anesthesia. Emphasis has repeatedly been placed on the importance of the chronic pregnant model for the purpose of investigating fetal and uteroplacental physiology.[12]

To date, the PEP and VET are two STIs that have been extensively investigated in the fetuses. Reports on other STIs have been limited in number. For this reason, the following sections deal mainly with the PEP and VET of the fetal cardiac cycle.

A. Fetal Heart Rate and Systolic Time Intervals

Previous studies on infants, children, and adults demonstrated that the PEP shortens when the heart rate increases. Similarly, Organ et al have shown this inverse relationship between the PEP and heart rate[13,14] (Fig. F.X.3). The authors also demonstrated this relationship to be independent of gestational age.[14]

In contrast, Robinson et al[15] and Murata and Martin[10] observed the lack of a direct relationship between the PEP and

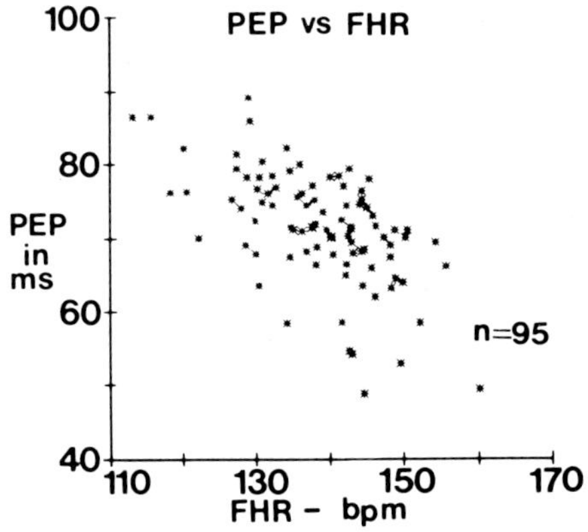

Fig. F.X.3. The relationship between preejection period (PEP) and fetal heart rate (FHR) from 95 normal fetuses. Gestational age ranged from 20 to 43 weeks. (From Organ et al.[13])

heart rate in human as well as monkey fetuses.[16] Their studies included the observation, during baseline fetal heart rate measurements, of average baseline variability, early decelerations, transient accelerations, and the initial slowing phases of mild variable decelerations. Lack of a relationship between PEP and heart rate has also been reported in separate studies when the heart rate change resulted from vagal stimulation or cardiac pacing.[17] Interestingly, Murata et al observed no change in the PEP during descending rims of the variable deceleration.[10] The same investigators also demonstrated that the inverse correlation between PEP and heart rate existed only in fetal monkeys receiving an intravenous infusion of epinephrine.[16] These observations suggest that changes in heart rate itself do not affect the PEP. Adrenergic stimulation, however, having both chronologic and inotropic stimulations at the same time, increases both heart rate and myocardial contractility, thus shortening the PEP. It may therefore be clinically important to observe fetal heart rate simultaneously for the interpretation of the PEP changes.

A clear positive relationship between the VET and R-R interval has been demonstrated in normal human fetuses during labor[10] (Fig. F.X.4) and also in antepartum fetal monkeys[18] (see Fig. F. X. 7). This relationship was observed between 330 and 530 msec (115–180 bpm) in the human fetus and between 240 and 400 msec (150–250 bpm) in the monkey fetus. Above these ranges, R-R intervals in both species were encountered with no further lengthening of the VET. Other studies from adults and infants also indicate the strong effect of the R-R interval on the VET.

B. Gestational Age of the Fetus

A consistent finding by all investigators is that the PEP lengthens as gestational age of the fetus advances. This is seen in the human,[10,14,19] monkey,[16] and sheep fetus.[20] In the normal antepartum human fetus, Murata and associates[6] calculated an increment of the PEP to be 1.52 msec per week between 33 and 42 weeks, and Wolfson et al[19] reported a value of 0.85 msec per week between 20 and 40 weeks. A similar value, 0.84 msec per week, was reported by Bärtling et al.[21] Organ and co-workers[14] demonstrated that the value of the weekly increment was 1.4 msec.

Murata and associates concluded that the physiologic lengthening of the PEP associated with advancing gestational age was due to a concurrent increase in QRS duration secondary to increasing myocardial volume.[16] This conclusion was based upon two isolated observations: the first that there were identical increments in the lengthening of the PEP (Q-Ao), ICT (Q-Mc), and QRS duration with advancing gestational age,[16] as shown in Figure F.X.5; the second, that there was a statistically better correlation between the PEP and newborn body weight than between PEP and gestational age of the fetus. Later, Organ and his associates[14] substantiated the above findings, reporting the identical findings of increasing PEP and QRS duration with advancing gestational age of human fetuses.[22]

Following the lengthening of the PEP until 41 weeks, Bärtling et al[21] reported a shortening of the PEP between 41 and 43 weeks, with a decrement of 0.76 msec

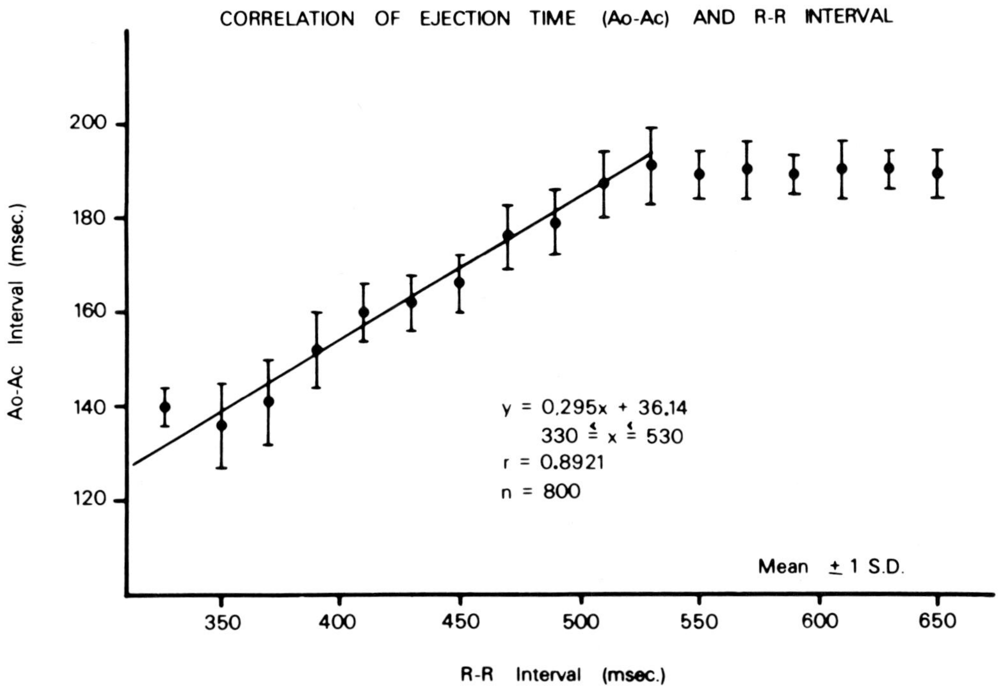

Fig. F.X.4. Relationship between the ventricular ejection time (Ao-Ac) and R-R intervals from 15 normal fetuses. The VET increases as R-R increases (heart rate decreases). No further lengthening was observed with R-R intervals greater than 530 msec (115 bpm). Mean ± SD (From Murata Y, Martin CB, Jr.[10])

per week. These observations were based on a rather small population and were not statistically significant.

There were no significant changes in the VET associated with the changes in gestational age either in the human[10,19] or the monkey fetus.[18]

C. Preload

Frank-Starling's law indicates that the ventricular muscle determines myocardial contractility; the higher the left ventricular end-diastolic pressure, the more the myocardial contractility. A study in which the left ventricle of the monkey fetus was catheterized demonstrated a strong inverse relationship between LVEDP and PEP.[16] Furthermore, clinical observation made on antepartum fetuses with supraventricular arrhythmia revealed that a short PEP was associated with a cardiac cycle preceded by long R-R interval—that is, an increase in preload. Conversely, a short R-R interval (decreased preload) was followed by prolonged PEP.[16] Hawrylyshyn et al[23] reported a similar case with the same findings.

D. Blood Pressure

The PEP was positively correlated with both systolic and diastolic pressure, whereas the EMLT and IVC were not significantly related to either blood pressure.[16] Increased diastolic pressure requires higher intraventricular pressure to exceed intraaortic pressure and open the aortic valve, as shown in Figure F.X.1. Thus, the PEP will be longer. The relationship between the PEP and systolic pressure is more complex and somewhat controversial, even in the adult subject.

Widening of pulse pressure is known to

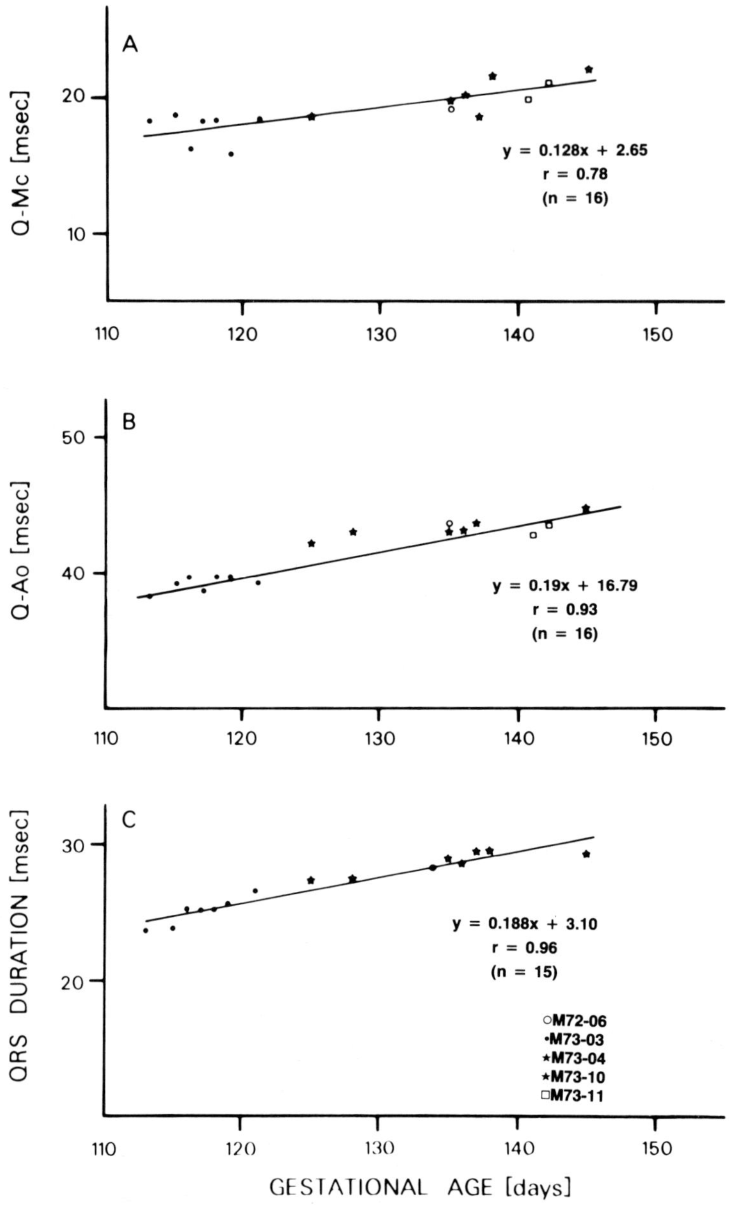

Fig. F.X.5. Correlations between systolic time intervals and gestational age in the normal fetal rhesus monkey. From the top, **A**: electromechanical latent time (Q-Mc); **B**: preejection period (Q-Ao); **C**: QRS duration of electrocardiogram. Increments in three intervals within observed range of gestational age are virtually identical.[16])

be associated with an increase in stroke volume and ventricle preload, other factors being equal.[24] The relationship between the PEP and the pulse pressure under physiologic conditions was not found to be significant because of the small range of aortic pulse pressure observed in the monkey fetus. Figure F.X.6 indicates that a clear inverse correlation between the PEP and the pulse pressure was observed in one distressed monkey fetus which had a wide range of pulse pressures.[16]

E. Coronary Blood Flow and the Preejection Period

There has been one study in which the PEP and coronary blood flow were measured using a radioactive microsphere in chronically catheterized fetal lambs. Observations were performed under normal physiologic conditions and experimentally stressed conditions. The data indicated a statistically significant inverse correlation between the PEP and coronary blood flow expressed in ml/kg/beat. The relationship, however, disappeared as the fetal lambs were exposed to the stress of hypoxemia or hypercapnia.[20]

V. PATHOLOGIC RESPONSES OF THE SYSTOLIC TIME INTERVALS

A. Hypoxemia

Reported evidence from different investigators has not been in total agreement concerning the fetal PEP response to hypoxemia. A significant shortening of the PEP was reported by Organ et al, [25] who determined the PEP using simultaneous recordings of fetal ECG and arterial blood pressure tracings in the exteriorized fetal lamb. The mothers were kept under intravenous chloralose anesthesia during the experiment. Shortening of the PEP was observed when an abrupt drop in the fetal PaO_2 was created by administering 100% nitrogen through an endotracheal tube to the pregnant ewe. The authors speculated that catecholamine release from the fetus due to acute hypoxia was responsible for this shortening of the PEP. Shortening of the PEP associated with a decrease in arterial PO_2 in chronically catheterized fetal lambs was also reported by Evers and co-wokers.[26] Morgenstern et al,[27] using fetal lambs in acute experimentation, not only demonstrated shortening of the PEP during fetal hypoxemia but also showed that the degree of shortening of the PEP was proportional to the severity of hypoxemia.

Contradictory results were reported by

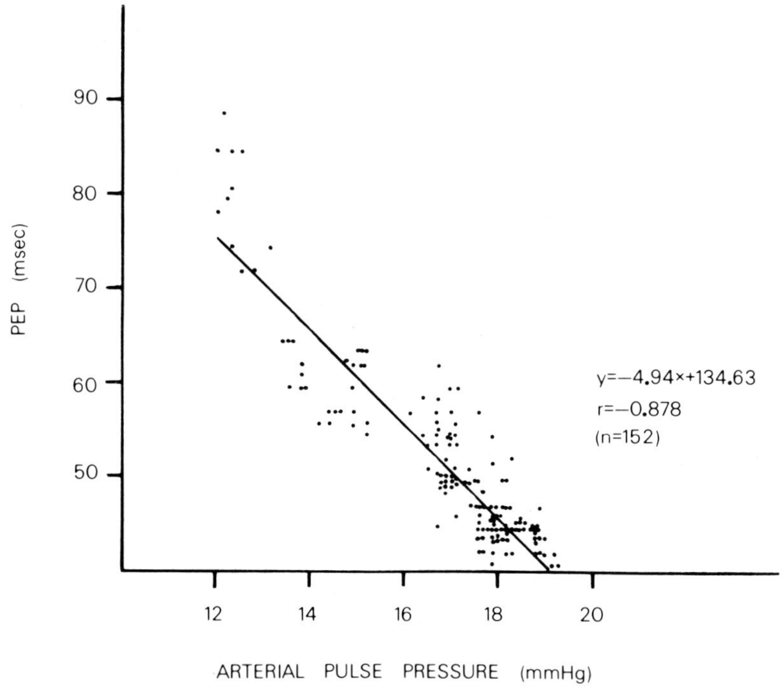

Fig. F.X.6. An inverse correlation between the preejection period (PEP) and arterial pulse pressure in one distressed monkey fetus. (From Murata et al.[16])

Goodlin and his associates,[7] who observed the prolongation of the R-S_1 interval in one severely depressed human fetus in labor. Murata and co-workers[16] demonstrated no direct relationship between the PEP and fetal arterial PO_2 in chronic preparations of the rhesus monkey. They found, however, that in addition to the prolongation of the PEP, which was proportional to the degree of acidemia, further prolongation was observed in rhesus monkey fetuses with combined acidemia and hypoxemia.

More recently, Organ and his associates,[14] observing an antepartum human fetus with prolonged PEP, which subsequently resulted in neonatal death, proposed that the PEP shortens during the acute phase of hypoxia due to the adrenal medullary secretion of catecholamine. When hypoxia becomes more severe, hypoxic depression of the myocardium overrides the catecholamine effect, and thus the PEP becomes prolonged.

Observations of the VET made by Murata et al,[18] using the chronically catheterized rhesus monkey fetus, demonstrated no significant changes due to hypoxemia in the fetus without the presence of acidemia. However, the VET, corrected for R-R interval, exhibited shortening in the fetuses with combined acidemia and hypoxemia. Similar shortening of the VET was also observed in chronically distressed fetuses.[18] Figure F.X.7 shows shortening of the VET of the monkey fetus with combined acidemia, hypoxia, and chronic stress.

B. Acidemia

A significant inverse correlation between the PEP and fetal pH was reported by Murata et al.[16] The prolongation of the PEP was essentially the same whether the decrease in arterial pH was of metabolic or respiratory origin (Fig. F.X.8). Figure F. X. 8 also indicates that the prolongation of the PEP was due to prolongation of both ICT and EMLT. This suggests that not only depression of myocardial contractility but also delay between electrical activation and the onset of mechanical con-

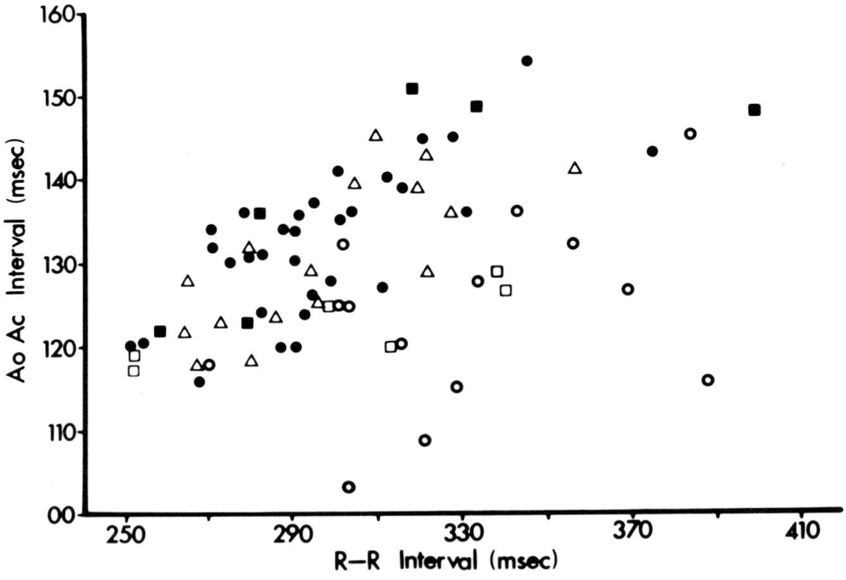

Fig. F.X.7. Relationship between the ventricular ejection time (Ao-Ac) and R-R intervals in rhesus monkey fetuses from the groups of control (●), hypoxemia only (△), acidemia only (■), combined hypoxemia and acidemia (□), and chronic distress (○). (From Murata et al.[18])

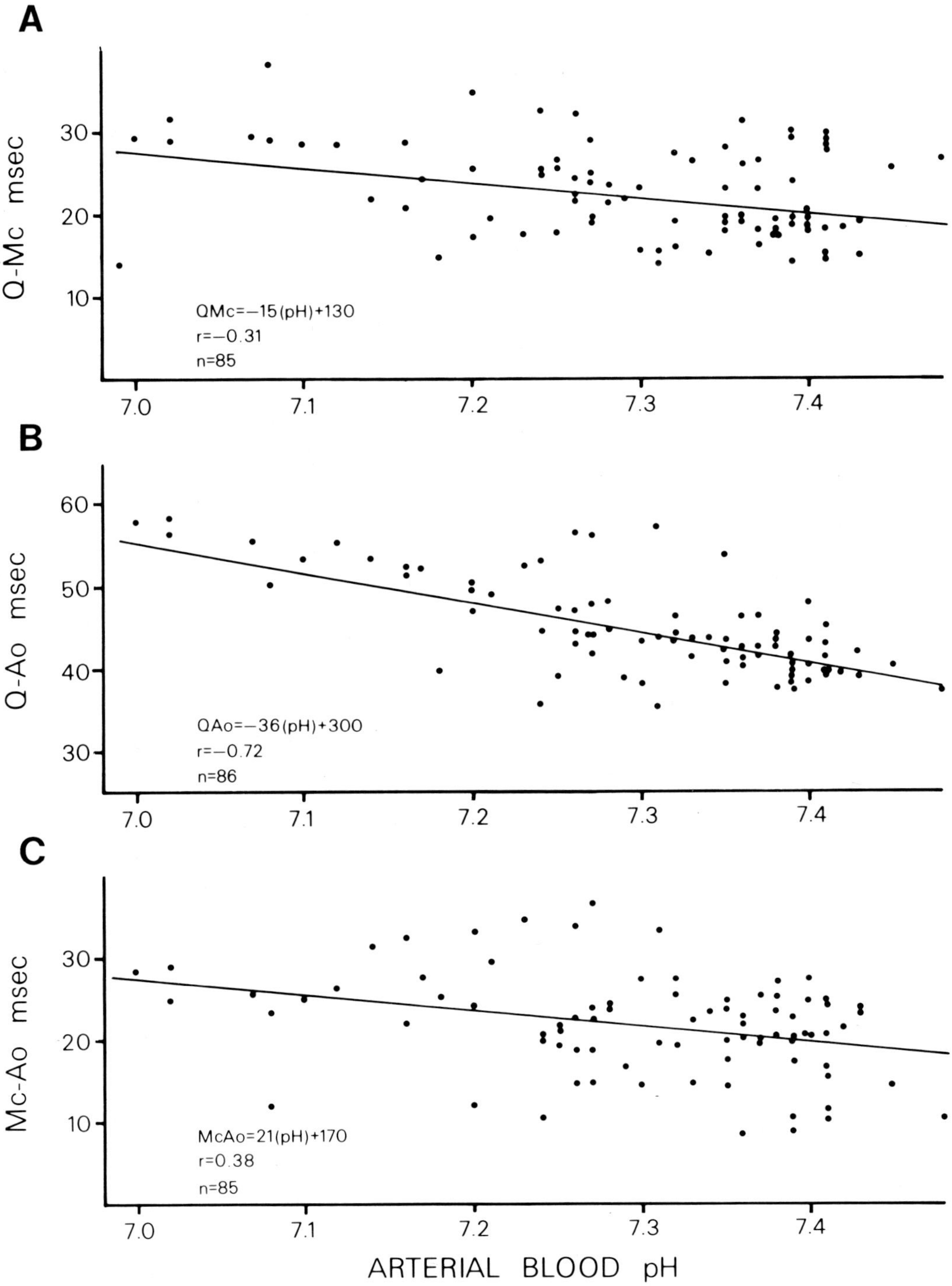

Fig. F.X.8. Systolic time intervals and arterial blood pH obtained from the chronically catheterized rhesus monkey fetus. From the top, **A**: electromechanical latent time (Q-Mc); **B**: preejection period (Q-Ao); **C**: isovolumic contraction time (Mc-Ao). (From Murata et al.[16])

traction are responsible for prolongation of the PEP. Similar relationships between the PEP and fetal arterial pH have been obtained from different species of laboratory animals[20] and by other investigators.[28] Bärtling et al[21] observed the PEP with simultaneous sampling of fetal scalp blood for pH determination during the intrapartum period. The studies showed that only a pH over 7.3 (normal) was associated with PEP values between 65 and 80 msec. Decrease in pH in linear fashion was accompanied by PEP values under 65 or over 80 msec. The same study also demonstrated a nonsignificant relationship between the PEP and base excess in fetal scalp blood.

The VET was shown to be not directly affected by arterial pH in the rhesus monkey fetus. Acidemia per se did not alter the VET, but combined acidemia and hypoxemia shortened the VET when corrected for fetal heart rate.[18]

VI. CLINICAL APPLICATION OF THE SYSTOLIC TIME INTERVALS

To date many investigators have made significant contributions to the understanding of the pathophysiology of the STIs. Present knowledge, however, is by no means sufficient to utilize these parameters in patient management. It is premature to make critical judgment of the fetal status based solely upon the STIs. It is, therefore, wise to wait for large, well-controlled prospective studies to evaluate clinical usefulness of the STIs.

In the following section, clinical application of the STIs is discussed in relation to reported studies, the majority of which have been performed retrospectively and have tested the PEP as a predictor of fetal status.

A. Systolic Time Intervals of Antepartum Fetuses

1. Observations on normal fetuses

The first description of the STI on the term fetus prior to labor was made in 1971 by Murata et al.[5] They reported a mean PEP (Q-Ao) of 71 msec, with a range from 60 to 80 msec. A mean VET (Ao-Ac) during normal baseline fetal heart rate of 177 msec, ranging from 170 to 190 msec, was reported in the same study. This study also included mean values and ranges of the EMLT (QMc), ICT (McAo), and isovolumic relaxation time (II Mo). Wolfson and coworkers,[19] using a computor processing technique, reported an average PEP value of approximately 60 msec from normal antepartum fetuses between 38 and 40 weeks of gestation.

In Murata and associates' report[6] the normal range of the PEP defined by the 5th and 95th percentile was determined from 33 to 42 weeks of normal gestation. This is shown in Figure F.X.9. The authors described normal PEP values from antepartum fetuses of 63.9 ± 3.7 msec. In the same report, a comparison was made between antepartum and intrapartum PEP values. The antepartum PEP values were approximately 9.5% shorter than the determination of PEP during the intrapartum period. There was also evidence that the PEP determined immediately after contraction stress testing (CST) exhibited lengthening of approximately 9.1% from the pretest (without significant uterine activity) values. The authors therefore speculated that slight hypoxemia and/or acidemia caused by uterine contractions were responsible for the prolongation.

Organ and his associates,[14] considering the physiologic lengthening of the PEP due to advancing gestational age and due to slowing of the heart rate, proposed the use of the $PEP_{140,40}$, which corrected the PEP values to a standard heart rate of 140 bpm and a gestational age of 40 weeks. They reported a $PEP_{140,40}$ value from 95 normal antepartum fetuses as 72.9 ± 2.8 msec.

2. Systolic time intervals as a predictor of fetal well-being

Weekly determination of the PEP was performed until delivery by Murata et al.[6] The last PEP values, obtained within a week before birth, were compared with the

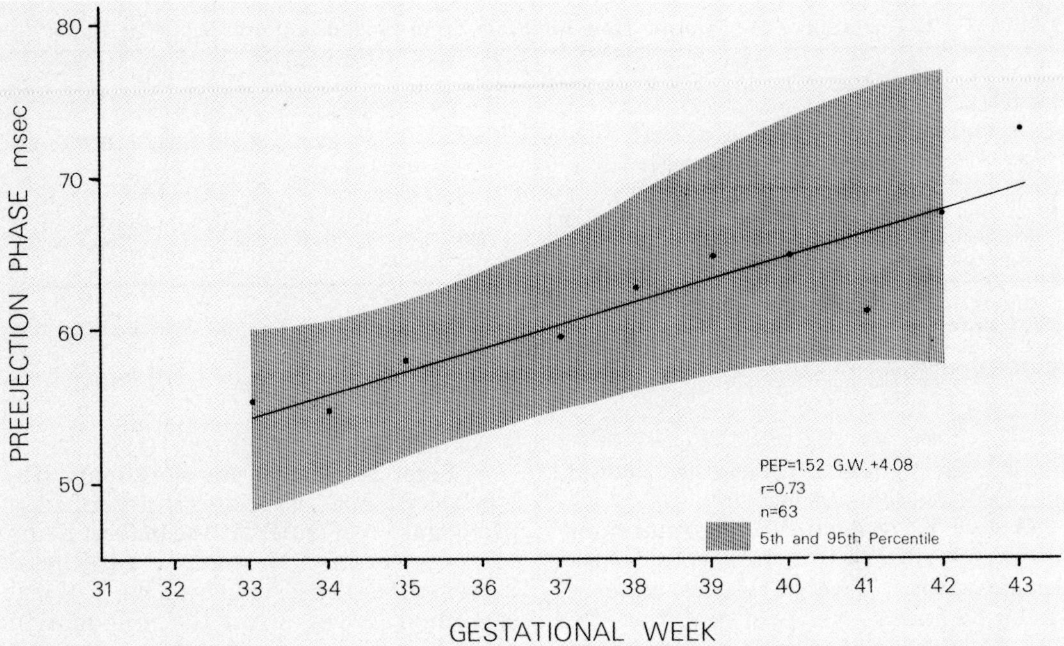

Fig. F.X.9. Normal range of the preejection period defined by 5th and 95th percentile from antepartum human fetuses between 33 and 42 weeks of gestation (From Murata et al.[6])

outcome of the infant. Definition of normal and abnormal fetuses in this report included the results of contraction stress test (CST), intrapartum fetal heart rate patterns, fetal scalp sampling results, Apgar scores at birth, and neonatal outcome. Twelve fetuses who had prolonged PEP greater than the 95th percentile at corresponding gestational ages exhibited a significantly higher incidence of perinatal abnormalities.

Organ et al[14] reported the PEP values of 13 fetuses who subsequently developed abnormal perinatal courses. The $PEP_{140,40}$ became shortened in eight cases and was prolonged in one fetus who died in the neonatal period. In four cases the $PEP_{140,40}$ remained within normal range. The authors, however, employed a nonreactive nonstress test (NST) as an additional criterion for abnormal, and at least four fetuses were included in the abnormal group because of a nonreactive NST.

One of the most difficult aspects of this type of study remains defining normal and abnormal fetuses. Clinical treatments given to either mother or fetus obscure pathological pictures and alter the outcome of the infant to some degree. The data provided thus far, however, suggest a high incidence of abnormal perinatal course outcome for the fetus with either a prolonged or shortened PEP.

There have been no studies reported to date that indicate the clinical usefulness of the VET in predicting fetal well-being.

B. Systolic Time Intervals of Intrapartum Fetuses

1. Observations on normal fetuses

Organ and his associates[29] employed the simultaneous fetal ECG and Doppler cardiogram to determine the PEP on the normal intrapartum fetuses at term and reported a PEP value of 73 ± 10 msec. Murata and Martin,[10] using the same technique, determined a PEP value of 70.0 ± 6.1 msec in similar patients. Later Bärtling et al,[21] also using the same tech-

TABLE F.X.2. Duration of the Systolic Time Intervals From 15 Normal Fetuses During Labor*

	EMLT	ICT	PEP	IRT
All fetuses (gestational age from 36 to 40 weeks)	41.2 ± 3.1	27.6 ± 6.8	67.3 ± 6.1	54.7 ± 6.8
12 fetuses between 38 and 40 weeks	41.3 ± 3.3	29.4 ± 5.6	70.0 ± 2.4	56.7 ± 3.7

*Numbers are means ± SD in milliseconds.
EMLT: electromechanical latent time; ICT: isovolumic contraction time; PEP: preejection time; IRT: isovolumic relaxation time (this interval is one of the diastolic time intervals).
Modified from Murata and Martin.[10]

nique, reported 72 ± 7.9 msec as the normal PEP value at term.

Table F.X.2 indicates the normal range of the STIs observed in 15 normal fetuses during labor.[10] Twelve fetuses were between 38 and 40 weeks of gestation, two fetuses were at 36 weeks, and one fetus was at 37 weeks of gestation.

The VET of the cardiac cycle from these 15 normal fetuses during labor was observed by Murata and Martin.[10] They found that the VET increased as the R-R interval increased from 330 msec (180 bpm) to 530 msec (115 bpm). No further prolongation of the VET was observed with R-R intervals greater than 530 msec. The authors suggested that maximal ventricular filling and stroke volume may be achieved in human fetuses near term at approximately 115 bpm and that the slowing of the heart rate below this point could be reflected by a decrease in cardiac output.

2. Detection of fetal distress by systolic time intervals: Observation of STIs with fetal heart rate patterns

Simultaneous display of fetal heart rate and STIs together with intrauterine pressure has become available with the aid of sophisticated electronic equipment and computer techniques. Comparative studies of fetal heart rate patterns and STIs have helped to elucidate pathophysiologic changes of the STIs that may appear concurrently with fetal heart rate changes of known etiology.

a. Fetal heart rate accelerations. Hawrylyshyn and associates[23] described a prolongation of the PEP due to fetal heart rate acceleration associated with fetal movement. By observing both the A-V and semilunar valves during the prolongation of the PEP, they found that this was caused by a prolongation in isovolumic contraction time (ICT) due to delay in semilunar valve opening.

b. Early decelerations. In an earlier study Organ and associates[13] developed a continuous photographic display of PEP and fetal heart rate patterns. They reported one fetus with early decelerations where an increase in the PEP was associated with uterine contractions. In contrast, Hon et al,[30] using a similar method developed separately, observed no significant changes in the PEP during early deceleration of the fetal heart. This lack of change in the PEP may have been a result of limited resolution in their technique, but it can also be well exlained by the fact that the PEP is not affected by the changes in heart rate due to vagal stimulation, as demonstrated by Harris et al.[17]

The VET was observed during early deceleration and was found to be slightly prolonged with prolongation of R-R intervals.[30]

c. Variable decelerations. Variable decelerations of the fetal heart rate have been observed with umbilical cord occlusions. Decrease in preload due to umbilical vein occlusion and increase in afterload due to umbilical artery occlusion both resulted in prolongation of the PEP.[25,26,28,30,31] Hawrylyshyn et al[23] observed delay in both the A-V closure and semilunar valve opening occlusion of the umbilical cord, thus explained the prolongation of the PEP.

d. Late decelerations. Prolongation of the PEP during the baseline fetal heart rate was observed in eight intrapartum fetuses who exhibited mild to moderate late decelerations, and none of these fetuses was clinically depressed at birth.[10] Organ et al[13] however, in their early study, noted shortening of the PEP associated with late deceleration. A proposed mechanism of the shortened PEP during late deceleration is an increase in myocardial contractility resulting from an adrenergic surge secondary to hypoxemia.

Organ later reported two different types of response in the PEP, depending upon whether the fetal hypoxia is acute or chronic in nature.[14] In acute hypoxemia, the authors described the same response in the PEP—shortening. The data exhibited by Hawrylyshyn[23] seem to substantiate this theory, but he demonstrated a marked shortening of the PEP obtained at the ascending rim of the late deceleration where a recovery of the fetal heart rate was almost complete (Fig. F.X.10).

Prolongation of the PEP in chronic hypoxia is seen as a reflection of impaired myocardium. Under this circumstance catecholamines are no longer effective in increasing myocardial contractility. Organ et al[14] hypothesized the causal mechanisms to explain fetal status. They based their judgment on a combination of the PEP and nonstress testing of the fetal heart rate. According to their hypothesis, shortened PEP with reactive NST indicated fetal stress where the fetal adrenal medulla is being stimulated by acute hypoxia. If the NST is nonreactive and the PEP is shortened, the fetus is thought to be in

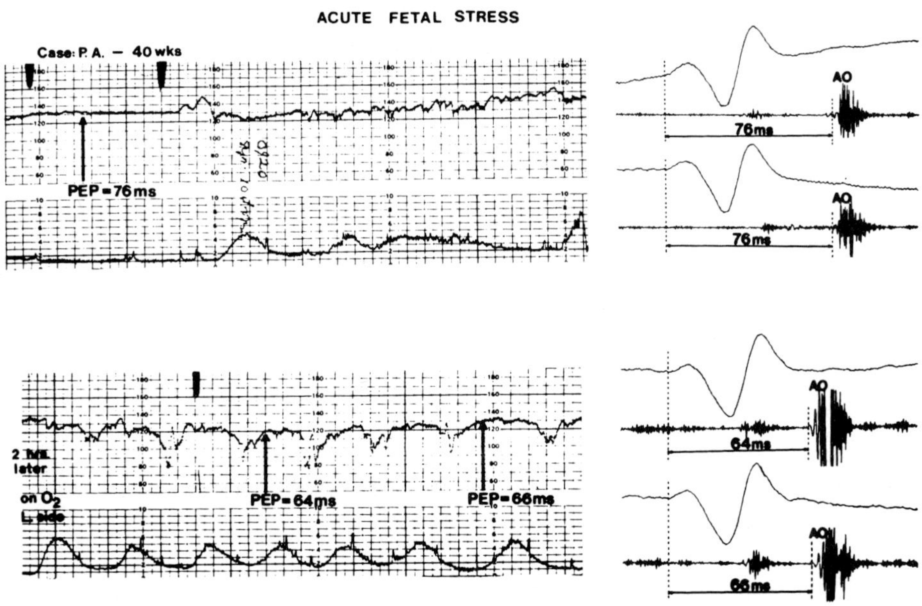

Fig. F.X.10. Shortening of the preejection period (PEP) with acute hypoxia resulting from uterine hyperstimulation by oxytocin. The PEP sampled at normal fetal heart rate was 76 msec (arrow on the top tracing). The PEP revealed shortening to 64 and 66 msec at the ascending rim of late decelerations (arrows on the bottom tracing). The ECG and Doppler cardiogram on the right demonstrate shortening in semilunar valve opening (Ao). (All PEP intervals are plotted at FHR of 130 bpm.) This fetus was subsequently delivered with normal blood gases. (From Hawrylyshyn et al.[23])

A

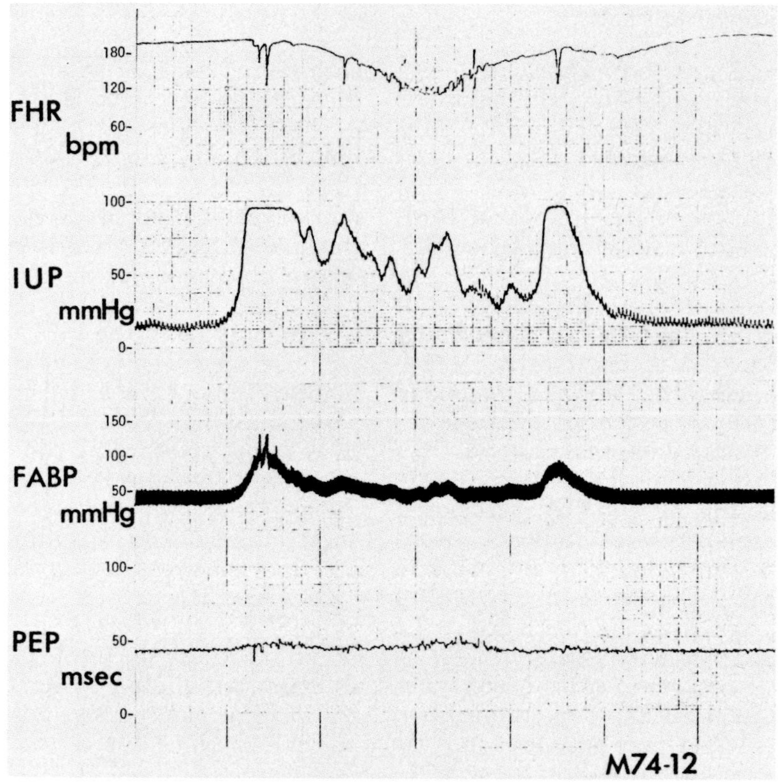
FHR
bpm
180-
120-
60-
IUP
mmHg
100-
50-
0-
FABP
mmHg
150-
100-
50-
PEP
msec
100-
50-
0-
M74-12

B

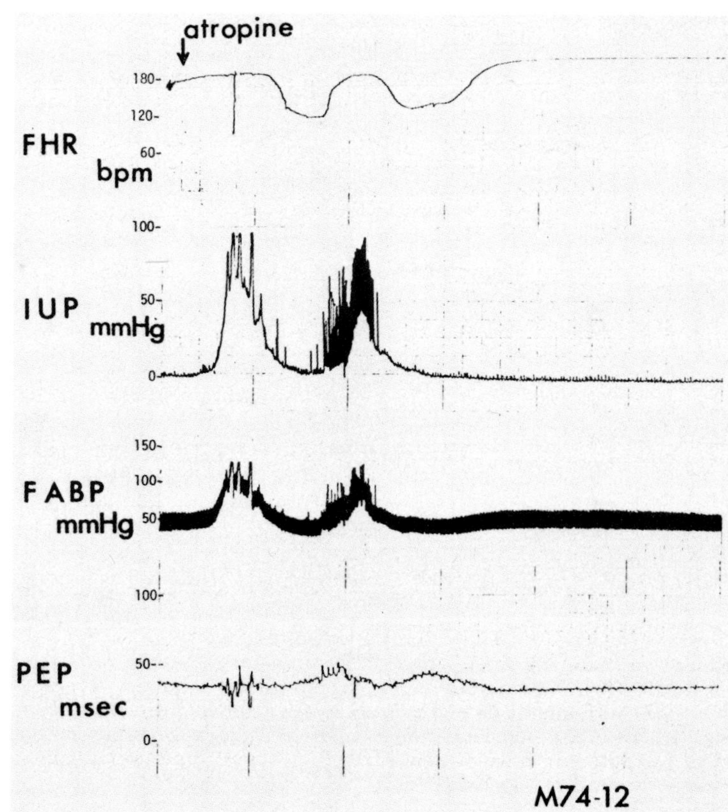
atropine
FHR
bpm
180-
120-
60-
IUP
mmHg
100-
50-
0-
FABP
mmHg
150-
100-
50
PEP
msec
100-
50-
0-
M74-12

distress, indicating central nervous system depression. The most ominous combination of prolonged PEP and nonreactive NST implies hypoxic depression of the fetal myocardium and potential fetal demise. A normal PEP with nonreactive NST can be regarded as normal fetal response to central nervous system depressants (eg, diazepam). Figure F.X.11-A demonstrates the prolongation of the PEP associated with a late deceleration that was not blocked by atropine injection in contrast to Figure F.X.11-B, where the prolongation of the PEP persists following atropine.

VII. REFERENCES

1. Wiggers CJ. Studies on the consecutive phases of the cardiac cycle, II The laws governing the relative duration of ventricular systolic and diastolic. Am J Physiol. 1921; 56:39–52.
2. Katz LN, Feil HS. Clinical division of the dynamics of ventricular systole. Arch Intern Med. 1923; 32:672–682.
3. Weissler AM, Peeler RG, Rochll W II, Durham NC. Relationship between left ventricular ejection time, stroke volume and heart rate in normal individuals and patients with cardiovascular disease. Am Heart J. 1961; 62:367–371.
4. Persianinov LS, Illyin IV, Karpman VL, Saveliera GM. The dynamics of fetal cardiac activity. Am J Obstet Gynecol. 1966; 94:367–377.
5. Murata Y, Takemura H, Kurachi K. Observation of fetal cardiac motion by M-mode ultrasonic cardiography. Am J Obstet Gynecol. 1971; 111:287–294.
6. Murata Y, Martin CB Jr, Ikenoue T, Lu PS. Antepartum evaluation of the pre-ejection period of the fetal cardiac cycle. Am J Obstet Gynecol. 1978; 132:278–284.
7. Goodlin RC, Girard J, Holman A. Systolic time intervals in the fetus and neonate. Obstet Gynecol. 1972; 39:295–301.
8. Dock W. Mode of production of first heart sound. AMA Arch Intern Med. 1933; 50:737–740.
9. Harris A, Sutton G. The second heart sound in normal subjects. Br Heart J. 1968; 30:739–742.
10. Murata Y, Martin CB Jr. Systolic time intervals of the fetal cardiac cycle. Obstet Gynecol. 1974; 44:224–232.
11. Murata Y, Takemura H, Mochizuki S, Kurachi K. The phase and frequency analysis of fetal placental Doppler signals by ultrasound. Med Ultrason. 1970; 8:1–16.
12. Assali NS, Brinkman CR III, Nuwayhid B. Comparison of maternal and fetal cardiovascular function in acute and chronic experiment in sheep. Am J Obstet Gynecol. 1974; 120:411–423.
13. Organ LW, Bernstein A, Smith KC. The pre-ejection period of the fetal heart: Pattern of changes during labor. Am J Obstet Gynecol. 1974; 120:49–55.
14. Organ LW, Bernstein A, Hawrylyshyn PA. The pre-ejection period as an antepartum indicator of fetal well-being. Am J Obstet Gynecol. 1980; 137:810–819.
15. Robinson HP, Adam AH, Flemming JEE, Huston A. Fetal electromechanical intervals in labor. Br J Obstet Gynecol. 1978; 172–176.
16. Murata Y, Martin CB Jr, Ikenoue T, Petrie R. Cardiac systolic time intervals in fetal monkeys: Pre-ejection period. Am J Obstet Gynecol. 1978; 132:285–293.
17. Harris WC, Schoenfeld CD, Wissler AM. The effect of adrenergic receptor activation and blockade on the systolic pre-ejection period, heart rate and arterial pressure in man. J Clin Invest. 1967; 46:1704–1712.
18. Murata Y, Martin CB Jr, Ikenoue T, Petrie R. Cardiac systolic time intervals in fetal monkeys: Ventricular ejection time. Am J Obstet Gynecol. 1980; 136:603–608.
19. Wolfson RN, Zador, IE, Pillay SK, Timor-Tritsch JE, Herz RH: Antenatal investigation of human fetal systolic time intervals. Am J Obstet Gynecol. 1977; 129:103–207.
20. Murata Y, Miyake K, Quilligan EJ. Pre-ejection period of cardiac cycle in fetal lamb. Am J Obstet Gynecol. 1979; 133:509–514.
21. Bärtling TH, Klöck FK. Die pre-ejektion periode des menschelichen fetalen herzens. Bedeutung des base-line-schwankung in der perinatal periode. Z Geturtsch Perinat. 1979; 183:202–211.
22. Murata Y, Pijls N, Miyake K, Schmidt P, Martin CB Jr, Singer J. Antepartum determination of the pre-ejection period of fetal cardiac cycle: Its relation to newborn body weight. Am J Obstet Gynecol. 1979; 133:515–518.
23. Hawrylyshyn PA, Organ LW, Bernstein A. A new computer technique for continuous measurement of the pre-ejection period in the human fetus: Physiologic significance of pre-ejection period patterns. Am J Obstet Gynecol. 1980; 137:801–109.

Fig. F.X.11. Polygraphic recordings from a chronically instrumented rhesus monkey fetus, during labor, exhibiting late decelerations. From the top, fetal heart rate (FHR), intrauterine pressure (IUP), fetal carotid blood pressure (FA BP) and preejection period (PEP). The PEP was obtained from the peak of the R wave to the onset of FABP upstroke. Note prolongations of the PEP associated with late decelerations (**A**), which were not alleviated by atropine administered to the fetus (**B**). Prolongation of the PEP became more significant with late decelerations of the fetal heart rate.

24. Wallence AG, Skinner NS, Mitchell JH. Hemodynamic determination of the maximal rate of rise of left ventricular pressure. Am J Physiol. 1963; 205:13–15.
25. Organ LW, Milligan JE, Goodwin JW, Bain MJ. The pre-ejection period of the fetal heart: Response to stress in the term fetal lamb. Am J Obstet Gynecol. 1973; 115:377–385.
26. Evers H. The cardiac pre-ejection period during pre-natal life. Nijmegan: Krips, Repro-Meppel, 1978.
27. Morgenstern J, Czerny H, Schmidt H, Schulz J, Wernicke K. Systolic time intervals of the fetal cardiac cycle. J Perinat Med. 1978; 6:173–196.
28. Schmidt H, Czerny H, Morgenstern J, Schulz J, Wernicke K. Verlaufe der pre-ejektion periode bei fetalen declerationen. Tierexperimentelle Untersuchungen an Schlafsfeten N. In: Schmidt JW, Dudenhansen, eds. Perinatale Medizin, Vol VII. Stuttgart; Thieme, 1978.
29. Organ LW, Bernstein A, Rowe, I. The pre-ejection period of the fetal heart. Detection during labor with Doppler ultrasound. Am J Obstet Gynecol. 1973; 115:369–373.
30. Hon EH, Murata Y, Zanini D, Martin CB Jr, Lewis D. Continuous microfilm display of the electromechanical intervals of the cardiac cycle. Obstet Gynecol. 1974; 43:722–728.
31. Bärtling TH, Klöck FK, Courtin E. Ein neues verfarhren zur on-line-registrerung der pre-ejection des menschlichen fetalen herzens parallel zum CTG. Z Guburtsch Perinat. 1978; 182–186.

F.XI

Echocardiography and Phonocardiography

Pradub Sukhum, MD

I. FETAL PHONOCARDIOGRAPHY

A. Introduction

Fetal heart sounds as detected through the maternal abdominal wall have quite low intensity. Sounds from fetal motion and, particularly, sounds from the maternal abdominal organs such as abdominal vessels and the gastrointestinal tract are usually louder and frequently interfere. Recording fetal heart sounds with conventional phonocardiographic equipment, even that equipped with a selective band pass filter suitable for fetal heart sound frequencies, is not an easy task. Due to overlapping frequencies, amplifying the fetal heart sounds creates the same effect on the undesirable sounds mentioned.

Phonocardiography from birth throughout adulthood is useful to demonstrate and define both normal and abnormal heart sounds. The phonocardiogram is often simultaneously recorded with some form of external impulse to acquire additional information. When used properly, the phonocardiogram aids the understanding of cardiovascular physiology and physical examination. It may also lead to the diagnosis and hemodynamic correlation of certain heart diseases.[1] Little work has been done in this regard with the fetus; fetal phonocardiography has been developed only for the detection and monitoring of fetal heart rate.

B. History

Fetal phonocardiography was introduced in 1908 by Hofbauer and Weis.[2] The early fetal phonocardiographic works were handicapped by a lack of understanding of the characteristics of sound signals and by underdeveloped equipment.[3–9] A partial solution of these problems led to the

Cardiac Problems in Pregnancy, pages 509–520

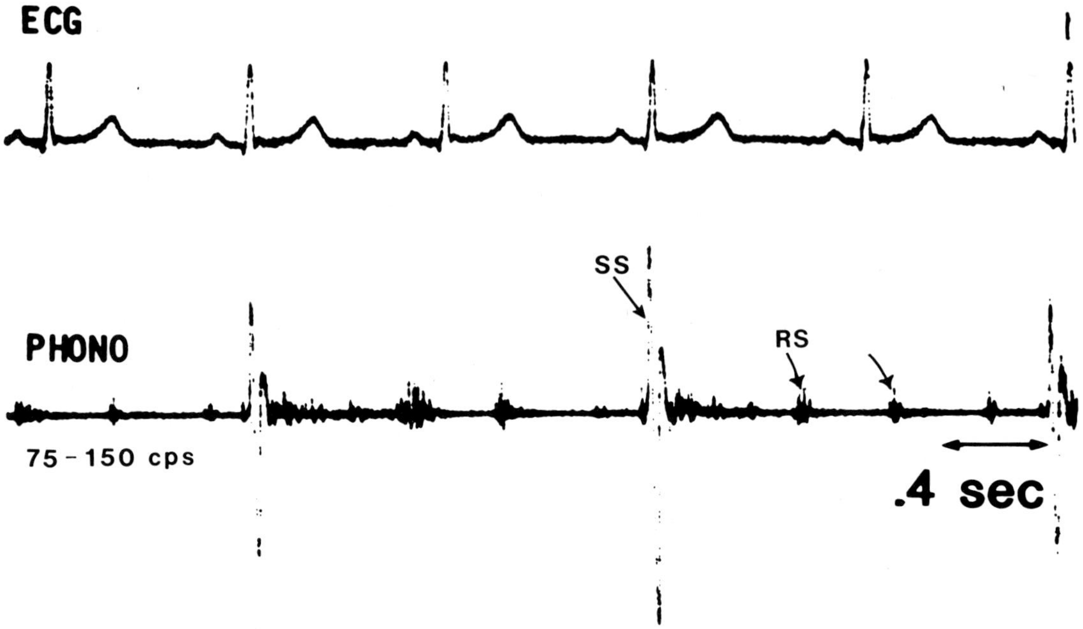

Fig. F.XI.1. Fetal Doppler phonocardiogram. ECG = maternal electrocardiogram; Phono = phonocardiographic recording of the Doppler sound signal at approximate frequency of 75–150 Hz; RS = repetitive sound signal; SS = slower rate sound signal (see text).

development by Hammacher of a monitor that derived fetal heart rate from fetal heart sounds.[10–11] Commercial equipment evolving from his principle (Hewlett-Packard 8020A Cardiograph, 1968) created some enthusiasm for this new, noninvasive technique, which offered both physical and electrical safety to the patient. At that time, the new technique appeared promising, and it was believed that further development might lead to its widespread use. However, the basic pitfalls could not be completely overcome, and the newer, more effective Doppler ultrasound technique (see Chapter F.VIII). enjoys greater popularity than phonocardiographic fetal heart rate monitoring.[12–14]

C. Current Application

A recent comparison among the three noninvasive methods for external fetal cardiography indicates that phonocardiography is inferior to abdominal electrocardiography and Doppler ultrasound cardiography.[14] A 1979 survey of fetal heart monitoring equipment revealed phonocardiographic capability in only three of seven models, whereas six of seven models were equipped with abdominal electrocardiography, and all with Doppler ultrasound capabilities.[15]

If the phonocardiographic application for fetal heart rate monitoring is declining, will there be any other use for this technique in the future? It may be possible that one could use a conventional phonocardiograph (or for that matter, other multipurpose recorders) to record a combination of signals such as the fetal electrocardiogram and Doppler ultrasound signal for measurement of fetal systolic time intervals (see Chapter F.VIII).[16–18]

We have attempted to use this combination technique to make the diagnosis of fetal heart block.[19] The diagnosis was substantiated by M-mode echocardiography and was confirmed after birth by electrocardiography. Figure F.XI.1 shows the phonocardiographic recording of the Doppler ultrasound signal through the loud speaker on which the phonocardiographic microphone was placed. The signals were derived from two groups of moving structures at different rates which were independent of each other. The repetitive signal (RS) is likely to be associated with atrial or atrioventricular valve(s) motion at the atrial rate. The slower rate signal (SS), is likely to be from ventricular or related structure(s) motion at the ventricular rate. Although the signal at the slower rate may appear to be related to every other maternal QRS complex on this record, a longer strip demonstrated no constant relationship. The M-mode echocardiogram (Fig. F.XI.2, upper panel) performed simultaneously, shows two groups of cardiac structures moving at different rates, compatible with the phono-Doppler ultrasound recording. The final diagnosis was confirmed by electrocardiogram and M-mode echocardiogram after birth (Fig. F.XI.2, lower panel).

II. FETAL ECHOCARDIOGRAPHY

A. Introduction

The past decade has brought a breakthrough for pulsatile ultrasound diagnostic technique. Ability to visualize, differentiate, and quantitatively measure

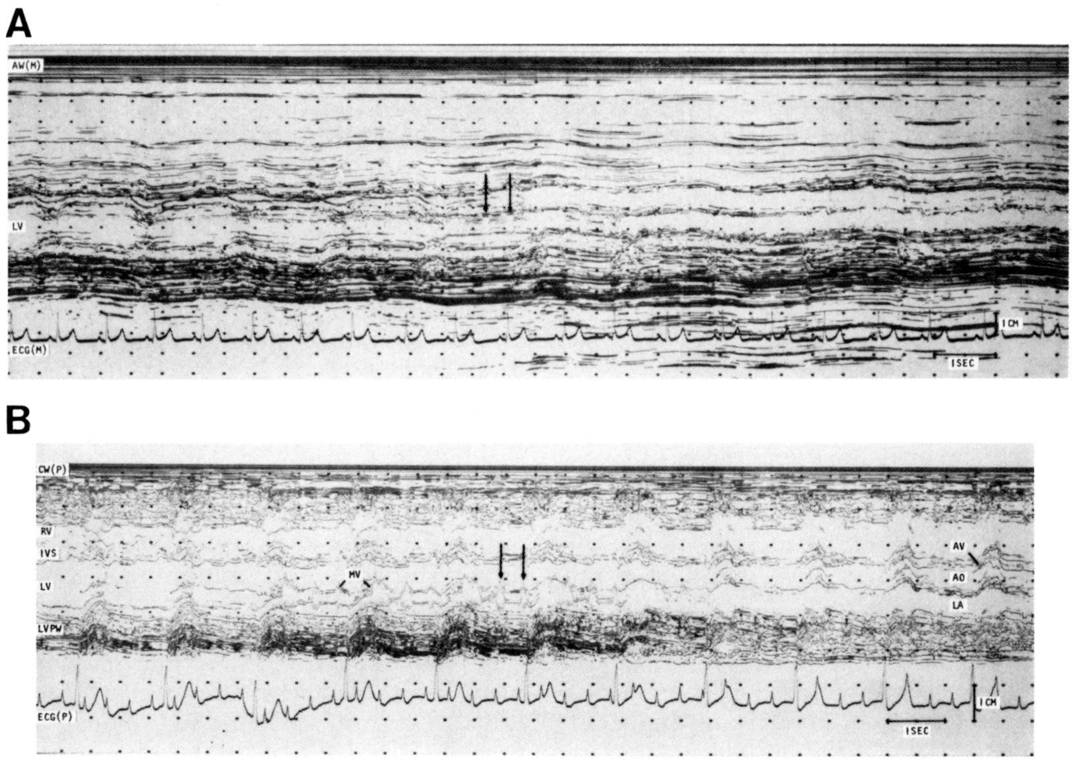

Fig. F.XI.2. **A**: Prenatal M-mode scan echocardiogram. AW(M) = maternal abdominal wall; V = fetal ventricle (probably left ventricle); ECG = maternal electrocardiogram. The two long arrows point at structures likely to represent an atrioventricular valve (possibly mitral valve) opening at the same rate as the repetitive sound signal (RS) of Figure XI.1. **B**: Postnatal M-mode scan echocardiogram. CW(P) = infant's chest wall; RV = right ventricle; MV = mitral valve; AV = aortic valve; AO = aortic root; LA = left atrium; LVPW = left ventricular posterior wall; ECG(P) = infant's ECG. The two long arrows point at mitral valve opening during atrial contraction at atrial (sinus) rate compatible with P wave on infant's ECG. Note the similarity of the prenatal and the postnatal M-mode echocardiographic scans.

certain human body internal organs harmlessly and conveniently encourages growth in this field. Rapid improvements in technology and technique have expanded the usefulness of this technique to several fields in medicine, including obstetrics, gynecology, and, particularly, cardiology. Adult and pediatric echocardiography has reached its mature state, while fetal echocardiography is just in the beginning stage. This is not too surprising because the fetal heart is so small, requiring better equipment with higher resolution, which was not available during the earlier period. The fetal lie in relationship to the maternal abdominal wall determining transducer placement differs from case to case. This makes the standard positional approach for identification, verification, and measurement of fetal heart structures more difficult, less consistent, and sometimes impossible. Other factors may relate to the separation of the echocardiographic and obstetric-gynecological ultrasound laboratories. Ultrasound specialists and ultrasound equipment commonly used in these laboratories are often not suitable for combination study.

B. History

Bang and Holm in 1968 were probably the first investigators who reported use of A-, B-, and M-mode echograms to examine fetal heart movement.[20] Fifty patients at various stages of pregnancy, from the tenth to the thirty-ninth week of gestation, were studied, and it was possible to demonstrate fetal heart movement accurately from the twelfth week on. The correct diagnoses of fetal death and false pregnancy were obtained. Bang and Holm commented that this method is superior to fetal electrocardiography, X-ray, and fetal heart sound auscultation in the diagnosis of fetal death. Robinson in 1972, using the same echocardiographic approach, was able to confirm and extend the sensitivity of the technique to as early as the forty-seventh amenorrhic day of pregnancy, which appeared to be superior to using abdominal Doppler ultrasound technique alone.[21]

Four years after the work of Bang and Holm, Winsberg (1972) published a remarkable, high-quality fetal echocardiographic study on fetuses over 30 weeks old.[22] He demonstrated many cardiac structures similarly obtained in adults and children. The method included application of the earlier real-time, two-dimensional equipment (Siemen Vidoson with rotating transducer and reflected parabolic mirror in water bath) to help locate the fetal lie and the heart position in its thorax. The M-mode echocardiogram was used, but only on the fetus that had its anterior thorax facing the maternal abdominal wall (or the transducer), simulating the echocardiographic position from which recordings are made in adults and children. The relatively high-quality fetal echocardiograms thus obtained allowed him to measure ventricular dimension, calculate stroke volume and cardiac output, and compare the results with previous data from other methods.

Using two-dimensional B-scans, Egeblad et al (1975), studying fetuses over 36 weeks of gestation, demonstrated that the fetal heart structures may be identified with fetal lie at various positions as long as the orientation could be identified by the B-scan ultrasound.[23] The transverse and long axis scans were done through the fetal thorax transversely and longitudinally, respectively, in relation to the fetal body. The vertebral column and lungs served as landmarks on the transverse view. The study included M-mode for motion characteristic display and measurement scale; however, the quality of the echocardiogram appeared not to have improved since the Winsberg study. Finally, an example of an M-mode scan taken from a position virtually opposite the standard postnatal echocardiographic study was shown.

A higher quality, long axis M-mode scan was published in 1979 by Madison et al, using B-scan and standard M-mode echocardiographic equipment with a high-resolution strip chart recorder. This application, together with phonocardiographic and Doppler ultrasound, permitted the diagnosis of fetal complete heart block[19] (Fig. F.XI.2).

Recent (1980) publications by Lange et al and Sahn et al probably represent the state of the art of fetal echocardiography at the time of this writing.[24,25] They used the standard B-scan examination for fetal lie and fetal heart position, and then performed a higher resolution, real-time, two-dimensional echocardiogram. Applying the commonly used echocardiographic views for adult and pediatric examination to the fetal heart, Lange et al were able to record detailed fetal cardiac anatomy at very high percentages in the second half of pregnancy. Sahn et al, from the same institution, carried the work further quantitatively. They were able to measure right and left ventricular dimensions, aorta, and pulmonary artery sizes. These measurements were correlated with the calculated fetal weight, and the fetal cardiac growth curve was derived. The idea of using fetal cardiac size and volume to help estimate fetal age is not new. Garrette et al (1970) and Suzuki et al (1973) have used the B-scan ultrasonic study to obtain this information.[26,27] The real-time, two-dimensional echocardiographic study should be superior by better identification of various moving cardiac structures, views and orientation, and changes during the cardiac cycle. Sahn et al also did serial fetal echocardiographic studies and immediate postnatal examinations for comparison and understanding of transitional circulatory change and fetal cardiac growth follow-up. There were no fetal M-mode echocardiographic studies in the Lange and Sahn reports. This may be due in part to the preferable two-dimensional echocardiographic equipment used; the linear array over the phased array, for certain reasons, was not capable of simultaneous M-mode recordings, while spatial orientation is displayed by two-dimensional echocardiography. The authors commented that gross congenital fetal cardiac or great vessel anomalies should be detectable by this method.

C. Current Instrumentation, Equipment, and Techniques

Although the A-mode presentation is available in many diagnostic pulsatile ultrasonic systems, its primary use in fetal echocardiography is limited. At present, the instruments required for fetal echocardiographic study should include B-scan, M-mode, and real-time two-dimensional capabilities.

1. B-scan ultrasonic equipment

B-scan equipment is usually designed for general ultrasonic diagnosis in various specialties, including obstetrics and gynecology. With this equipment, the experienced technician can quickly determine fetal lie and fetal parts. The scan through the fetal thorax can locate and record the fetal heart on different axes in relationship to the fetal lie or the fetal thorax. The more commonly performed axes are the transverse and long axis views (Fig. F.XI.3A and B). Using the orientation of the fetal thorax and other fetal structures such as the spine, lungs, and liver as landmarks, identification, and perhaps measurement, of certain fetal heart structures may be achieved.[20] B-scan equipment that has the capability of selective focal area enlargement may be beneficial, not only in providing a larger view of the fetal heart but also in recording the fetal heart motion better (Fig. F.XI.4A and B).

Despite the fact that the current B-scan gray scale ultrasonic equipment has quite good resolution, it has the major disadvantage of offering no real-time motion display or recording. Since the heart and its parts are moving structures, looking at the heart in still pictures causes a significant loss of information and characteristics. It has been shown clearly that complete adult and pediatric echocardi-

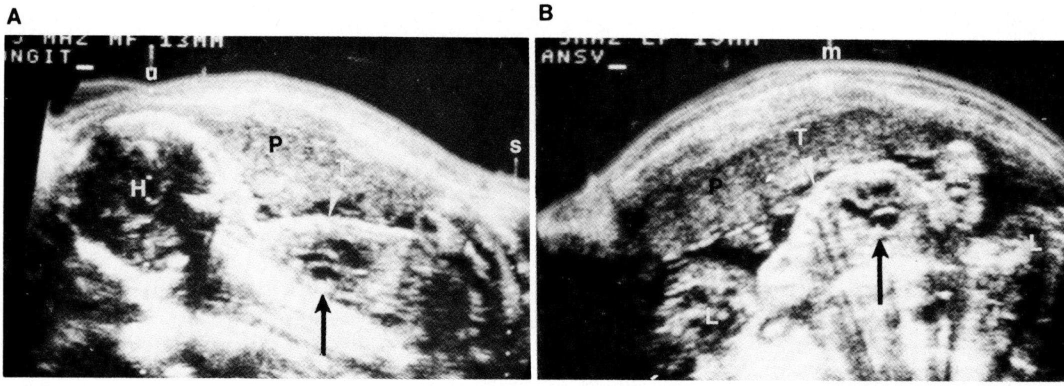

Fig. F.XI.3. Two-dimensional ultrasonic B-scans through a fetus demonstrating the fetal heart within its thorax (black arrow). **A.** Longitudinal axis through fetal head and fetal body—thorax. **B.** Transverse axis through fetal thorax and limbs. The fetus is in breech position. Its anterior thorax is facing anteriorly, the ideal position for real-time, two-dimensional and M-mode fetal echocardiographic study. H = fetal head; L = fetal limb; m = maternal abdominal midline on transverse plane; P = placenta; s = maternal symphysis pubis landmark; T (with white arrowhead) = fetal anterior thorax; u = maternal umbilical landmark.

ographic examinations can only be done with motion study in the form of time motion (M-mode) or real-time two-dimensional echocardiography.[28]

2. M-mode echocardiographic equipment

The M-mode fetal echocardiographic examination, in comparison to adult and pediatric studies, is considerably more difficult. With M-mode alone, it can be difficult to locate the fetal heart because the single beam visualizes one small area at a time. B-scan, or real-time two-dimensional examinations preceding the M-mode study are usually required to help determine fetal lie, fetal thorax, and fetal heart position. The M-mode recording of the fetal heart and fetal heart structures may be adequate if the information needed is fetal heart motion, fetal heart rate, or confirmation of fetal life. To acquire a detailed fetal heart anatomic and physiologic evaluation, the transducer must be placed in a position simulating that employed in the adult and pediatric approach. In order to accomplish this goal, the anterior fetal thorax has to face the anterior abdominal maternal wall.[22] Rolling the mother from side to side may be necessary when the fetal anterior thorax is facing sidewards or obliquely. Periodic reexamination for fetal thorax position by B-scan may be necessary, particularly if the fetus moves.

The high-quality M-mode scan of the left heart long axis, as done in the adult or pediatric patient, is difficult to obtain, and it may not be possible routinely. Such a scan requires precise and proper heart position in relationship to the transducer, and the M-mode echocardiogram by itself cannot determine the accurate position. Occasionally, multiple scans from the best position, detected by a preceding B scan, or real-time, two-dimensional ultrasound examination, may result in good M-mode scans.[19]

3. Real-time, two-dimensional ultrasonic equipment

Of the various types of real-time, two-dimensional equipment, the one most commonly used in obstetric-gynecological work is the multiple-element linear array system. The large transducer in this system does not create problems in abdominal or fetal examination. In fact, it appears to be easy to manipulate (and control) on the smooth abdominal wall, and it may give better orientation of the sound path axis or angulation.[24,25]

The adult chest wall has a small acoustic window for the ultrasound path in between the ribs. The equipment for the adult echocardiogram therefore requires a smaller transducer, which gives the arc-like two-dimensional picture with less display of near structures, compared to the rectangular picture of the linear-array system. The currently popular arc scanners are a mechanical rotating transducer and electronic phased array. There are certain advantages and disadvantages to all of these real-time systems.

It is important to have high-resolution equipment for the smaller and more difficult fetal echocardiographic study. Our impression is that both the multiple-element linear-array scanner and its larger transducer and the arc scanner with its smaller transducer will work adequately if the proper technique is mastered. A complete study should combine the real-time, two-dimensional and the M-mode techniques, with the latter giving better axial dimension, motion, and resolution. It is probably important that the equipment have the capability of simultaneous M-mode recording with the real-time, two-dimensional picture display. This capability is essential in fetal echocardiographic examination because of increased difficulty associated with fetal position and motion. All the motion studies may need simultaneous abdominal fetal ECG recording.

Figures F.XI.5, F.XI.6, and F.XI.7 are the stop frames of the real-time two-dimensional echocardiogram on the same fetus in long axis, short axis, and apical four-chamber views, respectively. These are the same important views as in adult and pediatric real-time, two-dimensional echocardiography.[29] The image is far better when viewed in real-time motion, and the resolution can be further improved with the development of better equipment. The examination shown in Figures F.XI.5 and F.XI.6 was performed with

A B

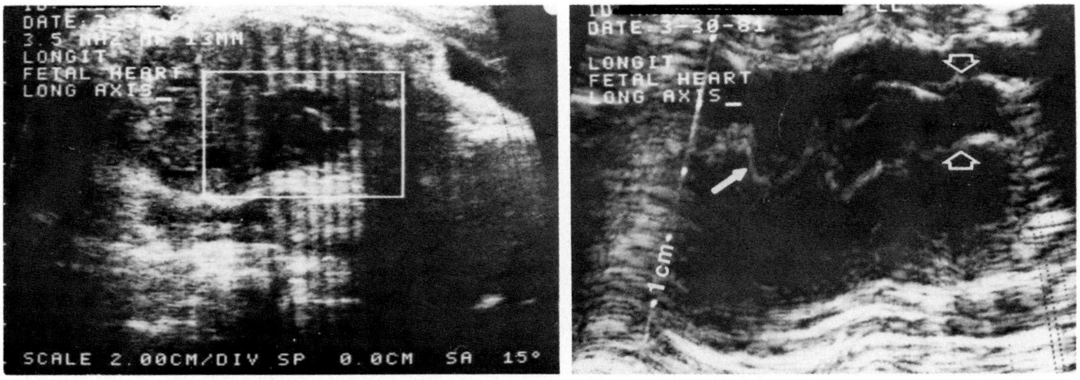

Fig. F.XI.4. **A**. Longitudinal axis B-scan through a fetal thorax. The fetal heart is within the white rectangular frame. **B**. The area in Figure XI.4A rectangular frame was enlarged on the next scan performed a few seconds later. The large open arrows are pointing at structures that may represent aortic root. The small solid arrows are pointing at more mobile structures, possibly the mitral valve. The fetal heart picture now looks like an M-mode echocardiographic scan of the left heart.

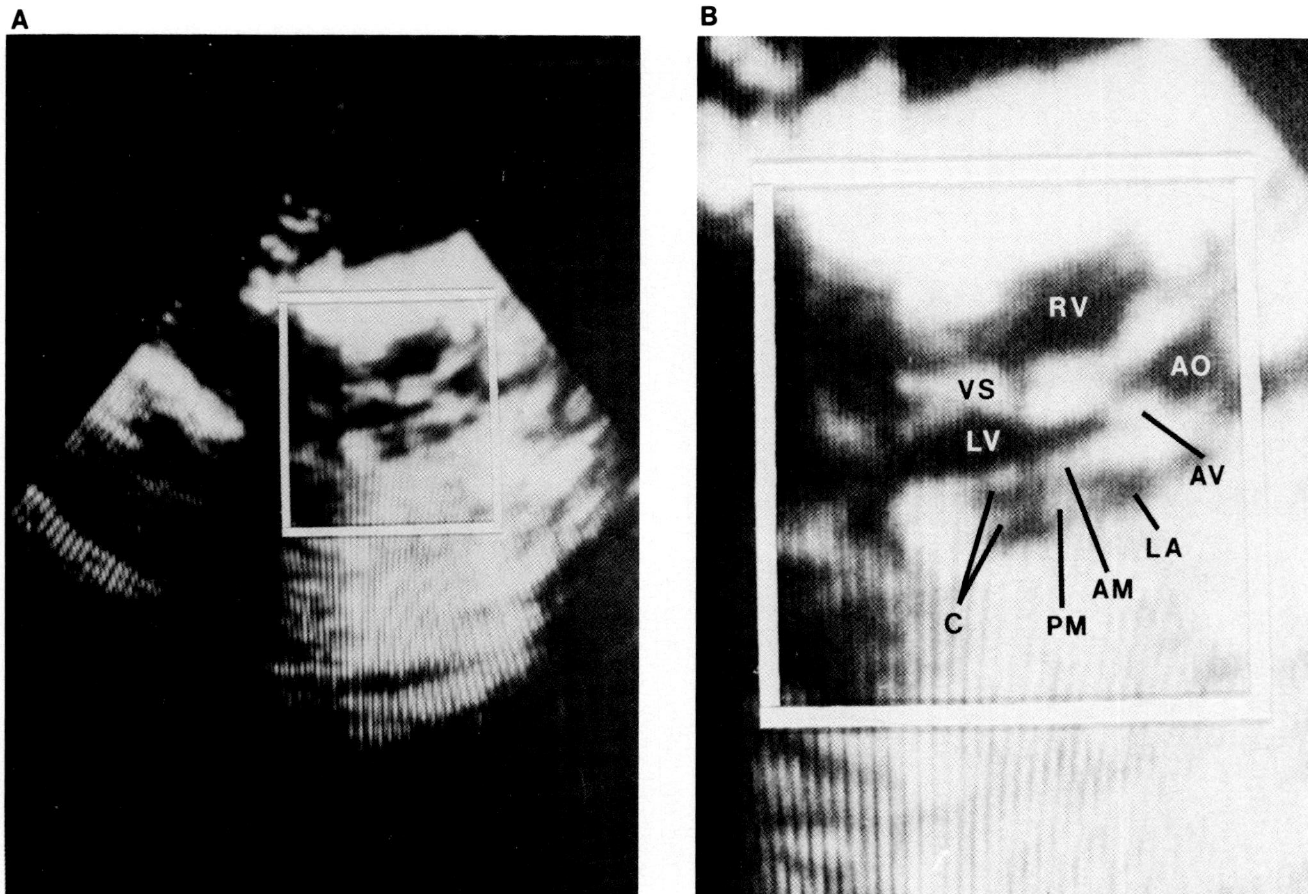

Fig. F.XI.5. **A**. A stop frame of the real-time, two-dimensional fetal echocardiogram on long axis. The fetus was on its side, and the study was done with the mother lying on the opposite side to expose the fetal anterior thorax to the transducer. **B**. Enlargement of the fetal heart seen within the white square frame of Figure XI.5A. AM = anterior leaflet of the mitral valve; AO = aortic root; AV = aortic valve; C = chordae tendineae; LA = left atrium; LV = left ventricle; PM = posterior leaflet of the mitral valve; RV = right ventricle; VS = interventricular septum.

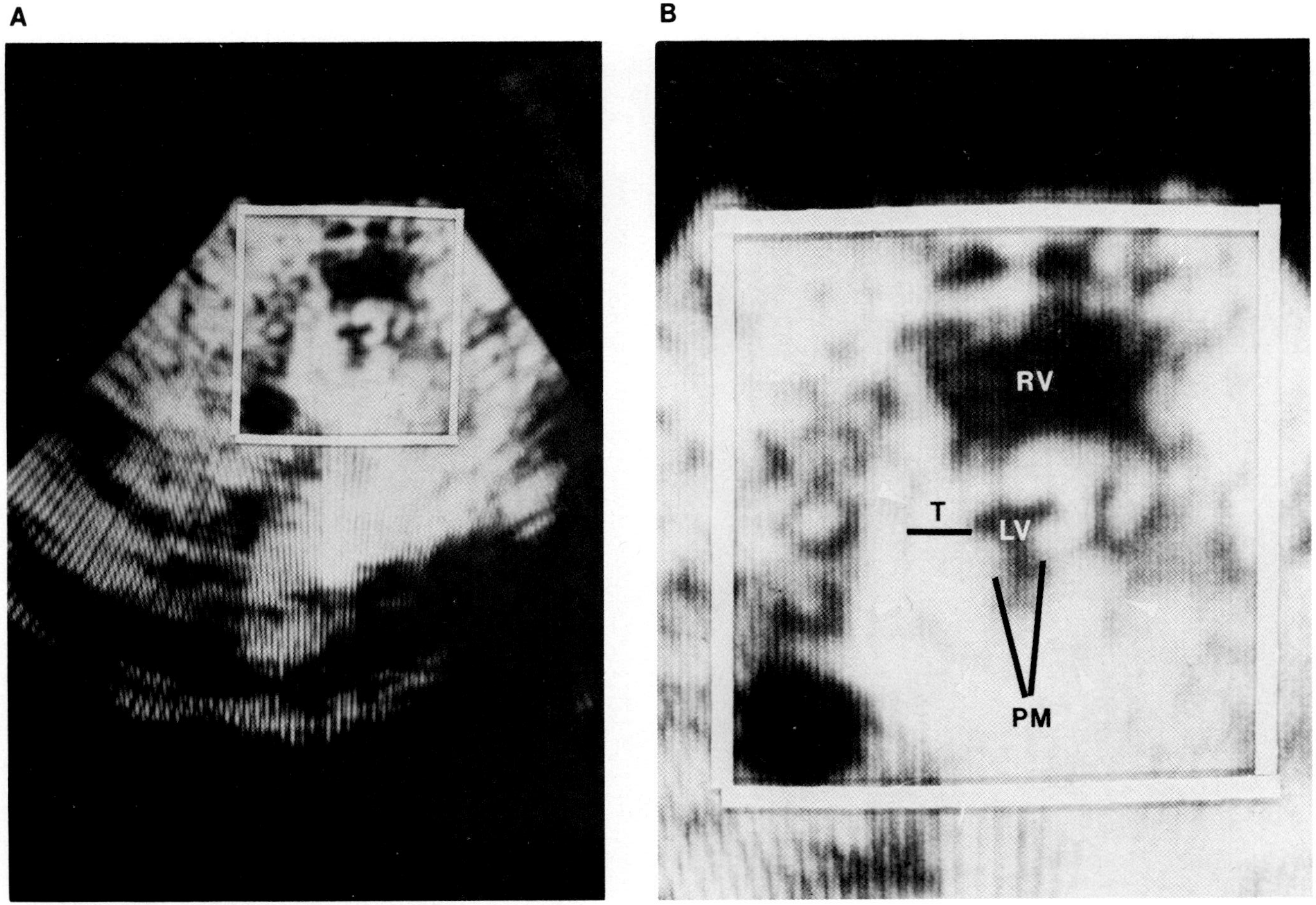

Fig. F.XI.6. **A**. A stop frame of the real-time, two-dimensional fetal echocardiogram on short axis at the level of the papillary muscles. This is the same patient, using the same studying technique, as shown in Figure XI.5. **B**. Enlargement of the fetal heart seen within the white square frame of Figure XI.6A. LV = left ventricular chamber; PM = papillary muscles; RV = right ventricle; T = left ventricular wall thickness at the level just above the posterior medial papillary muscle. The white arrowheads outline the left ventricular epicardial–pericardial border.

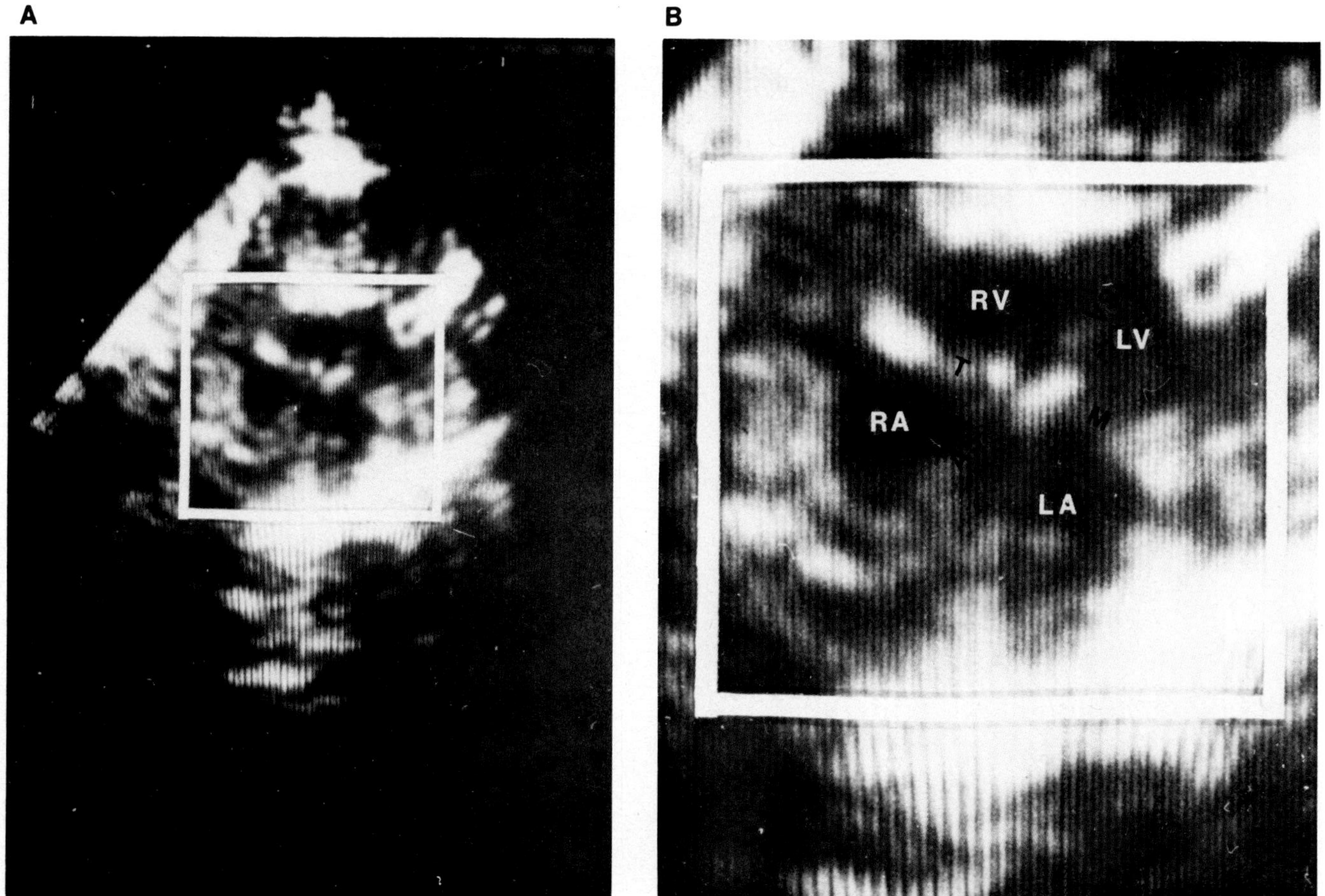

Fig. F.XI.7. **A**. A stop frame of the apical four-chamber view of the real-time, two-dimensional fetal echocardiogram. This is the same patient shown in Figures XI.5 and XI.6. The mother was in the supine position. **B**. Enlargement of the fetal heart shown within the white square frame of Figure XI.7A. The resolution and motion characteristic are significantly better on the real-time display. AS = interatrial septum; LA = left atrium; LV = left ventricle; M = mitral valve; RA = right atrium; RV = right ventricle; T = tricuspid valve; VS = interventricular septum.

the mother in the lateral position to expose the anterior fetal thorax to the transducer.

III. CONCLUSIONS

Fetal phonocardiographic technique has been developed and used mainly for fetal heart rate monitoring. The low intensity of the fetal heart sounds and problems created by multiple interference signals in the fetal and maternal environment are difficult to overcome. At present, among the noninvasive fetal heart rate monitoring techniques, the phonocardiographic technique appears to be inferior to the abdominal fetal ECG and Doppler ultrasound technique. With further improvement of the latter, it is possible that the phonocardiographic fetal heart rate monitoring technique will decline in use.

Using fetal phonocardiography for purposes other than fetal heart rate monitoring is possible. Here again, the recent emergence of fetal ultrasound and echocardiographic techniques may prove to be far superior.

Having made a major impact in adult and pediatric cardiology, echocardiography may now be entering the field of fetal cardiology. Continuing improvement of equipment and technique is expected. The firm background in adult and pediatric echocardiography and the ability of this technique to study anatomy and physiology of the heart should accelerate the growth of this field. Above all, it is noninvasive, which is most important when dealing with the fetus. Echocardiography has long been known to have no biological side effects at the level of energy used, and recent preliminary data in a one-year follow-up of infants exposed to ultrasound in utero seem to confirm that.[30] Our impression is that the combination of real-time, two-dimensional and M-mode echocardiography is the method of choice, as is true in adult and pediatric echocardiography. The ultrasonic two-dimensional B-scan may be used to help identify the fetal lie, fetal thorax, and fetal heart position; however, with experience, this information may be obtained from the real-time, two-dimensional examination. What echocardiography has contributed to adult and pediatric cardiology it is expected to contribute to fetal cardiology in the future. Anatomy and physiology of the fetal heart, fetal circulation, fetal development, and the transitional change after birth will be known in more depth. Detection of many fetal heart anamolies will be possible during gestation, which may lead to development of prevention and treatment plans.

IV. ACKNOWLEDGMENTS

The author is grateful to Karol Ann Kohorst and Marilyn Herrell for their technical assistance.

V. REFERENCES

1. Tavel ME. Clinical Phonocardiography and External Pulse Recording. Chicago: Year Book Medical Publishers, Inc., 1978.
2. Hofbauer J, Weis O. Photography Registrierung d fotalen Herztone. Zentralbl Gynaekol. 1908; 32:429–431.
3. Falls FH, Rockwood AC. Use of microphonic stethoscope in demonstration of fetal heart tones. JAMA. 1923; 81:1683–1684.
4. Smith AL, Hervert WJ. A method for recording and reproducing fetal heart sounds. Am J Obstet Gynecol. 1940; 40:102–110.
5. Wood MC. The amplification and recording of foetal heart sounds. Electronic Engineering. 1953; 25:90–93.
6. Smith DH. A foetal pulse rate recorder. Electronic Engineering. 1957; 29:132–135.
7. Gunn AL, Wood MC. The amplification and recording of foetal heart sounds. Proc R Soc Med. 1953; 46:85–91.
8. Sawyer HS. The design of a fetal phonocardiotachometer. IRE Natl Conv Rec. 1959; 9:64–72.
9. MacRae DJ. Monitoring the heart of the foetus and the newborn. Lancet. 1959; 2:266–269.
10. Hammacher K. The diagnosis of fetal distress with an electronic fetal heart monitor. In: Intrauterine Dangers to the Foetus. Proceedings of a Symposium, Prague, 10/11–14/1966. Amsterdam: Excerpta Medica Foundation, 1967: 228–233.
11. Hammacher K. The clinical significance of cardiotocography. In: Huntingford PJ, ed. Proceedings of the First Congress of Perinatal Medicine. Stuttgart: Georg Thieme, 1969:80–93.

12. Serr DM. Methods and problems of fetal heart monitoring. Int J Gynaecol Obstet. 1972; 10: 186–190.
13. Curran JT. Fetal Heart Monitoring. London: Butterworths, 1975.
14. Solum T. A comparison of the three methods for external fetal cardiography. Acta Obstet Gynecol Scand. 1980; 59:123–126.
15. O'Keeffe DF, Freeman RK. A survey of fetal monitoring equipment. Contemp Obstet Gynecol. 1979; 14:25–27.
16. Murata Y, Martin CB, Ikenoue T, Lu PS. Antepartum evaluation of the pre-ejection period of the fetal cardiac cycle. Am J Obstet Gynecol. 1978; 132:278–284.
17. Murata Y, Pyls N, Miyake K, Schmidt P, Martin CB, Singer J. Antepartum determination of pre-ejection period of fetal cardiac cycle: Its relation to newborn body weight. Am J Obstet Gynecol. 1979; 133:515–518.
18. Zador IE, Wolfson RN, Pillay SK, Timor-Tritsch IE, Hertz RH. Fetal cardiac time intervals and their potential clinical applications. Clin Obstet Gynecol. 1979; 22:651–663.
19. Madison JD, Sukhum P, Williamson DP, Campion BC. Echocardiography and fetal heart sounds in the diagnosis of fetal heart block. Am Heart J. 1979; 98:505–509.
20. Bang J, Holm HH. Ultrasonics in the demonstration of fetal heart movements. Am J Obstet Gynecol. 1968; 102:956–960.
21. Robinson HP. Detection of fetal heart movement in first trimester of pregnancy using pulsed ultrasound. Br Med J. 1972; 4:466–468.
22. Winsberg F. Echocardiography of the fetal and newborn heart. Invest Radiol. 1972; 7:152–158.
23. Egeblad H, Bang J, Northeved A. Ultrasonic identification and examination of fetal heart structures. J Clin Ultrasound. 1975; 3:95–105.
24. Lange LW, Sahn DJ, Allen HD, Goldberg SJ, Anderson C, Giles H. Qualitative real-time cross-sectional echocardiographic imaging of the human fetus during the second half of pregnancy. Circulation. 1980; 4:799–806.
25. Sahn DJ, Lothar WL, Allen HD, Goldberg SJ, Anderson C, Giles H, Haber K. Quantitative real-time cross-sectional echocardiography in the developing normal human fetus and newborn. Circulation. 1980; 3:588–597.
26. Garrett WJ, Robinson ME. Fetal heart size measured in vivo by ultrasound. Pediatrics. 1970; 46:25–27.
27. Suzuki K, Minei L, Schnitzer LE. Ultrasonographic measurement of fetal heart volume for estimation of birthweight. Obstet Gynecol. 1974; 43:867–871.
28. Feigenbaum H. Echocardiography, 3rd Ed. Philadelphia: Lea & Febiger, 1981.
29. Tajik AJ, Seward JB, Hagler DJ, Mair DD, Lie JT. Two-dimensional real-time ultrasonic imaging of the heart and great vessels: Technique, image orientation, structure identification, and validation. Mayo Clin Proc. 1978; 53:271–303.
30. Scheidt PC, Stanley F, Bryla DA. One year follow-up of infants exposed to ultrasound in utero. Am J Obstet Gynecol. 1978; 13:743–748.

F.XII

The Normal and Abnormal Fetal Heart Rate

Bruce K. Young, MD

I. INTRODUCTION

Over the past quarter of a century an enormous body of literature about fetal monitoring has appeared. The technological progress that has produced this extensive research has permittted the rapid incorporation of electronic fetal monitoring into clinical obstetrics. Despite the extensive research and widespread clinical use, electronic fetal monitoring has not been proved to be of substantial value, and has been accused of contributing unnecessary cesarean sections to an already high cesarean section rate.

Of course, electronic fetal monitoring is just a tool to be used by the obstetrician. It is not the technology that is responsible for either beneficial or harmful effects; the obstetrician bears the responsibility for the results of using electronic fetal monitoring, as he does for the results of forceps, or any other clinical tool. Just as skill in the use of forceps is necessary for the best results, so is a thorough knowledge of electronic fetal monitoring. However, this skill is much more difficult to maintain, since the field of fetal monitoring is evolving very rapidly. At present, electronic fetal heart rate monitoring provides the best guide to fetal status both antepartum and intrapartum.

II. FETAL MONITORING TECHNIQUES

Electronic fetal monitoring is performed by two different modalities. External monitoring is noninvasive. It uses a strain gauge to register the uterine contraction wave. The abdominal wall deformation caused by the contraction is measured by the strain gauge (tocodynamometer). The monitor processes the data and prints a nonquantitative curve that reflects the duration of the contraction accurately. The intensity of the contraction is not measured with this technique.

The external measurement of fetal heart rate is by a continuous beam of ul-

Cardiac Problems in Pregnancy, pages 521–534

trasound focused on the fetal heart. The ultrasound transducer uses the Doppler effect for counting the fetal heart rate. This requires extensive electronic processing of the complex signal produced by deformation of the ultrasound beam by the events of the fetal cardiac cycle. The peak of each complex wave is detected, and the interval between two peaks is measured, giving the instantaneous heart rate.

External heart rate monitoring thus can be seen to be associated with a considerable amount of artifact from the technique itself. First, the ultrasound beam may be inadequately focused, resulting in a poor signal for counting. Second, fetal movements may alter the sound wave and produce Doppler effects that affect counting. Finally, the complexity of the waveform introduces an increased variability in peak detection and counting. A result of this is increased variability of the baseline fetal heart rate when in the external mode. Whereas reduced variability seen with external monitoring may be considered reliable, increased variability most likely is artifactual.

Internal monitoring of uterine contractions requires the introduction of a sterile water-filled catheter into the uterus after rupture of the membranes. The outside end of the catheter is connected to a Statham gauge. The gauge must be calibrated in millimeters of mercury before each use. The result is a semiquantitative measurement of intrauterine pressure at the location of the catheter tip. The duration and frequency of uterine contractions are measured and recorded very accurately, and the intensity in mm Hg is relative to the height of the gauge but is otherwise quantitative.

Internal fetal heart rate monitoring is invasive, utilizing an electrode attached to the fetal scalp. The fetal electrocardiogram is detected, and the R wave is the signal used for peak detection and counting. This is a very "clear" signal for electronic processing and counting. As a result, the beat-to-beat and baseline variability are reasonably reliable compared to the data obtained by external monitoring. The artifacts encountered with the internal technique are few and infrequent; most common is a poor recording, with marked discontinuity and increased variability of the fetal heart rate. This is due to either poor attachment or a faulty electrode. Next is an unphysiologic variation in baseline with marked beat-to-beat abnormalities. Physiologic beat-to-beat changes rarely exceed 10 bpm, and beat-to-beat changes of 15 or greater are nearly always artifacts. Persistence of such changes usually indicates electrical interference or arrhythmia. This can be evaluated by obtaining a fetal electrocardiogram. If no fetal ECG is observed, the problem is electronic. If a clear fetal ECG is seen, the arrhythmia can be diagnosed. (see Chapter F.XIII). Finally, if the electrode is in contact with the cervix, maternal ECG interference may be the source of the artifactual pattern. Once again, examination of the fetal ECG complex will reveal the problem, with maternal QRS complexes visible on the electrocardiogram. In general, the occurrence of a persistent artifact is an indication for viewing the fetal ECG. For more detail concerning the technical and physical aspects of fetal monitoring, see chapters F.VIII and IX.

The fetal heart rate pattern is displayed on a printed paper record. The record has an upper channel for the heart rate and a lower channel for uterine activity, and is customarily run at a paper speed of 3 cm/min. The fetal heart rate pattern should be present for at least ten minutes if a meaningful interpretation is to be made. The relationship between fetal heart rate and changes in uterine and fetal activity as seen in the lower channel may be diagnostic of clinical conditions in the fetus. Correlation of intrapartum fetal heart rate patterns with neonatal outcome is greatest when these patterns are persistent, expecially if persistent until delivery. Antepartum observations are not well correlated with neonatal outcome when the fetal heart rate pattern is abnormal. Normal (reactive) patterns are correlated with fetal survival in utero for the ensuing seven days after either the nonstress or the contraction stress test.[1-3]

III. THE FETAL HEART RATE

Consideration of the normal and abnormal fetal heart rate should start with a description of the baseline heart rate. The baseline heart rate is the heart rate between contractions, with a normal range of 120–160 beats per minute (bpm). Rates below 120 bpm are classified as fetal bradycardia, and over 160 as tachycardia. Moderate bradycardia is a heart rate of 100–119 bpm, while marked bradycardia is a heart rate below 100 bpm.[4] Moderate bradycardia is a harmless pattern. It is not related to fetal acidosis or hypoxia and requires no intervention in the absence of other abnormalities. Moderate bradycardia is caused by the reflex response of the fetus to mild head compression. (Fig. F.XII.1). Usually, the continuous head compression is due to posterior or transverse positions of the vertex. When the moderate bradycardia is prolonged, lasting for an hour or longer, cephalopelvic disproportion or, rarely, brow presentation must be suspected.[5,6]

Marked bradycardia may be of serious concern when it persists for ten minutes or longer. Even short episodes of three to five minutes of marked bradycardia frequently are associated with a drop in tissue pH, most likely because fetal tissue perfusion is greatly reduced under such circumstances. Marked bradycardia may be caused by many etiologies, such as maternal hypotension, placental abruption, severe umbilical cord compression, and congenital fetal cardiac abnormalities. It is one of the few fetal heart rate patterns that is usually indicative of fetal distress.

Fetal tachycardia of 160–179 bpm is considered moderate, whereas a fetal heart rate of 180 or higher is marked tachycardia.[4] When either moderate or severe tachycardia is present for intervals less than ten minutes, they are not of clinical significance. Even prolonged tachycardia, lasting over an hour, may be innocuous when there is good baseline variability present. In such cases, the tachycardia may be associated with maternal agitation, autonomic dyssynergia as may be seen with maternal spinal cord lesions, sympathomimetic and atropine-like drugs, fetal factors producing activation of the fetal sympathetic nervous system, and fetal tachyarrhythmias. However, the combination of fever and fetal tachycardia is very strongly suggestive of chorioamnionitis. Fetal tachycardia with minimal base-

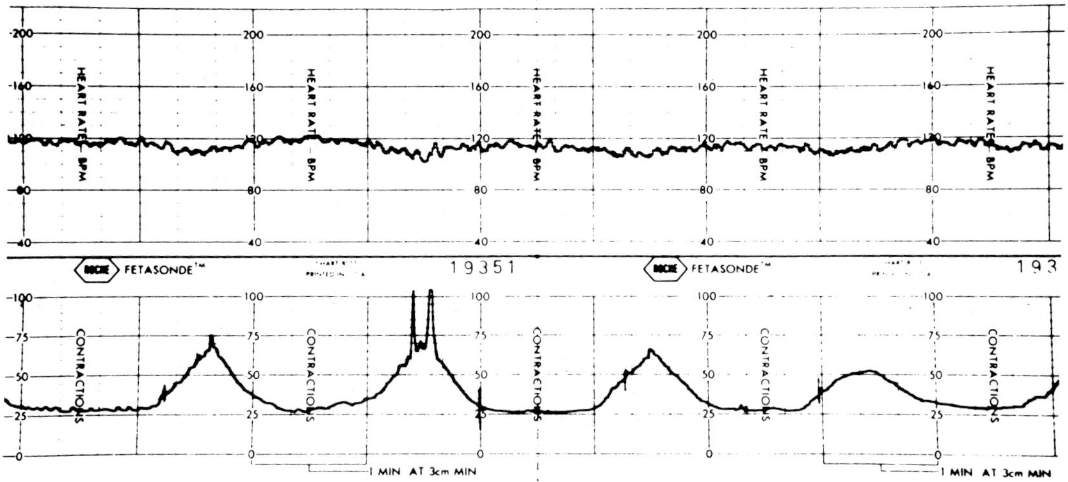

Fig. F.XII.1. Moderate fetal bradycardia.

line variability is associated with the development of fetal acidosis in labor and a lowered neonatal blood pH.[7,8] This pattern is of serious concern.

Thus, variability of the baseline heart rate is seen to be a key factor in the significance of fetal tachycardias. In fact, baseline variability is important in the analysis of all fetal heart rate patterns. Unfortunately, visual analysis permits an unacceptable variation in interpretation due to individual subjectivity, despite attempts to establish criteria. Visual criteria are not uniformly accepted at this time, nor are there quantitative criteria that have found general acceptance at present. The simplest numerical approach to baseline variability 1) should include both beat-to-beat and long-term variability, 2) should be applicable over any period of monitoring, 3) should be correlated with visual interpretation of baseline variability, and 4) should be comprehensible to the clinician.

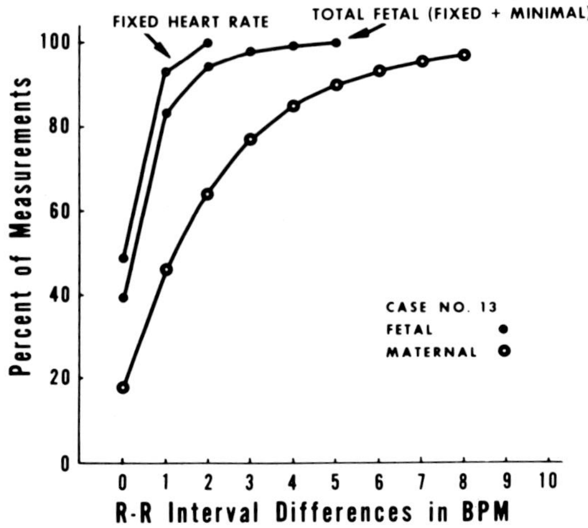

Fig. F.XII.2. Quantitative variability plot. The variability is minimal where 90% of the measurements show a 1 to 2 beat-to-beat difference. The maternal heart rate shows average variability, with 90% of the measurements with a 5 to 6 beat-to-beat difference.

Such an approach is employed for quantitative baseline variability analysis at New York University and has been incorporated into some of the new fetal monitors.[9] Choosing the simplest mathematical definition of baseline heart rate, it may be defined as the arithmetic sum of all the beat-to-beat changes. The variability visualized by the observer is the gross variation around an imagined baseline heart rate caused by the beat-to-beat changes on the fetal monitoring record. The beat-to-beat change in heart rate is the difference in the instantaneous rate calculated by measuring two consecutive two-beat intervals. Beat-to-beat changes cannot be seen by the observer because the paper speed is too slow. Therefore, the observer sees baseline variability. However, the quantitative expression of baseline variability may be derived from the beat-to-beat changes by computer analysis online. This may be expressed in terms of the percentage of beat-to-beat changes which are 1, then 2, then 3, etc, up to 10 bpm from the baseline. Beat-to-beat differences over 10 bpm are usually arrhythmias or artifact.[10] A convenient quantitative description of baseline variability may thus be given by the beat-to-beat difference, which includes 90% of all beat-to-beat changes observed in a given period of monitoring. For example, if 90% of all the beat-to-beat changes are 1 bpm or less, the variability is that of a fixed baseline. If 90% of all the beat-to-beat differences are 2 bpm or less, there is minimal baseline variability. However, if the 90% extends the range of beat-to-beat changes to 10 bpm, there is marked baseline variability present (Fig. F.XII. 2).[9]

Baseline variability is thought to reflect fetal autonomic nervous activity. It is reduced by fetal "sleep cycles"[11] and drugs such as barbiturates, meperidine, and magnesium sulfate.[12] However, when there is no apparent cause for a reduced baseline variability, and the fetus is unresponsive to stimulation, it is a poor prognostic finding in both antepartum and intrapartum fetal monitoring. At present, the prognostic significance of marked variability is unclear. The consensus is that it is benign, and mirrors an overactive fetal autonomic nervous system.

In the normal fetal heart rate record, a number of periodic changes may be superimposed on the underlying heart rate and variability. The mere occurrence of early or variable decelerations at some point in a fetal monitoring record does not indicate that the tracing is abnormal. In fact, together with accelerations, these are found occasionally in the majority of fetal heart rate recordings. A record should be considered abnormal only when there is an unusual pattern present, or when one pattern predominates for at least ten minutes without disappearing at all. Moreover, the brief appearance of one of the so-called ominous patterns is not very likely to be related to outcome when there are no other indications of fetal jeopardy. The growing tendency to catch a glimpse of an "ominous" fetal heart rate pattern and immediately perform a cesarean delivery must be decried. Fetal monitoring must be used as an early warning system. The clinician should be alerted by abnormal patterns. The proper diagnosis and conservative treatment should be sought before proceeding to rapid delivery. A persistent fetal heart rate abnormality, or one that shows progressive deterioration over 30 minutes or more, despite conservative treatment, may be a cause for prompt action. Neonatal outcome correlates best with the pattern present just before delivery, so that *intrauterine* resuscitative measures are the favored approach to abnormal patterns. If the baby's condition can be improved before delivery, that is much better than trying to improve it after delivery.

A. Benign Fetal Heart Rate Patterns

Certain periodic fetal heart rate patterns, despite their persistence for long periods, are not causes for treatment or strenuous diagnostic efforts. These include accelerations, which are brief rises of at least 10 bpm, due to increased activity of the fetal sympathetic nervous system. (Fig. F.XII.3) Another of these is early deceleration, which is a fall in the fetal heart rate exactly concurrent with the uterine contraction and resembling the mirror image of the contraction curve (Fig. F.XII.4). Early decelerations are believed

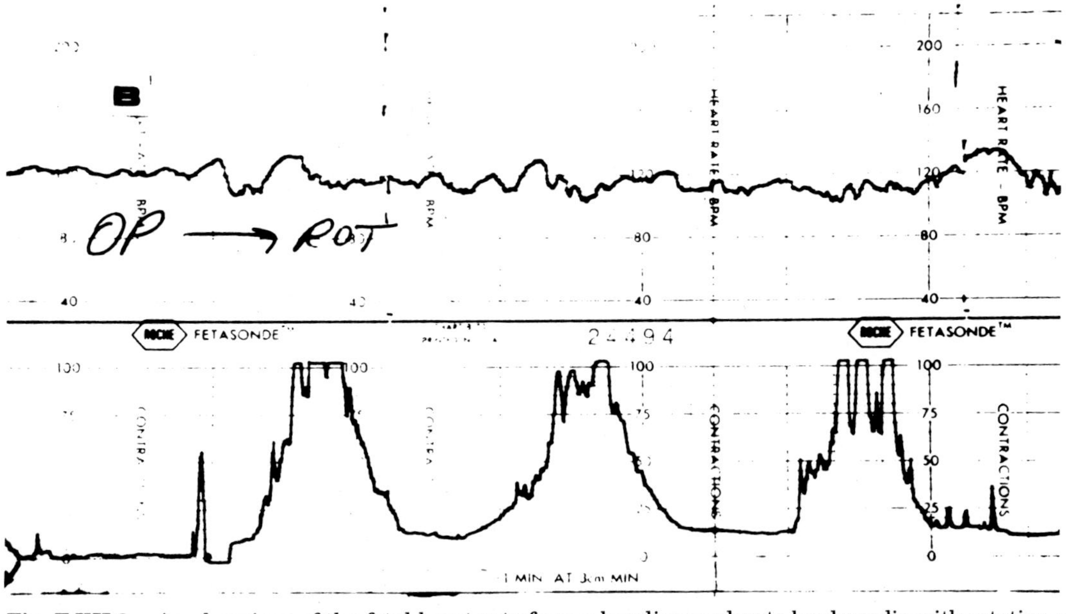

Fig. F.XII.3. Accelerations of the fetal heart rate from a baseline moderate bradycardia with rotation of the vertex from posterior to transverse. Following this, the heart rate rose to 120–140 as the rotation continued to ROA.

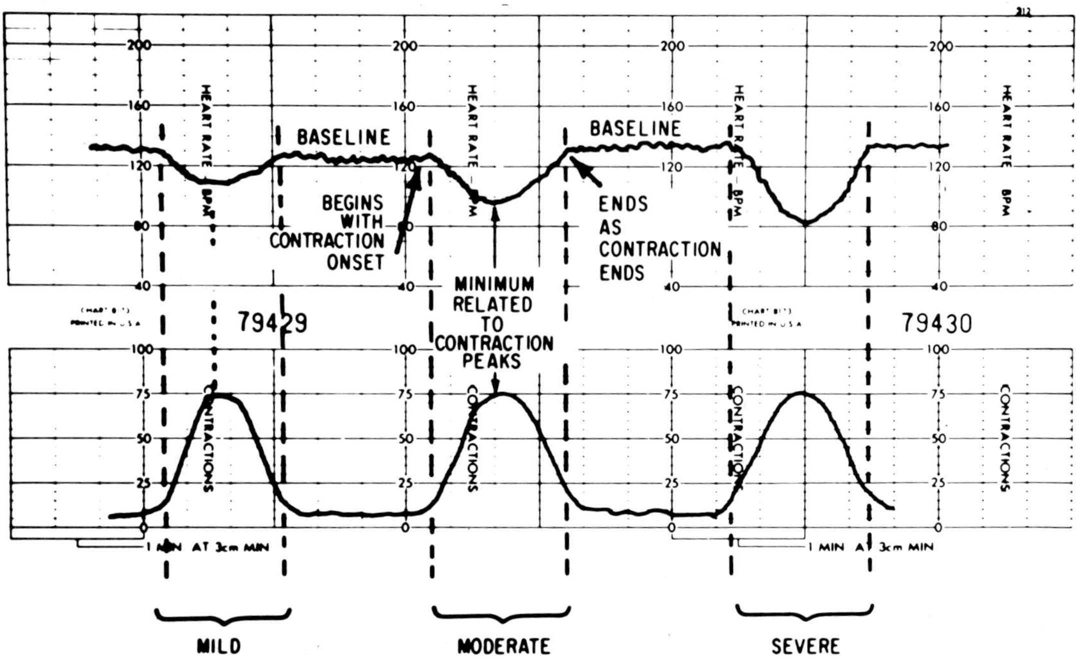

Fig. F.XII.4. Early deceleration of the fetal heart rate. Note the direct relationship to uterine contractions.

to be vagally mediated due to fetal head compression by the uterine contraction. They are harmless and not associated with fetal acidosis or poor neonatal results. Last among these innocuous patterns is that seen with fetal cardiac arrhythmias. Although there is no specific pattern for arrhythmias, there is generally an erratic heart rate, usually containing frequent episodes of artifact. This is the result of the intermittency of most arrhythmias and their usually exceeding the limits of physiological variability. Frequent and deep variable decelerations are common. The tachyarrhythmias are often seen with very high baseline heart rates and reduced variability. While there have been reports of neonatal and fetal heart failure with prolonged supraventricular tachyarrhythmias, the vast majority of them are benign and disappear spontaneously by 24 hours postpartum.[13,14] Bradyarrhythmias are more often associated with congenital cardiac anomalies, especially heart blocks due to endocardial cushion developmental defects. These neonates often do not fare well, although they seem to tolerate the fetal state and labor reasonably well.[14] The adaptation of the fetal electrocardiogram and sophisticated ultrasonography in the fetus, particularly in the presence of fetal cardiac arrhythmias, should open a new era in intrauterine diagnosis of cardiac disease. Congenital valvular disease already has been diagnosed from the fetal electrocardiogram,[15] and fetal electrocardiography should be available wherever internal fetal monitoring is practiced. For more detail on fetal arrhythmias see Chapter F.XIII.

B. Ominous Fetal Heart Rate Patterns

Still less reassuring to the clinician than bradyarrhythmias are the often associated variable deceleration patterns, as well as those of late deceleration and sinusoidal heart rate. Late deceleration is a smooth fall in heart rate beginning after the contraction has started and ending after the contraction is over (Fig. F.XII.5). Both hypoxic and reflex components are probably involved in the genesis of these

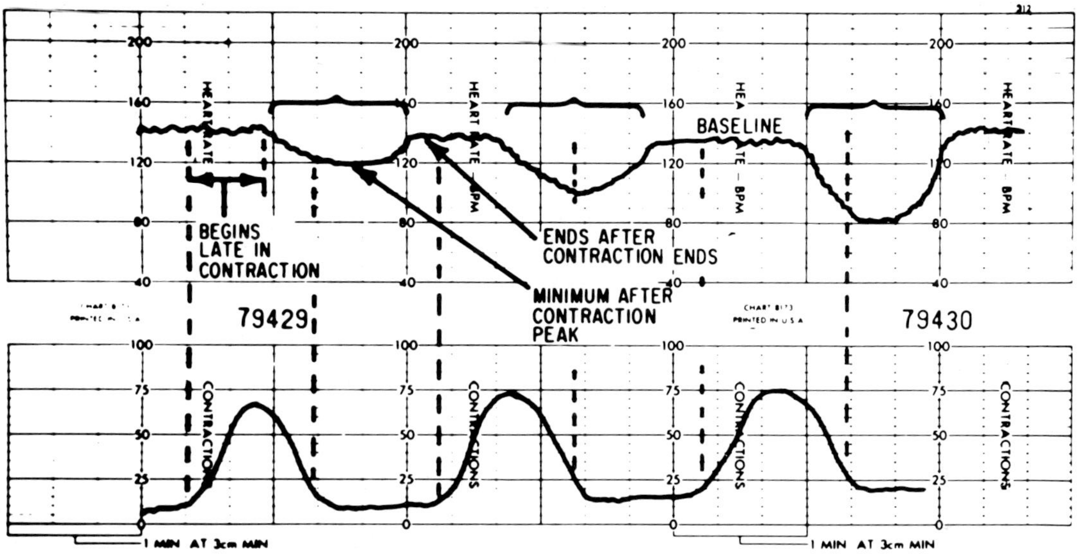

Fig. F.XII.5. Late deceleration of the fetal heart rate. Note the onset at least 20 seconds after the onset of the contraction and the relatively smooth deflection from the baseline heart rate.

decelerations. They are associated with falling fetal pH and a potential for perinatal morbidity and mortality.[16,17] However, late decelerations of up to 40 bpm depth may persist for hours without fetal death or a depressed newborn, and they may disappear during the course of labor or with cessation of oxytocin stimulation. Therefore, the late deceleration pattern should be regarded as indicative of fetal stress. It may be followed by fetal deterioration and demands further diagnosis. Biochemical assessment of fetal status is the appropriate procedure, using fetal scalp blood or tissue pH. Maternal pH must be considered as well, to interpret correctly the acid-base state of the fetus. Careful evaluation of fetal health by fetal heart rate and acid-base modalities in cases of fetal stress will permit more accurate diagnosis of fetal distress. When it is persistent until birth and other risk factors have not been excluded,[7,16] the pattern of late deceleration has been associated with a 40–60% incidence of fetal pre-acidosis or acidosis and Apgar scores below 7. This 40–60% risk is a maximum figure for estimating the hazards of continued labor with persistent late decelerations, emphasizing the need for biochemical information rather than immediate delivery.

Another fetal stress pattern is the sinusoidal heart rate (Fig. F.XII.6). This pattern was first recognized by Manseau and co-workers in patients with Rh isoimmunization in 1972. It has been thought to carry a perinatal mortality of 50–75% when present antepartum or intrapartum.[18–20] Sinusoidal heart rate may be defined as a pattern of regular variability resembling a sine wave, with a relatively fixed period of three to five cycles per minute and amplitude of 5–40 bpm from the baseline rate. Using this definition, and following 16 cases with scalp blood or tissue and umbilical artery pH, perinatal mortality was avoided in our series.[21,22] There was an incidence of 31% fetal pre-acidosis or acidosis, as well as Apgar scores below 7. There was no consistent cause of the pattern, although abruption and other causes of fetal hypoxemia were prominent. Biochemical evaluation of sinusoidal heart rate patients led to cesarean section in only four of 16 cases.[21]

The mechanism for the sinusoidal heart rate is unclear, but it probably is a response to moderate fetal hypoxemia. The

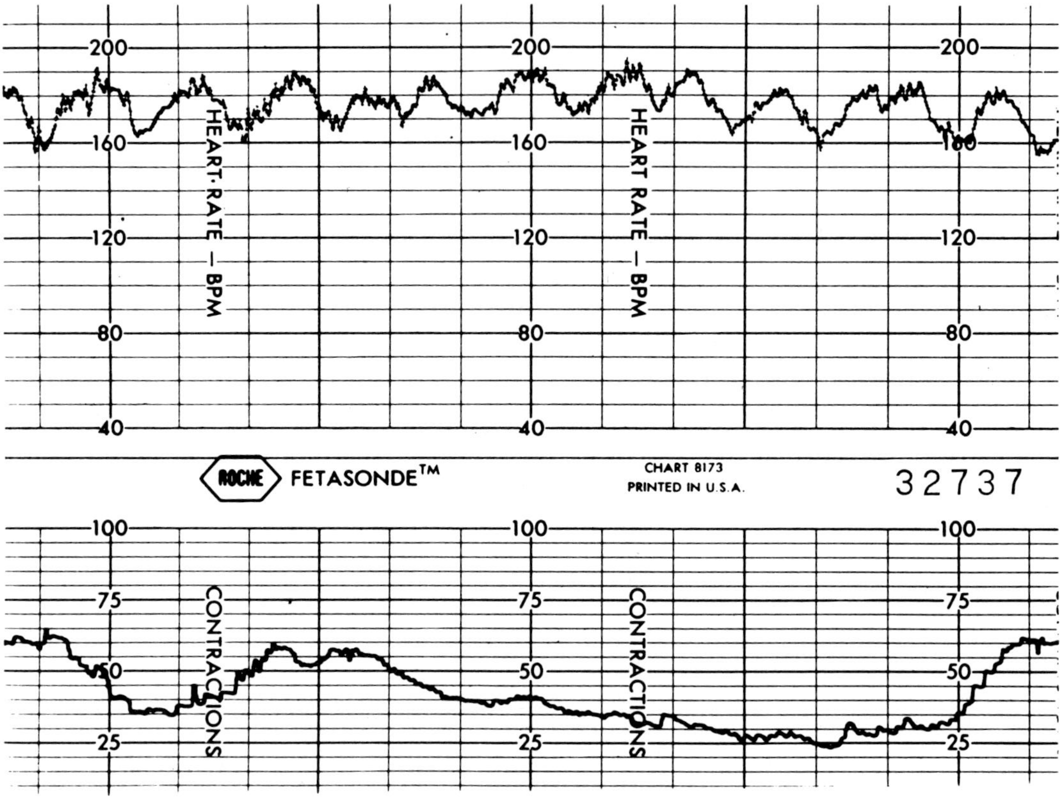

Fig. F.XII.6. Sinusoidal heart rate with a periodicity of 3 cycles per minute and an amplitude of 10–15 beats per minute.

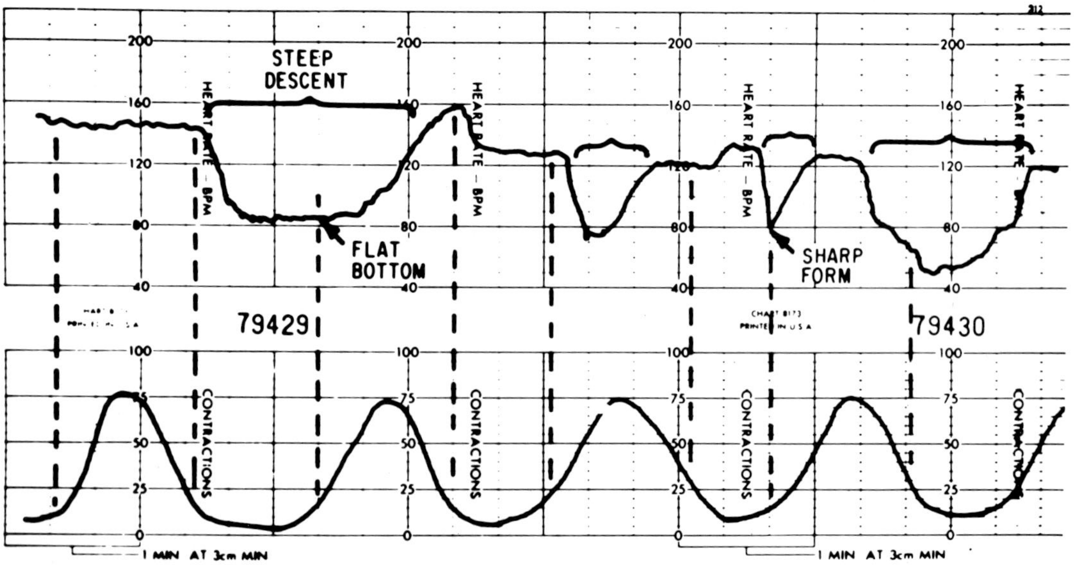

Fig. F.XII.7. Variable deceleration of the fetal heart rate. There is an inconstant relationship to the uterine contractions and a varying configuration of the decelerations, which usually resemble the letters U, V, or W.

fetal autonomic nervous system discharges alternately in a compensatory fashion. Increased sympathetic stimulation due to the fetal hypoxemia speeds up the heart rate. This improves the hypoxemia, and the parasympathetic nervous system is activated. The fetal heart then slows, and the hypoxemia recurs, beginning the cycle over again.

These investigations showed that fetal acidosis was not necessarily present during the sinusoidal heart rate. Continuous fetal tissue pH studies demonstrated that a falling pH followed the onset of the sinusoidal pattern, and the pH rose when the sinusoidal pattern disappeared.[22] Not only did the fetus tolerate the sinusoidal pattern without severe acidosis but also it compensated for the stress; the pattern disappeared, and there was a rise in pH as well. Nevertheless, the sinusoidal pattern is associated with fetal hypoxemia. When the amplitude exceeds 15 bpm, there is a significant incidence of low fetal scalp blood and tissue pH. There is also a significant risk of fetal distress with this pattern. Careful evaluation of patients with fetal pH analysis will clarify the need for prompt cesarean delivery and avoid operation whenever possible.

The third fetal stress pattern is that of variable decelerations (Fig. F.XII.7). The clinical significance of this fetal heart rate (FHR) pattern remains controversial despite intensive study for more than 20 years. Although some relationship between the morphology of the deceleration and fetal condition seems to be present,[16,23,24] the predictability and pathophysiology have remainded elusive. Application of continuous tissue pH measurement to this problem has overcome the technical difficulties inherent in the study of such a rapidly changing pattern.[25] The variable deceleration pattern may be subdivided into 1) variable deceleration without late component; 2) variable deceleration with late onset only, in which the deceleration begins at least 20 seconds after onset of the contraction, but recovers by the end of the contraction; and 3) variable deceleration with late recovery, in which the recovery to baseline heart rate is delayed until after the contraction (Fig. F.XII.8). The variable deceleration pattern without a late component is be-

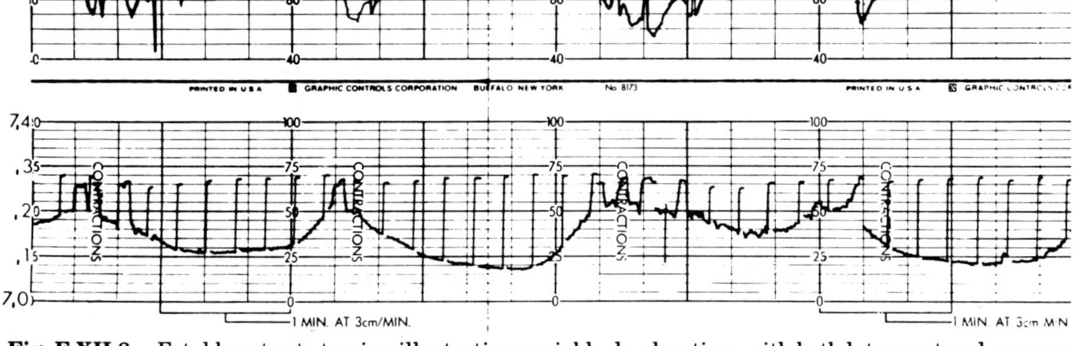

Fig. F.XII.8. Fetal heart rate tracing illustrating variable decelerations with both late onset and recovery with continuous TpH values falling from 7.28 to 7.25 during the decelerations. The tissue pH is shown at the left of the figure on the lower channel along with uterine contractions. Each vertical bar superimposed on the contraction curve indicates a TpH measurement. The upper channel shows continuous fetal heart rate by internal spiral electrode.

nign, no matter how deep the deceleration. These are not associated with acidosis or low Apgar scores to any significant degree. The variable deceleration with late recovery is not benign (Fig. F.XII.8). A falling pH during the period of decelerations was observed in every case, and the pH fell progressively and maximally in these patients. In these cases, the duration of the late component and the depth of deceleration were proportional to the degree of decrease in pH, when the deceleration exceeded 40 bpm. Acidosis or preacidosis was present with decelerations in excess of 60 bpm; however, this relationship was observed only with variables with late recovery, and not with the other forms of variable deceleration.

When the pattern of variable deceleration with late recovery persisted to delivery, 56% of the newborns had Apgar scores below 7, compared to only 8% of those with variable decelerations without late component. The pattern of variable deceleration with late onset showed a fall in pH in 31% of cases, and it probably is intermediate in pathogenesis between the late recovery pattern and that without a late component.[25]

Thus, the harmless variable deceleration pattern may be distinguished from the variable deceleration with late component. The latter is the most hazardous form of variable deceleration. It appears more troublesome than late decelerations or sinusoidal heart rate and must be evaluated and treated promptly for optimal neonatal outcome.

C. Fetal Distress Patterns

Considerable confusion surrounds the diagnosis of fetal distress. Much of that confusion stems from lack of consensus on the meaning of fetal distress. The condition may be defined as follows: Fetal distress is a pathological condition of the fetus that is likely to cause fetal or neonatal death or damage to the newborn if not corrected within one hour.

There are numerous causes for fetal distress, and multiple factors and phenomena are associated with it. However, only the following few fetal heart rate patterns are associated with fetal distress:

1) Undulating baseline—an alternating tachycardia and bradycardia with wide swings—often with reduced short-term variability
2) Severe bradycardia, with heart rates below 80
3) Severe tachycardia and reduced baseline variability unrelated to drugs
4) Severe tachycardia associated with periodic changes in fetal stress; eg, late decelerations, sinusoidal pattern, or variable decelerations with late component

These patterns demand careful diagnosis and prompt therapy.

The interpretation of these patterns requires biochemical data. A fetal scalp blood sample for pH, pO_2, pCO_2, HCO_3, base excess, and lactate is helpful, and may be done on 200 μl of fetal capillary blood. A maternal arterial or venous pH sample may be helpful in evaluating abnormal results. Continuous tissue pH may be useful as well, particularly for following trends. The determination of pH, at least, should be repeated in 15–30 minutes to establish a trend and to verify the initial sample. During this time, the mother should be placed in the lateral decubitus position, given oxygen and intravenous fluids, and oxytocin should not be used. Careful observation of the maternal vital signs and fetal heart rate should be continued. If the clinical picture and the diagnostic maneuvers indicate progressive fetal acidosis, the diagnosis of fetal distress is confirmed. Prompt delivery of the fetus must be accomplished by the appropriate route. If no preacidosis or acidosis is present, conservative management should be maintained, with careful evaluation of the trend. Only in this way can needless cesarean delivery be avoided, while protecting the fetus from the hazards of labor.

IV. THE FETAL MONITORING CONTROVERSY

Broad discussion of the benefits and risks of electronic fetal monitoring (EFM) has recently become the focus of the media, the government, and the medical profession. The public has been told that "electronic fetal monitoring may do more harm than good"[26] and that "the common practice of electronically monitoring a baby's birth is potentially dangerous to both mother and child"[27].

The basis for this viewpoint derives from a 1978 review of the literature on EFM by Banta and Thacker, two nonpracticing physicians working under the auspices of the National Center for Health Services Research, U.S. Department of Health, Education and Welfare.[28] Their review consisted of an epidemiological and statistical analysis of the data reported from the four randomized controlled scientific studies extant at the time and a statistical study by Neutra et al.[29] They dismissed the other data available, including a statistical analysis by Wood.[30] Banta and Thacker stated in their report that "the four controlled clinical trials have methodologic problems, and possibly conflicting conclusions as to the benefits and complications of EFM." They commented on Neutra's study: "The study does give evidence of some benefit in terms of mortality from EFM in selected patients." No mention is made of the fact that Neutra's study omitted intrapartum fetal deaths, perhaps the major problem that EFM is designed to prevent.

This complex issue has been carefully studied by an NIH task force, which concluded its discussions in March 1979. The conclusions reached have been published.[31]

The NIH consensus was that events occurring during labor account for one-fifth of all stillbirths and 30–50% of brain damaged newborns, although the true magnitude of these problems remains unknown. Such events during labor are more likely to occur in known high-risk pregnancy, but they may occur unpredictably in patients not known to be at increased risk, the task force concludes.

Despite these conclusions, the task force went on to recommend intermittent auscultation of the fetal heart as acceptable in low-risk patients, based on the absence of epidemiological data evaluating EFM in low-risk patients. They did endorse EFM when used with other information, including fetal scalp blood sampling, in high-risk patients. The questions of associated complications of monitoring and increased cesarean section rate due to monitoring were answered as being of minimal significance, although present. Thus, the NIH task force clearly favors EFM in high-risk patients and does not agree with the media statements that EFM "is potentially dangerous to both mother and child," or with the report of Banta and Thacker.

Several points in the NIH approach require amplification. While the task force did an outstanding job in grappling with the data, epidemiologic considerations, as well as consumer and other pressures, certain problems persist.

First is the fact that no system yet exists for accurate prediction of the high- and low-risk pregnancy. Many high-risk cases can be defined before the onset of labor, but how many are missed is not known. It is estimated that 25–35% of patients considered to be at low risk will become high-risk patients during labor by most authorities on high-risk pregnancy. These "high-risk converters" may go undetected without EFM until it is too late to prevent damage. The statistical approach to answering the question of benefit in low-risk cases would require controlled studies with thousands of patients in each group, since the perinatal mortality figure for such low-risk populations approximates 1–8 per thousand. Such studies cannot be done very readily. However, EFM can easily show fetal heart patterns correlated with fetal jeopardy that cannot be heard with a fetal stethoscope. These patterns include reduced heart rate variability, variable decelerations with late component, late decelerations, and sinusoidal heart rate. Demonstration of abnormal patterns in babies thought to be low-risk in labor is thus an obvious benefit of EFM, not needing statistical verification of significance. Reasonable as this conclusion may be, statistical verification could be found in terms of a comparison of auscultation findings with EFM findings, rather than neonatal mortality and cesarean section rates for the two groups.

A third consideration is the report from the Obstetrical Collaborative Project in 25,000 cases, which states that there is "no reliable auscultation indicator of fetal distress existing in terms of fetal heart rate, except in an extreme degree."[32] Thus, auscultation is of little value, except when an extreme situation of fetal distress is present, based on a statistical study of over 25,000 pregnancies. It seems difficult to argue with the idea that EFM might be better than auscultation under any circumstances, if the goal is the early diagnosis of fetal distress. The "risk" of cesarean section does appear to be greater in EFM patients than in patients having auscultation, but it was statistically significant in only two of the four controlled studies reviewed, according to the NIH task force. The wisdom of restraint in imputing an increased risk of cesarean is reinforced by a 1959 study comparing auscultation of the fetal heart with no auscultation or monitoring of any kind. The results were an increased cesarean section and forceps delivery rate in the auscultated group without an improvement in the perinatal mortality.[33] This demonstrates that it is very difficult to impose the epidemiologic model on clinical situations without either very large numbers or very strictly controlled groups. Perhaps no attention should be given to the fetal heart during labor at all, in order to keep down the cesarean section rate! Once again, if the goal is the early detection of fetal distress, some increase in cesarean section rate is likely and probably reflects appropriate early intervention.

The question of unnecessary intervention due to misinterpretation of EFM data must be considered as well. No clear accounting of such ill-advised judgments is possible. This does not alter the usefulness of the data obtained from EFM, but it does emphasize the need to educate all professionals who care for pregnant women in the use of EFM, and fetal scalp blood sampling, as well.

The risks of EFM in terms of infection with internal monitoring were accurately assessed as minimal, and no known risk was stated for external monitoring. It should be emphasized, nevertheless, that internal monitoring should be used only when external monitoring is not satisfactory, in order to avoid any risk of infection. External monitoring is advisable unless it is unsatisfactory for interpretation, since it is not invasive. If external EFM is unsatisfactory, the internal approach should be used, since the complication rate is acceptably low even with the internal techniques. Continuous monitoring and recording of the fetal heart rate and uterine activity can be achieved only with EFM. Auscultation cannot offer more than intermittent information and cannot recognize most of the key patterns of fetal stress. Auscultation of the fetal heart alone has been shown to be unsatisfactory as it is currently performed. It should be combined with EFM, and used alone only in low-risk situations when EFM is not available, in the manner described by the NIH task force.

A significant reduction in perinatal deaths has been demonstrated in high-risk patients followed by EFM. However, no proper study has been done to demonstrate such a reduction in low-risk patients. Nevertheless, since low-risk patients may become high-risk unpredictably in labor, there is good reason to expect some benefit from EFM in low-risk patients, although the information is not yet available to prove that expectation. EFM is a screening procedure for the early detection of possible fetal distress. It is not diagnostic by itself, and must be confirmed by such other means as fetal blood gases, pH studies, and clinical observations. EFM is analogous to the Papanicolaou smear; both are screening devices with a low yield in low-risk situations, and both require verification by more definitive means. Despite a yield of only one carcinoma in 2,000 cases screened, no one would advocate dispensing with the Pap test at the cost of one missed cancer. Should we be any more willing to accept dead or damaged babies?

V. REFERENCES

1. Bruce SL, Petrie RH, Yeh SY. The suspicious contraction stress test. Obstet Gynecol. 1978; 51:415.
2. Gauthier RJ, Evertson LR, Paul RH. Antepartum fetal heart rate testing II. Intrapartum fetal heart rate observation and newborn outcome following a positive contraction stress test. Am J Obstet Gynecol. 1979; 133:34.
3. Petrie RH. Stress and nonstress antepartum monitoring. In: Young BK (ed). "Perinatal Medicine Today." New York: Alan R. Liss, Inc., 1980: 151–169.
4. Hon EH. An Introdcution to Fetal Heart Rate Monitoring, Los Angeles: Harty Press, Inc. 1971.
5. Young BK, Weinstein HM. Moderate fetal bradycardia. Am J Obstet Gynecol. 1976; 126:271.
6. Young BK, Katz M, Klein SA, Silverman F. Fetal blood and tissue pH with moderate bradycardia. Am J Obstet Gynecol. 1979; 135:45–47.
7. Saling E, Schneider D. Biochemical supervision of the fetus during labor. J Obstet Gynecol Br Commonw. 1967; 74:799.
8. Young BK, Hirschl IT, Klein SA, et al. Continuous fetal tissue pH monitoring in labor with high risk pregnancies. Arch Gynecol. 1978; 226:169.
9. Young BK, Weinstein HM, Hochberg H, et al. Observations in perinatal heart rate monitoring I. A quantitative method of describing baseline variability of the fetal heart rate. J Reprod Med. 1978; 20:205.
10. Young BK, Hochberg H, George MED. An improved data display system for fetal heart rate monitoring. Obstet Gynecol. 1976; 47:496.
11. Read JA, Miller FC. Fetal heart rate accelerations in response to acoustic stimulation as a measure of fetal well-being. Am J Obstet Gynecol. 1977; 129:512.
12. Keegan KA, Paul RH, Broussard PM, et al. Antepartum fetal heart rate testing III. The effect of phenobarbital on the non-stress test. Am J Obstet Gynecol. 1979; 133:579.
13. Kerenyi T, Gleicher N, Meller J, et al. Transplacental cardioversion of intrauterine supraventricular tachycardia with digitalis. Lancet. 1980; 2:393–395.
14. Young BK, Klein SA, Katz M. Intrapartum fetal cardiac arrhythmias. Obstet Gynecol. 1979; 54:427.
15. Katz M, Valdes-Cruz LM, Greco MA, et al. Diagnosis of congenital mitral and aortic stenosis from the fetal electrocardiogram. Obstet Gynecol. 1979; 54:372.
16. Kubli F, Hon EH, Khazin AF, et al. Observations on heart rate and pH in the human fetus during labor. Am J Obstet Gynecol. 1969; 104:1190.
17. Myers RE, Mueller-Heubach E, Adamsons K. Predictability of the state of fetal oxygenation from a quantitative analysis of the components of late deceleration. Am J Obstet Gynecol. 1973; 115:1083.
18. Manseau P, Vaquier J, Chaviniu Y, et al. Le rhythme cardioque foetale "sinusoidal." J Obstet Gynecol Biol Rep. 1972; 1:343.
19. Kubli F, Ruttgers H, Haller U, et al. Die antepartale fetale Herz Frequenz II. Verhalten von Grundfrequenz, Fluktuation und Dezelerationen bei antepartalem Fruchttod. Z Geburtshilfe Perinatol. 1972; 176:309.
20. Baskett TF, Koh KS. Sinusoidal fetal heart rate pattern. A sign of fetal hypoxia. Obstet Gynecol 1974; 44:379.
21. Young BK, Katz M, Wilson SJ. Sinusoidal fetal heart rate I. Clinical significance. Am J Obstet Gynecol. 1980; 136:587.
22. Katz M, Wilson SJ, Young BK. Sinusoidal fetal heart rate II. Continuous tissue pH studies. Am J Obstet Gynecol. 136:594.
23. Cibils LA. Clinical significance of fetal heart rate patterns during labor. V. Variable decelerations. Am J Obstet Gynecol. 1978; 132:791.
24. Tejani NA, Mann LI, Sanghavi M, et al. The association of umbilical cord complications and variable deceleration with acid base findings. Obstet Gynecol. 1977; 49:159.
25. Young BK, Katz M, Wilson SJ. Fetal blood and tissue pH with variable deceleration patterns. Obstet Gynecol. 1980; 56:170.
26. Press release. National Center for Health Services Research, U.S. Department of Health, Education and Welfare, December 3, 1978.
27. Study finds risk in using electronic fetal monitors. Newsday, December 3, 1978.
28. Banta HD, Thacker SB. Costs and benefits of electronic fetal monitoring: A review of the literature. Washington, D.C.: U.S. Department of Health, Education, and Welfare. December 1978.
29. Neutra RB, Fienberg SE, Greenland S, et al. The effect of fetal monitoring on neonatal death rates. N Engl J Med 1978; 299:324–26.
30. Wood C. Gluck L ed. In: Intrauterine Asphyxia and the Developing Fetal Brain. Chicago: Year Book Medical Publishers, 1976.

31. III. Predictors of intrapartum fetal distress. In: Antenatal Diagnosis. Washington, D.C.: U.S. Department of Health, Education and Welfare. National Institutes of Health Publication No. 79-1973, April 1979.
32. Benson RC, Shubeck F, Deutschberger J, et al. Fetal heart rate as a predictor of fetal distress. Obstet Gynecol. 1968; 32:259–266.
33. Walker N. The case for conservatism in management of fetal distress. Br Med J. 1959; 2:1221–1226.

F.XIII

Intrauterine Dysrhythmias

Norbert Gleicher, MD, and Uri Elkayam, MD

I. INTRODUCTION

Cardiac dysrhythmias, including irregularities of the heart beat and disturbances of heart rate and conduction, may occur in utero in much the same way that they occur after birth.[1] The obvious impediments to attaining access to the fetus in utero, however, make diagnostic evaluations more difficult and lead to a delay in the application of commonly accepted medical procedures such as obtaining ECGs.

While the fetal heart rate, monitored by a variety of intrauterine and external monitoring devices, has been recognized as an important diagnostic tool in the perinatal follow-up of the fetus, more sophisticated evaluations of the fetal ECG have been performed in increasing numbers only recently. Normal and abnormal fetal heart rates are discussed in Chapter F.XII. The present chapter is restricted to the diagnosis and clinical relevance of intrauterine dysrhythmias.

II. THE FETAL ELECTROCARDIOGRAM

As noted in Chapters F.IX and F.XI a "fetal electrocardiogram" may be obtained by either external or internal means. The former in most instances do not provide a true ECG but represent the ultrasonic recognition of a moving portion of the fetal heart, frequently the mitral valve. In those instances a mildly M-shaped complex may be obtained, similar both to a regular QRS complex of an ECG and to the fairly typical echocardiographic picture of a mitral valve (Fig. F.XIII.1). With modern and sophisticated external fetal monitoring equipment, not only may a reliable fetal heart rate thus be obtained but also a representative picture for the cardiac cycle, at least concerning the timing of mitral valve motion. As mitral valve motion is relatively fixed within the typical cardiac cycle, the resulting external "ECG tracing," although not a true ECG, may provide reliable information about not only heart rate but also regu-

Cardiac Problems in Pregnancy, pages 535–564

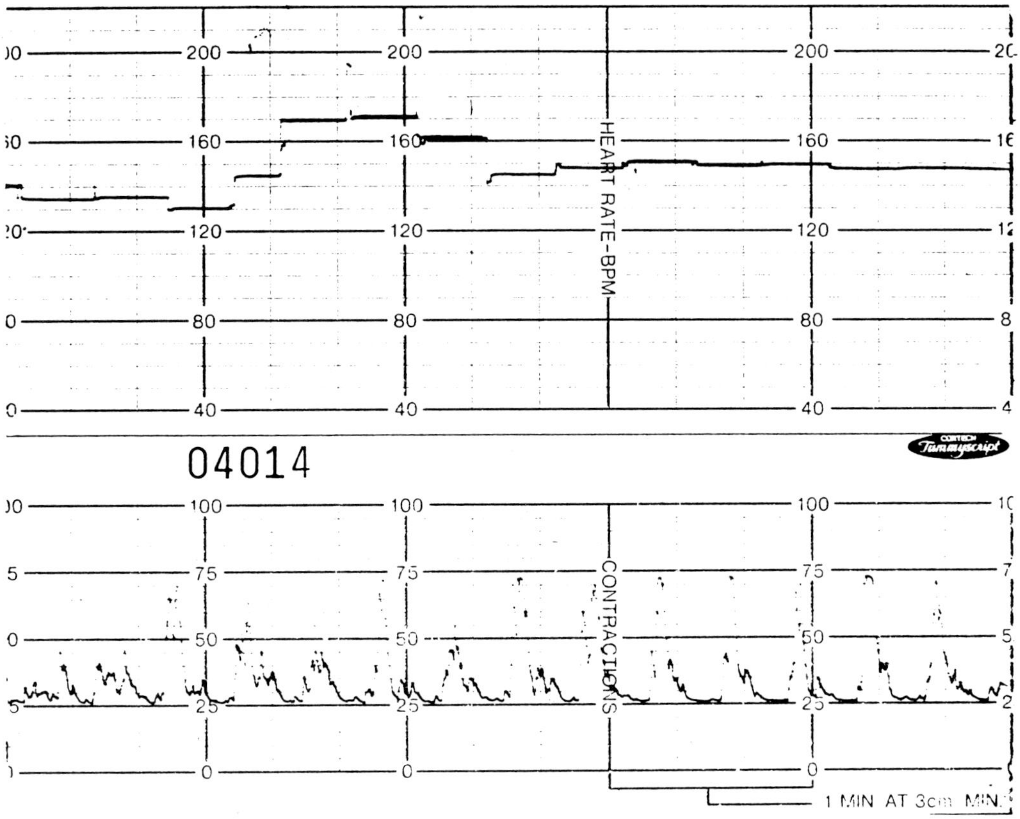

Fig. F.XIII.1. External fetal monitoring (Roche-Fetasonde®) M-shaped complexes on lower panel represent ultrasonic recognition of a moving fetal cardiac structure, most likely mitral valve. Upper panel represents beat-to-beat variability.

larity of heart rate, thus making the diagnosis of ectopic contractions and other heart rate irregularities feasible. However, utmost care should be taken to prevent overreading of externally obtained information. It must be recognized that external monitoring of this kind is, by far, more susceptible to artifacts, and therefore misinterpretation, than internal true ECG tracing, which will be discussed next. Moreover, as these tracings do not represent a real ECG tracing, no information other than rhythm-related information can be obtained, as may at times be derived from an internally obtained ECG. This is the reason why, in most of the illustrations in this chapter, special emphasis is placed on rate-related information.

Internally obtained ECGs of the fetus are derived from an internally attached electrode which, in accordance with Einthoven's original concept, records a fetal ECG in the form of a single lead. It is important to realize that only a single lead may be obtained, thus again severely restricting the use of the ECG for more sophisticated cardiac diagnosis than rhythm and rate disturbances. Only infrequently will such a single-lead ECG be adequate to make the unequivocal diagnosis of disturbances in conduction of the fetal heart. Even such simple evaluations as the estimation of the cardiac axis are impossible with a single-lead ECG. In fact, frequently the QRS complexes of the fetal ECG will be too small to allow accurate rhythm determinations. The repolarization of the maternal leg plate under such a circumstance may sometimes produce a larger QRS complex. However, the possibility of changing QRS size by such artificial means indicates that not many of the routine cardiac parameters that may be obtained from an ECG after birth will be available through an intrauterine ECG.

A prerequisite for an internal fetal ECG is rupture of fetal membranes. Consequently, a scalp electrode cannot and will not be attached to the fetus when rupture of membranes is medically contraindicated. In such instances an abdominal ECG (not to be confused with previously discussed external fetal monitoring based on the detection of cardiac motion by ultrasound) can be obtained. Under such circumstances, both maternal and fetal ECGs will be recorded on the same tracing. With appropriate axis conditions of the fetal heart, a fetal ECG tracing of adequate quality may be obtained (as a single lead) and may be clearly differentiated from maternal components. This technique is rarely used in clinical practice but has been used by a number of investigators (Fig. F.XIII.2).

The physical theory of the intrauterine ECG is discussed in detail in Chapter F. IX and is not repeated here. The purpose of this chapter is to demonstrate how, in spite of the severe restrictions to its use, a fetal ECG may be used as the major tool for the diagnosis and therapy of a large variety of intrauterine dysrhythmias. In a minority of instances, other noninvasive diagnostic modalities such as phonocardiography and echocardiography can be applied. Their use will be noted, with the appropriate indications, throughout this chapter.

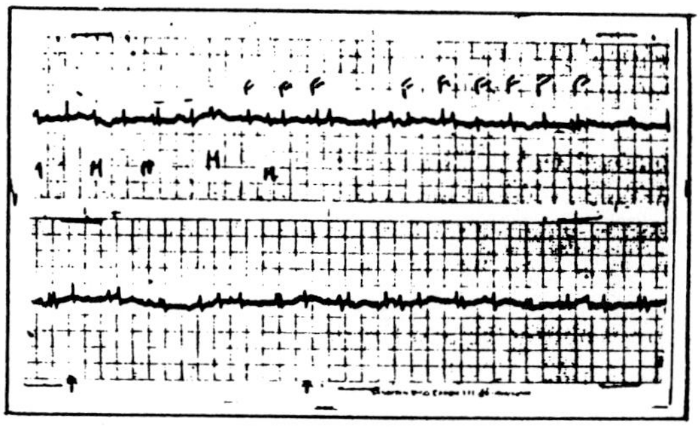

Fig. F.XIII.2. Abdominal ECG taken at 20 weeks gestation because of irregular heart rate. The upper tracing identifies the fetal complexes (F) and the maternal QRS complexes (M). The lower tracing at the arrows indicates two premature systoles with partial compensatory pauses. The relatively normal appearance of the QRS complex would indicate that it is of supraventricular origin. (From Shenker,[1] with permission of the author and the publisher.)

III. THE DIAGNOSIS OF INTRAUTERINE DYSRHYTHMIAS

Although fetal monitoring by electronic means has been in clinical use for more than a decade, only very recently have increasing numbers of intrauterine dysrhythmias been recognized and reported by a large number of different investigators. The late recognition of fetal arrhythmias as a rather frequent occurrence is due only in part to the more sophisticated monitoring equipment now at our disposition. The increased incidence of detection of intrauterine arrhythmias is probably more directly related to the efforts of observers to detect them. Although no studies have been reported confirming this belief, it has been our experience that the detection rate of intrauterine arrhythmias varies in proportion to the interest that hospital staff physicians show in these dysrhythmias. With staff physicians actively searching for intrauterine dysrhythmias for study purposes, short bursts of either tachy- or bradyarrhythmias were reported almost weekly on a labor floor with approximately 3,000 birth per year. An incidence of one per 50–100 patients in labor therefore does not seem exaggerated. Why, then, are intrauterine dysrhythmias still considered something of a curiosity?

The answer lies in the difficulty frequently involved in recognizing such dysrhythmias during routine external and/or internal monitoring. Dysrhythmias are frequently only shortlasting and therefore are considered artifacts or are overlooked. Otherwise, an abnormality of the fetal heart rate may be recognized; however, the necessary follow-up in obtaining a fetal ECG tracing may not occur, either because no adequate equipment is at the obstetrician's disposition or because the need for further work-up of the abnormal fetal heart rate is not recognized.

When, then, should a fetal ECG be obtained to rule out or confirm an intrauterine fetal dysrhythmia?

It was indicated in Chapter F.XII that the normal fetal heart rate changes with gestational age. A term infant has a normal heart rate between 120 and 160 bpm. Heart rates above 180 bpm should be considered suspicious for tachyarrhythmias; heart rates under 100 bpm should be viewed with suspicion until a bradyarrhythmia is ruled out. A large number of fetal arrhythmias will be identified with such a screening system; however, others will be missed, as the heart rate may be within the normal range and still be arrhythmic or dysrhythmic. Further recognition of heart rate or conduction abnormalities must rely on fetal ECGs or, as built into some monitoring apparatus, beat-to-beat variability recording. ECG abnormalities are discussed in more detail later. They are divided into the same subgroups as in the adult. Beat-to-beat monitoring is an unusual exercise in the adult and, therefore, it deserves some additional attention at this point.

The beat-to-beat variability monitoring capability and its clinical importance in the monitoring process of the fetus are discussed in detail in other chapters. The importance of beat-to-beat variability monitoring for the detection of intrauterine arrhythmias lies in its graphic representation of heart rate patterns that are more difficult to recognize in fetal ECGs. Thus, short bursts of fetal tachyarrhythmias may be lost in regular ECG tracings, either because of a wandering baseline of the fetal ECG or because of other artifacts of ECG monitoring. The beat-to-beat mon-

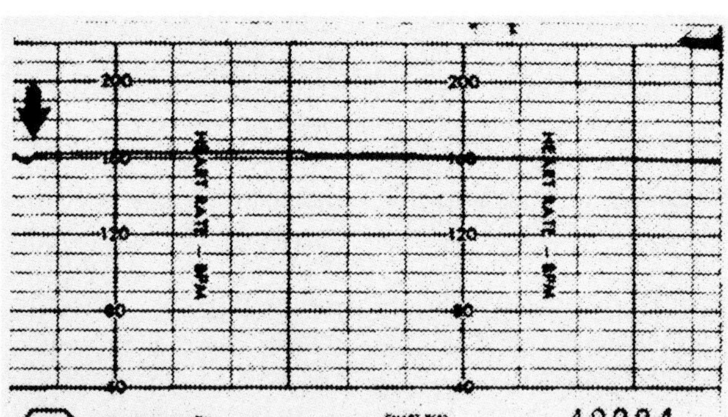

Fig. F.XIII.3. Intrapartum fetal monitoring with scalp electrode (Corometrics) attached. The lower panel demonstrates a wandering baseline which may prevent, in certain instances, the appropriate recording of the fetal heart rate. Small QRS complexes, representing the fetal ECG, are demonstrable. The upper panel represents the recording of the fetal heart rate, which in this tracing is approximately 160 bpm (arrow). Note the straight line, which indicates no beat-to-beat variability as otherwise a step-wise pattern would be seen (Roche-Fetal monitor).

itoring capability, which is based on the summation of the fetal heart rate during three cardiac cycles, may still be recordable and may present as a straight line (Fig. F.XIII.3), depending on the monitoring equipment employed. Even short bursts of tachyarrhythmias may thus be recognized.

In summary, if a rule were to be established for the obstetrician monitoring a fetus in utero, it would read: *"Push the ECG button whenever in doubt and check the beat-to-beat variability in order to get an accurate fetal heart rate."* Much of today's modern monitoring equipment records beat-to-beat variability at the upper panel of the monitoring strip whenever a direct fetal ECG is obtained in place of the routine fetal heart rate monitor strip. When this is the case, the beat-to-beat recording replaces the heart rate strip on the upper panel, while the fetal ECG recording replaces the uterine contraction recording on the lower panel (Fig. F.XIII.3). Variations of this arrangement may occur with different manufacturers and are of no significant importance if they simply represent placement differences of the varying recordings. No equipment, however, should be purchased that does not allow the monitoring and recording of fetal ECGs and beat-to-beat variability in graphic form. For more technical detail, see Chapter F.IX.

IV. SPECIFIC DYSRHYTHMIAS

A. Disorders of Rate and Rhythm

Most disorders of rate and rhythm that have been described after birth may be recognized in utero. However, limitations exist, and differences in the diagnosis of these disorders will be outlined by classifying them according to point of origin within the fetal heart.

The embryology of the developing conduction system is extensively reviewed in Chapter F.I. Pertinent to this chapter is a short recollection of the fact that the fetal conduction system is functionally "mature" by the 16th week of gestational life. At six weeks, a sinus node can be recognized, and by ten weeks it develops its own artery and is histologically almost identical to its adult counterpart. The major difference at this stage is a relative lack of collagen in the fetal node. The atrioventricular (A-V) node and the bundle of His originate separately but are united at approximately eight weeks gestational age. Their separate origin explains some of the congenital conduction disturbances, such as congenital heart block, which will be discussed later. The A-V node itself is completely formed by ten weeks gestational age.[2]

1. Derangements arising in the sinus node

a. Sinus bradycardia (Fig. F.XIII.4) In the adult, sinus bradycardia is defined as a slow but normal heart rate under 60 bpm with a normal spread of the atrial excitation. With the normal fetal heart rate defined as between 120 and 160 bpm, a diagnosis of sinus bradycardia can be made under 100 bpm. However, as in the adult, an ECG has to be obtained to confirm whether the excitation is originating in the sinus node and is normal in its spread throughout the atrium.

Whereas sinus bradycardia in the adult is sometimes a sign of excellent physical

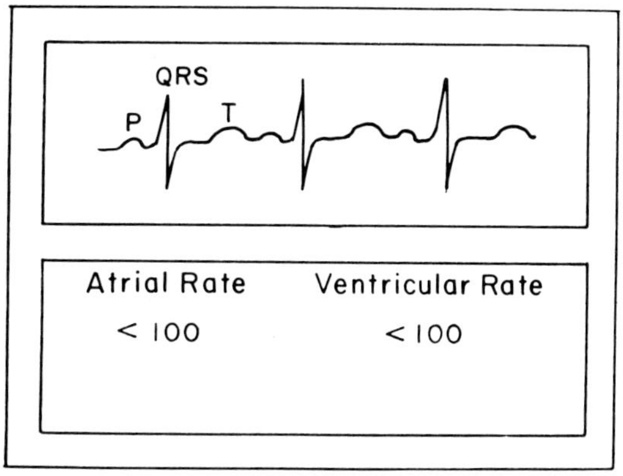

Fig. F.XIII.4. Sinus bradycardia.

fitness, as demonstrated by its frequent occurrence in athletes, in the fetus, its occurrence may be ominous. As discussed earlier, fetal heart rate has been used extensively in antepartum fetal evaluation. For more detail, see Chapter F.XII.

Even in the adult, not all sinus bradycardias are benign. Mainly in elderly patients, sinus bradycardias may be manifestations of sinus node dysfunction. In others, it may indicate latent or overt A-V conduction abnormalities, increased intracerebral pressure, myxedema, and hypothermia. In the fetus, only limited information is available concerning these causes. Among known causes of sinus bradycardia, the following have been reported in the literature: fetal head and umbilical cord compression, maternal hypotension, maternal seizures, maternal voiding, paracervical block anesthesia, and drugs such as propranolol and reserpine.[1,3–6]

In the fetus, it is also necessary to differentiate between "short-term" fetal heart rate deceleration and more "long-term" fetal bradycardia. Such a differentiation will not be difficult when the fetal heart rate remains under 100 bpm for more than a few minutes. A clear definition may be more difficult, however, when the fetal heart rate decelerates to under 100 bpm for a very limited time. It is the clinician's tendency to classify every fetal heart rate deceleration that lasts longer than one minute as "bradycardia." These "bradycardias" do, in fact, represent prolonged decelerations and have to be differentiated in their etiology from more classic sinus bradycardias, which may last for hours and may not have as ominous an implication as shorter-lasting ones.

Whenever a fetal heart rate under 100 bpm is recognized by either external or internal fetal monitoring, it is essential to obtain a fetal ECG. The differential diagnosis of sinus bradycardia includes heart block and blocked atrial ectopic beats.[7] It also should always be remembered that the maternal ECG may be transmitted through the fetus (Chapter F.IX). Under such circumstance, a situation may arise in which either external or internal fetal monitoring gives a picture indicative of persistent fetal sinus bradycardia (Fig. F.XIII.5). Even an intrauterine fetal ECG may transmit the picture of sinus bradycardia when, in fact, the fetus is dead and the maternal ECG is read as the fetal one. A number of such inci-

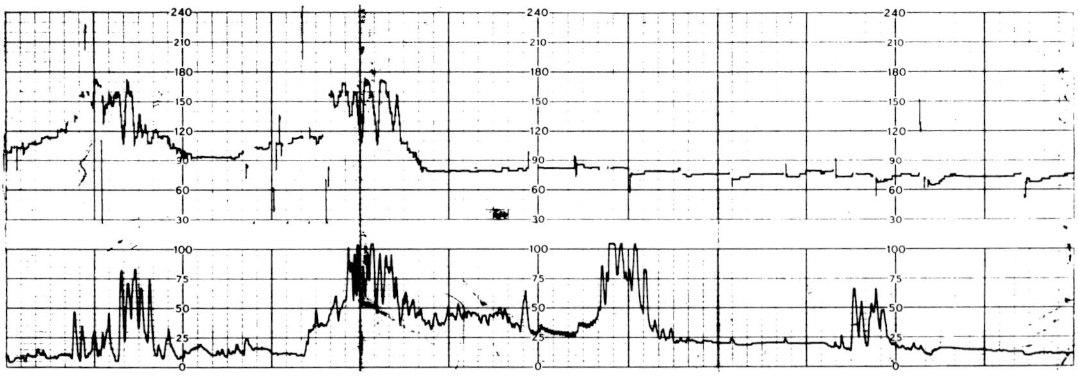

Fig. F.XIII.5. Terminal phase of fetal monitoring in fetus with sudden loss of fetal heart rate after uneventful pregnancy in a 27-year-old G1 PO at term. The preceding labor had been normal when, after three variable decelerations, a sudden persistent "bradycardia" of approximately 80 bpm occurred (upper panel). This heart rate turned out to correspond to the maternal rate, and fetal death was diagnosed. Shortly thereafter, a stillborn infant with multiple congenital abnormalities, including a large omphalocele, was delivered.

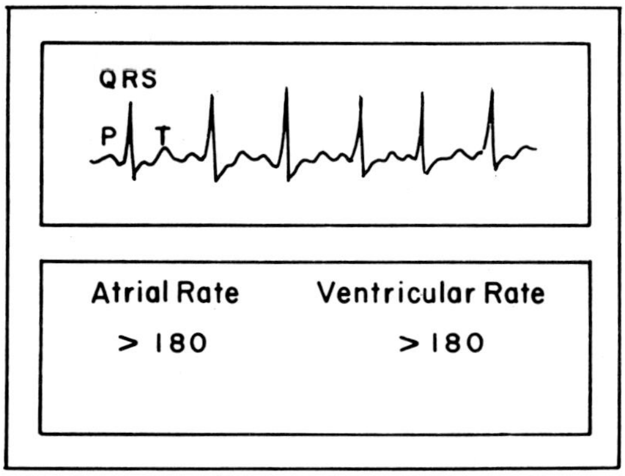

Fig. F.XIII.6. Sinus tachycardia.

dences have been reported in the literature and have, at times, presented as the basis for legal implications. It is therefore imperative to check the maternal heart rate against the fetal heart rate whenever a persistent fetal sinus bradycardia is recognized. Idially, simultaneous maternal and fetal ECGs should be obtained to rule out maternal transmission through the dead fetus.

b. Sinus tachycardia (Fig. F.XIII.6) Whereas in the adult tachycardia is defined as a sinus heart rate faster than 100 bpm, in the fetus sinus tachycardia is defined as a sinus initiated heart rate over 180 bpm. As with the adult, fetal sinus tachycardia must be distinguished from a number of different ectopic tachycardias. A clinical differentiation is important because the underlying condition causing sinus tachycardia, which is usually systemic, has to be treated, whereas in most ectopic tachycardias, a direct attempt at treatment of the heart can be made. In the adult, it has been stated that a rate less than 140 bpm favors the diagnosis of sinus tachycardia whereas a rate above 170 bpm is almost invariably caused by ectopic excitations.[8]

In the fetus, beat-to-beat variability will almost always be noticed and will remain in the range of 5–15 bpm.[1] Similar to sinus bradycardia, sinus tachycardia may occur in short bursts or as a persistent state. The type of tachycardia present frequently depends on the underlying cause. Among known causes of sinus tachycardia in the fetus, the following have been reported: cytomegalovirus disease, administration of drugs such as isoxsuprin, atropine, and scopolamine, maternal fever, amnionitis, early fetal hypoxia, and even maternal anxiety states.[1,9,10] Additional causes that can be extrapolated from the adult experience may include severe thyrotoxicosis, profound circulatory prolapse, and electrolyte imbalances. It is interesting to note that in the adult patient with severe advanced chronic airway disease, a sustained sinus tachycardia frequently can be observed. We reported the occurrence of sinus tachycardia in the fetus where the presumptive diagnosis of intrauterine meconium aspiration was made during labor (Fig. F.XIII.7).[11] It is tempting to speculate that in intrauterine meconium aspiration pathophysiologic mechanisms similar to those in the adult may cause the sinus tachycardia in the fetus.

The main differential diagnosis when sinus tachycardia is suspected is supraventricular tachycardia. It cannot be overemphasized, however, that whenever the presence of sinus tachycardia is observed in utero, an underlying cause must be searched for. It is especially noteworthy that sinus tachycardia may frequently be the first sign of amnionitis, long before the known occurrence of either fever or leukocytosis with a shift to the left.

c. Sinoatrial arrest In the adult, this is a rare derangement in the sinus node that is characterized by sporadic failure of the sinus node to generate an impulse. Consequently, a prolonged pause may be observed on the ECG between two P waves. Sinoatrial arrest may be caused in the adult by vagostimulation and vagostimulation occurs rather frequently in utero, so an ECG picture suggestive of sinoatrial arrest might be expected rather frequently in the fetus. However, an extensive review of the published literature and the per-

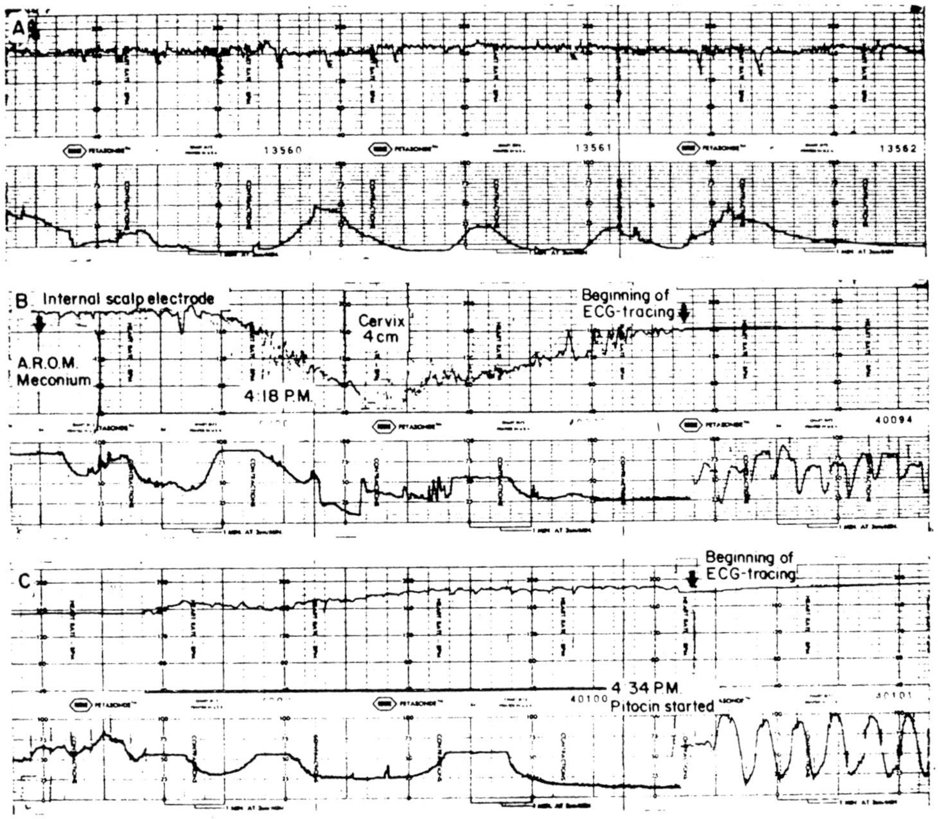

Fig. F.XIII.7. Intrauterine meconium aspiration: Fetal heart rate tracing: **A**) external monitor; **B**) internal scalp electrode placed; prolonged bradycardia after amniotomy; **C**) internal scalp electrode; slow rise of fetal heart rate to a sinus tachycardia of 180 bpm. In panels B and C, the mother was positioned on her left side. Uterine contractions were recorded by external monitor. The elevated baseline therefore does not represent an elevated resting pressure, but solely an artifact. (From Gleicher et al,[11] with permission of the publishers.)

sonal experience of the authors did not reveal a single incidence of sinoatrial arrest diagnosed in utero.

d. Sinus arrhythmia As in the adult, where this kind of dysrhythmia may be observed in almost all healthy young persons at rest, it represents a physiologic occurrence and indicates well-being of the fetus in utero. As noted earlier, the variation in a fetal heart rate is used extensively in fetal monitoring by evaluating the so-called beat-to-beat variability. This is discussed extensively in other chapters of the fetal section of this book and is not repeated here. It should, however, be noted at this point that beat-to-beat variability may be influenced by a large number of parameters, among which are drugs that the mother receives such as scopolamine, atropine, morphine derivatives, and other sedatives. It is also influenced by fetal stimulation, either by movement or by external stimulation. The latter observation is used in non-stress testing.

e. Sinoatrial block This dysrhythmia is characterized by the fact that a sinus impulse is generated; however, neither atrial nor ventricular depolarization occurs because the sinus impulse is prevented from reaching either atrium or ventricle. In the fetus, it is most frequently seen in cases of severe umbilical cord compression and may also be observed in instances of head compression. Fetal heart rate will drop significantly and may reach levels as low as 40–60 bpm. As a consequence of the blockage of the sinus impulse, the P-P interval of the ECG will be prolonged, most frequently to some multiple of the regular interval. If a sinoatrial Wenckebach exit block is present in addition, the ECG picture may be somewhat different; in such instances, the P-P interval may progressively and periodically shorten prior to a dropped P wave. Wenckebach blocks are discussed later under the section on abnormalities of conduction. Under the same heading, A-V blocks in general are reviewed in some detail. Sinoatrial blocks are only infrequently accompanied by an A-V block.

Although ECG changes thus may vary with associated conditions, a number of ECG abnormalities may be found rather consistently. Thus, the ECG will show either decreased amplitude of P waves or changes in the morphology of the P waves as the blockage of the sinus impulse leads to an arrest followed by an escape beat. These escape beats may originate anywhere along the atrial conduction pathway but most frequently will be nodal in origin. It will be obvious that these escape beats are essential in these situations and have to be considered life-saving until normal sinus excitation resumes.[1,8,12] The etiology of sinoatrial block in the fetus is still not completely understood. It is believed that strong parasympathetic input at the sinus node may result in sinoatrial blockage. As in the adult, hyperkalemia has been implicated; however, other associated etiologies in the adult such as drug therapy with digitalis and quinidine or acute myocardial damage have not been reported in the fetus.[1,8,9]

Frequently, an intrauterine ECG will not allow the unequivocal diagnosis of sinoatrial block because P wave changes cannot be adequately evaluated due to technical deficiencies. In such cases, all that can be noted are shorter or longer fetal heart rate decelerations that require obstetrical intervention. The mode of intervention, however, remains controversial. It is generally accepted, however, that whenever there is doubt, a fetal scalp pH should be obtained. If values are in the acidotic range (pH less than 7.25), immediate delivery is indicated. Some investigators, however, have suggested treating this dysrhythmia in utero with atropine. These investigators suggest that they succeed in increasing fetal cardiac output by inhibiting the parasympathetic input on the sinus node. Those who oppose pharmacologic intervention with atropine suggest that the slow rate reflects a protective reflex of the fetal heart and should not be changed.[4,13]

2. Derangements arising in the atrium

a. Ectopic atrial beats (Fig. F.XIII.8) This arrhythmia may represent the most frequent in utero arrhythmia. It has been estimated to occur with an incidence between 3 and 5% during labor.[14]

Premature atrial beats originate from an abnormal focus, which may lie anywhere within the atrium. In the adult, such ectopic atrial beats are generally considered benign but they may precede more serious cardiac dysrhythmias such

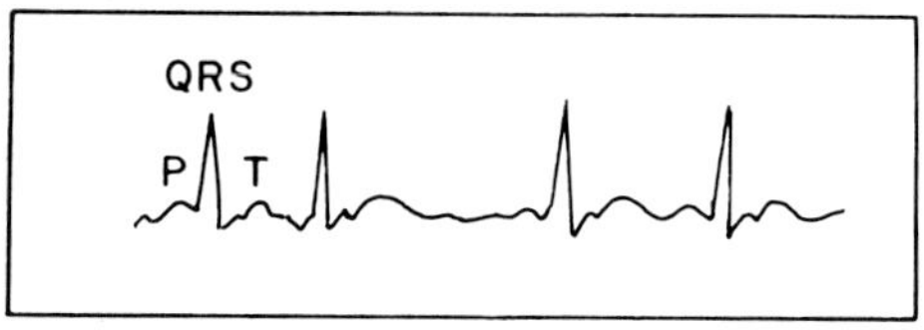

Atrial Rate	Ventricular Rate
Irregular and varying	Normal; following atrial excitation and therefore irregular

Fig. F.XIII.8. Ectopic atrial beats.

as atrial fibrillation or flutter or atrial tachycardia. By listening to the fetal heart, a situation may arise similar to the auscultation of the adult heart in that premature atrial beats may be confused with the significantly more serious ectopic ventricular beats. In most cases, it will be necessary to perform an ECG to differentiate between the two. On a purely statistical basis, in the majority of cases premature beats will be atrial in origin. However, because of the potential seriousness of ventricular ectopic beats, a clear differentiation between these two forms of ectopic excitation has to be made.

The classical sign of an atrial ectopic beat is a P wave preceding the QRS complex, which is usually normal both in configuration and duration. In the majority of cases, these P waves will occur prematurely and will be followed by an incomplete compensatory pause; thus the name "premature atrial beat." However, in a few cases, they may occur on time, and therefore the term "ectopic atrial beat" is generally preferred.[8] As noted, whenever ectopic atrial beats do occur prematurely, they are followed by incomplete compensatory pause (Fig. F.XIII.8). In some instances, the QRS complex may be distorted, both in amplitude and configuration. This will happen in association with an aberrant conduction through the cardiac conduction system. Under such conditions, the QRS complex looks wide and in most cases is similar to that seen with right bundle branch block. The differentiation between ectopic atrial beats and aberrant conduction from ventricular ectopic beats may be difficult and sometimes is impossible without the help of a His bundle electrocardiogram. The chance for aberrant conduction increases with an increase in prematurity of the ectopic atrial beat.[8]

As already noted, these arrhythmias represent the most frequently counted arrhythmias in the fetus. In general, the diagnosis should not be made unless confirmed by an internal fetal electrocardiogram or an abdominal electrocardiogram (Fig. F.XIII.2). Ectopic atrial beats have been described in the fetus before 20 weeks gestational age.[15] Also, as early as 1930, some authors described extrasystoles, which they identified by phonocardiographic techniques.[16] The total incidence of antepartum fetal heart rate arrhythmias at that time was estimated at approximately 10% (which represents an even higher number than the incidence recorded in our own experience). An increasing number of cases with ectopic atrial beats in the antepartum period has been reported ever since.[17–20] The consensus has been that ectopic atrial beats in the antepartum period represent a benign arrhythmia that usually will disappear during the first week of life in those neonates in whom extrasystoles were still detectable after birth. A number of cases have been reported in which ectopic atrial

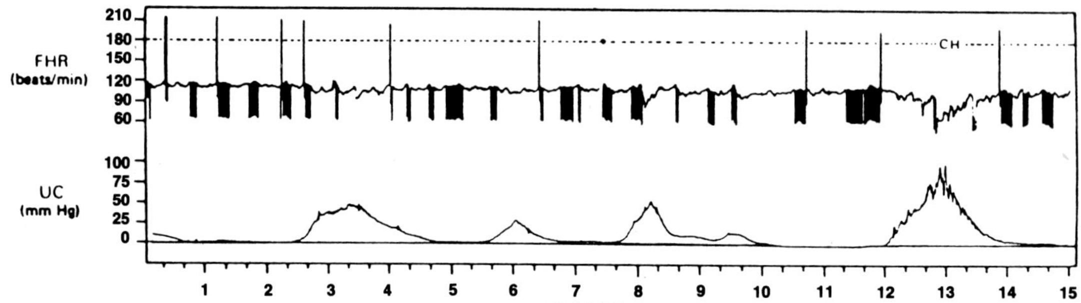

Fig. F.XIII.9. Direct fetal monitoring strip chart showing intermittent bursts of bigeminal rhythm. (From Sugarman et al,[23] with permission of the authors and the publisher.)

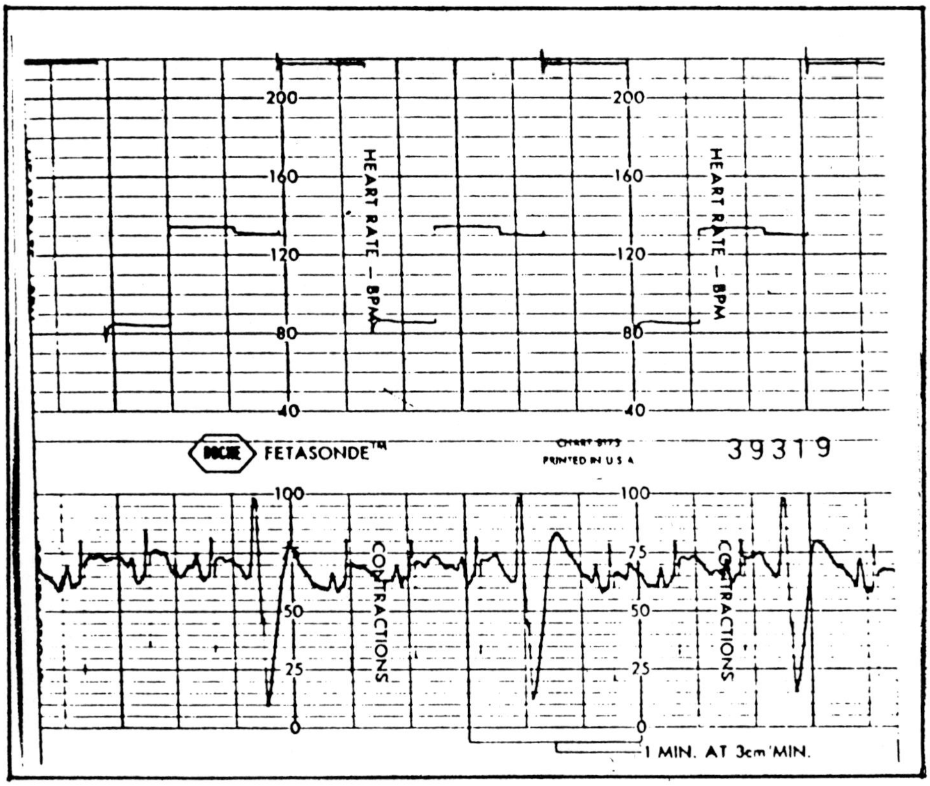

Fig. F.XIII.10. Fetal monitoring record at 25 mm/sec. Upper trace shows beat-to-beat FHR from the direct ECG obtained from the fetal scalp electrode during atrial trigeminy with ventricular extrasystoles. Three different heart rates are present. Lower trace clearly shows atrial trigeminy with ventricular extrasystoles by direct ECG. (From Young et al,[20] with permission of the authors and the publisher.)

beats occurred either in the form of a bigeminus or trigeminus (Figs. F.XIII.9 and F.XIII.10).[21–23] The terms "bigeminus" and "trigeminus" are used in the obstetrical literature in the context of atrial ectopic beats, but they should not be confused with the same terminology in association with ventricular ectopic beats, where the occurrence of bigeminus may have more significant clinical implications. It is generally believed that there is no increased incidence of congenital heart disease in fetuses with ectopic atrial beats unless such beats occur in association with other arrhythmias or unless fetal heart murmurs are detectable.[1,5] It should be noted, however, that single cases of supraventricular ectopic beats have been reported in association with severe fetal decompensation and even death.[24] The recognition of ectopic atrial beats should therefore not be considered alarming, but it should form the basis for a reevaluation of the pregnancy. It remains unknown whether the presence of ectopic atrial beats in the fetus may precede the onset of sustained atrial dysrhythmias such as atrial tachycardia, flutter, or fibrillation.

The diagnosis of ectopic atrial beats involves differentiation from ventricular ectopics. It should also be noted that when premature atrial beats are blocked, the diagnosis of complete heart block can be made erroneously.[6] The resulting fetal bradycardia may then falsely indicate fetal distress.[7]

b. Wandering atrial pacemaker In the discussion of sinoatrial block, we mentioned the occurrence of atrial escape beats. With a wandering atrial pacemaker, such escape beats occur because of an underlying sinus bradycardia. Pacemakers within the atrium and the A-V junction generate such escape beats. Consequently, the ECG will show a characteristic picture of late P waves, which may have varying forms, and varying PR intervals. Atrial fusion complexes may occasionally occur when QRS complexes overlap as a result of excitations in either the atria or the sinus or A-V nodes. In some instances, the pacemaker may "wander" through the atrium, starting out at the sinus node, and proceeding through the atrium to the A-V node and back again.[8] In adults, this is most often considered a benign disorder, but it may also occur as a sign of the sick sinus syndrome. Only one case has been reported in the literature that eventually could represent such an ECG pattern in the fetus.[23] Therefore, at this stage, no significant clinical importance can be attached to a wandering atrial pacemaker in the fetus. It should be reiterated, however, that escape beats, especially in association with sinoatrial block, do fulfill a life-preserving function.[1]

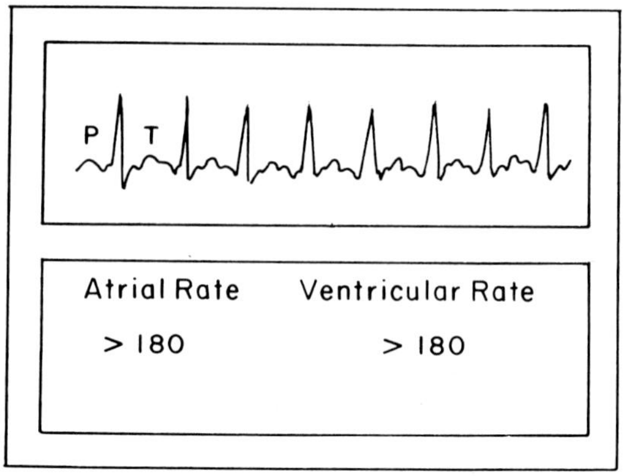

Fig. F.XIII.11. Paroxysmal supraventricular tachycardia.

c. Paroxysmal supraventricular tachycardia (Fig. F.XII.11) Although supraventricular tachycardia represents one of the most frequently diagnosed arrhythmias in the neonate, only 27 documented cases of supraventricular tachycardia have been reported in utero (Table F.XIII.1). In 1979 Shenker reviewed 19 of those cases.[1] Since then, seven additional cases have been reported, three from our own experience.[23,25–27]

In order to make the diagnosis, the ECG

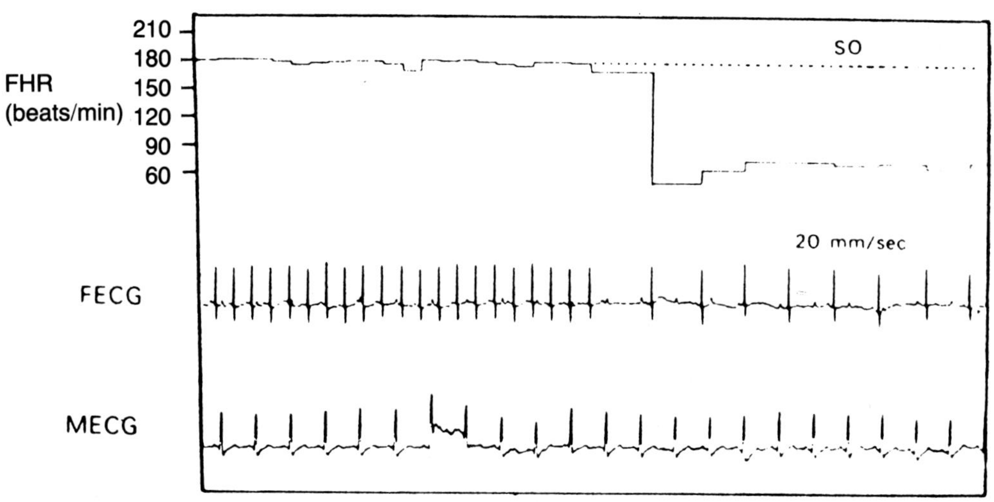

Fig. F.XIII.12. Direct fetal ECG showing spontaneous conversion from supraventricular tachycardia to sinus rhythm. (From Sugarman et al,[23] with permission of the authors and the publisher.)

has to show a rate of at least 180 bpm (Fig. F.XIII.12), but it will frequently show a rate significantly above 200 bpm (Fig. F.XIII.13).

Paroxysmal supraventricular tachycardia is classically called "paroxysmal atrial tachycardia." This name is derived from the fact that this dysrhythmia has been believed to be due to rapid discharges from an abnormal atrial pacemaker. More recent investigations indicate that frequently, although not in all instances, paroxysmal supraventricular tachycardia results from reciprocating rhythm; in

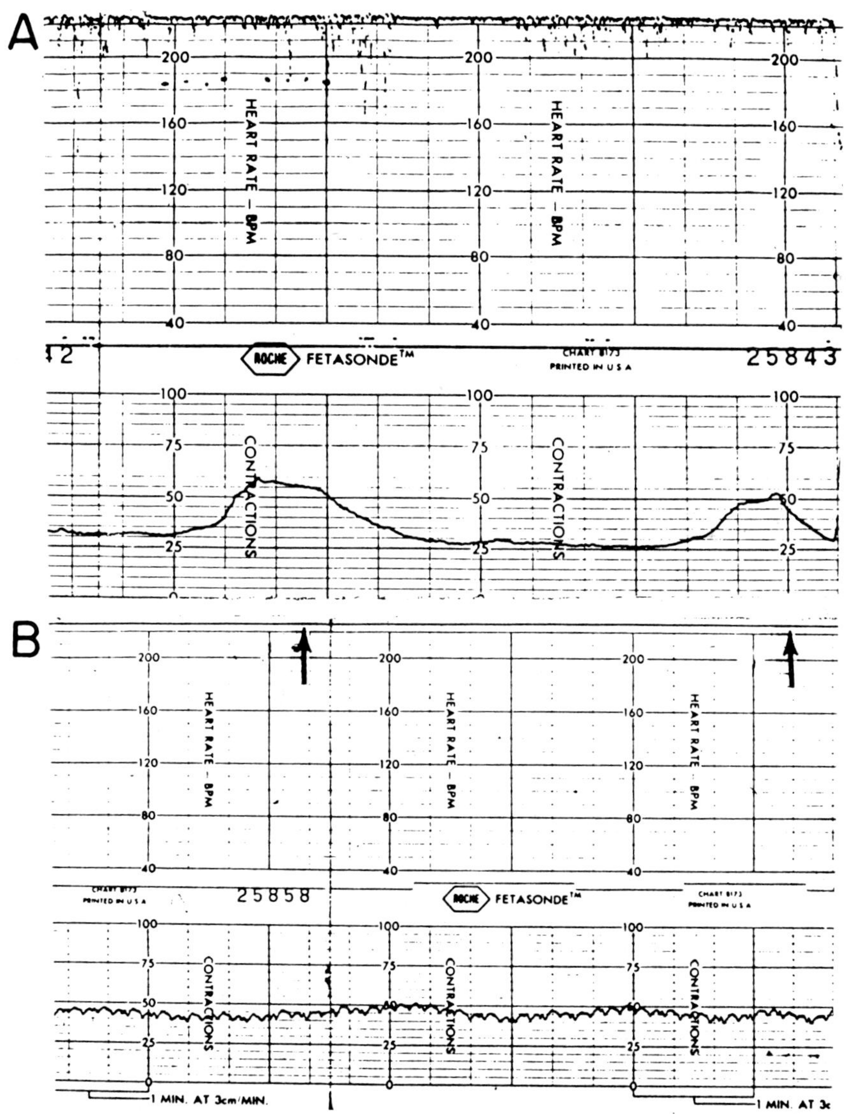

Fig. F.XIII.13. Supraventricular tachycardia in a fetus monitored with internal scalp electrode. **A**) A fetal heart rate of over 220 bpm can be seen on upper panel while the lower panel shows uterine contractions. **B**) The same fetus; the lower panel now exhibits the fetal ECG, indicative of supraventricular tachycardia, while the upper panel demonstrates the heart rate of above 220 bpm (arrows) and an absolute lack of beat-to-beat variability.

TABLE F.XIII.1. Supraventricular Tachycardia in Utero*

	Time of onset	Rate	Congestive failure	Congenital heart disease	No dysrhythmia after birth	Dysrhythmia disappeared at age	Postpartum therapy
1. Levkoff[31]	Labor	250	+	0		7 hours	Digitalis
2. Silber & Durnin[32]		240	+	0		10 days	Digitalis, quinidine
3. Tuxen et al[36]	Labor	260–280	0	0	+	?	—
4. Symonds[34]	Labor	190	+	0		7 days	Digitalis
5. Hedvall[37]	34 weeks	240	+	0		2 days	Digitalis
6. Hedvall[37]	38 weeks	240	+	0		1 day	Digitalis, diuretics
7. Hedvall[37]	36 weeks	250	+	0		1 day	Digitalis
8. Herin & Thoren[30]	Antenatal	160–200	+	0		?	Digitalis
9. Herin & Thoren[30]	Antenatal	140	+	0		Died[a]	Digitalis
10. Herin & Thoren[30]	Antenatal	180 (2:1 block)	0	0		?	Digitalis
11. Herin & Thoren[30]	Antenatal	100–180	0	0		nt?	—
12. Herin & Thoren[30]	Antenatal	200–250	+	+		Died[b]	Digitalis
13. Herin & Thoren[30]	Antenatal	120–200	+	+		Died[c]	Digitalis
14. Carretti et al[38]	Labor	300	0	0	+	8 hours	Atrial fibrillation
15. Klapholz et al[14]	Labor	180	0	0		Present 7 weeks	Paroxysmal tachycardia
16. Wildemeersch & Raven[35]	Labor	300–400	?	0		8 weeks	Digitalis

17. Jones[39]	Labor	200 (2:1 block)	0	0		Present 15 months	Digitalis
18. Hochberg et al[40]	Labor	300	0	0	+		Paroxysmal
19. Hughey & Elesh[41]	Labor	320	0	0		4 hours	
20. Newburger & Keane[25]	Antenatal	200–240	0	?		Died[d]	Digitalis, propranolol
21. Newburger & Keane[25]	36 weeks	240	+	WPW		4 days	Digitalis, diuretics
22. Sugarman et al[23]	Labor	250	0	0		4 minutes	Questionable if also antepartum
23. Wells et al[26]	Labor	200–220	+	0		Electric cardioversion, digitalis	
24. Klein et al[29]	28 weeks	140	+	WPW		4 days	Digitalis, propranolol
25. Chitkara et al[27]	35 weeks	220	+	WPW		Electric cardioversion	
26. Chitkara et al[27]	Labor	220	+	0	Flutter with variable block	10 hours	Digitalis, electric cardioversion
27. Chitkara et al[27]	30 weeks	240	+	WPW		10 hours	Digitalis, diuretics

[a]Ventricular fibrillation during cardiac catheterization.
[b]Eight weeks; necropsy—fibroelastosis.
[c]Necropsy—rhabdomyoma of heart.
[d]Died sudden death at five months after refractoriness of arrhythmia; "unusually shaped left atrial appendage."
*Modified from Shenker L: Fetal cardiac arrhythmias.[1]

other words, from sustained reentry of the excitation.[8] This concept is discussed in more detail in conjunction with the Wolff-Parkinson-White syndrome later in this chapter.

The clinical significance of supraventricular tachycardia may vary in importance. It is generally accepted that the vast majority of cases will be, similar to the adult experience, benign in nature. Also, the causes of supraventricular tachycardia will not be known in the majority of cases since most of the patients will not show any signs of organic heart disease after birth. However, also similar to the adult, a number of underlying causes should be considered. Thus, atrial septal defects, congenital mitral valve disease, and the Wolff-Parkinson-White syndrome should be considered.[8,28] We recently reported two fetuses who developed intrauterine supraventricular tachycardia and were found, after birth, to exhibit a Wolff-Parkinson-White syndrome.[28] A third and fourth case were reported by others,[25,29] thus establishing an incidence of four of 27 reported cases with intrauterine supraventricular tachycardia that were later found to have an underlying Wolff-Parkinson-White syndrome. The association between supraventricular tachycardia in the neonatal period and the Wolff-Parkinson-White syndrome was recognized earlier.[30] The association between Wolff-Parkinson-White and paroxysmal supraventricular tachycardia in utero seems therefore to be as well established as in the adult. Congenital heart disease, on the other hand, is, as may be seen from Table F.XIII.1, exceedingly rare as a cause of supraventricular tachycardia. The importance of atrial ectopic beats in the pathogenesis of idiopathic supraventricular tachycardia remains to be determined.

So what is, then, the clinical significance of supraventricular tachycardia in utero? It has become apparent that supraventricular tachycardia may occur in utero in two different ways: paroxysmal and short-lived, and persistent. Two factors appear most important for the eventual prognosis of the newborn. First, congenital heart disease in association with supraventricular tachycardia, which has been reported by Shenker to occur in 5–10% of cases,[1] is associated with high neonatal mortality. Second, the appearance of congestive cardiac failure, either in utero or in the neonate, may indicate an increase in neonatal morbidity. Intrauterine congestive heart failure is discussed in more detail in Chapter F.XIV. A few additional comments seem in place under the present heading, however. It is interesting to note that among the 19 cases that were reviewed by Shenker, seven of nine diagnosed in the antepartum period were found at birth to have varying degrees of congestive heart failure. In contrast, only three of ten cases that were first detected intrapartum showed congestive failure at birth. These findings indicate that prolonged presence of supraventricular tachycardia may predispose to intrauterine congestive heart failure. This notion is not shared by all investigators. Thus, some have clearly stated that supraventricular tachycardia by itself is not predictive of either the development or the severity of congestive heart failure in the newborn.[25,31] It is our belief, on the basis of published experience as well as our own,[27] that the duration of supraventricular tachycardia and the presence of a persistent pattern of supraventricular tachycardia determines whether congestive failure will or will not develop. We have speculated that the heart that is allowed to recover, with normal sinus rhythm patterns interposed between bouts of supraventricular tachycardia, has a lesser risk of failing than one that is subjected to persistent tachycardia over a prolonged period.[27] It has also been reported that the neonate who has had this dysrhythmia in utero will exhibit an increased birth weight, will have a heavier placenta, and will diurese more significantly during the first few days of life than neonates with normal heart rate.[1] All of these findings indicate that some degree of congestive heart failure may be present in the majority of cases of intrauterine supraventricular tachycardia. It has been suggested that supraventricular tachycardia in the fetus is better tolerated than in the newborn. The newborn, consequent to tachycardia, frequently develops significant heart failure. This is explained by the heavier load on the neonatal ventricles, which act in series and not in parallel as in the fetus.[1] It should be noted, however, that very severe fetal hydrops has been reported in association with antenatal supraventricular tachycardia.[29,32,33]

The management of the fetus with intrauterine supraventricular tachycardia will therefore be dependent on a number of observations. They include not only the diagnosis of the dysrhythmia but also such factors as duration and persistence of dysrhythmia and fetal condition. The latter will be evaluated by the parameters we use for routine fetal antepartum monitoring, such as non-stress testing, stress testing, ultrasonographic evaluation of the fetus for signs of scalp edema, ascites, and other signs of intrauterine congestive heart failure, intrauterine echocardiography, and fetal movements. The management of intrauterine congestive heart failure consequent to supraventricular tachycardia is discussed in more detail in Chapter F.XIV. Under the present heading, we will concentrate on some preliminary aspects of the clinical management of less severe cases of supraventricular tachycardia.

Until very recently, the general advice to obstetricians who recognize supraventricular tachycardias in utero had been to ignore it as a benign condition. More recently, however, a more aggressive approach to the fetus with recognized supraventricular tachycardia in utero has been suggested.[1,30] If supraventricular tachycardia is thought to cause overt congestive heart failure in almost all infants, then a more aggressive approach to management seems indicated. All cases will have to be individualized. Gestational age at the time of diagnosis and fetal maturity will play a significant part in the management of those infants. Assuming a term infant with proven lung maturity, it may be suggested to deliver the infant by the most appropriate means within a reasonably short time once supraventricular tachycardia is recognized. This advice will be followed by most clinicians without much hesitation if signs of impending intrauterine congestive heart failure can be found by any of the more sophisticated methods of intrauterine investigation already discussed. Such management will, however, seem more controversial when no such signs of fetal decompensation can be detected. This will be the case in most instances where supraventricular tachycardia appears for short periods only, interrupted by very long-lasting periods of normal sinus rhythm. It is still questionable if active management in these cases is indicated. Therefore, individualization has to remain the ground rule for successful management in every case. This approach will be found especially valid when supraventricular tachycardia occurs in a gestational stage at which the fetus is not expected to have mature lung function. At such a stage, delivery has to be evaluated and judged in reference to the risk for respiratory distress in the neonate. Again, a more aggressive approach will be indicated when signs of fetal decompensation and/or congestive heart failure can be found. However, more conservative management should be implemented when no such signs can be detected. It should always be recognized that the majority of fetuses with intrauterine supraventricular tachycardia will do well without aggressive management. However, the few who are in need of aggressive management will only be detected if each of the infants with supraventricular tachycardia enters a very rigorous investigative protocol. We have proposed such a protocol[27] requiring the following: A fetal electrocardiogram from maternal abdominal leads should be obtained whenever a fetal tachycardia over 180 bpm is noted. A fetal intrauterine echocardiogram will make it possible to rule out major congenital heart abnormalities. Serial sonographic investigations of the fetus at weekly intervals have to be performed to look for signs of congestive heart failure. These signs would include the presence of fetal ascites, fetal scalp edema, polyhydramnios, and an enlarged edematous placenta. In addition, a sonographic attempt can be made to look for an enlargement of the fetal heart and liver size. Treatment in utero will never be indicated unless fetal congestive heart failure is present at the gestational age at which delivery does not seem indicated due to severe lung prematurity. When delivery seems feasible and signs of congestive failure of the fetus are evident, delivery should be attempted by the most reasonable route. In cases with clearly established congestive heart failure in utero, it may be prudent to delivery the fetus by cesarean section in order to avoid the superimposed stress of labor on an already compromised fetus. All infants diagnosed in the antepartum period to exhibit supraventricular tachycardia should be cared for in an intensive neonatal care unit setting. Close observation of these infants is essential, as it is for all neonates who were found to have any kind of intrauterine dysrhythmia.

The role of supraventricular tachycardia in unexplained antepartum stillbirth is still highly controversial.[1] In the adult experience, supraventricular tachycardia rarely causes death. Extrapolating from that experience, a sudden death syndrome due to supraventricular tachycardia in utero seems highly unlikely. Although sudden death due to this dysrhythmia does not seem very likely, it has to be acknowledged that severe prolonged fetal congestive heart failure may lead to fetal decompensation as noted by any of the available fetal monitoring techniques. Interestingly, it has been suggested by one investigator that fetal acidosis in itself may contribute to fetal arrhythmias.[34]

In summary, supraventricular tachycardia in utero will, in the majority of cases, represent a benign condition. However, because of those few cases that may go on to a more serious fetal decompensation, close supervision of all cases is indicated. Intrauterine therapy, which is discussed in Chapter F.XIV, is not indicated unless signs of fetal decompensation are seen at the time where delivery seems contraindicated because of fetal immaturity. In all other instances, the fetus will remain under close observation in utero or will be delivered at that time in the most appropriate way.

d. Atrial tachycardia with block (Fig. F.XIII.14) This tachyarrhythmia resembles supraventricular tachycardia but has certain characteristics of atrial flutter. It resembles atrial flutter in the adult in that it responds to vagal stimulation, and it resembles supraventricular tachycardia in that its atrial rate is slower than that occurring in association with atrial flutter (usually between 120 and 250 bpm). The exact mechanisms by which it occurs are still unknown.[8] In the adult, this condition is frequently caused by either digitalis intoxication or potassium depletion. Both of these causes are highly unlikely in the fetus. This may be the reason why blocks in association with supraventricular tachycardia have been reported only twice.[30,35]

e. Atrial fibrillation (Fig. F.XIII.15) This dysrhythmia is probably underrecognized in utero.[1] The contraction of the atria is not defective and the A-V node, as well as

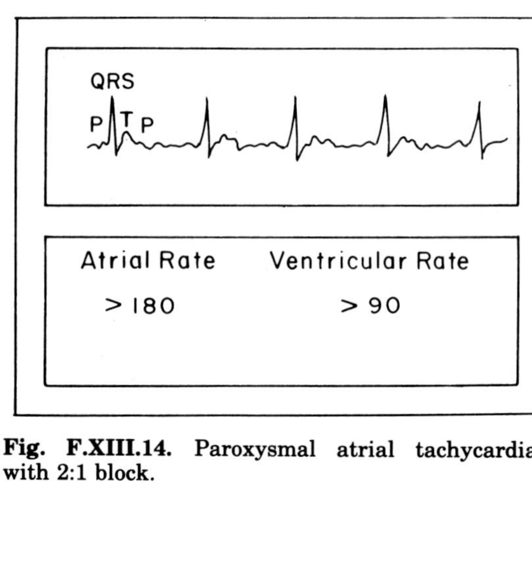

Fig. F.XIII.14. Paroxysmal atrial tachycardia with 2:1 block.

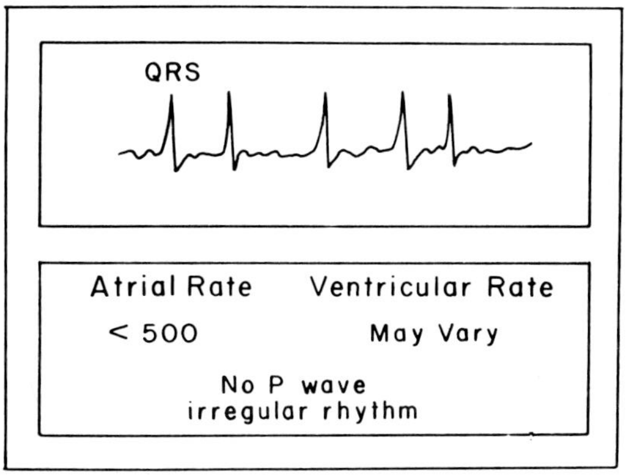

Fig. F.XIII.15. Atrial fibrillation.

the ventricles, is exposed to very rapid and very irregular stimuli from the atria. Consequently, many of these stimuli will be blocked at the A-V node, and others may pass through into the lower-lying conduction, resulting in rapid and irregular ventricular contractions. The clinical effect of atrial fibrillation will depend on the ventricular rate and the extent of the pulse deficit, which represents the proportion of ineffective and wasted ventricular beats.[8]

Only two cases of antepartum diagnosis of atrial fibrillation have been reported in the literature.[18,38] One of the infants also showed supraventricular tachycardia but did not require any neonatal therapy and did not exhibit any congenital heart disease.[38] The other, however, was diagnosed with Eisenmenger's syndrome and died soon after birth.[18]

The reported clinical experience with the intrapartum diagnosis of atrial fibrillation is therefore too small to allow any significant conclusions. It remains to be determined if an association with congenital heart disease will become apparent. Paroxysmal atrial fibrillation in the adult is most frequently seen in association with thyrotoxicosis, mitral stenosis, or in elderly persons with no obvious reasons.[8] Extrapolation to the fetal experience is impossible. However, a possible association with thyrotoxicosis or congenital mitral stenosis deserves further investigation.

The diagnosis is difficult to make and necessitates in all instances a fetal electrocardiogram. On simple heart rate auscultation, similar to the adult experience, atrial fibrillation with a normal ventricular rate, or at slightly increased ventricular rate, can easily be misdiagnosed as sinus rhythm with numerous extrasystoles. The diagnosis is especially difficult in the fetus because a heart rate of 120, considered to represent tachycardia in the adult, is normal. Thus, the diagnosis should never be made unless clear documentation with a fetal ECG can be obtained.

f. Atrial flutter (Fig. F.XIII.16). In the adult, atrial flutter is less common than atrial fibrillation. In the fetal experience, however, slightly more cases of atrial flutter have been reported than cases of atrial fibrillation.[1,25,31,34,42,43] The total of only seven reported cases to date clearly indicates the underreporting of this condition, as only half of all cases that are recognized in the neonatal period are recognized in one form or the other during the antepartum period.[44]

The mechanism of this dysrhythmia is still poorly understood and highly controversial. At present, the most likely mechanism is believed to be a reciprocating rhythm or circus current movement. The atria, in contrast to atrial fibrillation, contract at a rate of 250–350 bpm in the ma-

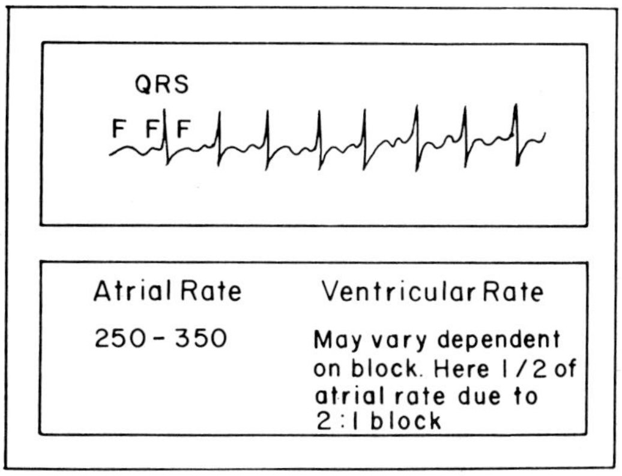

Fig. F.XIII.16. Atrial flutter.

jority of cases. An accompanying A-V block is almost always present, and its ratio usually follows even numbers. Consequently, the ventricular rate will be in the range of approximately 150 bpm or 75 bpm, depending on whether a 2:1 or a 4:1 block is present. However, the ventricular rate does not necessarily have to follow that rule. On occasion, two sites of block may occur at the A-V junction. For example a high junction 2:1 and a lower 3:2 block may exist and result in a ventricular rate that is not a constant multiple of the atrial rate. An additional variance occurs when the A-V block is constant but does not exhibit even-numbered atrioventricular ratios but rather odd-numbered ones such as 3:1, 5:1, etc. In such circumstances, ectopic ventricular beats with concealed retrograde conduction and antegrade A-V block have to be suspected.[8]

As in cases of atrial fibrillation, an ECG is essential for the accurate diagnosis of atrial flutter. This may be obtained either abdominally from the mother or through a scalp lead electrocardiogram. With a variable A-V block, an irregularity of the heart rate will be detectable by auscultation alone. However, with a fixed degree of block, the fetal heart rate may be regular and in the normal range for term pregnancy, and the abnormality may thus be easily overlooked.

Among the seven reported cases of atrial flutter diagnosed in the antepartum period, one was found to have congenital heart disease, namely tetralogy of Fallot.[42] One other case was found to be hydropic at birth.[43] Among the survivors, most neonates required intensive therapy, which included either pharmacologic cardioversion with digitalis or electric cardioversion. One infant was found to be acidotic at birth.[31] In addition to these seven cases that have been summarized by Shenker,[1] our own experience includes two cases with short bouts of atrial flutter, which were diagnosed in the antepartum period. Both cases represented infants who showed prolonged periods of intermittent supraventricular tachycardia that was interrupted by very brief episodes of atrial flutter. One of the infants also exhibited flutter in the neonatal period (Table F.XIII.1) and required both digitalis therapy and electric cardioversion.[27]

The experience with atrial flutter in the antepartum period is still very limited. Its clinical significance in the antepartum period therefore remains to be determined. Shenker, however, has suggested that atrial flutter may represent a potentially serious arrhythmia.[1] As evidenced by one case, atrial flutter can cause intrauterine congestive heart failure and result in fetal hydrops.[44]

g. Complex atrial dysrhythmias A number of additional, more complex atrial dysrhythmias have been reported in adults, but not as yet in the fetus. These include multifocal atrial tachycardia (MAT), sick sinus syndrome associated arrhythmias, chaotic atrial mechanism, and repetitive paroxysmal tachycardia. Only the last may have some relevance to intrauterine diagnosis in the near future. Repetitive paroxysmal tachycardia is a dysrhythmia that frequently appears in childhood (Parkinson-Pap syndrome) where it is characterized by a large number of brief bursts of tachycardia interspersed with brief episodes of sinus rhythm and multiple atrial premature beats. The brief bursts of tachycardia are most frequently paroxysmal supraventricular tachycardia, atrial fibrillation, or atrial flutter.[8] We noted earlier that we have seen patients who had different forms of supraventricular tachycardias diagnosed in utero. Similar observations have been reported by others. With a syndrome representing a dysrhythmia that mainly appears in childhood, it would not be surprising to see some cases of it occurring in utero.

3. Derangements arising in the A-V junction

These dysrhythmias refer to excitations that originate in the A-V junction, which includes fibers that are close to the A-V node in the lower right atrium, the A-V node, and the His bundle. Dysrhythmias that may originate in the area include ectopic junctional beats and A-V junctional tachycardias, which may be of *three* types: idiojunctional tachycardia (ventricular rate 100–140 bpm), paroxysmal A-V junctional tachycardia (ventricular rate 140–200 bpm), and A-V junctional rhythm, an escape mechanism that occurs when sinus impulses do not arrive at the A-V junction because of the sinus node dysfunction (ventricular rate 40–60 bpm). Intrauterine fetal electrocardiography has not yet achieved the capacity to describe electrocardiographic patterns of such sophistication. It is, however, expected that with progressive knowledge and recording of fetal intrauterine electrocardiograms, these patterns will sooner or later be recognized.

4. Derangements arising in the ventricles

a. Ectopic ventricular beats (Fig. F.XIII.17) In the adult patient, ventricular ectopic beats are relatively more frequent in patients with structural heart disease than are ectopic atrial beats. However, because they are so common in normal healthy adults, their presence rarely has any clinical significance unless accompanied by additional very specific findings.[8] Although the intrauterine fetal experience is still very limited, a similar statement can be made about the clinical significance of premature ventricular ectopic beats in utero. Shenker summarized 16 reported cases in 1979.[17,18,45–47] Since then, one additional case has been reported.[23] All of these cases took an uneventful course and did not exhibit long-term sequelae after delivery. The only case of associated neonatal death was also associated with complete congenital fetal heart block.[48] Thus, in summary, it may be stated that, like atrial ectopic beats, the ventricular ectopic beat is probably benign in most instances. It should, however, result in a reevaluation of the pregnancy. It must be assumed that the small number of reported cases is due to underreporting and underrecognition of this condition in utero.

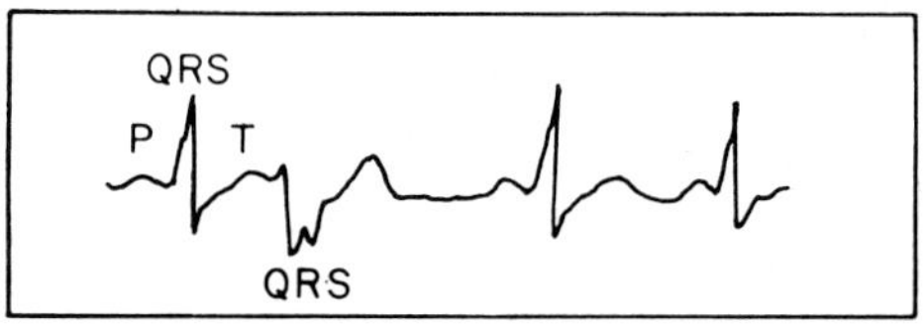

Atrial Rate	Ventricular Rate
Varies, dependent on ventricular impulses	Grossly normal but irregular

Fig. F.XIII.17. Ectopic ventricular beats.

b. Bigeminal rhythm Bigeminal rhythm is characterized by the prematurity of every alternate beat. Shenker states that ventricular premature systoles may cause bigeminy and trigeminy.[1] What he probably means is that there is a theoretical possibility as no ventricular case of either bigeminus or trigeminus in utero has been reported. As noted earlier, cases of associated supraventricular and ventricular extrasystoles that gave the picture of trigeminy have been reported. It should, however, be reiterated that the term "bigeminal rhythm," if applied in association with ventricular ectopic beats, possesses a different meaning than in association with atrial ectopic beats. After birth, "bigeminus" and "trigeminus" are terms reserved for ventricular ectopy. The obstetrical literature has made wide use of those terms in association with atrial ectopic beats. A clear differentiation, however, must be made as ventricular premature beats in true bigeminal or trigeminal fashion may have different clinical significance than similarly appearing atrial beats. In the adult, bigeminy has been associated with electrical instability of the ectopic pacemaker during repolarization, reentry, and enhancement of spontaneous depolarization of the ectopic pacemaker by the preceding beat.[8]

c. Ventricular tachycardia (Fig. F.XIII.18) In the adult experience, this dysrhythmia will be found significantly less frequently than its atrial counterpart. However, it must be noted that if it occurs, the clinical implications are far more serious.

Ventricular tachycardia is defined as three or more consecutive ventricular premature beats. Until very recently, only one case was reported in the literature.[49] Shenker added two cases of antepartum diagnosis of ventricular tachycardia to the published experience.[1] Since his report, one additional case has been reported,[20] increasing the total published experience to four cases. One of the cases reported by Shenker died at age 12 hours with a ventricular and atrial septal defect and bilateral hydronephrosis. The other case showed no evidence of congenital abnormalities, and the neonate improved after treatment with propranolol for ventricular premature contractions in the neonatal period.[1] The most recently reported case had a completely uneventful postpartum course and showed no abnormalities.[20] The experience with ventricular tachycardia in the antepartum period is, therefore, still limited. It would seem premature to come to any conclusions concerning the clinical implications of ventricular tachycardia in the antepartum period. It may, however, be stated, as with other intrauterine dysrhythmias, that the general principle should be upheld which suggests that the occurrence of any kind of intrauterine dysrhythmia should result in a reevaluation of the pregnancy. The dysrhythmia by itself should not be the basis for intervention. The association of the dysrhythmia with additional abnormalities may, however, form the basis for a change in management.

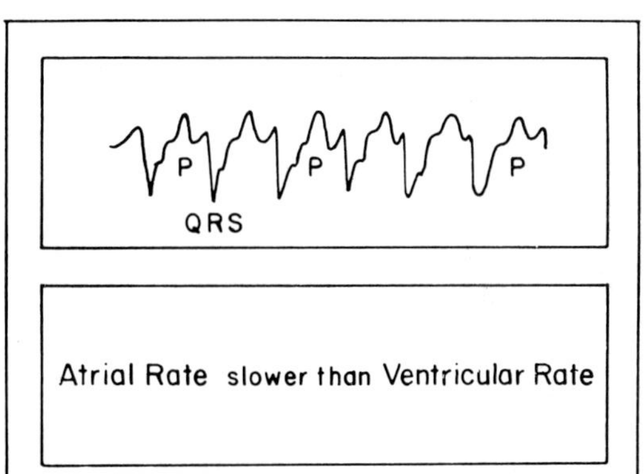

Fig. F.XIII.18. Ventricular tachycardia.

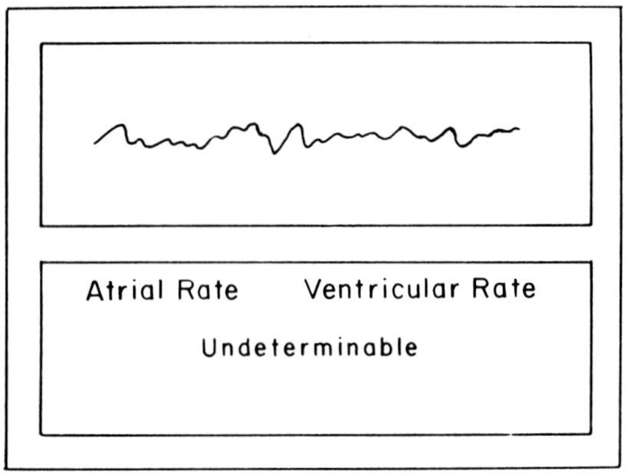

Fig. F.XIII.19. Ventricular fibrillation.

d. Ventricular fibrillation (Fig. F.XIII.19) Ventricular fibrillation lasting for longer than a few seconds is synonomous with instant death. Treatment in utero therefore does not seem possible even if the condition is recognized. To our knowledge, no case of ventricular fibrillation in a fetus has been reported. It remains to be determined however, if that is so because ventricular fibrillation does not occur in utero or because it has not been recognized and recorded. It is tempting to speculate that some of the unexplained death in utero may be due to this kind of dysrhythmia.

5. A-V dissociation

The name of this dysrhythmia already indicates that both atria and ventricles contract following two independent pacemakers. There are basically two different forms of A-V dissociation possible: the first, A-V dissociation with heart block, is caused by an excitation of a pacemaker in the A-V junction or the Purkinje system because all the impulses from the sinoatrial node or the atria are blocked in the area of the A-V conduction system. Contrary to that, A-V dissociation does occur without an antegrade block in the second type, called A-V dissociation due to interference. In this second form of A-V dissociation, the automaticity of the A-V junction or the ventricle exceeds that of the supraventricular pacemaker.[8]

The antepartum diagnosis of A-V dissociation was made for the first time in 1975.[50] The two cases reported by Platt and associates indicate the difficulties in reaching this diagnosis in utero. In the first case, the diagnosis was not made by abdominal or intrauterine fetal electrocardiogram but by demonstrating a different contraction rate of atria and ventricles by ultrasonography. Sonography was performed because fetal bradycardia of 60–80 bpm was recognized in the antepartum period. This infant was delivered by cesarean section because of obstetrical indications and was found to have multiple congenital abnormalities that were incompatible with life, including a persistent left superior vena cava, partial anomalous pulmonary venous return, a single atrium, mitral atresia, hypoplastic left ventricle, high muscular membrane with ventricular septal defect, and an overriding aorta. The pattern was considered consistent with the polysplenia syndrome. In the second case, the diagnosis was also made because of fetal bradycardia of 50 bpm. Real-time ultrasonography confirmed cardiac dynamics that suggested complete A-V dissociation. At term, simultaneous maternal and fetal ECGs confirmed the diagnosis. After a normal delivery, the infant became septic on day three of life, went into congestive heart failure, and died. No congenital abnormalities of the heart were detected on postmortem examination. Interestingly, this fetus also showed multiple ventricular ectopic beats both antepartum and postpartum. Because of the associated abnormality of A-V dissociation, this case was not included in our discussion of ventricular ectopic beats.

A-V dissociation thus represents an atrio-ventricular interruption of conduction, which in turn represents an abnormality of excitation. This is to be differentiated from heart block, which is discussed under the next heading, and which is characterized by the fact that the wave of excitation from the atria is either delayed pathologically or blocked at the junctional tissues represented by the A-V node and His bundle.[8]

B. Abnormalities of conduction

1. A-V block

The PR interval in an ECG represents the time that it takes for the excitation to pass through the atrium, the A-V node, the His bundle, and the bundle branches. In the adult, the PR interval should not exceed 0.2 seconds. In children, the PR interval is somewhat shortened, and in the fetus it has been only unsatisfactorily defined but seems, as discussed in other chapters, to be dependent on gestational age, similar to other fixed intervals in the fetal ECG. Heart block or atrioventricular block may exist in one of three forms: first-degree A-V block, second-degree (partial) A-V block, or third-degree (complete) A-V block.

a. First-degree A-V block (Fig. F.XIII.20) This is defined as a PR inter-

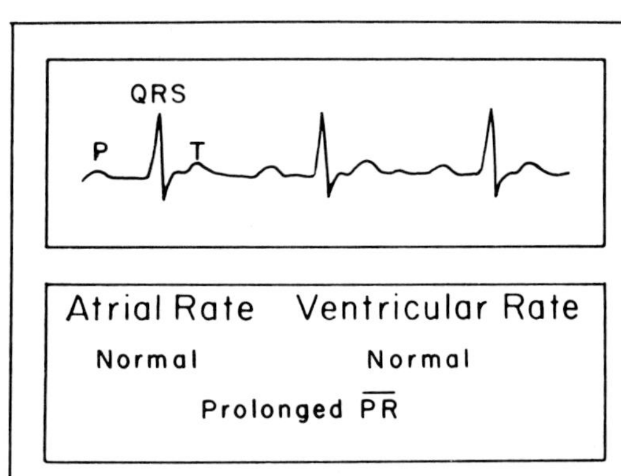

Fig. F.XIII.20. First-degree A-V block.

val that exceeds the normal duration. It is essential that all atrial beats be followed by ventricular beats, thus indicating normal (even if delayed) progression of the excitation from the atria toward the ventricles. This form of A-V block is usually caused by impaired conduction in the A-V junction but may also be due to a trifascicular block. The latter is rare.

Surprisingly, no case of first-degree heart block has been reported in the fetus. As first-degree heart block may be recognized in the neonatal period, it must be assumed that the condition has been overlooked and is clearly underdiagnosed.

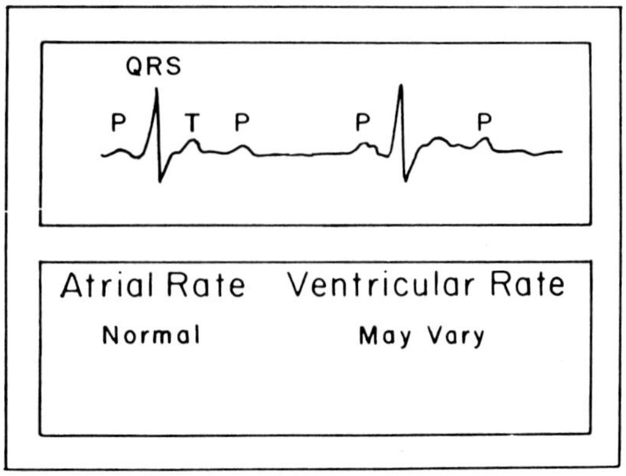

Fig. F.XIII.22. Mobitz type I (Wenkebach) block.

b. Second-degree (partial) A-V block (Fig. F.XIII.21) Second-degree A-V block is characterized by the fact that, intermittently, atrial impulses are not capable of penetrating the conduction system and therefore do not excite the ventricles. This form of A-V block can appear in two forms: Mobitz type I block (Wenkebach block) and Mobitz type II block.

Wenkebach block (Fig. F.XIII.22) is defined by an increasing PR interval. Finally, an atrium-derived impulse will be completely blocked, resulting in nonoccurrence of the corresponding ventricular beat. In the majority of cases, but not always, His bundle studies have shown an impaired conduction proximal to the His bundle.[8] In the adult, Wenkebach block frequently appears in association with heightened vagal tone, or it may occur spontaneously. Other etiologies include drug therapy such as with morphine and digitalis. In general, a Mobitz type I block is considered benign if not associated with other known pathology and will be transient in the majority of cases.[8] Figure F.XIII.23 demonstrates a Wenkebach block recognized in the immediate neonatal period in a viable male delivered after uneventful labor.

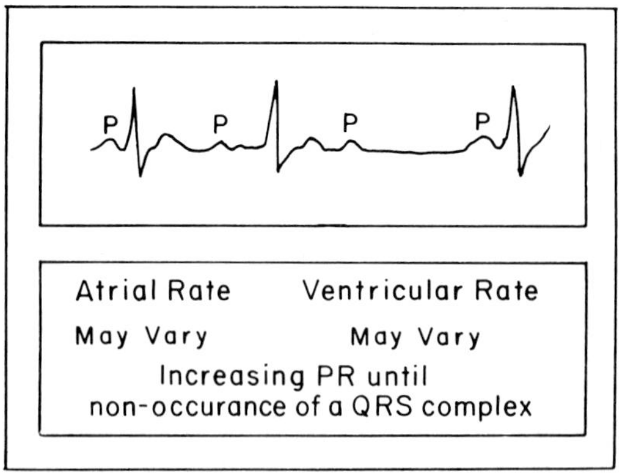

Fig. F.XIII.21. Second-degree (partial) A-V block.

Mobitz type II block is considered a more serious disorder in the adult. In the fetal experience, this is the kind of second-degree A-V block that will be present in most fetuses with very rapid atrial rates, as may be observed in supraventricular tachycardia.[1] This form of second-degree A-V block is characterized by a normal or increased PR interval, which is fixed except when beats are dropped. Contrary to Mobitz type I, where the QRS duration is usually normal, the QRS in Mobitz type II block may be prolonged. Complexes may exhibit bizarre patterns, similar to those discussed under bundle branch block. Varying forms of block, either 2:1, 3:1, 4:1, or irregular ratios may occur.[8] The origin of Mobitz type II block is usually in either the His bundle or a trifascicular block.

Only six cases of second-degree block in utero have been reported.[8,51]

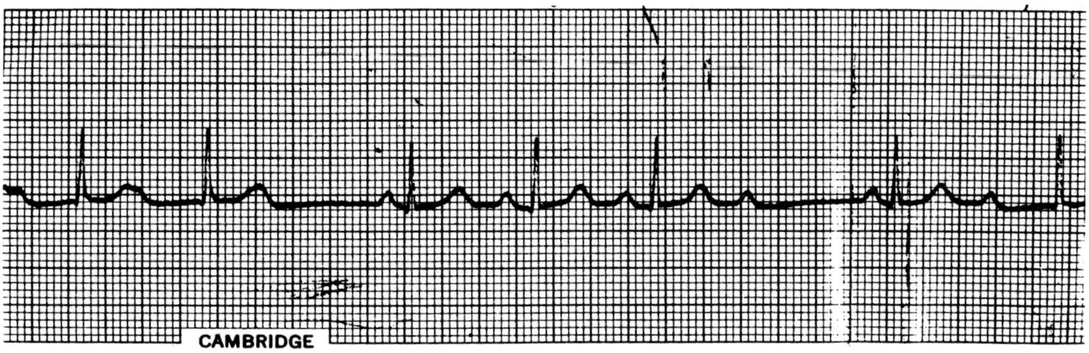

Fig. F.XIII.23. Wenkebach block diagnosed in a viable male infant shortly after delivery. Maternal history was negative and labor had been uneventful.

c. Third-degree (complete) A-V block (Fig. F.XIII.24) This form of A-V block represents the most frequently diagnosed entity in the antepartum period. At the turn of the century, it had already been recognized that congenital heart blocks in neonates were commonly associated with a large variety of cardiovascular problems. The incidence of major cardiovascular malformations in children with congenital third-degree (complete) A-V block has been estimated to be over 50%.[52,53] Children with congenital complete heart block exhibit the same complications as adults. Follow-up studies have suggested that children with complete heart block as their only cardiac problem who have a ventricular rate above 55 bpm do, in general, show a satisfactory prognosis, with normal growth and development. Children who have additional cardiac problems and/or a heart rate under 55 bpm exhibit severe complications such as Stokes-Adams attacks or syncope, congestive heart failure, and death in infancy or early childhood. The reported incidence of complete block is 1/20,000 live births. The first diagnosis prior to birth was made by Plant and Stevens in 1945.[56] Since then, an increasing number of cases has been reported, and different methodologies have been employed in the antepartum diagnosis. The first review of the subject was published by Teteris and associates in 1968.[57] In their report, 15 of 29 infants died with congenital heart disease. Shenker reviewed that experience and added an additional 13 cases more recently.[1] Among those 13 infants, five were found to have congenital heart disease, and six died, either from congenital heart disease or with a pacemaker in situ.[1,18,47,48,58–64] The very high incidence of major cardiovascular congenital abnormalities in association with congenital heart block is confirmed by more recent studies.

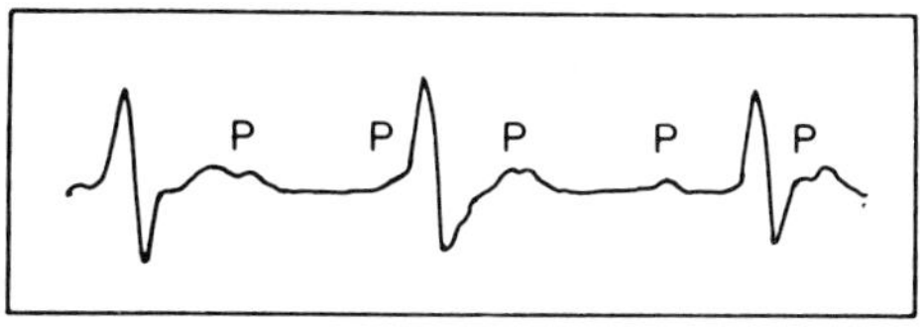

Atrial Rate	Ventricular Rate
Normal	Significantly slower than atrial rate

Fig. F.XIII.24. Third-degree (complete) A-V block.

Increasing attention has focused on the association between congenital A-V block and maternal collagen vascular disease, especially systemic lupus erythematosus (SLE). In 1966 Hull and associates reported congenital heart block and widespread fibrosis due to maternal SLE.[65] After a lull of some years, this association received some additional supportive evidence through newer studies. Thus, McCue and associates were able to show that 14 of 22 children who were born to 11 mothers with clinical or overt connective tissue disease exhibited a congenital complete heart block.[66] This association was confirmed in the same year by Chameides and associates,[67] and the following year by Berube and co-workers.[64]

The importance of this association cannot be overemphasized. It allows the prospective search for congenital fetal heart block in offspring of mothers with known connective tissue disease and, vice versa, the search for dormant connective tissue disease in mothers of infants with congenital A-V block. These principles have been applied since those original publications, and some investigators have reported the diagnosis in utero of complete A-V block in a fetus from a mother with SLE by means of echocardiography and phonocardiography.[68] These noninvasive modalities seem thus to attain increasing importance in the antepartum diagnosis of fetal heart disease. For more detail, see Chapter F.XI.

The suspicion and correct diagnosis in utero of a complete A-V block is of major clinical importance. The resulting fetal bradycardia may be falsely interpreted as fetal distress and lead to unnecessary maternal morbidity from cesarean section. Recently these implications have been extensively discussed by Reid and associates.[69] These authors were also able to report the first documented case of fetal congenital third-degree block in a seemingly healthy mother who, after extensive investigation, turned out to be positive in an antinuclear factor test, showing the speckled variety with a titer of 1:80 and a rising rheumatoid factor. Mothers of infants born with congenital complete A-V block should therefore be thoroughly investigated for overt disease.

The pathophysiology of congenital third-degree A-V block is poorly understood. Both the A-V node and the His bundle seem to develop separately and join early in fetal development.[2] It has been suggested that failure of union between A-V node and His bundle may explain the presence of congenital A-V block, at least in some cases.[70] The reasons for congenital A-V block in the offspring of mothers who have connective tissue disease are unknown. Antibodies and, possibly, immune complexes may cross the placenta to the fetus. Immune complexes, especially in association with viral disease, are believed to be able to induce fetal tissue damage.[71] This could represent one of the mechanisms of A-V block. However, it remains unexplained why the tissue damage is restricted to the conduction system, and specifically to the area of junction between A-V node and His bundle. It is also interesting to note that, although a small percentage of offspring of mothers with systemic lupus erythematosus exhibit transient lupus after birth, only a small minority will have congenital A-V block. The majority even of those infants that show passive transfer of maternal disease will have a completely normal heart.

In summary, the antepartum diagnosis of third-degree A-V block will be one of the most frequently made diagnoses among any of the dysrhythmias in utero. Compared to most of the earlier discussed dysrhythmias, it also has the most ominous prognostic significance, indicating a very high incidence of congenital cardiac disease in the fetus, which may involve either morphologic structures of the heart or the conduction system. In addition, the maternal implications in reference to connective tissue disease may be important.

How, then, is the diagnosis in utero made? As noted, a high degree of suspicion should exist if the mother is known to have a connective tissue disease. Otherwise, the presenting symptom will be fetal bradycardia. It is important to differentiate fetal bradycardia from fetal distress in those situations. With complete A-V block, none of the excitation passes from the atria into the ventricles. The ventricles contract due to excitations in an infranodal pacemaker, which is usually located in the His bundle. Most cases of complete heart block are infra-A-V nodal, caused by a block in the bundle of His or by bilateral bundle branch block.[8] Additional characteristics of the ECG include a PP interval that is shorter than the RR interval and a sometimes distorted QRS complex. The QRS complex may or may not be distorted, depending on the site from which the ventricular signal originates. According to Shenker, fetal heart rates as low as 20 bpm have been reported; however, the majority of fetuses will exhibit heart rates in the range of 50–70 bpm.[1] The in utero diagnosis of complete block will depend on the proper utilization of antepartum fetal ECG, phonocardiography, and echocardiography.[68,69]

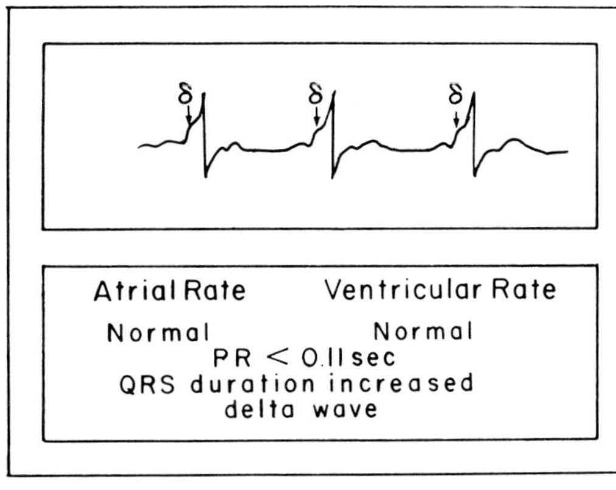

Fig. F.XIII.26. The Wolff-Parkinson-White syndrome.

2. Bundle branch block disorders (Fig. F.XIII.25)

Bundle branch block disorders represent impaired conduction in specific areas of the conduction system. The accurate diagnosis of either left or right bundle branch block is dependent on a complete ECG (Fig. F.XIII.25). As intrauterine ECGs are limited to a single lead, the diagnosis of bundle branch block disorders in utero by means of electrocardiography does not seem feasible. It is therefore not surprising that no case has been reported. Nevertheless, a widened QRS complex should be considered with suspicion and should be followed in the neonatal period.

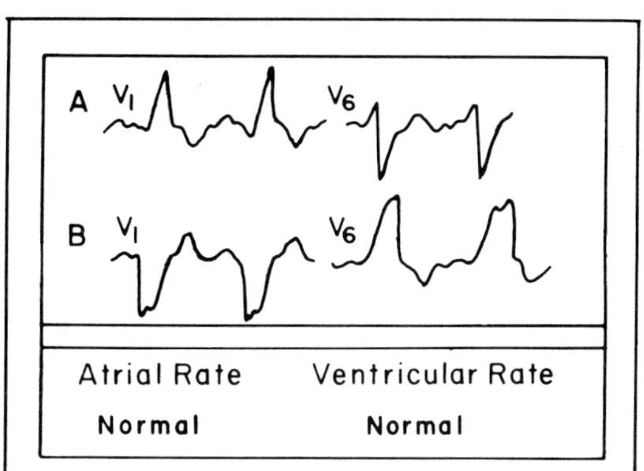

Fig. F.XIII.25. A. right bundle branch block; B. left bundle branch block.

3. The Wolff-Parkinson-White syndrome (anomalous atrioventricular excitation) (Fig. F.XIII.26)

As in the adult experience, the Wolff-Parkinson-White syndrome has been recognized in neonates to be associated with a pronounced tendency for the occurrence of atrial tachyarrhythmias such as paroxysmal atrial tachycardia, atrial flutter, and atrial fibrillation.[72] Only recently has the same association been made for the situation in utero. We noted earlier in this chapter that two fetuses that exhibited supraventricular tachyarrhythmias in utero were found to have a classical Wolff-Parkinson-White pattern after birth (Table F.XIII.1).[28] Two additional cases were reported in the literature.[25,29]

The Wolff-Parkinson-White syndrome is characterized by a typical ECG appearance: P waves are normal, the PR interval is 0.11 seconds or less, and the QRS duration is increased and shows a slur on the initial phase of the QRS complex, which is called the delta wave.[8] From this description, it will be evident that the diagnosis in utero cannot be made with available ECG technology. What can be made, however, is the presumptive association of the syndrome with intrauterine tachyarrhythmias. This association has been retrospectively estimated by us to represent approximately 10% of all cases with supraventricular tachyarrhythmias in utero.[28] This estimation needs confirmation through a larger number of reported cases. It seems obvious, however, that cases of intrauterine tachyarrhythmias should always be suspected to have an underlying Wolff-Parkinson-White pattern. It also should be remembered that Wolff-Parkinson-White may be associated with the Epstein anomaly and other congenital abnormalities, as well as mitral valve prolapse and hypertrophic cardiomyopathy. Hyperthyroidism has also been associated with the preexcitation syndrome.[8] We recently suggested that pregnancy may predispose to arrhythmias in females with Wolff-Parkinson-White syndrome.[73] It is tempting to speculate that in both mother and fetus hormonal factors of pregnancy may influence and increase the incidence of symptomatic Wolff-Parkinson-White, which results in arrhythmias. It must be understood, however, that this suggestion represents pure speculation.

V. SUMMARY

In our introduction we outlined the theoretical difficulties in obtaining a reliable fetal intrauterine electrocardiogram, either abdominally or by internal fetal scalp electrode. Shenker, one of the most knowledgeable investigators in the field, recently stated that knowledge of fetal cardiac arrhythmias diagnosed during pregnancy and labor is incomplete.[1] He summarized the necessity for the antepartum diagnosis of cardiac fetal arrhythmias as follows: 1) the need to distinguish fetal dysrhythmias from fetal distress; 2) the need to recognize the coexistence of congenital heart disease and varying forms of dysrhythmias; 3) the need to be able to recognize (and treat[34]) congestive heart failure both in utero and immediately after birth; 4) the need to be able to prepare for immediate cardiac work-up and treatment at time of delivery; 5) the need to recognize the relationship between maternal collagen vascular disease and congenital third-degree A-V block.

Increasing sophistication of intrauterine electrocardiography will undoubtly result in a major advancement of antepartum cardiac diagnosis in the fetus. Thus, the diagnosis of mitral and aortic stenosis based on a fetal electrocardiogram was recently made by Katz and associates.[74] Nobody will doubt that the early diagnosis of congenital lesions not only will benefit the fetus immediately after birth but also will prevent unnecessary maternal morbidity due to cesarean section performed for falsely diagnosed fetal distress. It can be concluded that fetal electrocardiography, although still in a rather early stage of its development, in combination with other means of noninvasive cardiac diagnoses such as phonocardiography and intrauterine echocardiography, will significantly enhance the antepartum diagnosis of the abnormal fetal heart.

VI. REFERENCES

1. Shenker L. Fetal cardiac arrhythmias. Obstet Gynecol Surv. 1979; 34:561–572.
2. James TN. Cardiac conduction system: Fetal and postnatal development. Am J Cardiol. 1970; 25:213–226.
3. Budnick IS, Leikin S, Hoeck LE. Effects in the newborn infant of reserpine administered antepartum. AMA Am J Dis Child. 1955: 90:286–289.
4. Goodlin RC, Haesslein HC. Fetal reacting bradycardia. Am J Obstet Gynecol. 1977; 129:845–856.
5. Redman TF. The significance of some unusual foetal cardiac arrhythmias. J Obstet Gynaecol Br Emp. 1958; 65:304–309.
6. Webster RD, Codmore DW, Gray J. Fetal bradycardia without fetal distress. Case presentation and review of the literature. Obstet Gynecol. 1977; 50(Suppl):50s–53s.
7. Dgani R, Borenstein R, Levavi E, Feigl A, Kauli N, Lancet M. Prenatally diagnosed blocked atrial premature beats. Obstet Gynecol. 1978; 51:507–509.
8. Sobel BE, Braunwald E. Cardiac arrhythmias. In: Isselbacher KJ, Adams RD, Braunwald E, Petersdorf RG, Wilson JD eds. Harrison's Principles of Internal Medicine, 9th Ed. New York: McGraw-Hill, 1980: 1044–1063.
9. Ferrer PL. Arrhythmias in the neonate. In: Roberts NK, Gelband H eds. Cardiac Arrhythmias in the Neonate, Infant, and Child. New York: Appleton-Century-Crofts, 1977: chapter 17.
10. Odendaal HJ, Crawford JW. Fetal tachycardia

and maternal pyrexia during labor. S Afr Med J. 1975; 49:1873–1875.
11. Gleicher N, Chin JM, Brown BL, Kerenyi TD. Intrauterine meconium aspiration syndrome. Diagnost Gynecol Obstet. 1980; 2:151–155.
12. Yeh SY, Zanini B, Petrie RH, Hon EH. Intrapartum fetal cardiac arrest: A preliminary observation. Obstet Gynecol. 1977; 50:571–577.
13. Queenan JT. Discussion of Ref. 4. Am J Obstet Gynecol. 1977; 129:845.
14. Klapholz H, Schifrin BS, Rivo E. Paroxysmal supraventricular tachycardia in the fetus. Obstet Gynecol. 1974; 43:718–721.
15. Nielsen JS, Moestrup JK: Foetal electrocardiographic studies of cardiac arrhythmias and the heart rate. Acta Obstet Gynecol Scand. 1968; 47:247–256.
16. Hyman AS. Irregularities of the fetal heart. Phonocardiographic study of fetal heart sounds from fifth to eighth month of pregnancy. Am J Obstet Gynecol. 1930; 20:332–347.
17. Hon EH, Huang HS. The electronic evaluation of fetal heart rate: VII Premature and missed beats. Obstet Gynecol. 1962; 20:81–90.
18. Komaromy B, Gaal J, Lampe L. Fetal arrhythmia during pregnancy and labour. Br J Obstet Gynecol. 1977; 84:492–496.
19. Itskovitz J, Timor-Tritsch I, Brandes JM. Intrauterine arrhythmia: Atrial premature beats. Int J Gynaecol Obstet. 1979; 16:419–421.
20. Young BK, Katz M, Klein SA. Intrapartum fetal cardiac arrhythmias. Obstet Gynecol. 1979; 54:427–432.
21. Harrigan JT, Acerra D, LaMagra R, Hoeveler J, Chandra N. Fetal cardiac arrhythmia during labor. Am J Obstet Gynecol. 1977; 128:693–694.
22. Schneider H, Weinstein HM, Young BK. Fetal trigeminal rhythm. Obstet Gynecol. 1977; 50(Suppl):58s–61s.
23. Sugarman RG, Lawlinson KF, Schifrin BS. Fetal arrhythmia. Obstet Gynecol. 1978; 52:301–307.
24. Schlotter CM, Kunz S: Fetale Parasystolie—Eine seltene Form fetaler Arrhythmie bei Hydramnion und Hydrops Fetalis. Z Geburtshilfe Perinatol. 1978; 182:371–375.
25. Newberger JW, Keane JF. Intrauterine supraventricular tachycardia. J Pediatr. 1979; 95:780–786.
26. Wells DH, Shaw GG, McNeal RM, Ronslov S. Neonatal paroxysmal supraventricular tachycardia. Cin Pediatr. 1979; 17:581–583.
27. Chitkara U, Gleicher N, Longhi R, Gergely RZ, Kerenyi TD. Persistent supraventricular tachycardia in utero. Diagnost Gynecol Obstet. 1980; 2:291–298.
28. Gleicher N. The Wolff-Parkinson-White syndrome predisposes to intrauterine arrhythmias. in preparation.
29. Klein AM, Holzman IA, Austin EM. Fetal tachycardia prior to the development of hydrops. Attempted pharmacologic cardioversion. Case report. Am J Obstet Gynecol. 1979; 136:347–348.
30. Herin P, Thoren C. Congenital arrhythmias with supraventricular tachycardia in the perinatal period. Acta Obstet Gynecol Scand. 1973; 52:381–386.
31. Levkoff AH. Perinatal outcome of paroxysmal tachycardia of the newborn with onset in utero. Am J Obstet Gynecol. 1969; 104:73–79.
32. Silber DL, Durnin RE. Intrauterine atrial tachycardia, associated with massive edema in a newborn. Am J Dis Child. 1969; 117:722–726.
33. Kerenyi TD, Gleicher N, Meller J, Brown E, Steinfeld L, Chitkara U, Raucher H. Transplacental cardioversion of intrauterine supraventricular tachycardia with digitalis. Lancet. 1980; 2:393–394.
34. Symonds EM. Fetal cardiac arrhythmias and fetal acid base status. NZ J Obstet Gynaecol. 1972; 12:170–175.
35. Wildemeersch D, Raven E: Fetal atrial arrhythmia: Case report. Z Geburtshilfe Perinatol. 1975; 179:57–60.
36. Tuxen P, Kaplan EL, Ueland K. Intrauterine paroxysmal atrial tachycardia. Am J Obstet Gynecol. 1971; 109:958–960.
37. Hedvall G. Congenital paroxysmal tachycardia: A report of three cases. Acta Paediatr Scand. 1973; 62:550–552.
38. Carretti NG, Galli PA, Pellegrino P. Fetal paroxysmal supraventricular tachycardia: Report of a case documented by trans-vaginal electrocardiogram during fetal distress in labour. Acta Obstet Gynecol Scand. 1974; 53:275–277.
39. Jones JB. Accelerated rhythm causing intrapartum fetal tachycardia. Br J Obstet Gynaecol. 1976; 83:986–988.
40. Hochberg HM, Poppers PJ, George ME. Fetal paroxysmal supraventricular tachycardia recorded by intrauterine scalp electrocardiography. J Perinat Med. 1976; 4:51–54.
41. Hughey M, Elesh R. Profound atrial tachycardia in utero. Am J Obstet Gynecol. 1977; 128:463–465.
42. Pearl W. Cardiac malformations presenting as congenital atrial flutter. South Med J. 1977; 70:622–624.
43. Van der Horst RL. Congenital atrial flutter and cardiac failure presenting as hydrops foetalis at birth. S Afr Med J. 1970; 44:1037–1039.
44. Moller JH, Davachi F, Anderson RC. Atrial flutter in infancy. J Pediatr. 1969; 75:643–651.
45. Freistadt H. Fetal bigeminal rhythm. Report of a case. Am J Obstet Gynecol. 1962; 84:13–14.
46. Eibschitz I, Abinader EG, Klein A, Sharf M. Intrauterine diagnosis and control of fetal ventricular arrhythmia during labor. Am J Obstet Gynecol. 1975; 122:597–600.
47. Sorland S, Torp KH, Jenssen J. Hjerte-arytmier hos foster og nyfdt. En oversikt og omtale av 5 kasus. T Norsk Laegeforen. 1963; 83:1654–1659.
48. Armstrong DH, Murata Y, Martin Jr CB, Ikenoue T. Antepartum detection of congenital complete fetal heart block: A case report. Am J Obstet Gynecol. 1976; 126:291–292.

49. Müller-Schmid P. Die paroxysmale Tachikardie in utero. Geburtshilfe Frauenheilk. 1959; 19:401–407.
50. Platt LD, Manning FA, Gray C, Guttenburg M, Turkel SB. Antenatal detection of fetal A-V dissociation utilizing real-time B-mode ultrasound. Obstet Gynecol. 1979; 53 (Suppl):59S–61S.
51. Chan TS, Potter RT, Liu L. Congenital intraventricular trifascicular block. Am J Dis Child. 1973; 125:82–87.
52. Morquio L. Sur une maladie infantile et familiale caraterisee par des modificatieus permanentes du pouls des attaques syncopales et epileptiformes et la morte subite. Arch Med Enfant. 1901; 4:462–467.
53. Griffiths SP. Congenital complete heart block (editorial). Circulation. 1971; 43:615–617.
54. Michaelsson M, Engl MA. Congenital complete heart block: An international study of the natural history. Pediatr Cardiol. 1972; 4:86.
55. Hochberg SH. Congenital heart block. Am J Obstet Gynecol. 1964; 88:238–241.
56. Plant RK, Stevens RA. Complete A-V block in a fetus. Case report. Am Heart J. 1945; 30:615–618.
57. Teteris NJ, Chisholm JW, Ullery JC. Antenatal diagnosis of congenital heart block. Report of a case. Obstet Gynecol 1968; 32:851–853.
58. Smith JJ, Schwartz ED, Blatman S. Fetal bradycardia fetal distress or cardiac abnormality? Obstet Gynecol. 1960; 15:761–764.
59. Dunn HP. Antenatal diagnosis of congenital heart block. J Obstet Gynaecol Br Emp. 1960; 67:1006–1007.
60. Sokol RJ, Hutchinson P, Krouskop RW, Brown EG, Reed G, Vasquez H. Congenital complete heart block diagnosed during intrauterine fetal monitoring. Am J Obstet Gynecol. 1974; 120:1115–1117.
61. Abdulla U, Charters DW. Congenital heart block diagnosed antenatally associated with multiple fetal abnormality. Br Med J. 1975; 4:263.
62. Altenburger KM, Jedziniak M, Roper WL, Hernandez J. Congenital complete heart block associated with hydrops fetalis. J Pediatr. 1977; 9:618–620.
63. Hamilton LA Jr, Fisher E, Horn C, DuBrow I, Vidyasagar D. A new prenatal cardiac diagnostic device for congenital heart disease. Obstet Gynecol. 1977; 50:491–494.
64. Berube S, Lister Jr G, Toews WH, Creasy RK, Heymann MA. Congenital heart block and maternal systemic lupus erythematosus. Am J Obstet Gynecol. 1978; 130:595–596.
65. Hull D, Binns BA, Joyce D. Congenital heart block and widespread fibrosis due to maternal lupus erythematosus. Arch Dis Child. 1966; 4:688–690.
66. McCue CM, Mantakas ME, Tingelstad JB, Ruddy S. Congenital heart block in newborns of mothers with connective tissue disease. Circulation. 1977; 56:82–90.
67. Chameides L, Truex RC, Vetter V, Raskind WJ, Galiolo FM Jr, Noonan JA. Association of maternal systemic lupus erythematosus with congenital complete heart block. N Engl J Med. 1977; 297:1204–1207.
68. Madison JP, Sukhum P, Williamson DP, Campion BC. Echocardiography and fetal heart sounds in the diagnosis of fetal heart block. Am Heart J. 1979; 98:505–509.
69. Reid RL, Pancham SR, Kean WF, Ford PM. Maternal and neonatal implications of congenital complete heart block in the fetus. Obstet Gynecol. 1979; 54:470–474.
70. Carter JB, Blieden LC, Edwards JE. Congenital heart block: Anatomic correlation and review of the literature. Arch Pathol. 1974; 97:51–57.
71. Gleicher N, Theofilopoulos AN. Immune complexes (ICs) and pregnancy: Pregnancy as an IC-state or IC-disease and the influence of IC-diseases on pregnancy. Diagnost Gynecol Obstet. 1980; 2:7–31.
72. Lubbers WJ, Losekoot TG, Anderson RH, Wellens HJJ. Paroxysmal supraventricular tachycardia in infancy and childhood. Eur J Cardiol. 1974; 2:91–99.
73. Gleicher N, Meller J, Sandler RZ, Sullum S. Wolff-Parkinson-White syndrome in pregnancy. Obstet Gynecol. (In press.)
74. Katz M, Valdes-Cruz LM, Greco MA, Yanagawa Y, Klein SA, Mufarrij A, Young BK. Diagnosis of congenital mitral and aortic stenosis from the fetal electrocardiogram. Obstet Gynecol. 1979; 54:372–374.

F.XIV

Intrauterine Congestive Heart Failure

Norbert Gleicher, MD, and Uri Elkayam, MD

I. INTRODUCTION

Until very recently, intrauterine heart failure has attracted only very limited attention in the medical literature. In fact, to our knowledge, the subject has never been summarized before. Consequently, a large amount of relevant information will have to be extrapolated from the adult experience, starting with the definition of heart failure. According to the textbook definition, heart failure is a "pathophysiologic state in which an abnormality of cardiac function is responsible for the failure of the heart to pump blood at the rate commensurate with the requirement of the metabolizing tissues."[1] The acceptance of this definition for the fetal situation implies that the same mechanisms may lead to heart failure in both fetus and adult. The biophysics of the developing heart are still incompletely understood, although recent work has shed some light on the topic (see Chapter F. II).[2,3]

In the adult experience, a distinction is made between heart failure due to myocardial damage associated with abnormal ventricular function and congestive state due to other causes that are not dependent on myocardial function. Congestive heart failure is subdivided in the adult experience into high-output failure and low-output failure, acute versus chronic, right-sided versus left-sided, and backward versus forward heart failure.[1] But even in the adult situation, a clear distinction between opposite terms cannot always be made. In the fetal experience, that kind of differentiation is even more difficult and has rarely been used in published case reports. Braunwald describes these terms as useful in a clinical setting but stresses the fact that they are solely descriptive and do not signify fundamentally different disease states.[1] Extrapolating from

Cardiac Problems in Pregnancy, pages 565–576

the adult experience, low-output failure could arise in a fetus in one of the following reported and/or presumptive etiologies: myocardial disease, valvular disease, pericardial disease, hypertension, and coronary artery disease. High-output failure, on the other hand, could be associated with fetal anemia, hyperthyroidism, and atrioventricular (A-V) fistula. Acute heart failure in the adult usually is a result of a large myocardial infarction or valve rupture; neither has been reported in fetuses. Chronic heart failure in the adult is frequently due to multiple valvular heart disease. In the fetal experience, a distinction between these forms of heart failure has not been made. Heart failure is referred to as right-sided or left-sided according to which of the ventricles is affected by an excessive fluid accumulation. Again, the distinction between these two forms of heart failure in the fetal experience is more difficult, because the fetal circulation clearly is different from the adult. Thus, conditions that primarily affect the right ventricle, such as valvular pulmonic stenosis or pulmonary hypertension, will play little or no role in utero, as most of the blood returning to the heart is shifted through the foramen ovale into the left atrium and bypasses the fetal lungs. It must be recognized, however, that when an excessive load is applied to one of the ventricles for prolonged periods, failure of the whole heart may occur. There has been speculation that this may occur because the muscle bundles that compose both ventricles are continuous. Another cause is given by the fact that the ventricles share the interventricular septum.[1] In the adult experience, it is believed that a rigid differentiation between backward heart failure and forward heart failure is artificial. Both mechanisms seem to appear and are operative in most patients who show signs and symptoms of chronic heart failure.[1]

The differential diagnosis of heart failure in the adult is given by the clinical situation in which abnormal salt and water retention occurs consequent to renal failure or excessive parenteral administration of fluids and electrolytes. This situation is termed "the congested state."[1] It is unknown if a similar situation occurs in utero. It may be assumed, however, that congestive heart failure secondary to excessive intrauterine transfusion therapy may occur.

II. CAUSES OF INTRAUTERINE HEART FAILURE

Some authors differentiate between "underlying" and "precipitating" causes of heart failure. Such a distinction may be important where a chronic condition that does not lead to decompensation of the heart exists and where a precipitating cause in addition to the underlying cause is necessary to lead to heart failure. In the fetal situation, such a distinction has not yet been made. Also, such a distinction probably is not necessary because long-lasting chronic conditions rarely occur in the fetus. Only a few etiologies of intrauterine congestive heart failure have been recorded, but others can be extrapolated from the adult experience, and in this discussion, these are termed "presumed" causes of heart failure. A large group of other possible etiologies of heart failure in the adult are irrevelant to the fetal experience and are not discussed here. Table F.XIV.1 gives a list of causes of heart failure and is subdivided into causes that have been reported in the fetal experience

TABLE F.XIV.1. Causes of Heart Failure*

Reported in fetus
Anemia
Dysrhythmias
Presumed to occur in fetus (although probably very rare)
Infections
Thyrotoxicosis
Myocardial infarction
Pulmonary embolism
Congenital heart lesions
Systemic hypertension

*This list was compiled from a presentation of the adult experience[1] and subdivided according to reported and/or presumptive fetal occurrence.

and those that are presumed to occur in the fetus.

A. Fetal Anemia

Anemia is associated with a decrease in the oxygen-carrying capacity of the fetal blood. In order to maintain proper oxygenation of the different tissues, cardiac output increases. A normal heart will be able to sustain an increasing cardiac output. A compensated heart, however, that for various reasons is either overloaded or diseased may not be able to do so. Such a situation may arise in utero in a number of conditions, which are discussed in the sections that follow.

1. Hemolytic disease

Hemolytic disease of the fetus occurs when fetal red blood cells possess an antigen against which there are circulating maternal alloantibodies that are capable of crossing the placenta.[4] Rh-disease, the presence of anti-D, represents the most important of the maternal-fetal blood group incompatibilities. Before the routine administration of Rho-immunoglobulin became available as a method for the prevention of immunization, 90% of all reported cases of severe hemolytic disease of the fetus were caused by the interaction of D-positive fetal red blood cells and maternal anti-D alloantibodies.[5] Since the wide clinical introduction of immune prophylaxis, other causes of hemolytic disease of the fetus, such as incompatibility of the ABO system, of antigens other than D in the Rh system, and so-called irregular antibodies have increased in relative importance.

Hemolytic disease of the fetus, if severe, can lead to a hydropic fetus. Interestingly, a very specific fetal heart rate pattern has been associated with severe hemolytic disease. This pattern, which is called *sinusoidal* (Fig. F.XIV.1), represents a modulatory pattern lacking beat-to-beat variability. This pattern of fetal heart rate was originally thought to be associated mainly with hemolytic disease of the fetus,[6] but it was later found to occur in a number of fetal distress situations and, in fact, to be one of the fetal heart rate patterns preceding death in utero.[7] Since then, a large number of clinical situations have been associated with sinusoidal fetal heart rate.[8] Nevertheless, hemolytic disease of the fetus still represents the large majority of reported cases.

Some investigators suggested that sinusoidal fetal heart rate may be due to

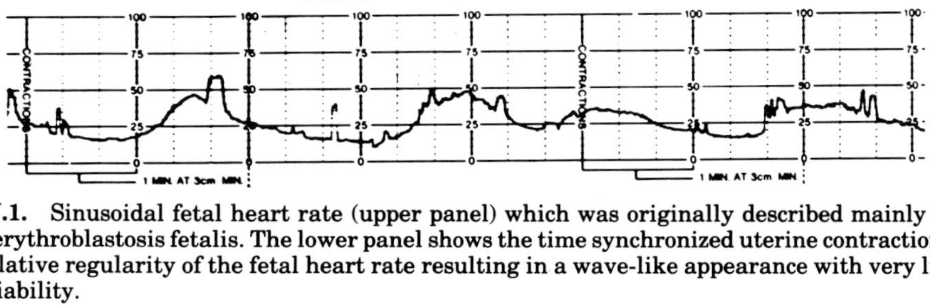

Fig. F.XIV.1. Sinusoidal fetal heart rate (upper panel) which was originally described mainly in association with erythroblastosis fetalis. The lower panel shows the time synchronized uterine contraction pattern. Note the relative regularity of the fetal heart rate resulting in a wave-like appearance with very little beat-to-beat variability.

high-output fetal cardiac failure.[9] Such an explanation, however, does not explain the occurrence of sinusoidal fetal heart rate in the terminal patterns seen in some asphyxiated fetuses.[10] Most recent evidence suggests that sinusoidal fetal heart rate may be due to a loss of autonomic nervous system control over the heart.[6,8]

Hemolytic disease of the fetus is a slowly progressing state. Congestive heart failure and fatal hydrops will be found in only the most severe cases. In general, the situation does not reach such a serious stage in a first pregnancy. With subsequent pregnancies, the severity of the disease tends to increase. If the presence of antibodies capable of producing hemolytic disease has been confirmed, the pregnancy has to be followed with serial amniocenteses. Fetal hemolysis results in an elevated bilirubin content in the amniotic fluid. Spectrophotometric measurements of bilirubin in amniotic fluid allow an exact determination of severity of fetal involvement. Most institutions use the method developed by Liley,[11] which reports optical density rises at 450 mμ (ΔOD 450) in specific grafs, allowing accurate comparison of results between laboratories in three levels of severity. The rise in optical density at 450 mμ is proportional to the degree of severity of Rh-disease in the hemolytic infant. Twenty to twenty-five percent of fetuses with erythroblastosis have such severe hemolysis that they ultimately develop universal edema with extreme ascites (hydrops). The mechanisms that lead to hydrops fetalis are multiple and are discussed in detail elsewhere.[12] Heart failure will develop only in a small percentage of hydropic fetuses and rarely, if ever, represents the primary cause of hydrops fetalis.[12] Earlier, it was believed that all hydrops fetalis was due to fetal heart failure, which, in turn, was caused by progressive anemia. More recent evidence indicates that the causative mechanisms for hydrops are much more complex and variable.[12] Once fetal involvement in the severe zone (zone 3) of the Liley graft has been determined by amniocentesis, intervention is indicated. If the fetus at that stage of pregnancy is too immature for delivery, intrauterine transfusion of the fetus represents the most appropriate form of therapy. In successful cases, fetal well-being clearly improves after such therapy. Among the recorded changes is the resolution of fetal sinusoidal heart rate after intrauterine transfusion.[13] It should be noted, however, that the opposite has also been reported. In at least two instances, sinusoidal fetal heart rate was noticed for the first time shortly after intrauterine transfusion.[14,15]

2. Twin transfusion syndrome

The twin transfusion syndrome may cause intrauterine heart failure in two forms. First, the twin that is hypertransfused by its co-twin may show signs of intrauterine heart failure due to the hypertransfusion. Second, the twin that is losing blood to the other twin may become severely anemic and, as a consequence, may develop intrauterine heart failure. Both of these instances are exceedingly rare. Although the twin transfusion syndrome represents a rather frequent entity, especially in monozygotic twin pregnancies, only rarely have significant cardiovascular consequences been reported.[16]

3. Fetal/maternal transfusion

Minor fetal-maternal transfusions probably occur in most pregnancies. Massive (greater than 30 ml) fetal-maternal transfusion, however, occurs in only about 0.3–0.7% of all cases.[17] If a prolonged fetal-maternal transfusion leads to severe intrauterine anemia, intrauterine heart failure may result. Similar to the experience outlined above in association with hemolytic disease of the fetus, a sinusoidal fetal heart rate may develop.[9]

4. Acute fetal blood loss

Acute fetal blood loss has not been reported in association with intrauterine heart failure. However, sinusoidal fetal heart rate patterns in association with acute fetal blood loss have been reported.[18,19] Similar to the adult experience, the rapid loss of large amounts of blood results in shock rather than in heart failure. Sinusoidal fetal heart rate will then result, not as an indicator of intrauterine heart failure but as a preterminal event, as noted above.

B. Intrauterine Dysrhythmias

In the adult experience, patients with underlying but compensated cardiac problems will decompensate and go into heart failure because of cardiac arrhythmias more often than any other precipitating cause.[1] Table F.XIV.2 presents a summary of mechanisms of heart failure in association with various dysrhythmias. That summary is based on the adult experience, but it can be assumed that at least some of the same mechanisms will be active in utero. Again, the fetal experience is rather limited and more or less confined to descriptive reports rather than explanations of cardiac physiology in utero.

1. Supraventricular dysrhythmias

Supraventricular dysrhythmias are discussed in detail in Chapter F.XIII. It is known that intrauterine heart failure due to supraventricular tachycardia may be related to the length and persistence of the tachyarrhythmia. From published reports, as well as our own experience, we have concluded that fetuses with persistent supraventricular tachycardia have a significantly higher chance of intrauterine heart failure than those with short bursts only.[20] It is also noteworthy that neonates who exhibit supraventricular tachycardia in utero and are not born with clinically apparent signs of intrauterine heart failure still exhibit signs that indicate partial decompensation such as heavier placentas, increased diuresis over the first few days of life, and increased birth weight.[21] Other supraventricular arrhythmias that may lead to intrauterine heart failure are atrial flutter and, possibly, atrial fibrillation. The experience with these two supraventricular arrhythmias is even smaller than that with supraventricular tachycardia. Neverthe-

TABLE F.XIV.2. Mechanisms of Heart Failure in Association With Dysrhythmias*

Dysrhythmia	Mechanism of heart failure
Tachyarrhythmias	Reduced time for ventricular filling
Supraventricular and ventricular arrhythmias	Dissociation between atrial and ventricular contractions results in loss of atrial booster pump mechanism
Ventricular tachycardia and arrhythmias with abnormal intraventricular conduction	Further impairment of myocardial performance because synchronicity of ventricular contractions is lost
Complete A-V block (with marked bradycardia)	Requires large increase in stroke volume to prevent reduction in cardiac output

*The mechanism for heart failure in association with dysrrhythmias may be multifactorial. For example, dissociation between atrial and ventricular contractions interferes with the atrial booster pump mechanism and results in a loss of the atrial contribution to ventricular filling and at the same time produces an increase in atrial pressure. Shortness of the diastolic period due to tachycardia is also a contributing factor resulting in diminution of left ventricular filling. In cases of ventricular tachycardia and arrhythmias with abnormal intraventricular conduction an impairment of myocardial performance may be seen due to the loss of synchronicity of ventricular contractions. Heart failure can also be caused by bradyarrhythmias where a marked decrease in the number of heart beats per minute may result in a significant decline in cardiac output.
Modified from Braunwald.[1]

less, atrial flutter is considered an especially dangerous arrhythmia in utero and seems to predispose to intrauterine congestive heart failure.[22] All of the reported cases of supraventricular arrhythmias have been discussed in detail in the preceding chapter.

2. Ventricular dysrhythmias

As shown in Table F.XIV.2, it is theoretically possible that heart failure may be caused by ventricular arrhythmias. The reported fetal experience to date (see Chapter F.XIII) is so small that no statement in reference to the etiologic association with congestive heart failure can be made.

3. Abnormal conduction

A complete atrioventricular block, especially if associated with very marked bradycardia, will require a large increase in stroke volume if the reduction in cardiac output is to be prevented.[1] As discussed in the preceding chapter, third-degree (complete) A-V block represents the most frequently diagnosed entity in the antepartum period. It does represent one of the best studied intrauterine dysrhythmias. As indicated earlier, this dysrhythmia is associated with a very high incidence of major congenital cardiovascular malformations, with systemic lupus erythematosus, and can result in intrauterine heart failure.

Another conduction abnormality that may be associated with intrauterine heart failure is represented by the Wolff-Parkinson-White syndrome. We noted earlier that approximately 10% of all fetuses with intrauterine supraventricular tachycardia, with or without associated heart failure, will show a Wolff-Parkinson-White pattern after birth.[23] It remains to be established if other intrauterine arrhythmias are associated with an underlying Wolff-Parkinson-White syndrome as well. As discussed in Chapter F.XIII, Wolff-Parkinson-White syndrome has been associated in the adult experience with an increase in the number of varying arrhythmias.

C. Intrauterine Infections

Intrauterine infections may be either bacterial or viral. Late in pregnancy, when the intrauterine infection of the fetus presumably may lead to heart failure, most of the well-recognized infections will be bacterial. Like the precipitating causes of intrauterine heart failure discussed earlier, in most instances, infections will not lead to failure. Only in a small percentage of cases, especially those where an underlying compensated cardiac process is present, will the additional precipitating cause of an infection result in heart failure. The mechanisms by which infections may do so are variable. In the adult experience, it has been stated that fever, tachycardia, hypoxemia, and the increased metabolic demands due to all of the factors may represent an intolerable additional burden on a borderline compensated heart muscle.[1] If the infectious process involves the heart, either pericarditis, myocarditis, or endocarditis may result. All of these considerations, however, have to remain theoretical, because, to our knowledge, no cases of heart failure in conjunction with fetal infection in utero have been reported. It should, however, be noted that, at present, therapy for the occurrence of intrauterine infection, if diagnosed, is immediate delivery. This fact may explain why more severe sequelae in the fetus have not been seen.

D. Presumptive Causes

Table F.XIV.1 lists presumed causes of heart failure in utero. As in the experience with infectious causes, all of the presumed etiologies listed in Table F.XIV.1 are based on the adult experience. None of these precipitating causes has been reported to have caused heart failure in utero.

III. CLINICAL MANIFESTATIONS

The clinical manifestations of intrauterine heart failure will be dependent on the underlying cause. This is especially true of the early stages of heart failure, before the full-blown picture develops. However, once intrauterine congestive heart failure has become evident, the diagnosis will not be too difficult to make, although some of the signs may not be pathognomonic of heart failure, and exclusion of other causes will have to be made. Table F.XIV.3 summarizes the most significant diagnostic findings in fetuses with intrauterine heart failure. Polyhydramnios will be frequently found. Its presence can be determined by any of the classical means, including routine clinical evaluation, sonographic determination of amniotic fluid volume, and volume determination by any of the dilution techniques commonly employed. Obviously, polyhydramnios does not represent a pathognomonic entity for heart failure. It is a very frequent finding in both normal and abnormal pregnancies. Similarly, fetal scalp edema does not necessarily indicate intrauterine congestive heart failure. It can be found with a large variety of conditions, not the least of which are the immunologic and nonimmunologic forms of hydrops fetalis which, as mentioned earlier, in the majority of cases are not based on intrauterine congestive heart failure. Fetal ascites also represents a very complicated finding. It has been recently recognized that fetal ascites occurs in utero much more frequently than earlier noted. The large majority of cases represent an idiopathic form of fetal ascites and have little or no clinical significance once the fetus is delivered. In those cases, it will disappear spontaneously after delivery. Only a few cases have an underlying cause, infectious, operative, or cardiac. We recently had an opportunity to evaluate two patients with cardiac ascites. Those cases led us to develop a very detailed management and evaluation protocol for fetuses with intrauterine ascites, which includes the use of intrauterine paracentesis for the investigation of the ascites fluid.[24] Figure F.XIV.2 shows a sonographic picture of a fetus with intrauterine congestive heart failure exhibiting a large amount of ascites fluid. Very small amounts of ascites can be detected with modern sonography, and intrauterine paracentesis can be accomplished rather easily under proper sonographic control. Increased placental size and hydropic consistency can also be diagnosed in utero by sonography. More than the above-mentioned signs, increased placental size is a very common finding in a number of conditions that can be summarized under the term "hyperplacentosis." With the exception of congenital cardiac lesions, intrauterine heart failure represents the most likely cause of changes in fetal heart size. The evaluation of fetal cardiac size is very difficult. Most recent advances in intrauterine echocardiography allow a detailed description of the fetal heart. Intrauterine echocardiography is discussed in detail in

TABLE F.XIV.3. Diagnostic Findings in Intrauterine Congestive Heart Failure

Finding	Method of detection
Polyhydramnios	Clinical evaluation Sonography Volume determination (dilution techniques)
Fetal scalp edema	Sonography
Fetal ascites	Sonography Intrauterine paracentesis
Increased placental size	Sonography
Fetal cardiomegaly	Intrauterine echocardiography

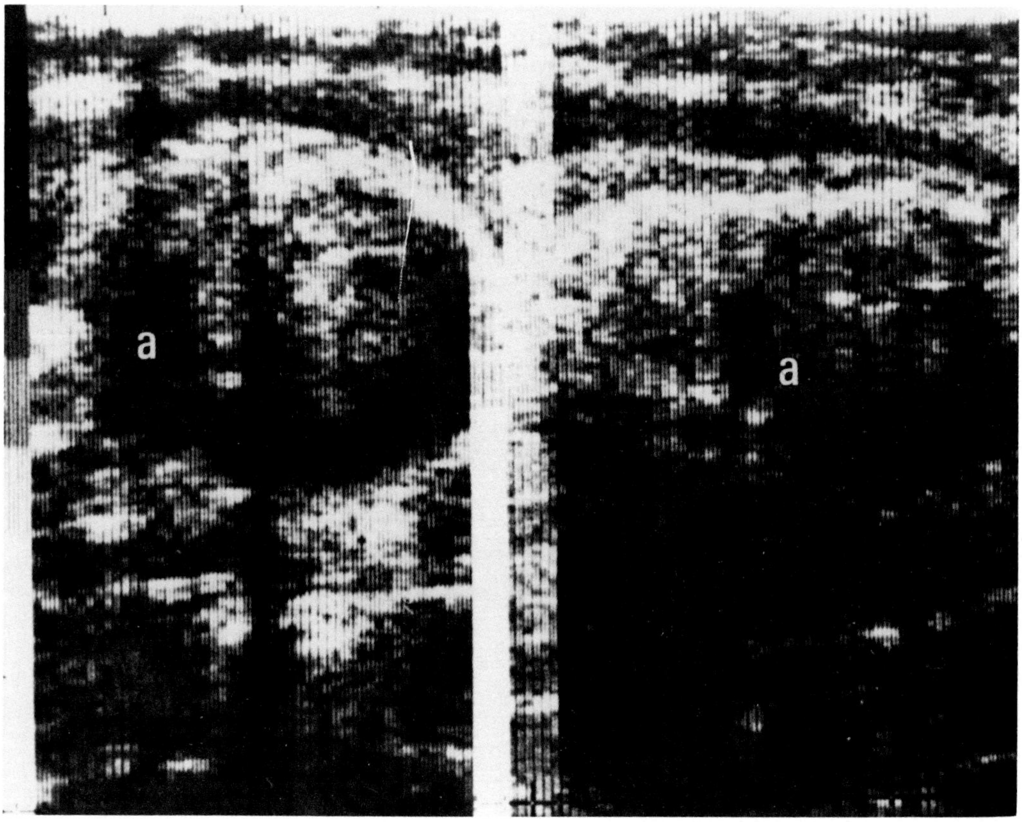

A B

Fig. F.XIV.2. Sonographic picture of fetus with cardiac ascites. **A.** Transverse scan of fetal abdomen. **B.** Longitudinal scan of fetal abdomen; "a" denotes ascites. The amount of intraabdominal fluid is clearly increased, as may be seen in the large echo-free areas of the sonogram.

Chapter F.XI. Under the present heading, it seems appropriate to mention that echocardiography has been used in the diagnosis of intrauterine congestive heart failure. We had the opportunity to investigate a fetus with severe intrauterine congestive heart failure due to persistent supraventricular tachycardia.[25] Figure F.XIV.3, demonstrates that, through the use of intrauterine echocardiography in this very specific case, we were able to demonstrate enlargement of the left atrium as the only abnormality of the fetal heart in utero. Immediately obtained neonatal echocardiograms confirmed our echocardiographic findings in utero (Fig. XIV.3). A similar case was later reported by Harrigan et al.[26]

In summary, clinical manifestations of intrauterine heart failure are nonspecific and frequently difficult to obtain. Whenever intrauterine heart failure is suspected, the diagnosis will be made by actively searching for any of the findings listed in Table F.XIV.3 and by investigating the possible precipitating causes for heart failure. If, as an example, an intrauterine dysrhythmia is recognized in association with any of the listed findings, the diagnosis of an intrauterine heart failure will appear more likely. The same is true if the cause of anemia can be iden-

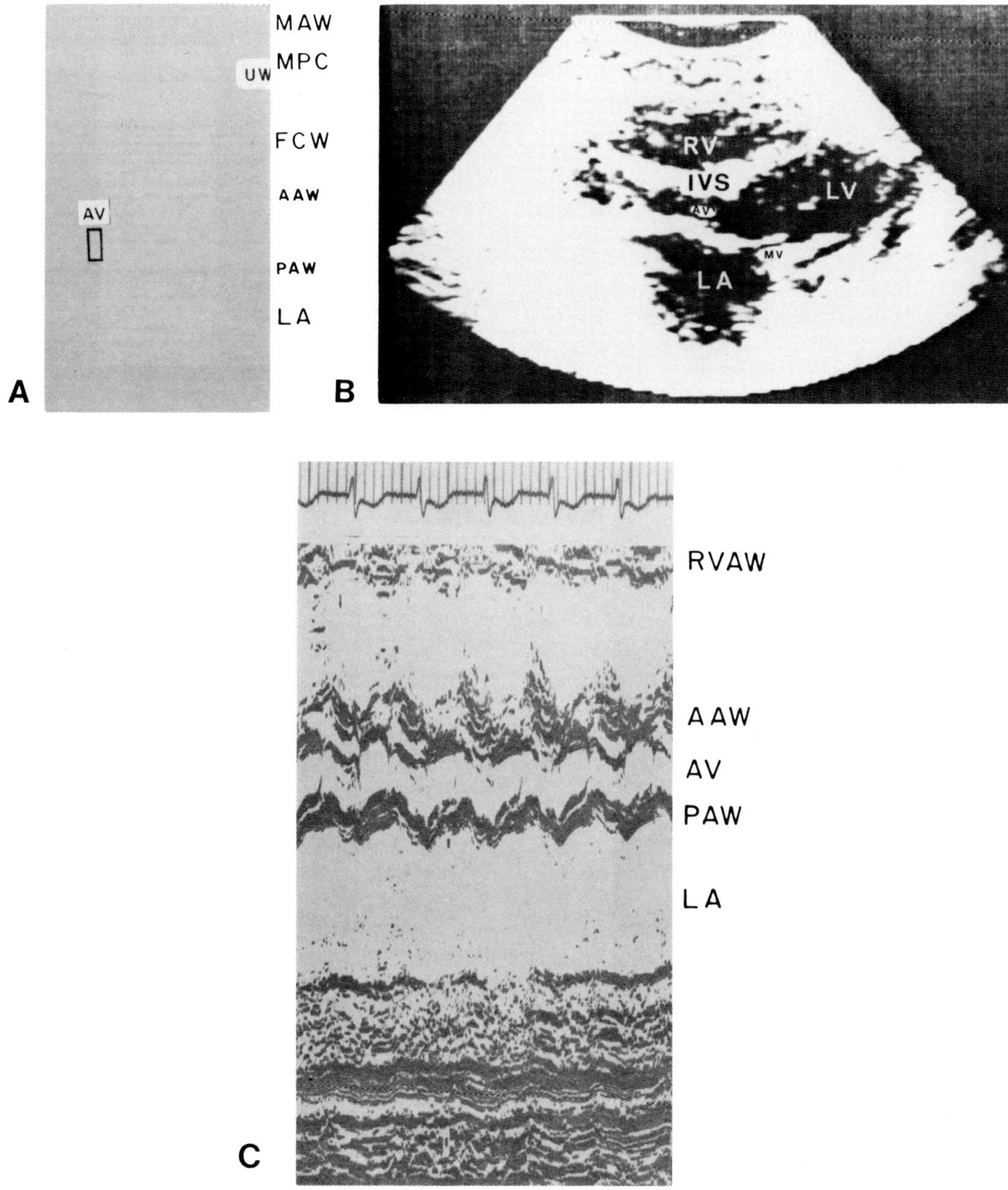

Fig. F.XIV.3. A. Intrauterine fetal echocardiogram showing normal cardiac structures with the exception of an enlarged left atrium due to intrauterine heart failure on the basis of supraventricular tachycardia. **B.** Confirmatory findings in immediate postpartum period by neonatal echocardiography, utilizing bidimensional (realtime) echocardiography. **C.** Neonatal echocardiogram with almost identical picture as obtained in utero (A) utilizing M-mode in both instances. MAW = maternal abdominal wall; FCW = fetal chest wall; AAW = anterior aortic wall; PAW = posterior aortic wall; AV = aortic valve; LA = left atrium; RV = right ventricle; RVAW = right ventricular anterior wall; LV = left **ventricle;** IVS = interventricular septum; MV = mitral valve. Fetal heart rate 240 beats/min. By permission from Kerenyi TD, Gleicher N, Meller J, et al.[25]

tified. In other words, the diagnosis of heart failure will frequently have to be made by exclusion of other causes for similar or identical findings on evaluation of the fetus in utero.

IV. TREATMENT OF INTRAUTERINE HEART FAILURE

It is apparent from the preceding discussion that intrauterine heart failure occurs only rarely. Once intrauterine heart failure is suspected or diagnosed, however, clinical action has to be taken in order to save the fetus. Once a diagnosis of heart failure is made, the precipitating cause has to be established. Obviously, therapy will have to be directed to that precipitating cause. As noted earlier, if fetal anemia is present, immediate action seems indicated. If the fetus has a reasonable survival chance after delivery, delivery itself is the appropriate treatment. However, if the fetus is too immature to survive when intrauterine heart failure is recognized, then intrauterine therapy has to be established. In association with fetal anemia, whatever the cause may be, intrauterine transfusion, as noted above, is an adequate course of action.

In the case of intrauterine dysrhythmias, the management is less clear. The rule that delivery is appropriate therapy when the fetus is mature or close to maturity applies to this situation as well. Nobody will argue with immediate delivery if the fetal survival chances are considered reasonable. In the case of intrauterine dysrhythmias in a situation where the fetus is far from maturity, intrauterine therapy will have to be considered. Such situations will be few and far between; however, several attempts at intrauterine treatment of congestive heart failure due to dysrhythmias have been reported. The first successful attempt was made with the involvement of one of the authors.[25] We succeeded in the transplacental cardioversion of a fetus with persistent supraventricular tachycardia, which had led to intrauterine congestive heart failure. Transplacental cardioversion was achieved by giving digitalis to the mother. Digitalis, like some other medications, crosses the placental barrier and reaches adequate levels in the fetal circulation. Figure F.XIV.4 demonstrates how, with increasing digitalization, the supraventricular tachycardia that was originally found to be at a rate of approximately 240 beats per minute, decreased. After a dose of 2 mg of digoxin to the mother, the fetal heart rate decreased to 120–160 beats per minute. It was found to be irregular, and was believed to represent atrial fibrillation. After 2.5 mg digoxin to the mother, the fetal heart rate was regular at 140 beats per minute and was considered to represent sinus rhythm. Soon after this successful cardioversion, unfortunately, a placental abruption occurred, which necessitated an emergency cesarean section. The delivery of the infant within a short time after cardioversion allowed us to obtain fetal digitalis levels. Maternal digitalis levels at the time of cesarean section were 2.7 ng/ml, umbilical cord levels were 0.7 ng/ml, and amniotic fluid levels were 1.7 ng/ml. Other attempts,[27] with the exception of one case very similar to our own,[26] to convert in utero utilizing digitalis and/or propranolol have remained largely unsuccessful. Nevertheless, it seems appropriate, based on these experiences, to recommend in selective cases the attempted intrauterine therapy of fetal congestive heart failure associated with intrauterine dysrhythmias. At present, this form of therapy represents only the last resort if delivery does not seem appropriate, and it has to be considered experimental.

V. PROGNOSIS

The prognosis of infants who developed heart failure in utero is, in the majority of cases, very satisfactory. Assuming that the precipitating cause of intrauterine heart failure is reversible the long-term prognosis is entirely satisfactory. Should the condition that resulted in intrauterine

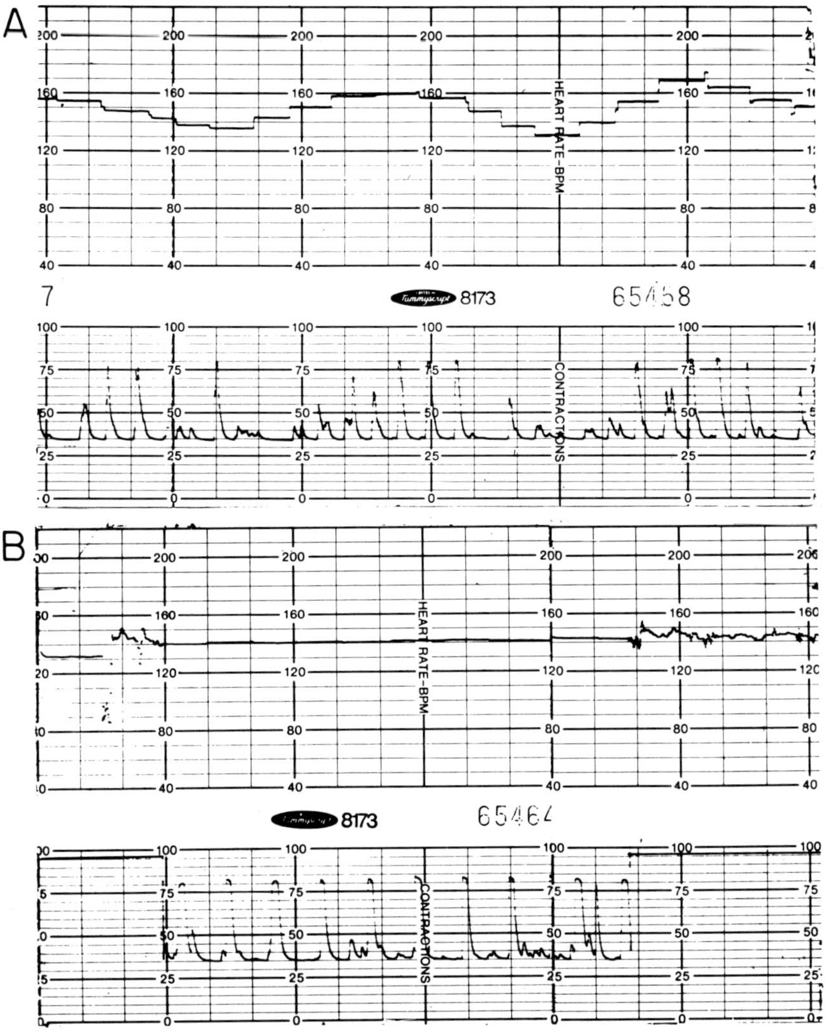

Fig. F.XIV.4. External fetal heart rate tracing. **A**. Irregular rate of 120–160 bpm, most likely atrial fibrillation, obtained after maternal dose of 2 mg of digoxin. **B**. Regular fetal heart rate at 140 bpm, most likely sinus rhythm, obtained after a cumulative dose of 2.5 mg digoxin. For details, see text. By permission from Kerenyi TD, Gleicher N, Meller J, et al.[25]

heart failure, however, persist into the neonatal period and thereafter, the prognosis may change. Such may be the case with congenital A-V block, where the long-term prognosis is not always satisfactory. The long-term sequelae in infants who required intrauterine transfusion because of anemia are not fully known. Bowman indicated that approximately one-third of affected infants have neurological sequelae, including low IQ.[12]

In summary, intrauterine heart failure represents a rarely occurring entity that, in the majority of cases, will be treated by immediate delivery of the fetus. However, in a minority of instances, especially when the fetus is considered too immature for delivery, intrauterine therapy may be indicated. In situations of fetal anemia, this therapy may be represented by intrauterine transfusion. When dysrhythmias are the cause of intrauterine heart failure, transplacental pharmacological intervention may be appropriate. With proper therapy, most infants will survive and have a satisfactory prognosis.

VI. REFERENCES

1. Braunwald E. Heart failure. In: Isserbacher KJ, Adams RD, Braunwald E, Petersdorf RG, Wilson JD, eds. Harrison's Principles of Internal Medicine, 9th Ed. New York: McGraw-Hill Book Company, 1980:1035–1044.
2. Anderson PAW, Manring A, Crenshaw C Jr. Biophysics of the developing heart. I. The force-interval relationship. Am J Obstet Gynecol. 1980; 138:33–43.
3. Anderson PAW, Manring A, Crenshaw C Jr. Biophysics of the developing heart. II. The interaction of the force-interval relationship with inotropic state and muscle length (preload). Am J Obstet Gynecol. 1980; 138:44–54.
4. Cherry SH. Current concepts in hemolytic disease and blood group incompatibility. Mt Sinai J Med (NY). 1980; 47:454–460.
5. Smith BD, Haber JM, Queenan JT. Irregular antibodies in pregnant women. Obstet Gynecol. 1967; 29:118–124.
6. Rochard F, Schifrin BS, Goupil F, et al. Nonstressed fetal heart rate monitoring in the antepartum period. Am J Obstet Gynecol. 1976; 126:699–706.
7. Cetrulo CC, Schifrin BS. Fetal heart rate patterns preceding death in utero. Obstet Gynecol. 1976; 48:521–527.
8. Gleicher N, Runowicz CD, Brown BL. Sinusoidal fetal heart rate pattern in association with amnionitis. Obstet Gynecol. 1980; 56:109–112.
9. Modanlov H, Freeman R, Ortiz O, et al. Sinusoidal fetal heart rate pattern and severe fetal anemia. Obstet Gynecol. 1977; 49:537–541.
10. Elliott JP, Modanlov HD, O'Keefe DF, Freeman RK. Significance of fetal and neonatal sinusoidal heart rate patter: Further clinical observations in Rh incompatibility. Am J Obstet Gynecol. 1980; 138:227–232.
11. Liley AW. Liquor amnii analysis in the management of the pregnancy complicated by rhesus sensitization. Am J Obstet Gynecol. 1961; 83:1359–1364.
12. Bowman JM. The management of Rh-isoimmunization. Obstet Gynecol. 1978; 52:1–16.
13. Hatjis CG, Mennum M, Sacks LM, Schwarz RH. Resolution of a sinusoidal fetal heart rate pattern following intrauterine transfusion. Am J Obstet Gynecol. 1978; 132:109–111.
14. Mueller-Heubach E, Caritis SN, Edelstone DI. Sinusoidal fetal heart rate pattern following intrauterine transfusion. Obstet Gynecol (Suppl). 1977; 52:435s–465s.
15. Verma V, Tejani N, Weiss RR, et al. Sinusoidal fetal heart rate patterns in severe Rh disease. Obstet Gynecol. 1980; 55:666–669.
16. Oxorn H. Multiple pregnancy. In: Oxorn H, ed. Human Labor & Birth, 4th Ed. New York: Appleton-Century-Crofts, 1980:275–279.
17. Zipursky A. The universal prevention of Rh immunization. Clin Obstet Gynecol. 1971; 14:869–884.
18. Caspi B, Lancet M, Kessler I. Sinusoidal pattern of uterine contractions in abruptio placentae. Int J Gynaecol Obstet. 1980; 17:615–616.
19. Young BK, Katz M, Wilson SJ. Sinusoidal fetal heart rate. I. Clinical significance. Am J Obstet Gynecol. 1980; 136:587–593.
20. Chitkara U, Gleicher N, Longhi R, et al. Persistent supraventricular tachycardia in utero. Diagnost Gynecol Obstet. 1980; 2:291–298.
21. Shenker L. Fetal cardiac arrhythmias. Obstet Gynecol Surv. 1979; 34:561–572.
22. Van der Horst RL. Congenital atrial flutter and cardiac failure presenting as hydrops foetalis at birth. S Afr Med J. 1970; 44:1037–1039.
23. Gleicher N. The Wolff-Parkinson-White syndrome predisposes to intrauterine arrhythmias. In preparation.
24. Kerenyi TD, Gleicher N. Intrauterine fetal paracentesis in the management of ascites. In preparation.
25. Kerenyi TD, Gleicher N, Meller J, et al. Transplacental cardioversion of intrauterine supraventricular tachycardia with digitalis. Lancet 1980; 2:393–395.
26. Harrigan JT, Kanpos JJ, Sikka A, Spisso KR, Natarajan N, Rosenfeld D, Leiman S, Korn D. Successful treatment of fetal congestive heart failure secondary to tachycardia. N Engl J Med. 1981; 304:1527–1529.
27. Klein AM, Holzman IR, Austin EM. Fetal tachycardia before the development of hydrops–attempted pharmacologic cardioversion: Case report. Am J Obstet Gynecol. 1979; 134:347–348.

The Neonatal Period

F.XV

Recognition of a Congenital Cardiac Anomaly at Birth

Burton W. Fink, MD

I. INTRODUCTION

It is the aim of this chapter to assist the physician caring for the newborn infant in recognizing a congenital cardiac anomaly at the time of birth. The approach is based upon the symptoms; namely, cyanosis, arrhythmias, congestive heart failure, and cardiac murmurs. Where appropriate, treatment is discussed, but it is important to note that such treatment is based upon current standards and may well change with time. There are several publications that offer more detailed discussion of the subject.[1–5]

II. CYANOSIS

Cyanosis implies decreased oxygen delivery to tissues. It must be remembered that all cyanosis is not cardiac in origin, and before a congenital cardiac lesion is considered as the etiology, noncardiac causes must be eliminated. Acrocyanosis of the newborn, a self-limiting natural phenomenon, is well known and recognizable as cyanosis of the hands and feet. Central nervous system depression can cause cyanosis, and the neurologic system must be carefully evaluated. Apparent cyanosis can also be caused by abnormal hemoglobinopathies, as well as by polycythemia of the newborn. The latter may be caused by either fetal–fetal or maternal–fetal transfusions. A hematocrit in excess of 75% is virtually diagnostic. Respiratory distress syndrome, atelectasis, pneumothorax, and other intrinsic pulmonary pathology probably present the most important differential diagnostic considerations in the presence of cyanosis.

Once cyanosis is recognized an arterial blood gas study should be performed and

Cardiac Problems in Pregnancy, pages 579–590

the partial pressure of oxygen (pO_2) determined. If the pO_2 is abnormally low, an oxygen atmosphere of 80–100% should be created for 15 minutes, after which the arterial blood gas study should be repeated. If the cyanosis is noncardiac in origin, an increase in the pO_2 in excess of 150 Torr would be expected. The persistence of a pO_2 in the vicinity of the baseline depressed value strongly indicates a cardiac origin of the cyanosis.

Once it has been established that the newborn has cyanotic congenital heart disease, the differential diagnosis includes tricuspid atresia, total anomalous pulmonary venous connection, truncus arteriosus, tetralogy of Fallot, and transposition of the great arteries. Although other lesions such as Ebstein anomaly, persistent fetal circulation, and complex cardiac abnormalities may also cause cyanosis, the first five lesions mentioned are, by far, the major considerations. Work-up should include a chest roentgenogram, electrocardiogram, and two-dimensional echocardiogram. Although the work-up will take place beyond the immediate newborn period, it seems prudent to discuss some of the specifics of the more common congenital defects.

III. TRICUSPID ATRESIA

This lesion is characterized by the absence of a tricuspid valve. It is subclassified as shown in Figure F.XV.1. Regardless of the anatomic variation, the basic blood flow is from the vena cavae to the right atrium, left atrium, left ventricle,

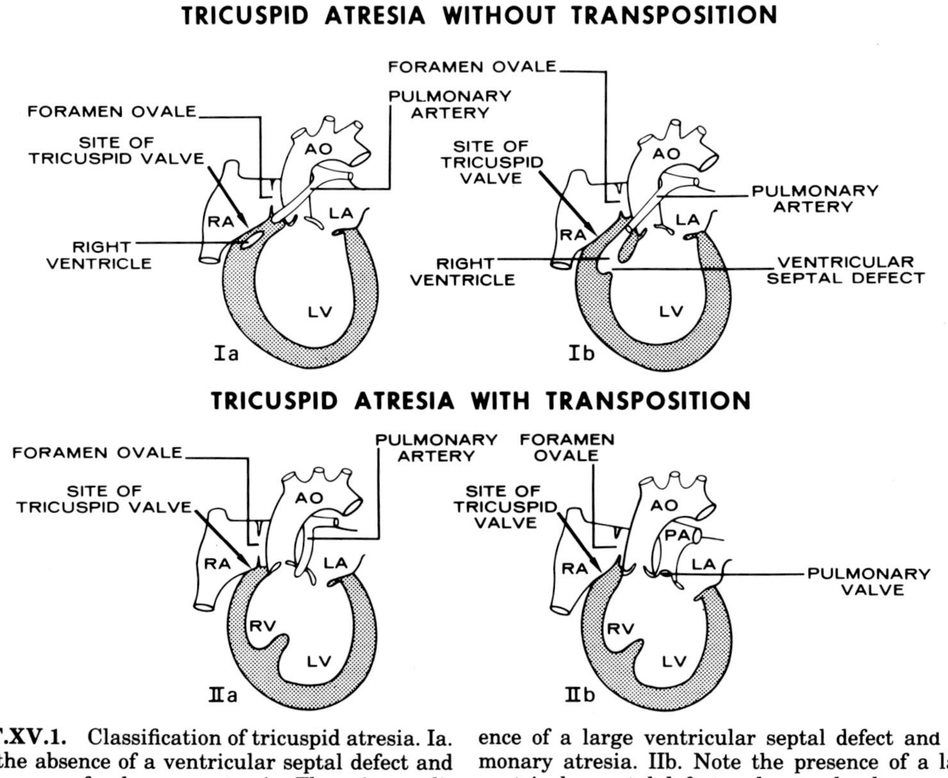

Fig. F.XV.1. Classification of tricuspid atresia. Ia. Note the absence of a ventricular septal defect and the presence of pulmonary atresia. There is a rudimentary right ventricle. Ib. Note the presence of a small ventricular septal defect and pulmonary stenosis. The right ventricle is small. IIa. Note the presence of a large ventricular septal defect and pulmonary atresia. IIb. Note the presence of a large ventricular septal defect and normal pulmonary artery. RA = right atrium; LA = left atrium; LV = left ventricle; AO = aorta; PA = pulmonary artery. (From Fink,[1] p 94.)

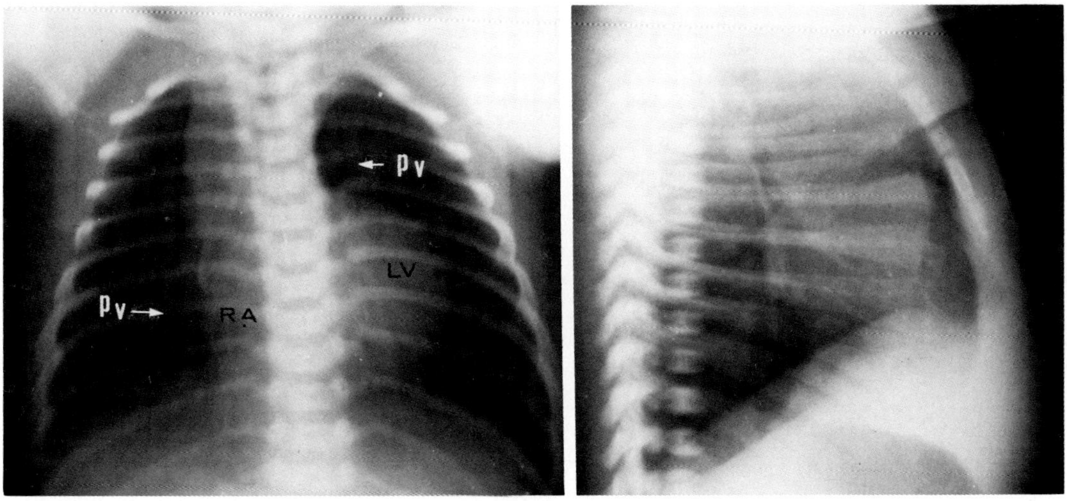

Fig. F.XV.2. Chest roentgenograms of a patient with tricuspid atresia. Note the cardiomegaly, elevated apex due to left ventricular enlargement, and prominent right atrium. The pulmonary markings are diminished. Pv = pulmonary vessels. (From Fink,[1] p 95.)

and then either to the aorta alone or through the right ventricle to the pulmonary artery, as well as to the aorta. On physical examination the patient will be deeply cyanotic. The precordium may not be particularly prominent, but a left ventricular thrust can be expected. The first heart sound will be single, as will the second sound. The murmurs heard are variable. A diastolic flow murmur across the mitral valve might be present. If a significant ventricular septal defect is present, a holosystolic murmur at the left sternal border would be expected. If pulmonary stenosis is present, an ejection systolic murmur at the second left interspace will be heard. However, and most commonly, no murmur is audible. The chest x-ray film will show a heart generally within normal limits in size, or slightly enlarged, but the vascular markings would be diminished (Fig. F.XV.2). The electrocardiogram will show left ventricular hypertrophy with left axis deviation (Fig. F.XV.3). The echocardiogram is of major importance in that it is capable of demonstrating the very large left ventricle with a normal mitral valve and a miniscule right ventricle with no tricuspid or pulmonary valve. This can be accomplished in either the 2-D or M-modes (Fig. F.XV.4).

Survival is, in the main, dependent upon flow through the ductus arteriosus. Infusion of prostaglandin E_1 through an umbilical arterial, central venous, or peripheral venous line is useful in preserving flow through that vessel pending establishment of a definitive diagnosis and, when indicated, surgical intervention.[2] Cardiac catheterization serves to confirm the clinical diagnosis and to demonstrate the intracardiac anatomy and the size of the great arteries and their branches.

The purpose of surgical therapy is to increase pulmonary blood flow, and this can be accomplished by any one of a number of systemic-to-pulmonary shunts. These carry the eponyms Blalock-Taussig—a subclavian artery to a pulmonary artery; Waterston—the ascending aorta to the right pulmonary artery; and Potts—the descending aorta to the left pulmonary artery. In addition, an artificial graft material, Gortex, can be used to connect any available systemic and pulmonary vessel.

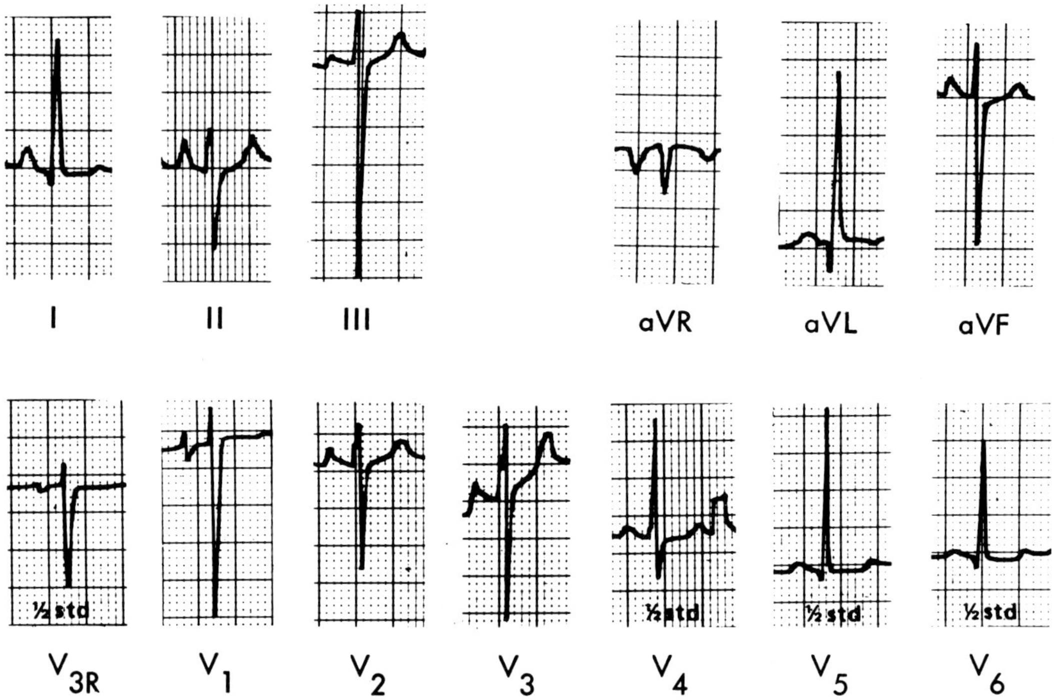

Fig. F.XV.3. Electrocardiogram of a patient with tricuspid atresia. The salient features are a tall P wave in lead II due to right atrial hypertrophy. The deep S wave in V_1 and tall R waves in leads V_5 and V_6 are interpretable as left ventricular hypertrophy. The negative P wave in lead V_{3R} suggests left atrial hypertrophy. The dominant R_1 and S_{aVF} are due to left axis deviation.

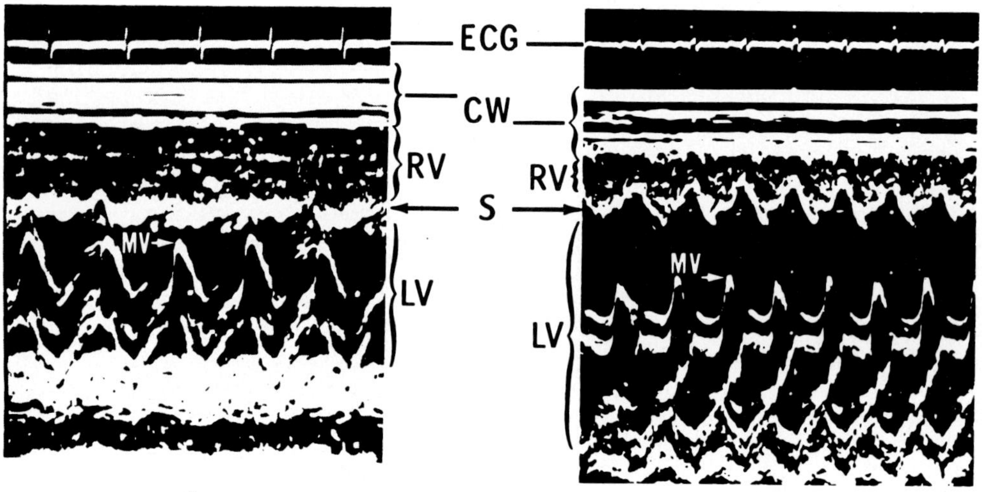

Fig. F.XV.4. Echocardiograms of a normal newborn (**A**) and a patient with tricuspid atresia (**B**). Note the relatively small right ventricle (RV) and very large left ventricle (LV) in the patient with tricuspid atresia. ECG = electrocardiogram; CW = chest wall; S = septum; MV = mitral valve. (Modified from Meyer RA, Kaplan S. Cardiovasc Dis. 15:341, 1973.)

IV. TOTAL ANOMALOUS PULMONARY VENOUS CONNECTION

This lesion occurs as a result of failure of appropriate absorption of the common pulmonary vein into the left atrium. This common vein can connect either the innominate vein, which drains into the superior vena cava, or the right atrium, the coronary sinus, or the hepatic system below the diaphragm (Fig. F.XV.5). Generally, only the variety complicated by obstruction to the common pulmonary vein causes the newborn to be in trouble. Because of the resulting pulmonary edema and congestive heart failure such an infant is not only cyanotic but also in severe respiratory distress. The chest roentgenogram will show a normal-sized heart with pulmonary edema (Fig. F.XV.6). The electrocardiogram will demonstrate right ventricular hypertrophy. An echocardiogram may show a second echo-free chamber behind the left atrium, representing the common pulmonary vein.

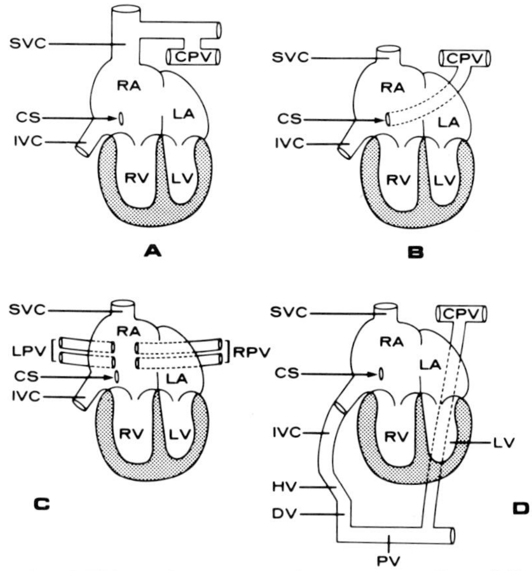

Fig. F.XV.5. Diagrammatic representation of the anatomic variations of total anomalous pulmonary venous connection. (See text for explanation.) SVC = superior vena cava; RV = right ventricle; LA = left atrium; LV = left ventricle. (From Fink,[1] p 146.)

V. TRUNCUS ARTERIOSUS

In the development of the heart, the truncus arteriosus normally is divided by a spiral septum delimiting the normal pulmonary artery and the aorta. If this septum fails to develop, there is left the common trunk, giving rise to this congenital entity. Since the ventricular septum requires the participation of the truncal

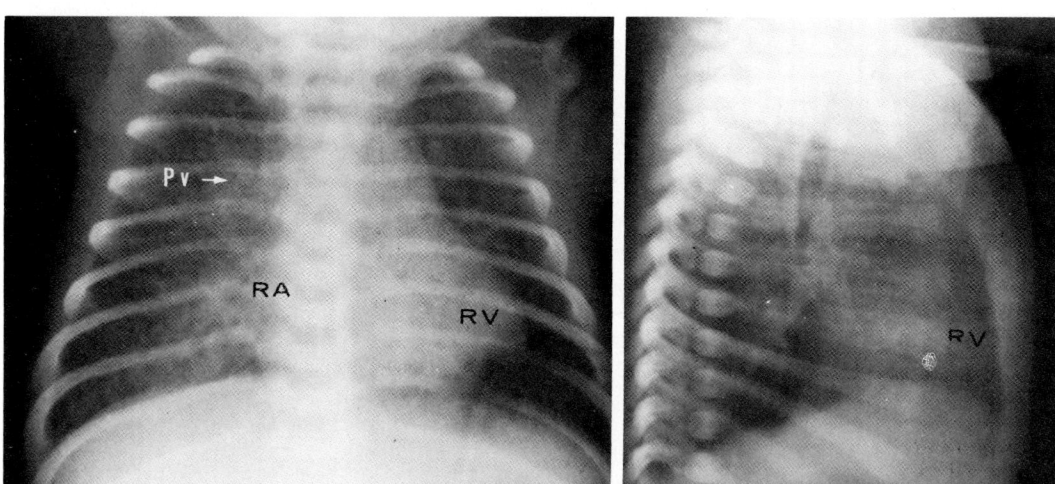

Fig. F.XV.6. Chest roentgenograms of an infant with total anomalous pulmonary venous drainage with obstruction. Note the over-small size of the heart and the punctate markings in the lungs representing pulmonary venous engorgement. RA = right atrium; RV = right ventricle; Pv = pulmonary venous engorgement. (From Fink,[1] p 148.)

septum, there is always a ventricular septal defect incorporated in the anatomy. The origin of the pulmonary arteries, or the bronchial arteries in the absence of any pulmonary artery, leads to the classification shown in Figure F.XV.7. It can be conceived that right and left ventricular flow will then leave the heart via the common trunk to be distributed through the pulmonary arteries in a degree dependent upon the relative resistances of the pulmonary and systemic circuits. This interplay dictates the degree of cyanosis. In type IV truncus, the cyanosis is maximal because of the gross restriction of pulmonary blood flow.

Cardiac murmurs vary depending upon the flow across the common valve or through the pulmonary arteries. One may hear either a simple ejection systolic murmur or a continuous one. Characteristically and consistently, the second sound is single. The chest roentgenogram will show increased cardiomegaly with increased vascular markings in types I, II, and III, and a smaller heart and decreased vascular markings in type IV. The electrocardiogram will be comparably variable, showing combined ventricular hypertrophy in the first three types and right ventricular hypertrophy in type IV. The echocardiogram will show a large single great artery overriding the ventricular septum. However, this finding is similar to that seen in tetralogy of Fallot and therefore is not totally diagnostic.

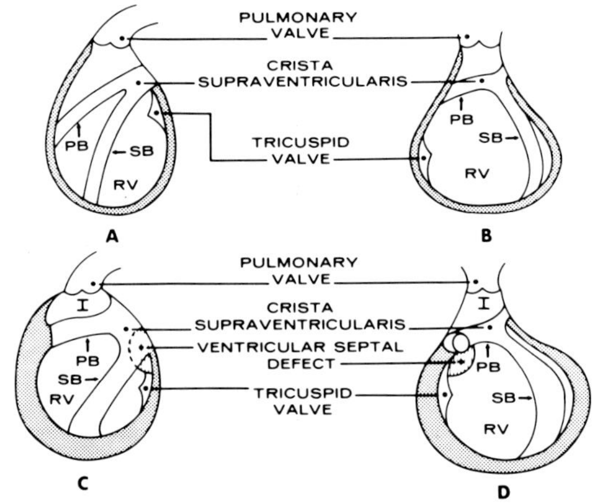

Fig. F.XV.8. Diagrammatic representation of the appearance of the crista supraventricularis and its parietal and septal bands in a normal patient and in a patient with tetralogy of Fallot. **A**, normal - lateral view; **B**, normal - AP view; **C** tetralogy of Fallot - lateral view; **D**, tetralogy of Fallot - AP view. Note the increased size in the parietal band and septal band and the presence of a ventricular septal defect in C and D. PB = parietal band; SB = septal band; RV = right ventricle; I = infundibulum. (From Fink,[1] p 83.)

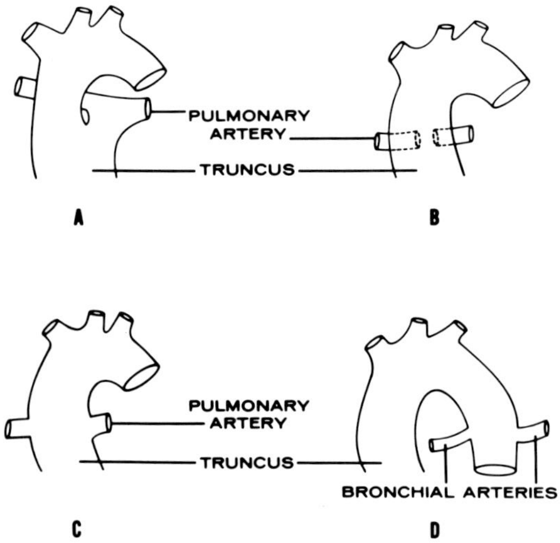

Fig. F.XV.7. Classification of truncus arteriosus. **A**: type I; note that the pulmonary arteries arise from the common trunk with an attempt at the division into a true main pulmonary artery. **B**: type II; note the origin of the pulmonary arteries from the posterior aspect of the truncus. **C**: type III; note the origin of the pulmonary arteries from the lateral aspect of the truncus. **D**: type IV; note the absence of any pulmonary artery and merely bronchial arteries. (From Fink,[1] p 116.)

VI. TETRALOGY OF FALLOT

Implicit in the definition of this entity is the presence of a ventricular septal defect, infundibular stenosis, overriding of the aorta, and right ventricular hypertrophy. However, a more physiologic definition would entail the presence of a ventricular septal defect that is the size of the aorta and progressive infundibular stenosis (Fig. F.XV.8). Parenthetically, the presence of right ventricular hypertrophy is then secondary to the outflow obstruction, and the overriding of the aorta is either anatomic or physiologic, but the end product is quite the same. In view of this definition, the symptoms are rather dependent upon the degree of pulmonary blood flow, which is influenced by the degree of subpulmonic stenosis. It is not at all uncommon for a child to be born with virtually normal pulmonary blood flow and be visually pink. As the infundibular hypertrophy progresses, the degree of right-to-left shunting increases, and cyanosis is then observed.

This lesion is not commonly observed in the newborn infant, but if the degree of infundibular stenosis is extraordinarily severe, it might be made apparent. Cyanosis would be expected. There would be a right ventricular heave. The second sound would be single. An ejection systolic murmur would be heard along the left sternal border. The chest roentgenogram would show a small heart, elevated apex, concave pulmonary artery, and diminished pulmonary blood flow (Fig. F.XV.9). Right ventricular hypertrophy would be seen on the electrocardiogram. An echocardiogram would demonstrate a large aorta overriding the ventricular septum. This would be supportive, but not diagnostic, because a truncus arteriosus would have similar findings.

VII. TRANSPOSITION OF THE GREAT ARTERIES

If in the development of a common trunk the septation fails to occur in a proper fashion, the great arteries may be transposed in such a way that the aorta will originate from the anterior right ventricle and the pulmonary artery from the posterior left ventricle (see Fig. F.XV.10). With this anatomic derangement, after birth systemic venous return will be delivered to the right ventricle, but then returned to the body via the aorta. At the same time pulmonary venous return will be delivered to the left ventricle and then

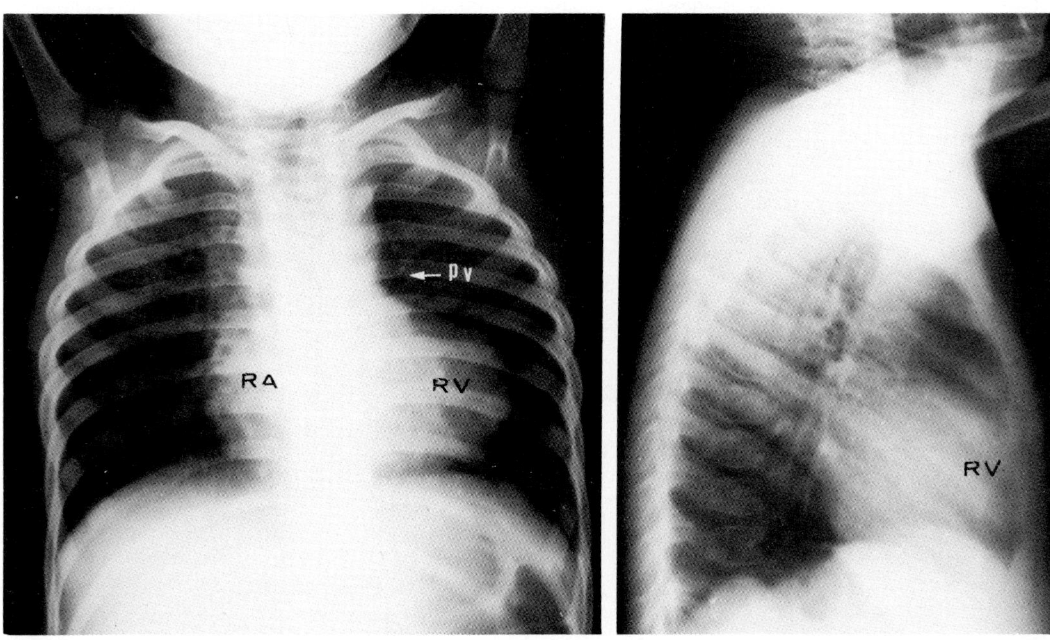

Fig. F.XV.9. Chest roentgenograms of a patient with tetralogy of Fallot. Note the enlarged right atrium and right ventricle and decreased pulmonary vessels. The overall appearance is that of a boot-shaped heart. RA = right atrium; RV = right ventricle; pv = pulmonary vessels. (From Fink,[1] p 85.)

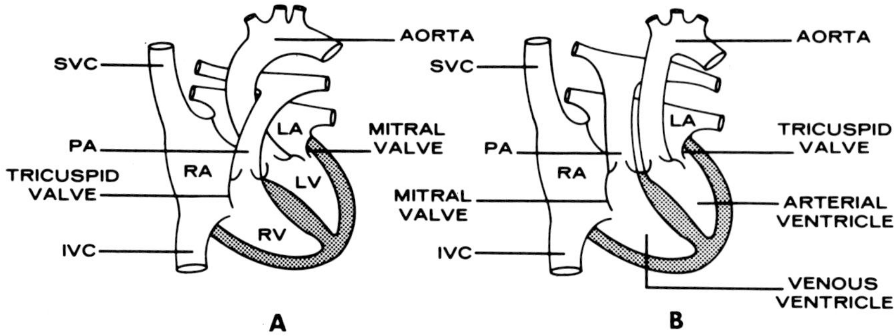

Fig. F.XV.10. Diagrammatic representation of the anatomy seen in a patient with transposition of the great arteries (**B**) as compared to the normal (**A**). (See text for explanation.) IVC = inferior vena cava: SVC = superior vena cava; RA = right atrium; RV = right ventricle; LA = left atrium; LV = left ventricle. (From Fink,[1] p 104.)

returned to the lungs via the pulmonary artery. Persistence of life is then dependent upon bidirectional flow through the ductus arteriosus.

This lesion can be suspected on the basis of cyanosis, which might be mild indeed. In the first hours of life no other symptom might be present, but with time tachypnea and congestive heart failure will follow. The heart on examination might be entirely normal with no thrust, heave, murmur, or single second sound. The chest roentgenogram, though frequently showing an enlarged heart with a narrow mediastinum and increased vascular flow, might be entirely normal (Fig. F.XV.11). The electrocardiogram would generally show right ventricular hypertrophy, but

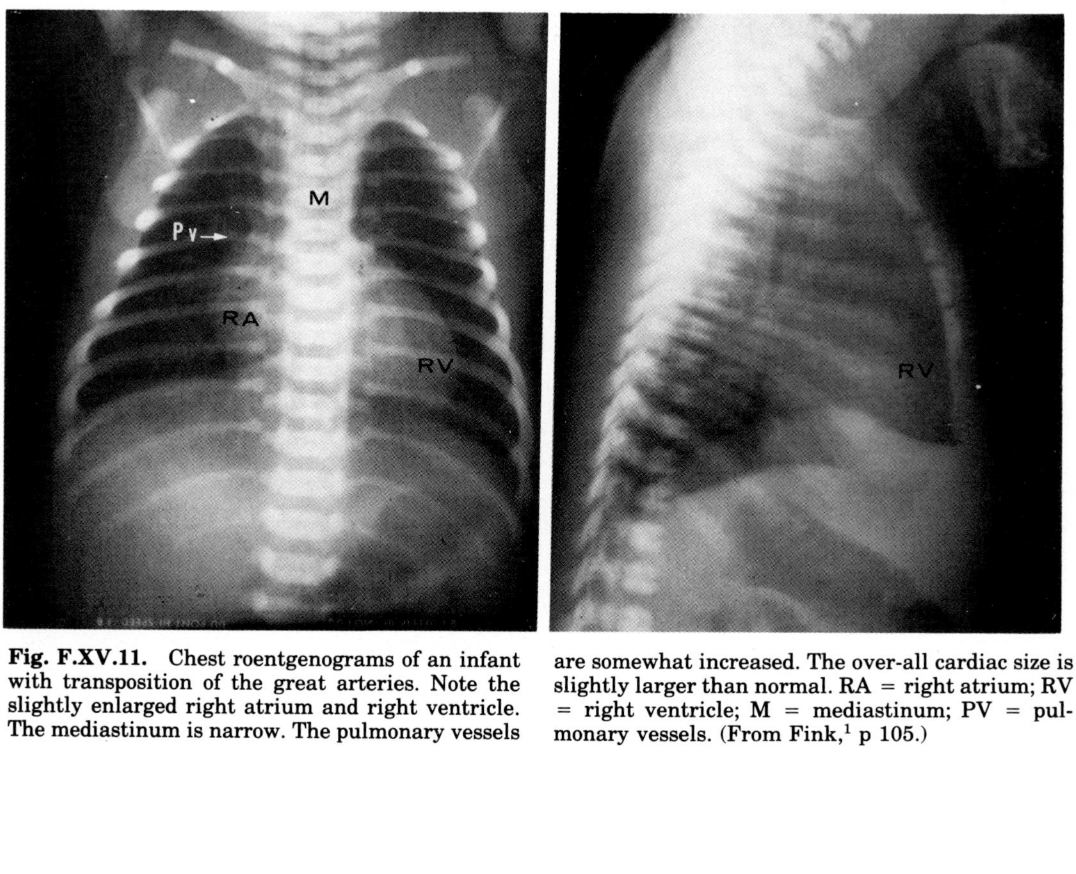

Fig. F.XV.11. Chest roentgenograms of an infant with transposition of the great arteries. Note the slightly enlarged right atrium and right ventricle. The mediastinum is narrow. The pulmonary vessels are somewhat increased. The over-all cardiac size is slightly larger than normal. RA = right atrium; RV = right ventricle; M = mediastinum; PV = pulmonary vessels. (From Fink,[1] p 105.)

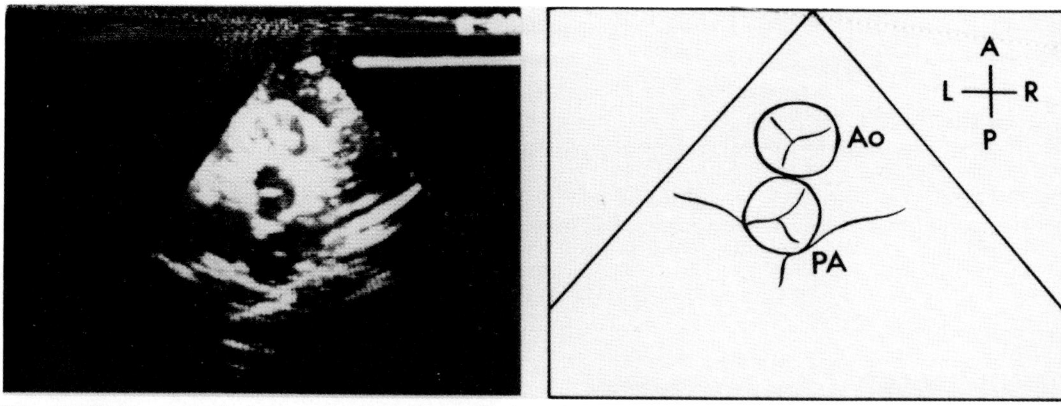

Fig. F.XV.12. Apical short axis view of a patient with d-transposition. The great vessels are seen, one above the other, with the aorta being the most anterior vessel. (From Duncan WJ: Atlas of Pediatric Two-Dimensional Echocardiography. Courtesy of Charles C Thomas, Publisher, Springfield, Illinois. 1981: 59)

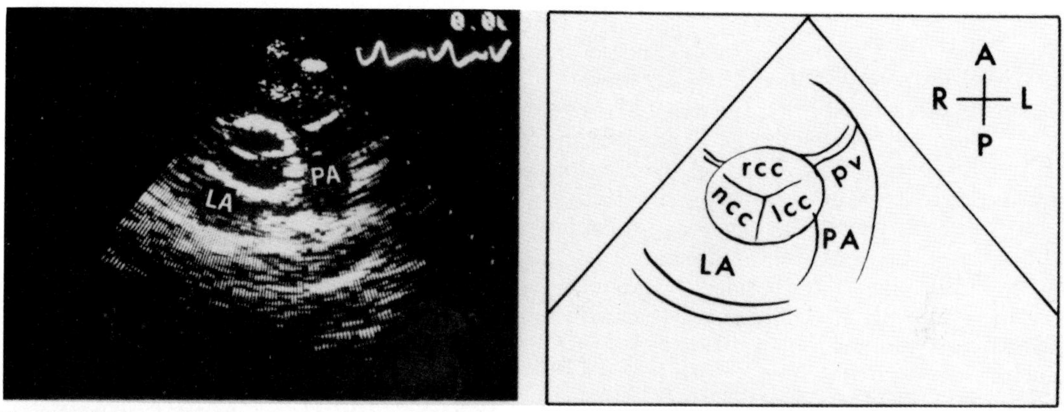

Fig. F.XV.13. Apical short axis view of a normal heart. The aorta is seen as a central circular image in cross section, with the pulmonary artery wrapping around that image. The pulmonary valve is seen. This is known as the "donut-and-sausage" image. (From Duncan WJ: Atlas of Pediatric Two-Dimensional Echocardiography. Courtesy of Charles C Thomas, Publisher, Springfield, Illinois. 1981: 25.)

it also might be entirely normal. A two-dimensional echocardiogram would show two circular echos with centrally located semilunar valves representing the two great arteries (Fig. F.XV.12). For reasons of comparison, a normal echocardiogram in the same view is demonstrated (Fig. F.XV.13).

VIII. ARRHYTHMIAS

An arrhythmia in the newborn will be heralded by either an irregular rhythm, an abnormally slow heart rate, or an abnormally fast heart rate.

A markedly slow rate (which, it must be added, may be recognized in utero; see Chapter F.XIII) may indicate a complete congenital heart block. If the intrinsic rate is adequate, such a block will offer no threat to the infant. An electrocardiogram should be done immediately after delivery to establish the rate and the source of the captured rhythm, be it junctional or ventricular (Fig. F.XV.14).

Tachyarrhythmias are potentially more troublesome. With a sinus tachycardia there is little consequence. However, supraventricular tachycardia due to reentry (Fig. F.XV.15) or chaotic atrial ectopy

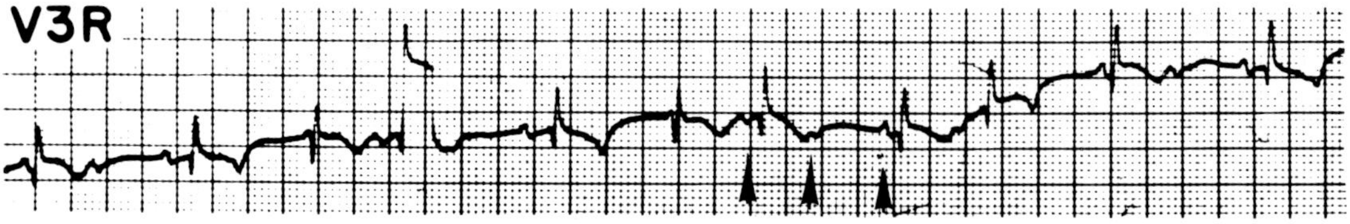

Fig. F.XV.14. An electrocardiogram in a patient with complete AV block and junctional escape rhythm. Note the regularly inscribed P waves as marked by the arrow.

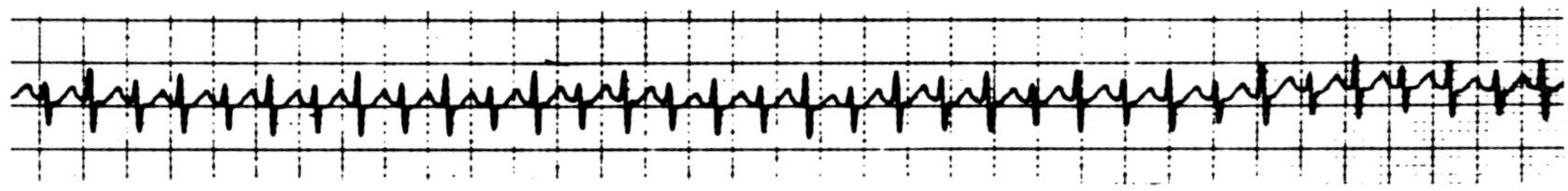

Fig. F.XV.15. An electrocardiogram in a patient with reentry supraventricular tachycardia. Note the rapid rate (300/minute), narrow ventricular complexes, and no P waves.

(Fig. F.XV.16) can occur. In each case if the rhythm has persisted for a prolonged period, congestive heart failure can follow. It must be stressed that supraventricular tachycardia can occur in utero and cause congestive heart failure prior to delivery. Such a patient might be hydropic at birth and present a considerable diagnostic challenge. If the tachyarrhythmia is still apparent, the diagnosis is easier. However, if conversion to a normal sinus mechanism occurs prior to delivery, or if the electrocardiogram does not demonstrate accelerated conduction, a grave diagnostic dilemma will be experienced.

Irregular rhythms require electrocardiography for definition. Sinus arrhythmia, though uncommon, can occur and is of no consequence. Ectopic complexes are frequently seen and tend to be transient in nature. They may present as premature atrial (Fig. F.XV.17), junctional (Fig. F.XV.18), or ventricular (Fig. F.XV.19) complexes. Atrial or junctional ectopy requires no therapy and generally resolves spontaneously. Ventricular ectopy, if unifocal and single, also requires no therapy. However, if runs of premature ventricular complexes are seen, lidocaine, quinidine, or in extreme circumstances, electrocardioversion, must be used.

IX. CONGESTIVE HEART FAILURE

Tachypnea (with or without dyspnea), tachycardia, and hepatomegaly, are generally accepted as the cardinal signs of congestive heart failure in an infant. It must be stressed that these findings can derive from a noncardiac lesion such as a large arteriovenous fistula in the great vein

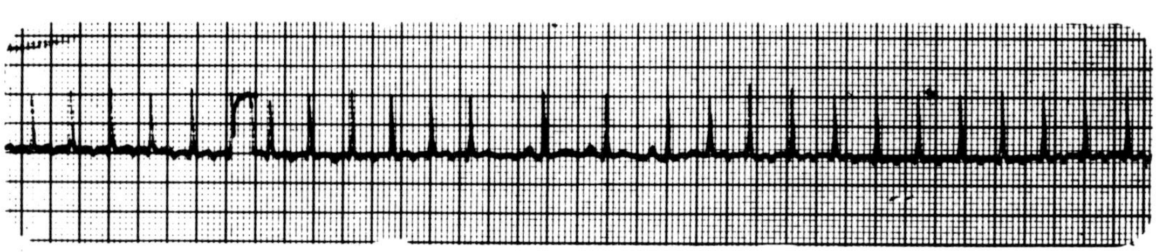

Fig. F.XV.16. An electrocardiogram in a patient with ectopic atrial tachycardia. Note the rapid rate, the narrow ventricular complexes, which are the same with or without a preceding P wave.

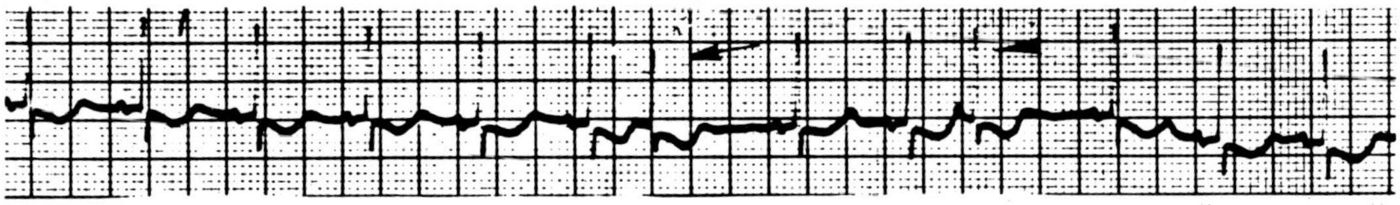

Fig. F.XV.17. An electrocardiogram in a patient with premature atrial complexes, as marked by the arrows.

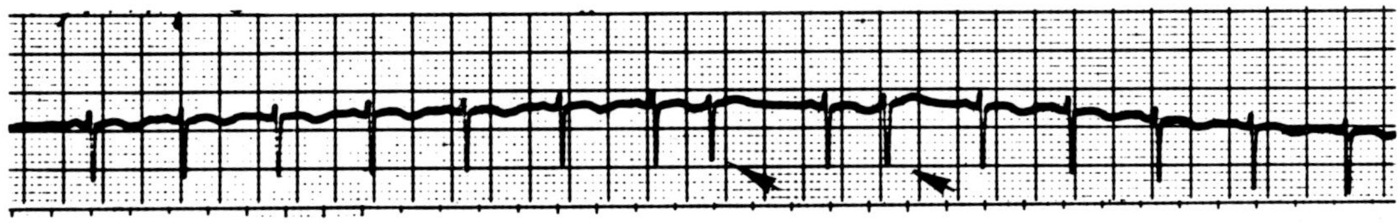

Fig. F.XV.18. An electrocardiogram in a patient with premature conjunctional complexes, as marked by an arrow.

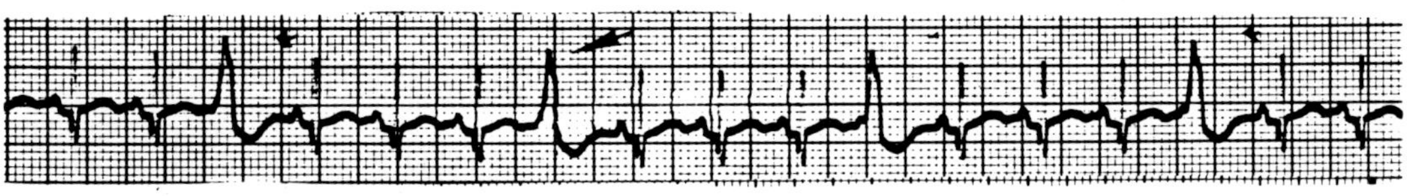

Fig. F.XV.19. An electrocardiogram in a patient with premature ventricular complexes, as marked with an arrow.

of Galen. It is also very rare for a newborn infant to have congestive heart failure due to cardiac causes. Congenital tricuspid insufficiency, premature closure of the foramen ovale, and intrauterine supraventricular tachycardia are the major causes of congestive heart failure in the newborn. The definitive diagnosis may not be possible until after congestive heart failure is controlled and laboratory studies utilized.

X. CARDIAC MURMURS

The recognition of a cardiac murmur at birth raises the possibility of congenital heart disease. It must be mentioned, however, that the ductus arteriosus may remain dynamic at birth for a few days. Short, ejection, systolic murmurs at the upper left sternal border may be heard transiently. If done, the chest roentgenogram, electrocardiogram, and echocardiogram would be entirely normal. The murmur should be expected to disappear before discharge.

The murmurs of aortic and pulmonary stenosis may be heard at the time of delivery. Each represents flow across a stenotic valve. The murmur of pulmonary stenosis will be heard at the second left interspace in the anatomic location of the pulmonary valve. It will be harsh, low pitched, and varying in intensity from grade 2 to Grade 4/6. Transmission through the pulmonary arteries into the back can be expected. A systolic ejection click might precede the murmur. A chest roentgenogram will be entirely normal, and the electrocardiogram will show right ventricular hypertrophy, the degree of which depends upon the severity of the stenosis.

The murmur of aortic stenosis will be heard at the fourth left interspace, the anatomic location of that valve. It is an ejection murmur and will vary from grade

2 to grade 4/6. It might transmit into the second right interspace and the neck. (It should be stressed that this transmission so commonly recognized in the older child and the adult is not at all common in the newborn.) The chest roentgenogram and electrocardiogram might be entirely normal. Echocardiography, though capable of demonstrating the aortic valve, is not capable, as of this writing, of predicting severity of stenosis.

Though not technically to be considered within the classification of cardiac murmurs, coarctation of the aorta is recognizable at the time of the first newborn examination in the delivery room. Radial pulses would be full and bounding, and femoral pulses would be either not felt at all or of significantly diminished intensity.

XI. REFERENCES

1. Fink BW. Congenital Heart Disease: A Deductive Approach to Its Diagnosis. Chicago & London: Year Book Medical Publishers, Inc., 1975.
2. Linday L, Engle M. Prostaglandin treatment of newborns with ductal dependent congenital heart disease. Pediatr Annu. 1981; 10:29–38.
3. Moss AJ, Adams FH (eds). Heart Disease in Infants, Children & Adolescents, 2nd Ed. Baltimore: The Williams & Wilkins Co., 1977.
4. Roberts NK, Fink BW. Arrhythmias in the pediatric patient. In: Mandel WJ (ed), Cardiac Arrhythmias—Their Mechanisms, Diagnosis and Management. Philadelphia & Toronto: J.B. Lippincott Co., 1900:454–479.
5. Roberts NK, Gelband H (eds): Cardiac Arrthymias in the Neonate, Infant & Child. New York: Appleton-Century-Crofts, 1977.

Index

B

C

E

I

J

K

L

N

O

S

U

V